TARGET JIPMER

(2010 – 2006)

(Model Questions with Solved Explanatory Answers)

"Get the inside edge! Authored by Jipmerites"

Fourth Edition (Volume 1)

Dr. T. ARUN BABU
MD Pediatrics (JIPMER), DAA (CMC, Vellore), MBA (HM)
Fellow in Neonatal Perinatal Medicine (Canada)
Associate Professor, Department of Pediatrics
Indira Gandhi Medical College and Research Institute (IGMC&RI)
A Government of Puducherry Institution
Puducherry – 605009
Website: www.drarunbabu.in

PEEPEE
PUBLISHERS AND DISTRIBUTORS (P) LTD.

TARGET JIPMER (Volume 1)

Published by
Pawaninder P. Vij and Anupam Vij

Peepee Publishers and Distributors (P) Ltd.
Head Office: 160, Shakti Vihar, Pitam Pura, Delhi-110 034 (India)

Correspondence Address:
7/31, First Floor, Ansari Road, Daryaganj
New Delhi-110 002 (India)
Ph: 65195868, 23246245, 9811156083
e-mail: peepee160@yahoo.co.in
e-mail: peepee160@rediffmail.com
e-mail: peepee160@gmail.com
www.peepeepub.com
join us on facebook.com/pp.publishers

First Edition: 2013

Fourth Edition: 2018

ISBN: 978-81-8445-230-3

Dedication

To my Parents, Teachers,
my wife Dr. Sharmila,
my kids Akshaya and Akash

Disclaimer:

This book fully complies with the non-disclosure agreement (NDA) levied by JIPMER. This book contains Model questions with solved explanatory answers. No questions included in this book have been obtained from any candidates registered for JIPMER exam. Any resemblance to the original JIPMER questions, if present, is purely coincidental. The author, contributors, publisher or sellers cannot be held responsible for any damage or loss caused to anyone, directly or indirectly.

PREFACE TO THE FOURTH EDITION (Volume 1)

I am glad to be meeting you with yet another supplement of TARGET JIPMER book. Big thanks for making TARGET JIPMER series the best book for JIPMER PGMEE preparation. This book series was started with the sole purpose of making model JIPMER questions accessible to PG aspirants. The questions have been solved by a team of subject experts from reputed academic backgrounds. This book is tailor-made for JIPMER PG entrance exam preparation. Most of our contributors are JIPMER alumni and have personally written JIPMER PG exams in the last few years and are well experienced and aware of the examination pattern. JIPMER questions are mostly taken from standard textbooks and articles. Though the pattern of JIPMER questions have changed in the last few years, the high yield area remains the same. You will understand this after going through all the volumes of 4th edition of TARGET JIPMER.

We have incorporated a systematic approach in solving each and every question which can be appreciated while reading this book. The schematic diagrams, tables, illustrations, bulleted key points and references are the highlights of this book and will make reading and understanding of the material easier and effective. Every solved question will have a valid reference citing a standard textbook or article in order to increase the credibility of the answers. The focused explanations should help you solve questions from same topics in the future easily.

I would like to thank all the contributors for their commitment and hard work that has led to the tremendous success of this book series. I wish to thank our publishers, Mr. Pawaninder Pal Vij and Mr. Anupam Vij, the Directors of Peepee Publishers and Distributors (P) Ltd., who have always been a pillar of support to our team. I would also like to thank our publishing team for their relentless efforts in releasing this book in a short notice. I am deeply indebted to students for their overwhelming support, feedback and critical appraisal. We are looking forward to hear your feedback and are fully committed in bringing out better editions in the future. For JIPMER students, a JIPMERITE tag is a matter of pride which they carry as a badge of honour throughout their professional life. For most others it is a dream. I believe and hope that this book will make your dream come true.

All the best!

T. Arun Babu

Website: *www.drarunbabu.in*

Email: *babuarun.t@gmail.com*

"Books are infinite in number and time is short. The secret of knowledge is to take what is essential."

–Swami Vivekananda

PREFACE TO THE FIRST EDITION

As an alumnus of the prestigious JIPMER Institute, I am always amazed at how much the institute has molded and influenced its students to great heights in their professional life. For JIPMER students, a JIPMERITE tag is a matter of pride and they always carry it as a badge of honour throughout their professional life. For most others it is a dream. As told by our former President Dr APJ Abdul Kalam, we should dream. If you don't dream, you have nothing to achieve. I truly believe that desire, self-belief, strategy, hard work and persistence is the hallmark for attaining success. PG entrance exams are unique. Your success depends on your performance and more importantly, your competitors on the D-day. Your aim should be to gather all information from all possible sources and stay ahead of the competition.

I have had the opportunity of closely working with numerous JIPMER PG exam aspirants over the years. From their feedback, it was obvious that there was an urgent need for a review book with genuine JIPMER PG entrance exam questions. This inspired and motivated me to come up with this book. I have taken extreme care to make sure that all the questions discussed in this book are genuine and authentic. The questions have been solved and scrutinised by a qualified and experienced team with reputed academic background. The schematic diagrams, tables, illustrations, bulleted key points and references are the highlight of this book.

I would like to thank all the PG aspirants who helped us by recollecting the questions. My sincere appreciation to all the contributors, for their hard work and effort. I would like to thank Mr. Pawaninder P. Vij, the Director of Peepee Publishers and Distributors (P) Ltd. for believing and supporting our work, along with his team for bringing out this book in record time.

Any suggestion or criticism about the book is welcome, it will help us strive harder to present better editions of the book in the years to come.

All the best!

T. Arun Babu

CONTRIBUTORS

Dr. Arun Babu T, MD Pediatrics (JIPMER), DAA (CMC), Fellow NPM (Canada)
Associate Professor, Department of Pediatrics
Indira Gandhi Medical College and Research Institute (IGMC&RI)
Puducherry – 605009
(Chief Editor)

Dr. Arul Varman, MD Psychiatry (JIPMER)
Assistant Professor, Department of Psychiatry
Indira Gandhi Medical College and Research Institute (IGMC&RI)
Puducherry – 605009
(Psychiatry)

Dr. Bharath Kumar VD, MD Pharmacology
Assistant Professor, Department of Pharmacology
BGS Global Institute of Medical Sciences
Bangalore, Karnataka
Dr. Bharath's Pharmacology MCQs and Discussion for PG Aspirants
(Pharmacology)

Dr. Dilip Kumar R, MD (JIPMER), MRCP (UK)
Consultant and Head, Department of Internal Medicine
Dr. Mehta's Hospitals, Chetpet, Chennai 31
(Medicine)

Dr. Dinesh Kumar, MD Pediatrics
Assistant Professor, Department of Pediatrics
Indira Gandhi Medical College and Research Institute (IGMC&RI)
Puducherry – 605009
(Pediatrics)

Dr. Karthikeyan Pethusamy
Senior Resident and PhD Scholar, Department of Biochemistry
All India Institute of Medical Sciences (AIIMS)
New Delhi
(Biochemistry)

Dr. Krishna Kumar S, MD Physiology (AIIMS)
Assistant Professor, Department of Physiology
SRM Medical College, Trichy Campus
Trichy–621105
(Physiology)

Dr. Mohd Khaleel Ahmed, MD Radiology
(Radiology)

Dr. Mugunthan N, MS Anatomy, DNB, FAIMS, MRSM, MBA
Associate Professor, Department of Anatomy
Mahatma Gandhi Medical College and Research Institute (MGMC&RI)
Puducherry – 607402
(Anatomy)

Dr. Mukul Mohindra, MS (Ortho), DNB, MNAMS, Dip. SICOT (Belgium)
Fellow National Board (Arthroscopy and Sports Medicine)
Sports Injury Center, Safdarjung Hospital and VMM College
New Delhi
(Orthopedics)

Dr. D. Pradeep, MS Gen Surg, MRCS (Edin)
Assistant Professor, Department of General Surgery
Shri Sathya Sai Medical College and Research Institute
Kancheepuram District, Tamil Nadu – 603108
(Surgery)

Dr. Prasanna S, MD Microbiology (AFMC, Pune)
Assistant Professor, Department of Microbiology
Shri Sathya Sai Medical College and Research Institute
Kancheepuram, Tamil Nadu – 603108
(Microbiology)

Dr. Rajamahendran, MS, MCh Gastro
Assistant Professor, Department of Surgical Gastroenterology
Government Villupuram Medical College
Villupuram – 605602
(Surgery)

Dr. Ranjith AR, MD Pathology (JIPMER)
Molecular Pathologist, Bangalore
(Pathology)

Dr. Sangeeta Dhanger, DA, DNB, MNAMS
Assistant Professor, Department of Anesthesiology
Indira Gandhi Medical College and Research Institute (IGMC&RI)
Puducherry – 605009
(Anesthesiology)

Dr. Satvinder Singh Bakshi, MS ENT (JIPMER), DNB
Assistant Professor, Department of Otorhinolaryngology
Mahatma Gandhi Medical College and Research Institute (MGMC&RI), Pillaiyarkuppam, Puducherry – 607 402
(ENT)

Dr. Sindhujha Sekar G, (JIPMER), DGO, DNB OG
Department of Obstetrics and Gynecology
Rajiv Gandhi Government Women and Children's Hospital
Puducherry
(OG)

Dr. Yogesh Bahurupi, MD PSM
Assistant Professor, Department of Preventive and Social Medicine
Indira Gandhi Medical College and Research Institute (IGMC&RI)
Puducherry – 605009
(PSM)

Dr. Udayashankar C, MD Dermatology (JIPMER), MBA (HM)
Professor and Head, Department of Dermatology
Indira Gandhi Medical College & Research Institute
(IGMC&RI)
Puducherry – 605 009
(Dermatology)

Dr. Venipriya, MS Ophthalmology
Assistant Professor, Department of Ophthalmology
Mahatma Gandhi Medical College and Research Institute
(MGMC&RI), Pillaiyarkuppam, Puducherry – 607 402
(Ophthalmology)

Dr. Vinoth Kumar S, MD General Medicine
Assistant Professor, Department of General Medicine
Indira Gandhi Medical College and Research Institute
(IGMC&RI)
Puducherry – 605 009
(General Medicine)

Dr. Yatiraj Singi, MD Forensic Medicine
Professor, Department of Forensic Medicine
Sree Mookambika Institute of Medical Sciences
Kulasekharam, District Kanya Kumari, TN
(Forensic Medicine)

ACKNOWLEDGEMENTS

Target JIPMER – Previous Edition Contributors

Dr. Balamurugan N, DCH, DNB, MRCPCH, Assistant Professor, Department of Pediatrics, SLIMS, Puducherry.
Dr. Tejswita Rajpal Hande, MBBS, DGO, MUHS, Nashik.
Dr. Saranya K, MD Physio (JIPMER), Assistant Professor of Physiology, JIPMER, Puducherry.
Dr. Abarna Devi S, DDVL (JIPMER), MD Medicine, Assistant Professor of Internal Medicine, SMVMCH.
Dr. Anshu Bahl, MD Anatomy (AIIMS), New Delhi.
Dr. Ankit Agarwal, MD RT (JIPMER), Senior Resident, GMCH, Sector 32, Chandigarh.
Dr. Dinesh Kumar, MD Pediatrics, Assistant Professor of Pediatrics, IGMC&RI, Puducherry.
Dr. Naga Dharshan Devendra, MD (JIPMER), Associate Professor and Course Director, Department of Biochemistry and Genetics, Trinity School of Medicine, Saint Vincent and Grenadines.
Dr. Saseendar S, MS (Ortho), DNB, Dip SICOT (Belgium), MNAMS, Care Sports Injury, Chennai.
Dr. Srirangaraj S, MD, Associate Professor, Department of Microbiology, MGMC&RI, Puducherry.
Dr. Sri Vengadesh Gopal, MS (JIPMER), Assistant Professor, Department of Surgery, IGMC&RI, Puducherry.
Dr. Sumanth MM, MD (JIPMER), DNB, Assistant Professor of Community Medicine, MMC&RI, Mysore, Karnataka.
Dr. Sentitoshi, (JIPMER) MD Forensic Medicine, Former Assistant Professor, MGMC&RI, Puducherry.
Dr. Asayas Bosco Chandrakumar, MS, Assistant Professor of Surgery, SLIMS, Puducherry.
Dr. Mahesh Nagappa, MD Anaes (JIPMER), DNB, MNAMS, Assistant Professor, SLIMS, Puducherry.
Dr. Sinhasan SP, MD, Associate Professor of Pathology, IGMC&RI, Puducherry.
Dr. Amiya Kumar Nath, MD (JIPMER), Assistant Professor of Dermatology, IGMC&RI, Puducherry.
Dr. Venkateswaran R, MD, Assistant Professor of Medicine, JIPMER, Puducherry.
Dr. Niranjan G, MD Biochem (JIPMER), Associate Professor of Biochemistry, MGMC&RI, Puducherry.
Dr. Vishnu Kanth, MD (JIPMER), Assistant Professor, Department of Respiratory Medicine, JIPMER, Puducherry.
Dr. Dilli Kumar, MD (JIPMER), Assistant Professor of Pediatrics, JIPMER, Puducherry.
Dr. Sachidananda Adiga, MD, Associate Professor of Pharmacology, IGMC&RI, Puducherry.
Dr. Usha Adiga, MD, Assistant Professor of Biochemistry, IGMC&RI, Puducherry.
Dr. Giriyanna Gowda, MD, Assistant Professor of Community Medicine, KIMS, Bangalore, Karnataka.
Dr. Gomathi Shankar V, MS (JIPMER), DNB, MNAMS, Assistant Professor of Surgery, JIPMER, Puducherry.
Dr. Karthik, MD Physiology (JIPMER), Assistant Professor of Physiology, JIPMER, Puducherry.
Dr. Lourdu Jafrin, MD, Associate Professor of Pharmacology, IGMC&RI, Puducherry.
Dr. Mahalakshmy T, MD PSM (JIPMER), Assistant Professor of PSM, JIPMER, Puducherry.
Dr. Melvin George, MD, DM Clin Pharm (JIPMER), Assistant Professor, Cardiac Clinical Trials and Research, Department of Cardiology, SRM Medical College and Hospital, Potheri, Tamil Nadu.
Dr. Naveen Nair, MS Orthopedics (JIPMER), Associate Professor of Orthopedics, IGMC&RI, Puducherry
Dr. Noyal Mariya Joseph, MD (JIPMER), Assistant Professor of Microbiology, JIPMER, Puducherry.
Dr. Raveendranath, MS Anatomy (St Johns), Assistant Professor of Anatomy, JIPMER, Puducherry.
Dr. Rupa Vani, DNB, Assistant Professor of Obstetrics and Gynecology, IGMC&RI, Puducherry.
Dr. Sindhujha Sekar G, MBBS, DGO (JIPMER), Assistant Surgeon, Puduchatram PHC, Cuddalore, TN.

Sincere Thanks to:

Dr. Zubaida Begum, MBBS (MGMC&RI), Junior Resident in Pediatrics, IGMC&RI, Puducherry.
Dr. Nandini Varman, MBBS (MGMC&RI), Junior Resident in Pediatrics, IGMC&RI, Puducherry.
Dr. Jeevitha, MBBS (IGMC&RI), Junior Resident in Pediatrics, IGMC&RI, Puducherry.
Dr. Nandini Varman, MBBS (MGMC&RI), Junior Resident in Pediatrics, IGMC&RI, Puducherry.
Dr. Piyush Singh, MBBS, BMCH, Chitradurga, Karnataka.
Dr. Ezhil Kugan, MBBS, IGMC&RI, Puducherry.
Dr. Raghu Ram, MBBS (IGMC&RI), MD Radiology (Stud), PGI, Chandigarh.
Dr. Pradeep Ravi, MBBS, IGMC&RI, Puducherry.
Dr. Dana Lakshmi, MBBS, IGMC&RI, Puducherry.
Dr. Bindu Monika, MBBS, IGMC&RI, Puducherry.
Dr. Vignesh Raja, MBBS, IGMC&RI, Puducherry.

Dr. Balamurugan, MBBS, IGMC&RI, Puducherry.
Dr. Vijayadevagaran, MBBS, Senior Resident, Department of Pediatrics, IGMC&RI, Puducherry.
Dr. Narayanan, MBBS, MS Anatomy, JIPMER, Puducherry.
Dr. Sandhiya Selvarajan, MD, DM, Senior Resident, Clinical Pharmacology, JIPMER, Puducherry.
Dr. Jude Antonio Raja, MBBS, Senior Resident, Department of Pediatrics, IGMC&RI, Puducherry.
Dr. Priyadarshini, MBBS, Senior Resident, Department of Obs and Gyne, IGMC&RI, Puducherry.
Dr. Vishwas K Vijayadev, MS, DOHNS (Eng), Commonwealth Fellow–Facial Plastic Surgery, UK.
Dr. Nilesh Rao, MD (JIPMER), Fellow in Neonatology, Vancouver, Canada.
Dr. Anil Kumar, MD (JIPMER), Assistant Professor of Pediatrics, BMC, Bengaluru, Karnataka.
Dr. Manish Kumar, MD (JIPMER), Resident in Pediatric Neurology, USA.
Dr. Renitha, MD (JIPMER), Assistant Professor of Pediatrics, JIPMER, Puducherry.
Dr. Yasser Soliman, Fellow, Neonatal Perinatal Medicine, University of Calgary, Alberta, Canada.
Dr. Arul Parithi, MD (ICH, Chennai), Assistant Professor of Pediatrics, KVMC, Tamil Nadu.
Dr. Tiroumourugane Serane, MD (JIPMER), DNB, MRCPCH, AG Padmavathy Hospital, Puducherry.
Dr. Rajkumar, MS (JIPMER), Assistant Professor of Surgery, JIPMER, Puducherry.
Dr. Pratap Kumar Patra, MD Pediatrics, Assistant Professor, Department of Pediatrics, AIIMS, Patna.
Dr. Barathy, C, MBBS (JIPMER), DCH, DNB Pediatrics, Assistant Professor of Pediatrics, IGMC&RI, Puducherry.
Dr. Sharath, MD Physiology (JIPMER), Puducherry.
Dr. Malathi, MD Dermatology (JIPMER), Assistant Professor, Department of Skin and STD, JIPMER, Puducherry.
Dr. Swetha, MBBS, SLIMS, Puducherry.
Dr. Kumaran, MBBS (JIPMER), Puducherry.
Dr. Sathish, MBBS (JIPMER), Puducherry.
Dr. Balachandar, Fellow PICU, JIPMER, Puducherry.
Dr. Johnson Reddy, DNB Ped, IGGHPGI, Puducherry.
Dr. Joseph, MBBS (JIPMER), Puducherry.
Dr. Kavitha, MBBS (JIPMER), Puducherry.
Dr. Arun Kumar, MBBS (JIPMER), Puducherry.
Dr. Maheswari, MBBS (JIPMER), Puducherry.
Dr. Sunil, MBBS (JIPMER), Puducherry.
Dr. Mugunthan, MD Micro (Stud), AFMC, Pune.
Dr. Madhumitha, MBBS, SVMCH, Puducherry.
Dr. Suvetha, Intern, MGMC&RI, Puducherry.
Mr. Thirunavukkarasu D, Government School English Lecturer (Retd), Puducherry.
Mrs. Sampurnam, Principal (Retd), SSVHSS, Puducherry.
Mr. Vijayan D, Cash Officer (Retd), SBI, Puducherry.
Mrs. Sagoundala, Under Secretary (Retd), Government of Puducherry.
Mr. Srinivasan Babu, PWD, Puducherry.
Mr. Dhinesh Shankar, MCA Team Leader, EDS Emphasis, Chennai.
Mr. Rajkumar, System Engineer, Apple, CA, USA.
Mr. Armin Nuhanovic, Calgary, Alberta.
Mr. Chezhian, Glori Offset Printers, Puducherry.

and

Dr. Govindaraj, MD, Director, IGMC&RI, Puducherry and
Dr. Shanthi AK, MD, PhD, HOD, Department of Pediatrics, IGMC&RI, Puducherry.

Write to Us

Any observations, suggestions, criticisms are welcome. Write to the author at *babuarun.t@gmail.com*

Errata

Please visit *www.drarunbabu.in and www.peepeepub.com*

Follow Author in Facebook: *www.facebook.com/targetjipmer/and* **Dr. Arun Babu's Pediatrics Discussion group**

CONTENTS

JIPMER–2010

ANATOMY

1. **Superficial inguinal ring is a defect in:**
   A. External oblique aponeurosis
   B. Internal oblique aponeurosis
   C. External oblique abdominis
   D. Internal oblique abdominis

   Ans: A. External oblique aponeurosis

   Ref: *Grays Anatomy 40th Ed*

   Explanation:
   - Inguinal canal extends from superficial inguinal ring to deep inguinal ring
   - It is **4 cm** in length
   - Inguinal canal situated above inguinal ligament which extends from anterior superior illiac spine to pubic tubercle
   - **Superficial inguinal ring** is a triangular space in external oblique aponeurosis lies medial to inferior epigastric artery
   - **Deep inguinal ring** is a defect in **fascia transversalis** which lies **lateral** to **inferior epigastric artery**

   Hesselbach's Triangle:
   - **Medially**-lateral border of rectus abdominis muscle
   - **Laterally**-inferior epigastric artery
   - **Base** –inguinal ligament

   Hernias occuring through the hesselbach's triangle are known as **Direct hernia.**

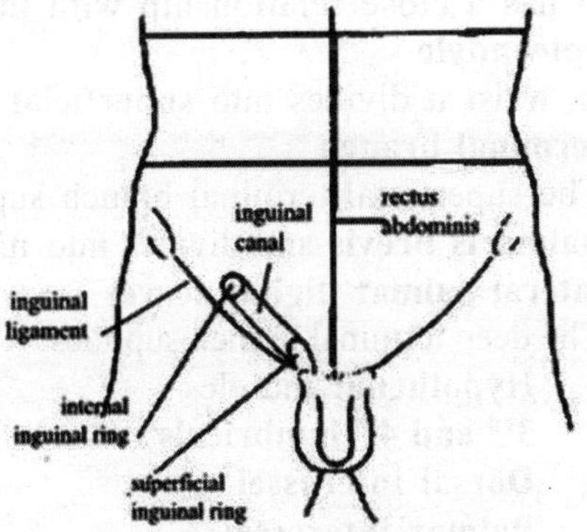

2. **All the following structures are related to carotid sheath *except:***
   A. Sympathetic trunk
   B. Vagus nerve
   C. Internal carotid artery
   D. Internal jugular vein

   Ans: A. Sympathetic trunk

   Ref: *Grays Anatomy 40th Ed*

   Explanation:

   Carotid sheath
   - It is the tubular investment of **deep cervical facsia**
   - The **anterior wall** of the sheath is formed by **pre-tracheal fascia**
   - The **posterior wall** is formed by **pre-vertebral fascia**
   - **Anca cervicalis** embedded in the **anterior wall** of carotid sheath
   - **Contents**:
     1. Common carotid artery
     2. Internal carotid artery
     3. Internal jugular vein
     4. Vagus nerve

3. **Left posterosuperior invagination of peritoneal cavity is known as:**
   A. Lesser Sac
   B. Hepato Renal Pouch
   C. Upper end of supra colic compartment
   D. Morrison's pouch

   Ans: A. Lesser sac

   Ref: *Grays Anatomy 40th Ed*

   Explanation:

   Lesser sac
   - Lesser sac is the **largest** of the **peritoneal recesses**
   - It is situated **behind the stomach** and **lesser omentum**
   - Through **formen of winslow** it communicate with **greater omentum**
   - **Hepato-renal pouch of morrison** is present in the **right side** between inferior surface of **liver** and **anterior surface** of **right kidney**

4. Which is not a branch of opthalmic artery?

A. Dorsal nasal artery
B. Superficial temporal artery
C. Supraorbital artery
D. Supratrochlear artery

Ans: B. Superficial temporal artery

Ref: *Grays Anatomy 40th Ed*

Explanation:

- Superficial temporal artery is terminal branch of external carotid artery

Opthalmic artery

- It is a branch of **internal carotid artery**
- The artery enter the orbit through the **optic canal** along with **optic nerve**
- It reaches the orbit **between medial rectus** and **superior oblique muscle**
- **Branches**
  1. Central artery of retina-(end artery)
  2. Posterior ciliary artery
  3. Anterior ciliary artery
  4. Lacrimal artery
  5. Posterior ethmoidal artery
  6. Anterior ethmoidal artery
  7. Medial palpebral artery
  8. Dorsal nasal artery
  9. Supra trochlear artery
  10. Supra orbital artery

5. All are derivatives of urogenital sinus *except:* (Repeat)

A. Bladder
B. Ejaculatory duct
C. Prostatic urethra
D. Membranous urethra

Ans: B. Ejaculatory duct

Ref: *Grays Anatomy 40th Ed*

Explanation:

- During 4th to 7th week of development, the cloaca divides into urogenital sinus anteriorly and anal canal posteriorly
- **Urorectal septum** present between them and its **lower part** will form **perineal body**
- Urogenital sinus
  - It has 3 parts
  - Upper part will form **urinary bladder**
  - Middle part (pelvic part) will **prostatic urethra** and **membranous urethra**
  - The third part is **Phallic part** which is flattened from side to side.

Note: Ejaculatory duct develops from **Mesonephric duct**

6. All are the following arise from mesonephric duct *except:*

A. Ductus deferens
B. Seminal vesicles
C. Epididymis
D. Rete testis

Ans: D. Rete testis

Ref: *Grays Anatomy 40th Ed*

Explanation:

Derivatives of mesonephric duct (Wolffian duct)

1. Kidney-Collecting tubules, pelvis & calyces
2. Ureter
3. Trigone of the bladder
4. Prostatic urethera
5. Epididymis
6. Vas deferens
7. Seminal vesicle
8. Ejaculatory duct
9. Part of prostate
10. Appendis of testis

Derivative of paramesonephric duct (Mullerian duct)

1. Uterus
2. Fallopian tube
3. Part of vagina

Note:

- **Scrotum** develops from **genital swelling**
- **Testis** and **ovary** develops from **genital ridge**

7. Superficial branch of ulnar nerve supplies:

A. Palmaris brevis
B. Abductor pollicis
C. Biceps brevis
D. Flexor carpi radialis

Ans: A. Palmaris brevis

Ref: *Grays Anatomy 40th Ed*

Explanation:

Ulnar nerve

- The ulnar nerve is formed from the **Medial Cord (C8, T1)**
- It has a close relationship with the **medial epicondyle**
- In **wrist** it divides into **superficial** and **deep terminal branch**
- The superficial terminal branch supplies the **palmaris brevis** and divides into **medial** and **lateral palmar digital nerves**
- The deep terminal branch supplies
  - **Hypothenar** muscles
  - **3rd and 4th lumbricals**
  - **Dorsal interossei**
  - **Palmar interossei**

8. Which is not a branch of posterior cord of brachial plexus?

A. Long thoracic nerve
B. Axillary nerve
C. Thoracodorsal nerve
D. Radial nerve

Ans: A. Long thoracic nerve

Ref: *Grays Anatomy 40th Ed*

Explanation:

Nerves arising from Brachial Plexus

Lateral cord	Lateral pectoral	C5, 6, 7
	Musculocutaneous	C5, 6 7
	Lateral root of median	C(5), 6, 7
Medial cord **(M4U)**	**M**edial pectoral	C8, T1
	Medial cutaneous of forearm	C8, T1
	Medial cutaneous of arm	C8, T1
	Ulnar	C(7), 8, T1
	Medial root of median	C8, T1
Posterior cord **(ULTAR)**	**U**pper subscapular	C5, 6
	Thoracodorsal	C6, 7,8
	Lower subscapular	C5, 6
	Axillary	C5, 6
	Radial	C5, 6, 7, 8, (T1)
Root	Dorsal scapular nerve	C5
	Long thoracic nerve of bell	C5,6,7
Trunk	Nerve to subclavius	C5,6
	Suprascapular nerve	C5,6

9. Nerve supply of tensor facia lata is:

A. Superior gluteal nerve
B. Inferior gluteal nerve
C. Femoral nerve
D. Sciatic nerve

Ans: A. Superior gluteal nerve

Ref: *Grays Anatomy 40th Ed*

Explanation:

Tensor fascia lata

- It is the **deep fascia of thigh**
- Superiorly it is attached to the **inguinal ligament** and **iliac crest**
- Inferiorly it is attached over the **knee anteriorly** and **laterally**
- Posteriorly it form **popliteal facsia**
- Its main insertion with **illio tibial tract**
- Actions are **medial rotation** and **flexion of thigh**
- **Nerve supply: Superior gluteal nerve (L5, S1)**

10. The afferent impulses of cremastric reflex are transmitted through:

A. Genitofemoral nerve **B.** Ilioinguinal nerve
C. Pudendal nerve **D.** Iliohypogastic nerve

Ans: A. Genitofemoral nerve

Ref: *Grays Anatomy 40th Ed*

Explanation:

Cremastreric reflex

- The cremaster muscle derived from **internal oblique** which suspend the testis and elevates it
- The reflex is elicited by lightly stroking the **superior and medial part of the thigh** in a **downward direction**
- The normal response is **contraction of cremaster** muscle that **pulls the testis** on the side stroked
- In **children** this reflex may be **exaggerated**
- In **spine injury** involving **L1, L2** and **torsion testis** this **reflex may be absent**
- **Afferent-Femoral** branch of **Genito femoral nerve**
- **Efferent-Genital** branch of **Genito femoral nerve**

11. Scala tympani and vestibuli is drained by:

A. Aqueduct of cochlea **B.** Perilymphatic duct
C. Enolymphatic duct **D.** Cochlear lymphatics

Ans: B. Perilymphatic duct

Ref: *Grays Anatomy 40th Ed*

Explanation:

Perilymph:

- It fills the **bony labyrinth (scala tympani & scala vestibule)**
- It is similar to **CSF**
- It is drained by **perilymphatic duct** into the adjoining subarachnoid space

Endolymph:

- It fills the **membranous labyrinth**
- Has **high K^+** and **low Na^+** similar to **intracellular fluid**
- It is produced by specialized cells in the **wall of cochlear duct**
- It is drained via **endolymphatic duct**

12. Cranial end of wolfian duct forms:

A. Epoophoron **B.** Paraepoophoron
C. Gartner cyst **D.** Bartholin cyst

Ans: A. Epoophoron

Ref: *Grays Anatomy 40th Ed*

Explanation:

Embryology of Reproductive System

Gonad	MALES (Testis)	FEMALES (Ovary)
Gubernacular cord	Gubernaculum testis	Ovarian and round ligaments
Mesonephros (Wolffian body)	Appendix of epididymis (?)	Appendices vesiculosae (?)
	Efferent ductules	Epoöphoron
	Lobules of epididymis	
	Paradidymis	Paroöphoron
	Aberrant ductules	
Mesonephric duct (Wolffian duct)	Duct of epididymis	Duct of epoöphoron (Gartner's duct)
	Vas deferens	
	Ejaculatory duct	
	Part of bladder and prostatic urethra	Part of bladder and urethra
Paramesonephric duct (Müllerian)	Appendix of testis	Uterine tube
		Uterus
	Prostatic utricle	Vagina
Allantoic duct	Urachus	Urachus
Cloaca:		
Dorsal part	Rectum and upper part of anal canal	Rectum and upper part of anal canal
Ventral part	Most of bladder	Most of bladder and urethra
	Part of prostatic urethra	
Urogenital sinus	Prostatic urethra distal to utricle	
	Bulbo-urethral glands	Greater vestibular glands
	Rest of urethra to glans	Vestibule
Genital folds	Ventral penis	Labia minora
Genital tubercle	Penis	Clitoris
	Urethra in glans	
Genital ridge	Testis	Ovary
Genital swelling	Scrotum	Labia majora

13. **Muscle not supplied by ansa cervicalis?**
A. Stylohyoid
B. Sternothyroid
C. Sternohyoid
D. Omohyoid

Ans: A. Stylohyoid

Ref: *Grays Anatomy 40th Ed*

Explanation:

Ansa cervicalis

- Ansa cervicalis is formed by a loop of two nerve fibres in cervical region
- ***Descendens hypoglossi*** (**superior** root) is formed from **C1** and this carries a fibre from **hypoglossal nerve**
- ***Descendens cervicalis*** (**Inferior** root) is formed by **C2, C3**
- Ansa cervicalis embedded in the **anterior layer of carotid sheath**
- The muscles supplied by the ansa cervicalis are (**Infrahyoid** muscles)
  1. ***Sternohyoid***
  2. ***Sternothyroid***
  3. ***Omohyoid***

14. **Sinus located in falx cerebelli is:**
A. Sigmoid sinus
B. Straight sinus
C. Occipital sinus
D. Inferior petrosal sinus

Ans: C. Occipital sinus

Ref: *Grays Anatomy 40th Ed*

Explanation:

Falx cerebelli

- It is a sickle shaped fold of duramater projecting forwards into the posterior cerebellar notch
- It separates the inferior surface of cerebrum and superior surface of cerebellum
- It **partitions** the **right** and **left cerebellar hemispheres**
- It is anchored to the **occipital crest** and contains **occipital sinus**

15. **Which of the following is not a content of adductor canal?**
A. Femoral artery
B. Femoral vein
C. Saphenous nerve
D. Nerve to vastus lateralis

Ans: D. Nerve to vatus lateralis

Ref: *Grays Anatomy 40th Ed*

Explanation:

Adductor canal/subsartorial canal/hunter's canal

- Located at the middle of the thigh
- Extends from **apex of the femoral triangle** to the **opening** of the **adductor magnus**
- Boundaries:
  1. **Roof** - Sartorius
  2. **Floor** - Adductor longus
  3. **Laterally** - Vastus medialis
- Contents:
  1. Femoral **artery**
  2. Femoral **vein**
  3. **Saphenous** nerve
  4. Nerve to **vastus medialis**
  5. Occasionally **posterior division of obturator nerve**

16. **The type of joint between epiphysis and diaphysis?**

A. Syndesmosis **B.** Synchondrosis
C. Fibrous joint **D.** Plain synovial joint

Ans: B. Synchondrosis

Ref: *Grays Anatomy 40th Ed*

Explanation:

Synchondrosis

- It is a **primary cartilagenous joint**
- The bones are united by a plate of hyaline cartilage, which is temporary in nature and is replaced completely by bone
- **No movement is possible** at this joint
- It is primarily designed for **bone growth**

Syndesmosis

- It is a type of **fibrous joint**
- Example-**Inferior tibio fibular joint**

17. **Which of the follwing is not present at birth?**

A. Malleus
B. Incus
C. Stapes
D. Petrous temporal bone

Ans: D. Petrous part of tempotal bone

Ref: *Grays Anatomy 40th Ed*

Explanation:

- **Ear ossicles** will be completely formed **before birth**

Development of Temporal Bone

- In neonate, the petrous and squamous parts of the temporal bone are usually partially separated by the petrosquamous fissure
- This opens directly into the mastoid antrum of the middle ear
- The **fissure** remains **open till 20 years** in **20–40% individuals**

18. **Short head of biceps attached to:**

A. Coracoid process
B. Supraglenoid tubercle
C. Acromion process
D. Bicipital groove

Ans: A. Coracoid process

Ref: *Grays Anatomy 40th Ed*

Explanation:

- Biceps brachii has two head-long head & short head
- **Long head** orginate from **supraglenoid tubercle**
- **Short head** orginate from **coracoid process**
- **Biceps tendon** inserted into the **radial tuberosity**
- The muscle is innervated by **musculo cutaneous nerve**
- The action of the muscles are **flexion** and **supinator**

19. **Anatomical snuff box not formed by:**

A. Extensor pollicis longus
B. Extensor pollicis brevis
C. Abductor pollicis longus
D. Abductor pollicis brevis

Ans: D. Abductor pollicis brevis

Ref: *Grays Anatomy 40th Ed*

Explanation:

Anatomical snuff box

- **Boundaries**
  Laterally - Tendon of Abductor pollicis longus (**APL**) & Extensor pollicis brevis (**EPB**)
  Medially - Tendon of Extensor pollicis longus (**EPL**)
  Roof - Skin, Fascia
  Floor - Styloid process of radius, Scaphoid, Trapezium & Base of first metatarsal
- **Contents-** ***Radial artery & cephalic vein***

(See Figure on the next page)

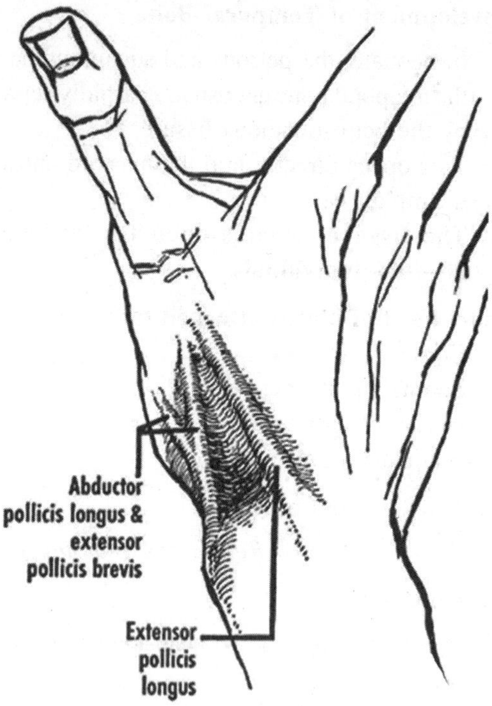

20. **Middle ear cavity is connected anteriorly to:**
A. Nasal cavity **B.** Nasopharynx
C. Mastoid antrum **D.** Mastoid air cells

Ans: B. Nasopharynx

Ref: *Grays Anatomy 40th Ed*

Explanation:

Middle ear cavity

- **Anterior wall** - Upper canal for tensor tympan muscle & lower canal for **auditory tube** which communicates to the **nasopharynx**
- **Posterior wall** communicates the **mastoid antrum** through **aditus**
- **Lateral wall** seperates the middle ear from **external ear**
- **Medial wall** separates the middle ear from **internal ear**

21. **Scarpa's fascia merges with:**
A. Inguinal ligament **B.** Conjoint tendon
C. Tensor fascia lata **D.** Pubic crest

Ans: C. Tensor fascia lata

Ref: *Grays Anatomy 40th Ed*

Explanation

Scarpa's facia is a **membranous fascia** of **abdomen** and it merges with **tensor fascia lata.**

Tensor fascia lata

- It is a **deep fascia of thigh**
- Encloses **entire thigh**
- It thickens on lateral side to form **illiotibial tract**

22. **Which is not a branch of facial nerve?**
A. Chorda tympani
B. Lingual nerve
C. Greater superficial petrosal nerve
D. Branch to stylohyoid muscle

Ans: B. Lingual nerve

Ref: *Grays Anatomy 40th Ed*

Explanation:

- **Lingual nerve** arises from **mandibular branch** of **trigeminal nerve**

Braches of Facial Nerve

A. Intra cranial branches
- **Greater petrosal nerve**
- **Nerve to stapedius**
- **Chorda tympani**
  - Submandibular gland
  - Sublingual gland
  - Special sensory taste fibers for the anterior 2/3 of the tongue.

B. Extra cranial branches
Distal to stylomastoid foramen, the following nerves branch off the facial nerve:
- **Posterior auricular nerve**
- Branch to **Posterior belly of Digastric muscle** and **Stylohyoid muscle**
- **Five major facial branches** (in **parotid** gland)
  - **Temporal** branch of the facial nerve
  - **Zygomatic** branch of the facial nerve
  - **Buccal** branch of the facial nerve
  - **Marginal mandibular** branch of the facial nerve
  - **Cervical** branch of the facial nerve

23. **Which is true regarding central retinal artery?**
A. Supplies optic nerve
B. End artery
C. Branch of ciliary artery
D. Course similar to central retinal vein

Ans: B. End artery

Ref: *Grays Anatomy 40th Ed*

Explanation:

The central retinal artery (retinal artery)
- Branch of **ophthalmic artery**, running **inferior to the optic nerve** within its **dural sheath** into the eyeball.

- It is an **end artery (No collaterals)**
- It supplies all the **nerve fibers that form the optic nerve** that carries the visual information to the lateral geniculate nucleus of the thalamus, including those that reach over the fovea.
- It divides into superior nasal, inferior nasal, superior temporal and inferior temporal branches.
- Each of these branches supply its corresponding quadrant in retina.

PHYSIOLOGY

1. **Vitamin B_{12} and folic acid absorption are:**
   A. Na^+ dependent process in colon
   B. Na^+ independent process in colon
   C. Na^+ dependent process in ileum
   D. Na^+ independent process in ileum

   Ans: D. Na^+ independent process in ileum

   Ref: *W F Ganong. Digestion, Absorption, & Nutritional Principles. In: Review of Medical Physiology. 24th ed. California: McGraw-Hill Companies; 2012, p485.*

   Explanation:

   - Most **vitamins** are absorbed in the **upper small intestine**, but **vitamin B_{12} is** absorbed in the terminal **ileum**
   - **Vitamin B_{12}** absorption and **folate** absorption are **Na^+-independent**, but other water soluble vitamins are absorbed by **Na^+ co-transporters** *(See Table 1)*

2. **Circadian rhythm is influenced by:**
   A. Supra optic nuclei
   B. Postero lateral nucleus
   C. Ventro-lateral nucleus
   D. Supra chiasmatic nucleus

   Ans: D. Supra chiasmatic nucleus

   Ref: *W F Ganong. Central and Peripheral Neurophysiology. In: Review of Medical Physiology. 24th ed. California: McGraw-Hill Companies; 2012, p278.*

   Explanation:

   Circadian rhythm is dependent on the **supra-chiasmatic nuclei (SCN)** located bilaterally above the **optic chiasm.** *(See Table 2 on the next page)*

3. **Stimulation of bipolar cells results in all *except:***
   A. Depolarisation
   B. Hyperpolarisation
   C. Neurotransmitter release
   D. Action potentials

   Ans: D. Action potentials

   Ref: *W F Ganong. Vision. In: Review of Medical Physiology. 23rd ed. California: McGraw-Hill Companies; 2010.*

   Explanation:

   *"Unlike most neurons, bipolar cells communicate via **graded potentials**, rather than **action potentials**"*

   Genesis of Electrical Responses in Retina

   - Electrical responses of most of the other neural elements in the **retina** are **local, graded potentials**
   - Only ***in the ganglion cells,*** all-or-none **action potentials** (transmitted over appreciable distances) are generated
   - Responses of the **rods, cones,** and **horizontal cells** are **hyperpolarizing**

Table 1 : Normal transport of substances by the intestine and location of maximum absorption or secretion

Absorption of:	Small Intestine: Upper (Duodenum & Jejunum)	Mid	Lower (Terminal ileum)	Colon
Sugars (glucose, galactose, etc.	++	+++	++	0
Amino acids	++	+++	++	0
Water-soluble and fat-soluble **vitamins** except vitamin B_{12}	+++	++	0	0
Long-chain fatty acid absorption and conversion to triglyceride	+++	++	+	0
Bile salts	+	+	+++	
Vitamin B_{12}	0	+	+++	0
Na^+	+++	++	+++	+++
K^+	+	+	+	Secreted
Ca^{2+}	+++	++	+	?
Fe^{2+}	+++	++	+	?
Cl^-	+++	++	+	+
SO_4^{2-}	++	+	0	?

Table 2 : Function of Hypothalamus

Region	Area	Nucleus	Function
Anterior	Medial	Medial preoptic nucleus	• Regulates the release of **gonadotropic** hormones from the adenohypophysis • Contains the sexually dimorphic nucleus, which releases **GnRH**, differential development between sexes is based upon in utero testosterone levels
		Supraoptic nucleus (SO)	• **Vasopressin** release
		Paraventricular nucleus* (PV)	• **Thyrotropin-releasing** hormone release • **Corticotropin-releasing** hormone release • **Oxytocin** release
		Anterior hypothalamic nucleus (AH)	• **Thermoregulation** • Panting • **Sweating** • Thyrotropin inhibition
		Suprachiasmatic nucleus(SC)	• **Circadian rhythms**
	Lateral	Lateral preoptic nucleus	
		Lateral nucleus (LT)	• **Thirst** and **hunger**
		Part of supraoptic nucleus (SO)	
Tuberal	Medial	**Dorsomedial hypothalamic nucleus (DM)**	• **Blood Pressure** • **Heart Rate** • **GI stimulation**
		Ventromedial nucleus (VM)	• **Satiety** • **Neuroendocrine** control
		Arcuate nucleus (AR)	• **Growth hormone-releasing hormone** (GHRH) • **Feeding** • **Dopamine**
	Lateral	**Lateral nucleus** (LT)	• **Thirst** and hunger
		Lateral tuberal nuclei	
Posterior	Medial	**Mammillary nuclei** (part of mammillary bodies) (**MB**)	• **Memory**
		Posterior nucleus (PN)	• Increase blood pressure • **Pupillary** dilation • **Shivering** • Vasopressin release
	Lateral	Lateral nucleus (LT)	

- Responses of the **bipolar cells** are either **hyperpolarizing** or **depolarizing**.
- **Amacrine cells** produce depolarizing potentials.

4. **Which of the following causes decrease in diastolic blood pressure?**
   A. Sympathetic stimulation
   B. Inhibition of Vasomotor center
   C. Stimulation of vagal center
   D. Stimulation of Vasomotor center

Ans: B. Inhibition of Vasomotor center

Ref: *Pal GK. Blood pressure and its regulation. In: Textbook of Medical Physiology.. Ahuja Publishing House. 2007; 80: 643*

Explanation:

- **Diastolic pressure** is mainly decided by **peripheral resistance**, which is mainly controlled by **sympathetic** system. (Remember: **No parasympathetic nerve supply to blood vessel**)
- **Vasomotor center** (rostral ventro-lateral medulla) is the higher center for **sympathetic** system. Inhibition of **VMC,** results in reduced **vaso-constrictor tone** (reduced sympathetic activity) which in turn **reduces diastolic BP**

Baroreceptor

↑ **BP**→stimulation (stretch) of baroreceptors (carotid sinus & aortic arch)→ through IX & X cranial nerve→ stimulation of NTS→**inhibition of VMC**→ ↓ sympathetic discharge→ ↓ **BP (↓ SBP by ↓ CO and ↓ DBP by ↓ vasoconstriction) and also ↓ HR.**

↓ **BP**→less/ no stimulation (stretch) of baroreceptors (carotid sinus & aortic arch)→ through IX & X cranial nerve→ less/ no stimulation of NTS→**disinhibition of VMC**→ ↑ sympathetic discharge→ ↑ **BP (↑ SBP by ↑ CO and ↑ DBP by ↑ vasoconstriction) and also ↑ HR.**

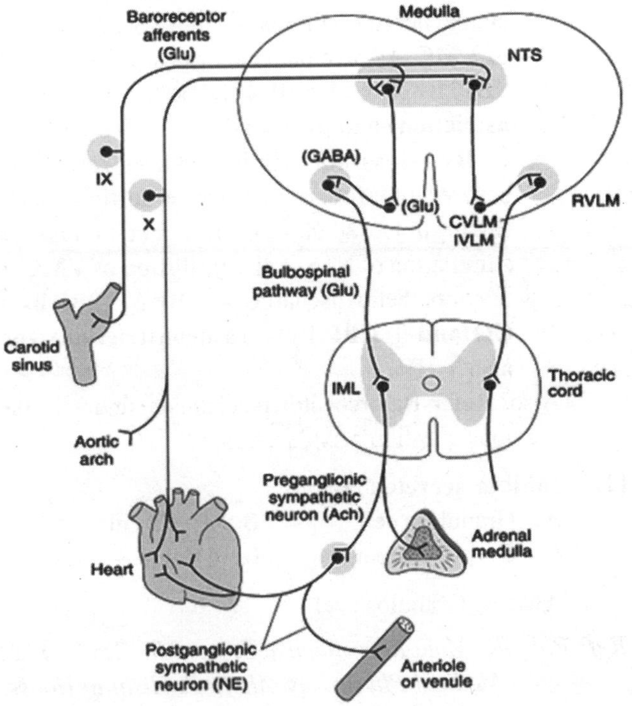

5. **Magnitude of action potential in neuron, is determined by:**
   A. Na^+ **B.** Mg^{2+}
   C. K^+ **D.** Ca^{2+}

   Ans: A. Na^+

Ref: *Pal GK. Nerve. In: Textbook of Medical Physiology. Ahuja Publishing House. 2007; 18: 158.*

Explanation:

- **Depolarization (upstroke) phase** of action potential in a neuron is due to **Na^+** influx
- **Repolarization** is due to **K^+** efflux
- **Mg^{2+}, Ca^{2+}** are not directly involved in generation of action potential in nerve

6. **Dopamine causes all, *except:***
   A. Decreases splanchnic circulation
   B. Increases cardiac output
   C. Decreases peripheral resistance
   D. Increases heart rate

   Ans: D. Increases heart rate

Ref: *KD Tripathi. Drugs Acting on ANS. In: Essentials of Medical Pharmacology. 6th Edn. Jaypee Brothers Medical Publishers (P) Ltd. 2008;126.*

Explanation:

Actions of Dopamine

- **D1 receptors** in **renal** and **mesenteric** blood vessels are the **most sensitive**: I.V. infusion of low dose of DA **dilates** these vessels
- Moderately high doses produce a **positive inotropic** (direct B1 and D1 action + that due to NA release), but **little chronotropic** effect on heart
- It raises **cardiac output** and **systolic BP** with **little effect on diastolic BP**

7. **The normal AV nodal delay is due to:**
   A. Junctional fibres are very small in size
   B. Decrease in amplitude of firing
   C. Resistance offered by myocytes
   D. Lack of tight junctions

   Ans: A. Junctional fibres are very small in size

Ref: *Pal GK. Functional Anatomy and Innervation of Heart. In: Textbook of Medical Physiology. Ahuja Publishing House. 2007; 69: 567*

Explanation:

- In **AV node**, fiber diameter is **small** and there are **multiple sub-branches**.
- Rate of impulse conduction is **slow (0.05 m/s);** delay of about **0.1** seconds
- As, impulse follows **all or none phenomenon**, there is **no change in amplitude**
- **AP** is an **electrical property** and, not affected by **mechanical factors**

8. **Testesterone secreted by:**
   A. Leydig cells **B.** Sertoli cells
   C. Cowper's gland **D.** Intermediate cells

   Ans: A. Leydig cells

Ref: *Pal GK. Male reproductive system. In: Textbook of Medical Physiology. Ahuja Publishing House. 2007; 54: 410.*

Explanation:

Sertoli Cell

1. Endocrine function

- Inhibin, Follistatin - ↓ FSH
- Activin - ↑ FSH
- MIS (Mullerian Inhibiting Substance) - 8th week of IUL
- Estrogen - from androgen by aromatase

2. Secretory functions
   - Androgen binding Protein (ABP) - binds with DHT, testosterone & transport to epididymis
   - H- Y antigen - development of gonads
   - Plasminogen activator

Leydig cells

- Secretes testosterone, DHEA, Androstenodione

Cowper's gland (Bulbourethral gland)

- homologous to Bartholin's glands in females
- Cowper's gland secretion helps to lubricate the urethra for spermatozoa to pass through, neutralizing traces of acidic urine in the urethra

9. Pitutary stalk damage can decrease the levels of all the following hormones *except:*

A. Prolactins
B. Growth hormone
C. Vasopressin
D. Follicular stimulating hormone

Ans: A. Prolactins

Ref: *Koeppen BM, Stanton BA. The Hypothalamus and Pituitary Gland In: Berne & Levy Physiology 6th ed. Mosby; 2008 p 724*

Explanation:

- Production and secretion of **PRL** are ***predominantly*** *under* ***inhibitory control*** *by the* ***hypothalamus.***
- Disruption of the **pituitary stalk** and the **hypothalamohypophysial** portal vessels (e.g., surgery or physical trauma) results in an ***increase in PRL*** (prolactin) levels but a decrease in ACTH, TSH, FSH, LH, and GH.

10. Decrease in BP causes:

A. Inhibition of vasoconstrictor center
B. Dis-inhibition of vasoconstrictor center
C. Increased stimulation of cardiac inhibitory center
D. Increased vagal stimulation

Ans: B. Dis-inhibition of vasoconstrictor center

Ref: *Pal GK. Blood pressure and its regulation. In: Textbook of Medical Physiology. Ahuja Publishing House. 2011; 42: 324.*

Explanation:

- Reduction in BP is perceived by baroreceptors and less nerve traffic (signals) is sent to cardiac inhibitory center (CIc) (Less stimulation to CIc)
- There will be **dis**-inhibition of **vasoconstrictor center** (Vasomotor center) by **CIC**
- **Increased VMC** activity **stimulates sympathetic** activity

Baroreceptor

↑ **BP**→stimulation (stretch) of baroreceptors (carotid sinus & aortic arch)→ through IX & X cranial nerve→ stimulation of NTS→**inhibition of VMC**→ ↓ sympathetic discharge→ ↓ **BP (↓ SBP by ↓ CO and ↓ DBP by ↓ vasoconstriction) and also ↓ HR**

↓ **BP**→less/no stimulation (stretch) of baroreceptors (carotid sinus & aortic arch)→ through IX & X cranial nerve→ less/no stimulation of NTS→**dis-inhibition of VMC**→ ↑ sympathetic discharge→ ↑ **BP (↑ SBP by ↑ CO and ↑ DBP by ↑ vasoconstriction) and also ↑ HR.**

Also, Refer Baroreceptor mechanism figure in the previous question's explanation.

11. Inhibin secreted by:

A. Granulosa cell **B.** Theca cell
C. Corpus leuteum **D.** Deciduas

Ans: A. Granulosa cell

Ref: *Pal GK. Male Reproductive System. In: Textbook of Medical Physiology. Ahuja Publishing House. 2007; 54: 451.*

Explanation:

Inhibin

Source
- **Male** – ***Sertoli*** cell
- **Female** – ***Granulosa*** cell

Structure
- Inhibin A Subunits - α, βA
- Inhibin B Subunits – α, βB

Function
- Inhibit FSH secretion

12. Gamma efferent motor neuron is influenced by:

A. Corticospinal tract
B. Tectospinal tract
C. Vestibulo spinal tract
D. Reticulospinal tract

Ans: D. Reticulospinal tract

Ref: 1.Pal GK. Regulation of Posture and Movement. In: Textbook of Medical Physiology. 114: 859.
2. Pal GK. Descending Pathways. In: Textbook of Medical Physiology. Ahuja Publishing House. 2007; 113: 845, 850.

Explanation:

- **Corticospinal tract** – 30% terminate in alpha motor neuron; 70% ends with interneurons in spinal cord
- **Tectospinal tract** – regulates contralateral movement of head to visual stimulus
- **Vestibulo** spinal tract – acts through á- motor neuron
- **Reticulospinal** tract – influences gamma motor neuron

13. **Preload of the heart depends on:**
   A. End diastolic volume
   B. End systolic volume
   C. Stroke volume
   D. Cardiac output

Ans: A. End diastolic volume

Ref: Pal GK. Blood pressure and its regulation. In: Textbook of Medical Physiology. Ahuja Publishing House. 2007; 80: 641.

Explanation:

- **Preload** is End Diastolic Volume (EDV)
- **Afterload** is the **peripheral resistance**. It is inversely related to **cardiac output**.

14. **Vestibulo-Ocular Reflex Mediated by:**
   A. Flocculonodular Lobe
   B. Vermal portion of Spinocerebellum
   C. Neocerebellum
   D. Paravermal region of Spinocerebellum

Ans: A. Flocculonodular Lobe

Ref: Pal GK. Cerbellum. In: Textbook of Medical Physiology. Ahuja Publishing House. 2007; 116: 871.

Explanation:

Functional Division of Cerebellum

Vestibulo cerebellum/ Arch-cerebellum (Flocculo-nodular lobe)

- Connections with vestibular apparatus
- Concerned with equilibrium and learning induced changes in vestibulo-occular reflex

Spino cerebellum

- Vermis - controls muscle movements of axial body
- Intermediate zone - controls muscle movements of limbs

Cerbrocerbellum (Ponto cerebellum/Neo cerbellum)

- Overall planning programming of motor activities

15. **Partial pressure of oxygen in room air at 760 mm of atmospheric pressure:**
   A. 160 mm of Hg **B.** 240 mm of Hg
   C. 580 mm of Hg **D.** 760 mm of Hg

Ans: A. 160 mm of Hg

Ref: Ganong's Medical Physiology, 21st ed.

Explanation:

- The atmospheric air mainly contains **79%** of nitrogen and **21%** of oxygen.
- Average sea-level pressure is **760 millimetres** of mercury (mmHg).
- **Each gas contributes** to the **total pressure** in **direct proportion** to their **concentration.**
- Therefore 79% of 760 is contributed by Nitrogen (approx 600 mm Hg) and the remaining by oxygen
- Oxygen is about 21% (21/100) in atmospheric air
- Partial pressure of O_2 (at sea level) is 0.21 x 760 = 159.6 = **160 mm Hg**

16. **True regarding blood pressure measurement with sphygmomanometer in comparison with intra-arterial pressure monitoring is:**
   A. Less than intravascular pressure
   B. Equal to intravascular pressure
   C. Depends on velocity of flow
   D. Greater than intravascular pressure

Ans: A. Less than intravascular pressure

Ref: Hunyor SN et al. Comparison of performance of various sphygmomanometers with intra-arterial blood-pressure readings. Br Med J. 1978 July 15; 2(6131): 159–162.

Explanation:

*"Systolic pressure was consistently **underestimated** (range 31-7 mm Hg) by sphygmomanometer when compared to simulataneous intra-arterial blood pressure measurement"*

BIOCHEMISTRY

1. **Which amino acid undergoes hepatic deamination?**
   A. Alanine **B.** Glutamate
   C. Aspartate **D.** Glycine

Ans: B. Glutamate

Ref: *Harper's Illustrated Biochemistry, 26th edition. Pg 244.*

Explanation:

*"Since **alanine** is also a **substrate for glutamate aminotransferase**, all the amino nitrogen from amino acids that undergo **transamination** can be concentrated in **glutamate**. This is important because **L-glutamate** is the **only amino acid** that undergoes **oxidative deamination** at an appreciable rate in **liver & kidney**." (Ref: Harper)*

BIOSYNTHESIS OF UREA

Urea biosynthesis occurs in four stages:
(1) Transamination
(2) Oxidative deamination of glutamate
(3) Ammonia transport
(4) Reactions of the urea cycle

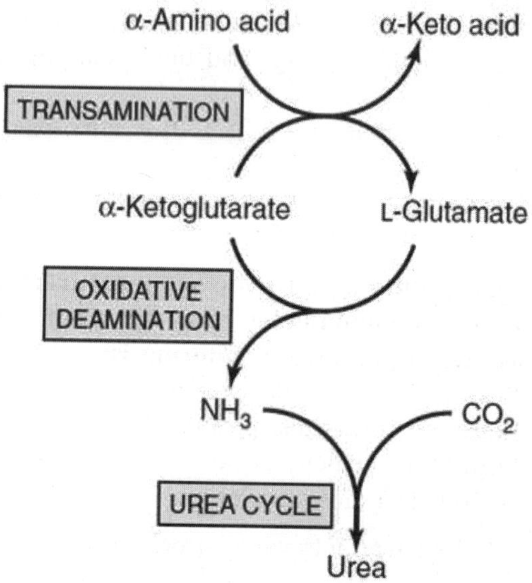

2. **Which of the following is a marker for peroxisomes?**
A. Glutamate dehydrogenase
B. Glucose 6 phosphatase
C. 5' nucleotidase
D. Uric acid oxidase

Ans: D. Uric acid oxidase

Ref: *Harper's Illustrated Biochemistry, 28th edition.*

Explanation:

Peroxisomes

- Also called **microbodies**
- Peroxisomes are found in many tissues, including liver
- They are rich in **oxidases & catalase**
- These organelles are involved in the
  - **Catabolism** of **very long chain fatty acids, branched chain fatty acids, D-amino acids & polyamines**
  - **Biosynthesis** of **plasmalogens**

Markers of Intracellular organelles

- **Plasma Membrane**: Na^+ K^+ ATPase & 5' Nucleotidase
- **Cytoplasm**: Lactate dehydrogenase
- **Mitochondria**: Glutamate dehydrogenase
- **Ribosome**: RNA
- **Endoplasmic reticulum**: Glucose-6-phosphatase
- **Lysosome**: Acid phosphatase
- **Golgi Apparatus**: Galactosyl transferase
- **Peroxisomes**: Catalase & Uric acid oxidase
- **Nucleus**: DNA

3. **Acetyl Co A carboxylase is stimulated by:**
A. Malonyl CoA **B.** Citrate
C. Palmitoyl CoA **D.** Acetoacetate

Ans: B. Citrate

Ref: *Harper's Illustrated Biochemistry, 26th edition. Pg 178. & Lippincott Illustrated Reviews Biochemistry, 3rd edition, Pg 182.*

Explanation:

*"**Acetyl-CoA carboxylase** is an allosteric enzyme and is **activated** by **citrate**, which increases in concentration in the well-fed state and is an indicator of a plentiful supply of acetyl-CoA" Ref: Harper*

- Acetyl-CoA Carboxylase Is the Most Important Enzyme in the regulation of **Lipogenesis (Fatty acid synthesis)**

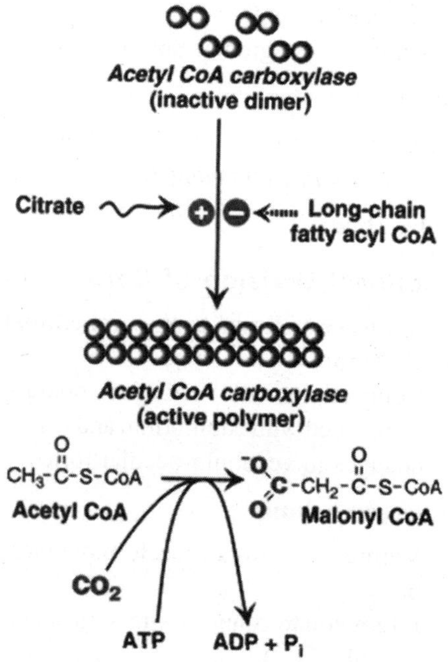

Short-term regulation of acetyl CoA carboxylase:

- This carboxylation is both the **rate-limiting** and the regulated step in **fatty acid synthesis**
- The inactive form of **acetyl CoA carboxylase** is a protomer (**Dimer**)
- The enzyme undergoes **allosteric activation** by **citrate**, which causes dimmers to polymerize.
- The enzyme can be allosterically inactivated by long-**chain fatty Acyl CoA** (the end product of the pathway), which causes its **depolymerization**.
- A second mechanism of short-term regulation is by reversible **phosphorylation**.
- In the presence of **counterregulatory hormones**, such as **epinephrine** and **glucagon**, acetyl CoA carboxylase is phosphorylated and, thereby, inactivated
- In the presence of insulin, acetyl CoA carboxylase is dephosphorylated and, thereby, activated.

Long-term regulation of acetyl CoA carboxylase:

- Prolonged consumption of a diet containing excess calories (particularly, high calorie, high-carbohydrate diets) causes an increase in **Acetyl CoA carboxylase synthesis**, thus increasing fatty acid synthesis.
- Conversely, a low-calorie diet or fasting causes a reduction acid synthesis by decreasing the synthesis of acetyl CoA carboxylase.

4. **Which of the following is required for glycogen phosphorylase in glycogenolysis?**

A. Thiamine pyrophosphate
B. Pyridoxal phosphate
C. FAD
D. Citrate

Ans: B. Pyridoxal phosphate

Ref: *Harper's Illustrated Biochemistry, 28th edition.*

Explanation:

Glycogen phosphorylase

- This enzyme catalyzes the **rate-limiting step in glycogenolysis** by releasing **glucose-1-phosphate** from the terminal **alpha-1, 4-glycosidic bond.**
- Glycogen phosphorylase has a **pyridoxal phosphate** (PLP, derived from Vitamin B6) at each catalytic site.

5. **Insulin acts through all *except:***

A. Tyrosine kinase receptor
B. Inhibition of membrane Na K ATPase
C. Inducing hexokinase activity
D. Increasing GLUT - 4 in cell surface

Ans: B. Inhibition of membrane Na K ATPase

Ref: *Harper's Illustrated Biochemistry, 28th edition. & Ganong's Physiology 21st ed.*

Explanation:

"Binding of insulin triggers the tyrosine kinase activity of the β subunits, producing autophosphorylation" Ref: Ganong

"GLUT 4 is the transporter in muscle and adipose tissue that is stimulated by insulin." Ref: Ganong

"Hexokinase IV, in beta cells of the pancreatic islets, serves as a glucose sensor to control insulin release, and similarly controls glucagon release in the alpha cells" Ref: Harper

"Insulin's increase in cellular potassium uptake lowers potassium levels in blood. This possibly occurs via insulin-induced translocation of the Na^+/K^+-ATPase to the surface of skeletal muscle cells" Ref: Harper

Effects of insulin on various tissues.

Adipose issue

- Increased glucose entry
- Increased fatty acid synthesis
- Increased glycerol phosphate synthesis
- Increased triglyceride deposition
- Activation of lipoprotein lipase
- Inhibition of hormone-sensitive lipase
- Increased K^+ uptake

Muscle

- Increased glucose entry
- Increased glycogen synthesis
- Increased amino acid uptake
- Increased protein synthesis in ribosomes
- Decreased protein catabolism
- Decreased release of gluconeogenic amino acids
- Increased ketone uptake
- Increased K^+ uptake

Liver

- Decreased ketogenesis
- Increased protein synthesis
- Increased lipid synthesis
- Decreased glucose output due to decreased gluconeogenesis and increased glycogen synthesis

6. **Nitric oxide acts by:**

A. cGMP **B.** cAMP
C. Calcium **D.** Kinase

Ans: A. cGMP

Ref: *Harper's Illustrated Biochemistry, 28th edition.*

Explanation:

Classification of Hormones by Mechanism of Action

I. Hormones that bind to intracellular receptors
• Androgens • Calcitriol (1,25[OH]$_2$-D$_3$) Estrogens • Glucocorticoids • Mineralocorticoids • Progestins • Retinoic acid • Thyroid hormones (T_3 and T_4)
II. Hormones that bind to cell surface receptors
A. The second messenger is cAMP • Alpha2 -Adrenergic catecholamines • Alpha-Adrenergic catecholamines • Adrenocorticotropic hormone • Antidiuretic hormone • Calcitonin • Chorionic gonadotropin, human • Corticotropin-releasing hormone • Follicle-stimulating hormone • Glucagon • Lipotropin • Luteinizing hormone • Melanocyte-stimulating hormone • Parathyroid hormone • Somatostatin • Thyroid-stimulating hormone
B. The second messenger is cGMP • Atrial natriuretic factor • Nitric oxide (EDRF)
C. The second messenger is calcium or phosphatidylinositols (or both) • Acetylcholine (muscarinic) • Alpha$_1$-Adrenergic catecholamines Angiotensin II • Antidiuretic hormone (vasopressin) • Cholecystokinin • Gastrin • Gonadotropin-releasing hormone • Oxytocin • Platelet-derived growth factor • Substance P • Thyrotropin-releasing hormone
D. The second messenger is a kinase or phosphatase cascade • Adiponectin • Chorionic somatomammotropin • Epidermal growth factor • Erythropoietin • Fibroblast growth factor • Growth hormone • Insulin • Insulin-like growth factors I and II • Leptin • Nerve growth factor • Platelet-derived growth factor • Prolactin

7. **Thyroid binding proteins is increased by:**

A. Androgens
B. Estrogens
C. Asparginase
D. Glucocorticoids

Ans: B. Estrogens

Ref: *Harper's Illustrated Biochemistry, 28th edition.*

Explanation:

Thyroid binding proteins

3 types of TBP

- **Albumin**
- **Transthyretin or thyroxine-binding pre-albumin (TBPA. or Prealbumin**
- **Thyroxine-binding globulin (TBG)**

Fluctuations in Binding

- When there is a sudden, sustained increa**se in the concentration of thyroid-binding proteins** in the plasma, the concentration of **free thyroid hormones falls.**
- This change is temporary, however, because the decrease in the concentration of free thyroid hormones in the circulation stimulates TSH secretion, which in turn causes an increase in the production of free thyroid hormones.
- A new equilibrium is eventually reached at which the total quantity of thyroid hormones in the blood is elevated but the concentration of free hormones, the rate of their metabolism, and the rate of TSH secretion are normal.
- Corresponding changes in the opposite direction occur when the concentration of thyroid-binding protein is reduced.
- TBG levels are elevated in **estrogen**-treated patients and during **pregnancy**.
- They are depressed by **glucocorticoids**, **androgens**, the weak androgen **danazol**, and the cancer chemotherapeutic agent L-**asparaginase**.

- A number of other drugs, including **salicylates**, the anticonvulsant **phenytoin**, and the cancer chemotherapeutic agents **mitotane** (*o,p*′-DDd) and 5-**fluorouracil** inhibit binding of T_4 and T_3 to TBG and consequently produce changes similar to those produced by a decrease in TBG concentration. *(See Table 3)*

8. During starvation, which organ doesn't use ketone bodies?

A. Brain **B.** Kidney

C. Heart **D.** Skeletal muscles

Ans: B. Kidney

Ref: *Harper's Illustrated Biochemistry, 28th edition.*

Explanation: *(See Table 4)*

Table 3 : Effect of variations in the concentrations of thyroid hormone-binding proteins in the plasma on various parameters of thyroid function after equilibrium has been reached

Condition	Concentrations of Binding Proteins	Total Plasma T_4, T_3, RT_3	Free Plasma T_4, T_3, RT_3	Plasma TSH	Clinical State
Hyperthyroidism	Normal	High	High	Low	Hyperthyroid
Hypothyroidism	Normal	Low	Low	High	Hypothyroid
Estrogens Methadone Heroin Major tranquilizers Clofibrate	High	High	Normal	Normal	Euthyroid
Glucocorticoids Androgens Danazol Asparaginase	Low	Low	Normal	Normal	Euthyroid

Table 4 : Summary of the Major Metabolic Features of the Principal Organs.

Organ	Major Pathways	Main Substrates	Major Products Exported	Specialist Enzymes
Liver	Glycolysis, gluconeogenesis, lipogenesis, Beta-oxidation, citric acid cycle, ketogenesis, lipoprotein metabolism, drug metabolism, synthesis of bile salts, urea, uric acid, cholesterol, plasma proteins	Free fatty acids, glucose (in fed state), lactate, glycerol, fructose, amino acids, alcohol	Glucose, triacylglycerol in VLDL, ketone bodies, urea, uric acid, bile salts, cholesterol, plasma proteins	Glucokinase, glucose 6-phosphatase, glycerol kinase, phosphoenolpyruvate carboxykinase, fructokinase, arginase, HMG CoA synthase, HMG CoA lyase, alcohol dehydrogenase
Brain	Glycolysis, amino acid metabolism, neurotransmitter synthesis	Glucose, amino acids, ketone bodies in prolonged starvation	Lactate, end products of neurotransmitter metabolism	Those for synthesis and catabolism of neurotransmitters
Heart	Beta-Oxidation and citric acid cycle	**Ketone bodies**, free fatty acids, lactate, chylomicron and VLDL triacylglycerol, some glucose	—	Lipoprotein lipase, very active electron transport chain
Adipose tissue	Lipogenesis, esterification of fatty acids, lipolysis (in fasting)	Glucose, chylomicron and VLDL triacylglycerol	Free fatty acids, glycerol	Lipoprotein lipase, hormone-sensitive lipase, enzymes of pentose phosphate pathway

Contd.

Contd.

Fast twitch muscle	Glycolysis	Glucose, glycogen	Lactate, (alanine and ketoacids in fasting)	—
Slow twitch muscle	Beta-Oxidation and citric acid cycle	**Ketone bodies**, chylomicron, and VLDL triacylglycerol	—	Lipoprotein lipase, very active electron transport chain
Kidney	Gluconeogenesis	Free fatty acids, lactate, glycerol, glucose	Glucose	Glycerol kinase, phosphoenolpyruvate carboxykinase
Erythrocytes	Anaerobic glycolysis, pentose phosphate pathway	Glucose	Lactate	Hemoglobin, enzymes of pentose phosphate pathway

9. In starvation, least common change seen is:

A. Depletion of buccal fat
B. Increased lipogenesis
C. Increased gluconeogenesis
D. Increased glycogenolysis

Ans: B. Increased lipogenesis

Ref: *Harper's Illustrated Biochemistry, 28th edition.*

Explanation:

Metabolic Fuel Reserves Are Mobilized in the Fasting State

- There is a small **fall in plasma glucose** in the **fasting state**, then little change as fasting is prolonged into starvation.
- **Plasma free fatty acids increase** in **fasting**, but then rise little more in starvation; as fasting is prolonged, so the plasma concentration of **ketone bodies** (acetoacetate and -hydroxybutyrate) **increases** markedly.

Plasma Concentrations of Metabolic Fuels (mmol/L) in the Fed and Fasting States

	Fed	40 Hours Fasting	7 Days Starvation
Glucose	5.5	3.6	3.5
Free fatty acids	0.30	1.15	1.19
Ketone bodies	Negligible	2.9	4.5

(See the following Figure)

- In the fasting state, as the concentration of glucose in the portal blood falls, so insulin secretion decreases, and skeletal muscle and adipose tissue take up less glucose. The increase in secretion of **glucagon** inhibits glycogen synthetase, and activates glycogen phosphorylase in the liver.
- The resulting glucose 6-phosphate is hydrolyzed by glucose 6-phosphatase, and glucose is released into the bloodstream for use by the brain and erythrocytes.

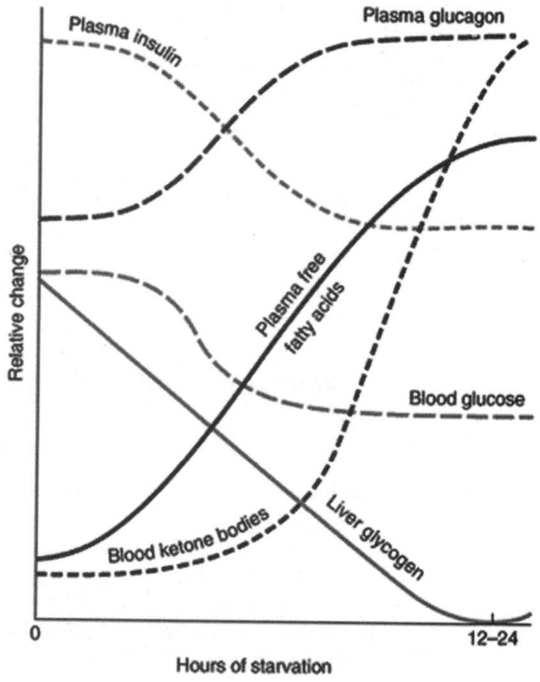

- Muscle glycogen cannot contribute directly to plasma glucose, since muscle lacks glucose 6-phosphatase, and the primary purpose of muscle glycogen is to provide a source of glucose 6-phosphate for energy-yielding metabolism in the muscle itself.
- However, acetyl-CoA formed by oxidation of fatty acids in muscle inhibits pyruvate dehydrogenase, leading to an accumulation of pyruvate.
- Most of this is transaminated to alanine, at the expense of amino acids arising from breakdown of "labile" protein reserves synthesized in the fed state.
- The alanine, and much of the keto-acids resulting from this transamination are exported from muscle, and taken up by the liver, where the alanine is transaminated to yield pyruvate.

- The resultant amino acids are largely exported back to muscle, to provide amino groups for formation of more alanine, while the pyruvate is a major substrate for gluconeogenesis in the liver.
- In adipose tissue the decrease in insulin and increase in glucagon results in **inhibition of lipogenesis**, inactivation of lipoprotein lipase, and activation of intracellular hormone-sensitive lipase
- This leads to release from adipose tissue of increased amounts of **glycerol** (which is a substrate for gluconeogenesis in the liver) and **free fatty acids**, which are used by **liver**, **heart**, and **skeletal muscle** as their preferred metabolic fuel, therefore **sparing glucose**.
- Although **muscle** preferentially takes up and metabolizes **free fatty acids** in the fasting state, it cannot meet all of its energy requirements by **beta-oxidation**.
- By contrast, the **liver** has a greater capacity for **beta-oxidation** than it requires to meet its own energy needs, and as fasting becomes more prolonged, it forms more **acetyl-CoA** than can be oxidized.
- This acetyl-CoA is used to synthesize the **ketone bodies** which are major metabolic fuels for skeletal and heart muscle and can meet some of the brain's energy needs.
- When there is no other source of glucose, liver and muscle glycogen would be exhausted after about 18 hours fasting.
- As fasting becomes more prolonged, so an increasing amount of the amino acids released as a result of protein catabolism is utilized in the liver and kidneys for gluconeogenesis.

10. Which of the following not a glycoprotein?

A. FSH **B.** LH

C. TSH **D.** ADH

Ans: D. ADH

Ref: *Harper's Illustrated Biochemistry, 28th edition.*

Explanation:

The Antidiuretic hormone (ADH) (vasopressin) is **peptide** consisting of **nine amino acids (non-apeptides)** and not a glycoprotein

Hormones that are glycoproteins include:

- Follicle-stimulating hormone (FSH)
- Luteinizing hormone (LH)
- Thyroid-stimulating hormone (TSH)
- Human chorionic gonadotropin (HCG)
- Alpha-fetoprotein (AFP)
- Erythropoietin (EPO)

(See Table 5)

Chemical Nature of Hormones

Insulin family

- Insulin • IGF • Relaxin

Glycoprotein family

- LH • FSH • TSH
- hCG

GH family

- GH • Prolactin • hPL

Secretin family

- Secretin • Glucagon • VIP
- GIP

Peptide hormones

- ANP • Calcitonin • CCK
- ADH • Inhibin • Somatostatin
- ACTH • PTH

Table 5 : Some important glycoproteins

Function	**Glycoproteins**
Structural molecule	**Collagens**
Lubricant and protective agent	**Mucins**
Transport molecule	**Transferrin, ceruloplasmin**
Immunologic molecule	Immunoglobins, histocompatibility antigens
Hormone	**HCG, TSH, FSH, LH, EPO, AFP**
Enzyme	Various, e.g., alkaline phosphatase, patatin
Cell attachment-recognition site	Various proteins involved in **cell–cell** (e.g., sperm–oocyte), **virus–cell, bacterium–cell**, and **hormone–cell interactions**
Interact with specific carbohydrates	**Lectins**, **selectins** (cell adhesion lectins), antibodies
Receptor	Various proteins involved in hormone and drug action
Affect folding of certain proteins	**Calnexin, calreticulin**
Regulation of development	Notch and its analogs, key proteins in development
Hemostasis (and thrombosis)	Specific glycoproteins on the surface membranes of platelets

PHARMACOLOGY

1. **Which of the following is not true regarding morphine?**
   A. Causes cerebral vasodilation
   B. Inhibits urinary voiding reflex
   C. Causes direct stimulation of chemoreceptor trigger zone in the medulla.
   D. Reduces muscle tone in high doses

   Ans: D. Reduces muscle tone in high doses

   Ref: *The Pharmacological basis of therapeutics by Goodman & Gilman - 12th edition, page no. 495-497*

   Explanation:

   *"**Morphine** in normal analgesic doses does not have any effect on the muscle tone. However when given in high doses especially in the anesthetic induction it can cause **muscle rigidity**" Ref: G&G*

   Morphine

   - **Filling of the urinary bladder** causes **activation** of the **voiding reflex** that causes contraction of the urinary bladder and **relaxation of the external urethral sphincter**. This process can be **inhibited** by **morphine** which **suppresses the voiding reflex** and **increases the tone of the external urethral sphincter** resulting in **increase in volume of the urinary bladder**.
   - Morphine does **not** directly cause cerebral vasodilation. However it causes **respiratory depression** which **results in carbon dioxide retention**. Increased CO_2 can cause **cerebral vasodilation**.
   - Morphine causes **direct stimulation of CTZ** in the **area postrema** in the medulla and thereby cause **nausea** and **vomiting**.

   Other actions of morphine

   - Morphine causes **Hitamine release** – this may cause ***vasodilation*** and ***bronchoconstriction***.
   - **Respiratory depression**
   - **Miosis**
   - **Suppresses cough reflex**
   - Reduces GI motility
   - Pruritus
   - Increased biliary pressure
   - Mental clouding
   - Dizziness

2. **Methotrexate is an example for which of the following class of drugs?**
   A. Antibiotic
   B. Alkylating agent
   C. Biologic response modifier
   D. Folic acid analogue

   Ans: D. Folic acid analogue

   Ref: *The Pharmacological basis of therapeutics by Goodman & Gilman - 12th edition, page no. 1669 -1671*

   Explanation:

   *"Methotrexate is an **anti-metabolite** which is a **folic acid analogue**." Ref: G&G*

   Classification of Anti-Cancer Drugs

   Anti-metabolites

   - Pemetrexed
   - 5 FU
   - Capecitabine
   - Cytarabine
   - Gemcitabine
   - 5-aza-cytidine

   Alkylating agents

   - Cyclophosphamide
   - Melphalan
   - Chlorambucil
   - Procarbazine
   - Busulfan
   - Dacarbazine
   - Cisplatin
   - Oxaliplatin

   Antibiotics

   - Doxorubicin
   - Daunorubicin
   - Dactinomycin

   Natural products include

   - Vinblastine
   - Vincristine
   - Paclitaxel
   - Irinotecan

   Biologic response modifiers include

   - Interferon alfa
   - Interleukin-2

   Other categories

   Tyrosine kinase inhibitors - imatinib, Sunitinib, Dasatinib
   mTOR inhibitors - Temsirolimus
   Proteasome inhibitors - Bortezomib

3. **Which is not true regarding disulfiram?**
   A. It irreversibly inhibits aldehyde dehydrogenase
   B. It has several active metabolites

C. It can be given to a patient who has abstained from alcohol for atleast 6 hours

D. Sensitization to alcohol can last as long as 14 days after last intake of disulfiram

Ans: C. It can be given to a patient who has abstained from alcohol for atleast 6 hours

Ref: *The Pharmacological basis of therapeutics by Goodman & Gilman - 12th edition, page no. 644*

Explanation:

Disulfiram can be given only to a patient who has abstained from alcohol for ***atleast 12 hours (not 6 hours).***

- Disulfiram **irreversibly** inhibits **aldehyde dehydrogenase**. However this action is brought about by several of its metabolites such as **diethylthiomethylcarbamate.**
- Patients taking **disulfiram** must **avoid alcohol** including disguised forms such as **fermented sugar, cough syrups**, after **shave lotions**.
- The daily dose of disulfiram is best taken in the **morning** since the urge to abstain from alcohol is **maximum** at that moment.
- Disulfiram can cause **acneiform eruptions, restlessness, and headache**.

4. **All the following drugs inhibit cytochrome P-450 *except:***

A. Alcohol **B.** Cyclophosphamide
C. Isoniazid **D.** Disulfiram

Ans: B. Cyclophosphamide

Ref: *The Pharmacological basis of therapeutics by Goodman & Gilman - 12th edition, page no.*

Explanation:

Cyclophosphamide is an enzyme **inducer**. All the others drugs mentioned in the choices are **enzyme inhibitors**. (Ref: Katzung)

Common enzyme inducers	Enzyme inhibitors
▪ Rifampicin	▪ Alcohol
▪ Phenytoin	▪ Cimetidine
▪ Phenobarbital	▪ Amiodarone
▪ Carbamazepine	▪ Erythromycin
▪ Dexamethasone	▪ Ketoconazole
▪ Fibrates	

5. **All are true regarding mifepristone *except:***

A. It is a pure antagonist
B. Ineffective against mineralocorticoids
C. No anti-estrogenic side effects
D. Anti androgenic action

Ans: A. It is a pure antagonist

Ref: *The Pharmacological basis of therapeutics by Goodman & Gilman - 12th edition, page no. 1184*

Explanation:

Mifepristone

- It is **not a pure antagonist** of progesterone receptors.
- It is considered to be a **modulator of progesterone receptors**.
- It also acts as a **competitive receptor antagonist** of progesterone and **glucocorticoid receptor antagonist.**
- Mifepristone in certain contexts has **agonistic activity** also whereas **onapristone** acts a **pure progesterone antagonist.**
- **Anti-androgenic effects** are common with mifepristone.
- High doses of mifepristone are known to cause **adrenal insufficiency** on account of its **anti-glucocorticoid action.**
- Most **severe adverse effect** with mifepristone is **vaginal bleeding**.

6. **Grey colour & yellow fluorescence in infant teeth is caused by:**

A. Phenytoin **B.** Porphyria
C. Tetracycline **D.** Barbiturate

Ans: C. Tetracyclines

Ref: *The Pharmacological basis of therapeutics by Goodman & Gilman - 12th edition, page no. 1526*

Explanation:

Tetracyclines

- Tetracyclines cause **grey colour & yellow fluorescence** in infant teeth.
- The discoloration is dependent on the **total drug dose** more than the number of days of exposure to drug therapy.
- The drug gets deposited in the **teeth** and **bones** as tetracyclines can bind with **calcium** to form **chelation complexes** in these tissues.
- **Children of mothers** exposed to **tetracyclines during pregnancy** are at high risk.
- The **greatest** time at which the **risk** is maximal is between **20 weeks gestation to 6 months post natal period.**

7. **Which of the following is a selective COX-2 inhibitor?**

A. Diflunisal **B.** Piroxicam
C. Sulindac **D.** Parecoxib

Ans: D. Parecoxib

Ref: *The Pharmacological basis of therapeutics by Goodman & Gilman - 12th edition, page no.962*

Explanation:

Parecoxib is a COX-2 selective inhibitor

- Other examples of **COX-2 selective inhibitors** include **celecoxib**, **etoricoxib**, **lumiracoxib**.
- **Sulindac**, **piroxicam** and **diflunisal** are **non selective NSAIDS**
- **Meloxicam** has COX-2 selective activity only at **lower** doses.
- Although etodolac is a non selective NSAIDS, it has also shown some COX-2 selectivity in vitro studies.
- **Ketorolac**, **flurbiprofen**, **ketoprofen** have maximal selectivity for **COX1**.

8. Which of the following is not a uricosuric drug?

A. Probenecid **B.** Benzbromarone
C. Sulfinpyrazone **D.** Febuxostat

Ans: D. Febuxostat

Ref: *The Pharmacological basis of therapeutics by Goodman & Gilman - 12th edition, page no. 997-998*

Explanation:

Febuxostat is an example for **non purine inhibitor** of **xanthine oxidase**. It **does not** have any **uricosuric action**

- Febuxostat should be given only in patients with acute gouty attacks and not in patients with asymptomatic hyperuricimia.
- The only three NSAIDs which have been approved by US FDA for treatment of gout are indomethacin, naproxen and sulindac.
- Sulfinpyrazone, benzbromarone and probenecid are examples of uricosuric drugs.
- Probenecid is the most common uricosuric drug used. However it can produce renal stones when prescribed alone. Consumption of adequate water can reduce the risk of stone formation. Addition of colchicine or NSAIDs can prevent the occurrence of gout.
- Rasburicase is a recombinant form of urate oxidase that catalyzes conversion of urate into allantoin, which is inactive. It has a special role in tumor lysis syndrome. May be used in pediatric leukemia/lymphoma.
- Losartan has mild uricosuric effect which may be used in hypertensive patients with hyperuricemia.

9. Dyslipedimia is least commonly seen with:

A. Amprenavir **B.** Atazanavir
C. Saquinavir **D.** Nelfinavir

Ans: B. Atazanavir

Ref: *The Pharmacological basis of therapeutics by Goodman & Gilman - 12th ed, page no. 1653*

Explanation:

Atazanavir is a **protease inhibitor** that does **not** cause **dyslipidemia** unlike **amprenavir**, **saquinavir**, **nelfinavir**.

Tipranavir is one of the **HIV protease inhibitors** that have a high incidence of **raised cholesterol** and **triglycerides**.

Adverse effects of Protease inhibitors

Common side effects seen with all protease inhibitors include:

- **Nausea**
- **Vomiting**
- **Diarrhea**
- Abdominal discomfort
- Lipodystrophy
- Hypercholesterolemia
- Hypertriglyceridemia

Specific ADR of different protease inhibitors

- **Ritonavir** – Perioral paresthesia
- **Fosamprenavir** – Skin eruption
- **Atazanavir** – Cholelithiasis, Cholecystitis
- **Darunavir** – Rash, hepatotoxicity
- **Indinavir** – Crystalluria, Nephrolithiasis, Hair loss, dry skin, Insulin resistance
- **Nelfinavir** – Chronic diarrhea
- **Tipranavir** – Fatal hepatotoxicity, intracranial hemorrhage.

10. Drug not acting on cell wall is:

A. Dactinomycin **B.** Cycloserine
C. Amoxicillin **D.** Bacitracin

Ans. A. Dactinomycin

Ref: *The Pharmacological basis of therapeutics by Goodman & Gilman - 12th ed, page no. 1669*

Explanation:

- **Dactinomycin inhibits RNA synthesis** reduces **mRNA production** and therby affects **protein synthesis**.
- It an **anti-cancer drug** which belongs to the **antibiotic class**.
- It is used in the treatment of **Choriocarcinoma**, **rhabdomyosarcoma**, **Wilm's tumor**, **Kaposi's sarcoma**.
- **Cycloserine**, **amoxicillin** and bacitracin are examples of **cell wall synthesis** inhibitors.

(See Table 6 on the next page)

Table 6

Mechanism of action	Examples
Cell wall synthesis inhibitors	▪ Beta lactams – Penicillins & Cephalosporins ▪ Glycopeptides such as vancomycin, teicoplanin, daptomycin
Protein synthesis inhibitors	▪ Aminoglycosides ▪ Tetracyclines ▪ Macrolides ▪ Linezolid ▪ Clindamycin ▪ Chloramphenicol ▪ Quinupristin, dalfopristin
Cell membrane inhibitors	▪ Polymyxin B ▪ Colistin
DNA synthesis inhibitors	▪ Quinolones ▪ Nitrofurantoin

11. **Which of the following is an example of a phase 1 Xenobiotic reaction? (Repeat)**

A. Acetylation **B.** Hydroxylation
C. Methylation **D.** Glucuronidation

Ans: B. Hydroxylation

Ref: *The Pharmacological basis of therapeutics by Goodman & Gilman - 12th ed, page no. 125*

Explanation:

- **Hydroxylation** is an example for **phase 1 reaction** while.
- **Acetylation, glucuronidation** and **methylation** are examples of conjugation reactions which are **phase 2 reactions.** *(See Table 7)*

12. **Sucralfate does not interfere with the absorption of:**

A. Phenoxy methyl penicillin
B. Ciprofloxacin
C. Phenytoin
D. Digoxin

Ans: A. Phenoxy methyl penicillin

Ref: *The Pharmacological basis of therapeutics by Goodman & Gilman - 12th ed, page no. 1315*

Explanation:

- **Sucralfate** forms a **viscous layer** in the **stomach** that prevents the absorption of other drugs such as **digoxin, phenytoin, quinolone antibiotics, ketoconazole** and **cimetidine.**
- Sucralfate comprises of **sucrose octasulfate** bound to **aluminium hydroxide.**
- In the presence of an **acidic environment, sucralfate** produces a **sticky polymer** which gets attached to the **ulcer crater for atleast 6 hours.**

Other indications for sucralfate besides acid peptic disease:

- **Oral mucositis** (Radiation and apthous ulcers)
- **Bile reflux gastropathy**

Side Effects

- Most common side effect of sucralfate is **constipation.**
- **Bezoar formation** can occur with consumption of sucralfate due to the sticky nature of the drug. Bezoar formation is more prone to occur in patients with **gastroparesis.**

13. **Which of the following is not seen with thiazide diuretics?**

A. Hypokalemia **B.** Hypercalcemia
C. Hyperuricemia **D.** Metabolic acidosis

Ans: D. Metabolic acidosis

Ref: *The Pharmacological basis of therapeutics by Goodman & Gilman - 12th edition, page no. 689*

Table 7

Type of reactions	Purpose	Examples of enzymes involved
Phase 1 reactions	To make the drug molecule inactive or active by oxidation, reduction or hydrolytic reactions	▪ Cytochrome P450 ▪ Flavin containing mono-oxygenases ▪ Epoxide hydrolases
Phase 2 reactions	To make the drug water soluble to facilitate excretion by reactions such as sulfation, methylation, glucuronidation, acetylation, glutathionylation.	▪ Sulfotransferases ▪ Glutathione –S-transferases ▪ UDP- glucuronyltransferase ▪ N-acetyltransferases ▪ Methyltransferases

Explanation:

- **Thiazide diuretics** are known to cause **hypokalemia, metabolic alkalosis, hypercalcemia** and **hyperuricemia**. Metabolic alkalosis occurs on account of the loss of hydrogen ions. They do not cause metabolic acidosis.
- Thiazide induced **hypokalemia** can cause **torsade de pointes**. Concomitant administration of **quinidine** in these patients can increase the risk of torsade de pointes.
- The major side effects associated with thiazide diuretics include:
  - **Hypotension**
  - **Hypokalemia**
  - **Hyponatremia**
  - **Hypochloremia**
  - **Metabolic alkalosis**
  - **Hypomagnesemia**
  - **Hypercalcemia**
  - **Hyperuricemia**.
- Other side effects are **vertigo**, **xanthopsia**, photosensitivity, **skin rash** and **erectile dysfunction.**
- An individual with **sulfonamides allergy** should avoid thiazide diuretics.
- Thiazides are known to **unmask latent diabetes** and **increase cholesterol** and **triglycerides**.

14. Ivermectin is indicated in all of the following *except:*

A. Ascaris **B.** Filariasis
C. Malaria **D.** Oncocerciasis

Ans: C. Malaria

Ref: *The Pharmacological basis of therapeutics by Goodman & Gilman - 12th edition, page no. 1455-1456* & Malaria Journal *2013;* ***12****:153*

Explanation:

Ivermectin has a beneficial therapeutic effect in

- Onchocerciasis
- Lymphatic filariasis
- Stronglyloidiasis
- Ascariasis
- Enterobiasis.

- Ivermectin is also effective in **head lice infection**, **cutaneous larva migrans** and **scabies**
- It does not have any proven beneficial effect in malaria.
- Since ivermectin can act on the **GABA receptors** in the **CNS**, it should be avoided in patients with **meningitis** and **African trypanosomiasis** that are associated with breached **blood brain barrier.**
- Ivermectin should **not be given to pregnant** and **lactating women**, **children less than 5 years of age** and **severely ill patient.**

Note:

- However ivermectin has been recently found to have a beneficial effect in reducing the risk of malaria transmission by its vector control activity by targeting the anopheles mosquito.
- However this is still needs to be verified with the help of large studies. (***Ref:*** *Malaria Journal* 2013; **12**:153)

15. Maximum bicarbonate loss occurs with:

A. Acetazolamide **B.** Furosemide
C. Thiazide **D.** Spirinolactone

Ans. A. Acetazolamide

Ref: *The Pharmacological basis of therapeutics by Goodman & Gilman - 12th edition, page no. 678 & Lippincott Illustrated Reviews Pharmacology, 2nd edition, page 226.*

Explanation:

- **Acetazolamide** causes maximum bicarbonate excretion upto **35%** of filtered load.
- **No other diuretic** causes **significant bicarbonate loss.**
- Loss of bicarbonate can result in **hypercholermic metabolic acidosis**.

(See Table 8)

Table 8

Diuretic	Mechanism of action	Site of action	Major ions lost in urine
Carbonic anhydrase inhibitors	Inhibition of carbonic anhydrase	Proximal convoluted tubule	HCO_3^-, $H_2PO_4^-$
Osmotic diuretic	Extract water from ICF, expand ECF, inhibit renin release, increased renal blood flow,	Osmotic effect in TAL of loop of Henle and proximal tubule	Na^+, Mg^{2+}
Loop diuretic	Inhibit Na^+-K^+-$2Cl^-$	Thick ascending limb of loop of Henle	Na^+, K^+, Ca^{2+}, Mg^{2+}, Cl^-,
Thiazides	Inhibit Na- Cl symport	Distal convoluted tubule	Na^+, K^+

16. **A drug which is an alpha agonist and orally used produg for autonomic insufficiency and postural hypotension is:**

A. Metamphetamine **B.** Midodrine
C. Phenylephrine **D.** Metaraminol

Ans. B. Midodrine

Ref: *The Pharmacological basis of therapeutics by Goodman & Gilman - 12th edition, page no. 295*

Explanation:

Midodrine

- It is an **alpha adrenergic receptor** agonist that has been approved for the treatment of **dysautonomia** and **autonomic failure**.
- It is also an example of a **pro-drug**.
- The active metabolite of **midodrine** is **desglymidodrine**
- As per the drug monograph, midodrine is indicated in **autonomic failure** in patients with **Bradbury-Eggleston syndrome, Shy Drager syndrome, diabetes mellitus disease** and **Parkinson's disease**.

Methamphetamine

- It is a **CNS stimulant** which is indicated only in the treatment of **Attention Deficit Hyperactivity Syndrom**e and **short term treatment of obesity**.
- It has no role in the treatment of autonomic failure.
- Methamphetamine is **not an alpha agonist**, but causes **neither release of nor adrenaline** from central nerve terminals.

Phenylephrine

- Although **phenylephrine** is an **alpha$_1$ selective agonist**, it is **not a pro-drug**.
- It is mainly used as **nasal decongestant** and as a **mydriatic agent**.
- It does not have any role in autonomic failure.

Metaraminol

- It is an **alpha$_1$ agonist** that is used in the treatment of **hypotension** especially as complication following **spinal anesthesia.**

17. **Drug contraindicated in severe hypertriglyceridemia is:**

A. Fibrates
B. Simvastatin
C. Niacin
D. Cholestyramine

Ans. D. Cholestyramine

Ref: *The Pharmacological basis of therapeutics by Goodman & Gilman - 12th edition, page no. 898-899*

Explanation:

- **Cholestyramine increases the triglyceride levels** and are hence **contraindicated** in patients with **hypertriglyceridemia**.
- **Cholestyramine** and **colestipol** are bile **acid sequestrants** or bile **acid resins.**
- **Colesevelam** is the most **recently developed agent** in this class.
- They are used as **second line therapy** in patients who do not show adequate lipid control with **statin therapy.**
- These drugs are **not absorbed from intestine** and hence **do not have systemic side effects.**
- **Gastrointestinal side effects** such as **bloating** and **dyspepsia** are common with bile acid resins.
- It can be reduced significantly if the drug is **dissolved in water** several hours before its intake.
- **Colesevelam** has less bloating effect
- Since bile acid resins interfere with the absorption of several drugs, it is better to administer all drugs **atleast 1 hour before or 4 hours after bile acid resin intake.**

Niacin

- It is effective in patients with **raised triglyceride levels**.
- **Niacin** is **contraindicated** in patients with **active peptic ulcer disease** and **pregnancy**.
- It can also cause **severe hepatotoxicity**.
- Patients with **diabetes** taking niacin can have **worsening of hyperglycemia** that warrants **insulin therapy**.

18. **Which of the following best depicts the mechanism of action of thiazolidinediones?**

A. Improving insulin sensitivity
B. Modifying receptors of beta cells
C. Increasing insulin secretion
D. Increasing number of GLUT -4

Ans. A. Improve insulin sensitivity

Ref: *The Pharmacological basis of therapeutics by Goodman & Gilman - 12th edition, page no. 1260*

Explanation:

Thiazolidinediones

- These are **insulin sensitizers** which enhance insulin mediated glucose uptake by **30-50%** through actions on the **PPARδ receptors** in **skeletal** muscle, **adipose** tissue and **liver**.

- They include **rosiglitazone** and **pioglitazone**.
- Thiazolidinediones decrease **hepatic gluconeogenesis** and **plasma levels of free fatty acids**.
- These drugs also **reduce triglycerides** and **raise the HDL levels**.
- **Rosiglitazone** has been withdrawn from the European markets and from several other countries including India due to increased risk of **myocardial infarction**.
- **Pioglitazone** has also been **withdrawn** in several countries due to the risk of **bladder cancer**.

PATHOLOGY

1. **Chronic myeloproliferative disorder includes all *except:***

A. CML
B. Polycythemia vera
C. Essential thrombocytosis
D. Erthyroleukemia

Ans: D. Erthyroleukemia

Ref: *Robbins Pathologic Basis of Disease, 8th edition*

Explanation:

List of Myeloproliferative Disorders

- Chronic myeloid leukemia CML
- Polycythemia vera
- Essential thrombocytosis
- Primary myelofibrosis
- Chronic eosinophilic leukemia
- Chronic neutrophilic leukemia
- Systemic mastocytosis (?)
  - In 2001, the World Health Organization classified "**chronic eosinophilic leukemia/hypereosinophilic syndrome**" and **chronic neutrophilic leukemia** under "Chronic myeloproliferative diseases"

Erythroleukemia

- It is a subtype of **AML**
- It is classified as an **M6 subtype of acute myelogenous leukemia (AML)** in the French-American-British (**FAb**) classification system on the basis of **morphologic** and **cytochemical** criteria.

2. **Lepidic cells are seen in:**

A. Lepromatous Leprosy
B. Rhabdomyoma
C. Glioblastoma
D. Cardiac myxomas

Ans: D. Cardiac myxomas

Ref: *Mallick SR. Right atrial myxoma with glandular differentiation: A rare entity in pediatric age group. Ann Pediatr Cardiol. 2010 Jul-Dec; 3(2): 159–162. & http://www.e-heart.org/*

Explanation:

*"**Lepidic cells** also called **myxoma cells** often form ring-like structures around capillaries or form small canaliculi or cords in the myxoid matrix". Ref: e-heart.org*

*"**Cardiac myxomas (CMs)** account for nearly half of the primary cardiac tumors in the elderly. They arise from **sub-endocardial "reserve"** or **lepidic" cells**, which may show divergent differentiation" Ref: Mallick*

*"Histologically, myxomas are composed of **stellate or globular myxoma cells** embedded within an abundant acid mucopolysaccharide ground substance. Peculiar vessel-like or gland-like structures are characteristic. Hemorrhage and mononuclear inflammation are usually present." Ref: Robbins*

Myxoma

- The **most common primary tumor of the heart** in **adults**
- They are **benign neoplasms**
- Associated with clonal abnormalities of **chromosomes 12 and 17**
- Arise from **primitive multipotent mesenchymal cells**.
- **90%** are located in the **atria (atrial myxomas)**
- **Left-to-right ratio** of approximately **4 : 1.**
- 10% of individuals with myxoma have a familial syndrome (Known as **Carney complex**) Characterized by:
  - Autosomal-dominant transmission
  - Multiple cardiac and extracardiac myxomas
  - Pigmented skin lesions
  - Endocrine overactivity.

3. **True regarding Hepatocellular carcinoma (HCC) is:**

A. NASH is a risk factor
B. OCPs are implicated
C. Focal Nodular Hyperplasia is premalignant
D. Chromosomal abnormalities are seen

Ans: A. NASH is a risk factor

Ref: *Robbins Pathologic Basis of Disease, 8th edition,*

Explanation:

Hepatocellular Carcinoma (HCC)

- Increasing incidence, mainly due to HCV and HBV chronic infection.
- Male predominance (2.4 : 1)

Pathogenesis

- Four major etiologic factors associated with HCC have been established:
  - Chronic viral infection (**HBV, HCV**)
  - Chronic **alcoholism**
  - Non-alcoholic steatohepatitis (**NASH**)
  - Food contaminants (primarily aflatoxins produced by Aspergillus flavus)
- Other conditions include
  - Tyrosinemia
  - Glycogen storage disease
  - Hereditary hemochromatosis
  - Non-alcoholic fatty liver disease
  - α1-antitrypsin deficiency
- The precise mechanisms of carcinogenesis are **unknown**.
- Progression to HCC might result from point mutations in selected cellular genes such as **KRAS** and **p53**, and constitutive expression of **c-MYC, c-MET** (the receptor for hepatocyte growth factor), **TGF-α**, and **insulin-like growth factor 2**.
- Recent global gene expression studies revealed that approximately 50% of HCC cases are associated with activation of **WNT or AKT pathways**.

Morphology

- HCC may appear grossly as
  - **Unifocal** (usually large) mass
  - **Multifocal**, widely distributed nodules of variable size
  - **Diffusely infiltrative** cancer
- All patterns of HCCs have a strong propensity for invasion of vascular structures.
- **Extensive intrahepatic metastases** ensue, and occasionally, **long, snakelike masses of tumor** invade the **portal vein** (with occlusion of the portal circulation) or inferior vena cava, extending even into the **right side of the heart**.
- HCC spreads extensively within the liver by obvious contiguous growth and by the development of **satellite nodules**, which can be shown by molecular methods to be derived from the parent tumor.
- Metastasis outside the liver is primarily via **vascular invasion**, especially into the **hepatic vein** system, but hematogenous metastases, especially to the lung, tend to occur late in the disease.

4. **Which of the following conditions is due to membrane receptor defect?**
   A. Beta thalassemia
   B. Familial hypercholesterolemia
   C. HSP
   D. Sickle cell disease

Ans: B. Familial hypercholesterolemia

Ref: *Robbins Pathologic Basis of Disease, 8th edition*

Explanation:

Familial hypercholesterolemia

Pathology: Mutations in the LDLR gene that encodes the **LDL receptor protein**, which normally removes LDL from the circulation, or apolipoprotein B (Apob), which is the part of LDL that binds with the receptor.
(See Table 9 on the next page)

5. **Which type of cell does not increase by steroid?**
   A. RBC **B.** Eosinophil
   C. Monocyte **D.** Netrophil

Ans: B. Eosinophil

Ref: *Robbins Pathologic Basis of Disease, 8th edition, Pg: & Ganong, Review of Medical Physiology, 21st edition.*

Explanation:

Effects of Glucocorticoids on the Blood Cells & Lymphatic Organs

- Glucocorticoids **decrease** the number of circulating **eosinophils** by increasing their sequestration in the spleen and lungs and also **lower** the number of **basophils** in the circulation
- Glucocorticoids **increase** the number of **neutrophils, platelets,** and **red blood cells**
- Glucocorticoids **decrease** the **circulating lymphocyte count** and the **size of the lymph nodes** and thymus by inhibiting **lymphocyte mitotic activity.**
- The reduced secretion of the **cytokine IL-2** leads to reduced proliferation of **lymphocytes**, and these cells undergo **apoptosis**.

Steroids -	**Increases** Neutrophils, RBCs & Platelets
-	**Decreases** Eosinophils, Lymphocytes and Basophils

6. **Auers rods are:**
   A. Condensation of granules within cytoplasm
   B. Aggregated ribosomes
   C. Aggregated globin chains
   D. Lysosymal granules

Ans: A. Condensation of granules within cytoplasm

Table 9 : Classification of Anemia According to Underlying Mechanism

Mechanism	Specific Examples
BLOOD LOSS	
Acute blood loss	Trauma
Chronic blood loss	Gastrointestinal tract lesions, gynecologic disturbances
INCREASED RED CELL DESTRUCTION (HEMOLYSIS)	
Inherited genetic defects	
Red cell membrane disorders	Hereditary spherocytosis, hereditary elliptocytosis
Enzyme deficiencies	
Hexose monophosphate shunt enzyme deficiencies	G6PD deficiency, glutathione synthetase deficiency
Glycolytic enzyme deficiencies	Pyruvate kinase deficiency, hexokinase deficiency
Hemoglobin abnormalities	
Deficient globin synthesis	**Thalassemia** syndromes
Structurally abnormal globins (hemoglobinopathies)	**Sickle cell disease**, unstable hemoglobins
Acquired genetic defects	
Deficiency of phosphatidylinositol-linked glycoproteins	Paroxysmal nocturnal hemoglobinuria
Antibody-mediated destruction	Hemolytic disease of the newborn (Rh disease), transfusion reactions, drug-induced, autoimmune disorders
Mechanical trauma	
Microangiopathic hemolytic anemias	Hemolytic uremic syndrome, disseminated intravascular coagulation, thrombotic thrombocytopenia purpura
Cardiac traumatic hemolysis	Defective cardiac valves
Repetitive physical trauma	Bongo drumming, marathon running, karate chopping
Infections of red cells	Malaria, babesiosis
Toxic or chemical injury	Clostridial sepsis, snake venom, lead poisoning
Membrane lipid abnormalities	Abetalipoproteinemia, severe hepatocellular liver disease
Sequestration	Hypersplenism
DECREASED RED CELL PRODUCTION	
Inherited genetic defects	
Defects leading to stem cell depletion	Fanconi anemia, telomerase defects
Defects affecting erythroblast maturation	Thalassemia syndromes
Nutritional deficiencies	
Deficiencies affecting DNA synthesis	B_{12} and folate deficiencies
Deficiencies affecting hemoglobin synthesis	Iron deficiency anemia
Erythropoietin deficiency	Renal failure, anemia of chronic disease
Immune-mediated injury of progenitors	Aplastic anemia, pure red cell aplasia
Inflammation-mediated iron sequestration	Anemia of chronic disease
Primary hematopoietic neoplasms	Acute leukemia, myelodysplasia, myeloproliferative disorders
Space-occupying marrow lesions	Metastatic neoplasms, granulomatous disease
Infections of red cell progenitors	Parvovirus B19 infection
Unknown mechanisms	Endocrine disorders, hepatocellular liver disease

D. Lysosymal granules >condensation of granules within cytoplasm

Ref: *Robbins Pathologic Basis of Disease, 8th edition & Ackerman GA. Microscopic and histochemical studies on the Auer bodies in leukemic cells. Blood. 1950 Sep;5(9):847-63.*

Explanation:

*"The **cytoplasm** often contains fine, **peroxidase-positive azurophilic** granules. Auer rods, distinctive **needle**-like **azurophilic** granules, are present in many cases; they are particularly numerous in **AML** with the **t(15;17) (acute promyelocytic leukemia)**"*

Ref: Robbins

- Auer rods are composed of **fused lysosomes/ primary neutrophilic granules** and contain peroxidase, lysosomal enzymes, and large crystalline inclusions. *(Ref: Acherman)*

7. **EBV causes all *except:* (Repeat)**

A. Kaposi sarcoma

B. Nasopharyngeal Ca

C. Burkitt lymphoma
D. Infecious mononucleosis

Ans: A. Kaposi sarcoma

Ref: *Robbins Pathologic Basis of Disease, 8th edition*

Explanation:

Diseases associated with Epstein-Barr virus

- Infectious mononucleosis
- Burkitt's lymphoma
- Hodgkin's lymphoma (Mixed cellularity, Lymphocyte rich & Lymphocyte depletion)
- Nasopharyngeal carcinoma
- Multiple sclerosis
- Extranodal NK/T-cell lymphoma
- X-linked lymphoproliferation syndrome (Duncan disease)
- Lymphoepithelioma-like carcinoma of Thymus
- Oral Hairy leukoplakia
- **Kaposi sarcoma** is associated with Human herpes virus-8 (**HHV-8**) infection.

8. **Defect in xeroderma pigmentosum (Repeat)**
A. Mismatch repair
B. Base excision repair
C. Nucleotide excision repair
D. Double strand break repair

Ans: C. Nucleotide excision repair

Ref: *Robbins Pathologic Basis of Disease, 8th edition, Pg: 275 & Frosina G. Commentary: DNA base excision repair defects in human pathologies Free Radic Res. 2004 Oct;38(10):1037-54.*

Explanation:

Types of defects in DNA-repair systems and conditions associated

DNA Repair Mechanisms	Diseases associated
Mismatch repair	• Hereditary Nonpolyposis Colon Cancer Syndrome • Muir-Torre Syndrome
Nucleotide excision repair	• Xeroderma pigmentosum • Cockayne's syndrome • Trichothiodystrophy
Base excision repair	• **Gross defects -** Not compatible with life • **Partial defects -** Colorectal cancer & Lung Cancers
Recombinational repair	• Ataxia Telangiectasia (ATM gene, genome instability syndrome) • Bloom syndrome (RecQ DNA helicase; BLM gene) • Fanconi anemia (BRCA-2) • Werner syndrome (WRNp protein- RecQ DNA helicase)
Direct Repair	—

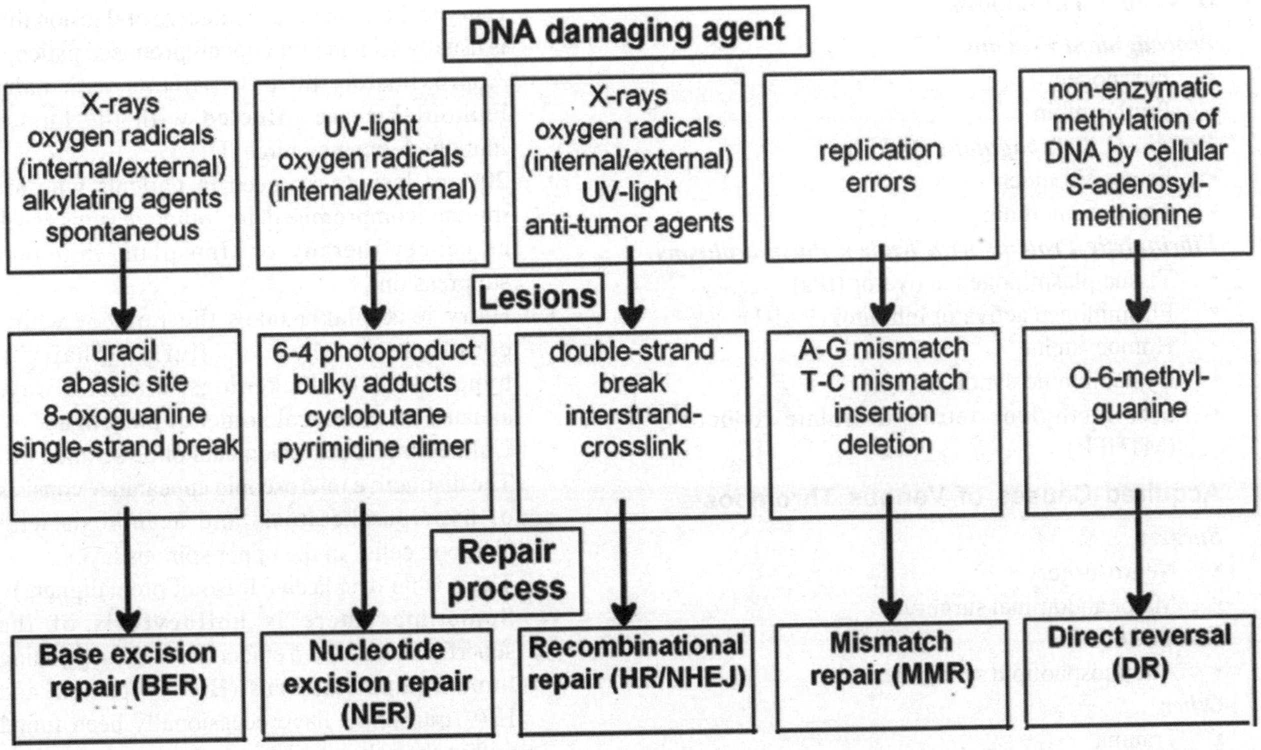

9. All the following disorders are inherited *except:*

A. Protein S deficiency
B. Antiphospholipid antibody syndrome
C. Protein C deficiency
D. Factor V Leiden mutation

Ans: B. Antiphospholipid antibody syndrome

Ref: *Robbins Pathologic Basis of Disease, 8th edition, Harrison's Online > Chapter 117. Arterial and Venous Thrombosis >*

Explanation:

Heritable Causes of Arterial and Venous Thrombosis

A. Arterial Thrombosis

Platelet Receptors
- Integrins
- PlA2 polymorphism
- GPIV
- GPIb
- Thrombin receptor

Redox Enzymes
- Plasma glutathione peroxidase
- Endothelial nitric oxide synthase
- Paraoxonase
- Homocysteine
- Cystathionine -synthase
- 5,10-methylene tetrahydrofolate reductase (MTHFR)

B. Venous Thrombosis

Procoagulant Proteins
- Fibrinogen
- Prothrombin

Protein C Anticoagulant Pathway
- Factor V Leiden
- Thrombomodulin

Fibrinolytic Proteins with Known Polymorphisms
- Tissue plasminogen activator (tPa)
- Plasminogen activator inhibitor (PAI-1)
- Homocysteine
- Cystathionine-synthase
- 5,10-methylene tetrahydrofolate reductase (MTHFR)

Acquired Causes of Venous Thrombosis

Surgery
- Neurosurgery
- Major abdominal surgery

Malignancy
- Antiphospholipid syndrome

Other
- Trauma
- Pregnancy
- Long-haul travel
- Obesity
- Oral contraceptives/hormone replacement
- Myeloproliferative disorders
- Polycythemia vera

10. Immune complex mediated hypersensitivity is classified as: (Repeat)

A. Type 1 Hypersensitivity reaction
B. Type 2 Hypersensitivity reaction
C. Type 3 Hypersensitivity reaction
D. Type 4 Hypersensitivity reaction

Ans: C. Type 3 Hypersensitivity reaction

Ref: *Robbins Pathologic Basis of Disease, 8th edition*

Explanation:

Refer 2011 Pathology question explanation

11. Oral hairy leukoplakia related to: (Repeat)

A. EBV
B. Candidiasis
C. Mucormycosis
D. Human papilloma virus

Ans: A. EBV

Ref: *Robbins Pathologic Basis of Disease, 8th edition*

Explanation:

ORAL HAIRY LEUKOPLAKIA (OHL)

- Hairy leukoplakia is a distinctive oral lesion that is usually seen in immunocompromised patients.
- Approximately 80% of patients with hairy leukoplakia are infected with the human immunodeficiency virus (HIV)
- 20% of lesions are seen in patients who are immunocompromised for other reasons, such as cancer therapy or transplant immunosuppression.
- Hairy leukoplakia takes the form of white, confluent patches of fluffy ("hairy"), hyperkeratotic thickenings, almost always situated on the lateral border of the tongue.
- Unlike thrush, the lesion cannot be scraped off. The distinctive microscopic appearance consists of hyperparakeratosis and acanthosis with "balloon cells" in the upper spinous layer.
- There is no dysplasia (It is not premalignant)
- Sometimes there is **koilocytosis** of the superficial, nucleated epidermal cells, suggesting **human papillomavirus (HPV)** infection, and HPV transcripts have occasionally been found within the cells.

- However, **EBV** is present in most cells and is now accepted as the cause of the condition.
- Sometimes there is superimposed **candidal infection** on the surface of the lesions, adding to the "hairiness."
- In HIV-positive individuals, with hairy leukoplakia, symptoms of AIDS follow in 2 to 3 years.

12. Medullary thyroid carcinoma occurs due to the mutation of: (Repeat)

A. RET oncogene
B. P53 gene
C. RAS H-RAS, K-RAS, N-RAS
D. BRCA-1

Ans: A. RET oncogene

Ref: Robbins Pathologic Basis of Disease, 8th edition

Explanation: (See table 10)

Table 10 : Selected Oncogenes, Their Mode of Activation and Associated Human Tumors

Category	Proto-oncogene	Associated Human Tumor
GROWTH FACTORS		
PDGF-β chain	***SIS* (official name *PBGFB.***	Astrocytoma
		Osteosarcoma
Fibroblast growth factors	***HST1***	Stomach cancer
	***INT2* (official name *FGF3*)**	Bladder cancer
		Breast cancer
		Melanoma
TGF-α	***TGFA***	Astrocytomas
		Hepatocellular carcinomas
HGF	***HGF***	Thyroid cancer
GROWTH FACTOR RECEPTORS		
EGF-receptor family	***ERBB1* (*EGFR*), *ERRB2***	Squamous cell carcinoma of lung, gliomas
FMS-like tyrosine kinase 3	***FLT3***	Breast and ovarian cancers
Receptor for neurotrophic factors	***RET***	Leukemia
		Multiple endocrine neoplasia 2A and B, familial medullary thyroid carcinomas
PDGF receptor	***PDGFRB***	Gliomas, leukemias
Receptor for stem cell (steel) factor	***KIT***	Gastrointestinal stromal tumors, seminomas, leukemias
PROTEINS INVOLVED IN SIGNAL TRANSDUCTION		
GTP-binding	***KRAS***	Colon, lung, and pancreatic tumors
	HRAS	Bladder and kidney tumors
	NRAS	Melanomas, hematologic malignancies
Nonreceptor tyrosine kinase	***ABL***	Chronic myeloid leukemia
		Acute lymphoblastic leukemia
RAS signal transduction	***BRAF***	Melanomas
WNT signal transduction	**β-catenin**	Hepatoblastomas, hepatocellular carcinoma
NUCLEAR-REGULATORY PROTEINS		
Transcriptional activators	**C-*MYC***	Burkitt lymphoma
	N-*MYC*	Neuroblastoma, small-cell carcinoma of lung
	L-*MYC*	Small-cell carcinoma of lung
CELL CYCLE REGULATORS		
Cyclins	**Cyclin D**	Mantle cell lymphoma
		Breast and esophageal cancers
	Cyclin E	Breast cancer
Cyclin-dependent kinase	***CDK4***	Glioblastoma, melanoma, sarcoma

13. Type of anemia seen in H.pylori infection: (Repeat)

A. Microcytic anemia
B. Megaloblastic anemia
C. Normocytic anemia
D. Aplastic anemia

Ans: A. Microcytic anemia

Ref: *Robbins Pathologic Basis of Disease, 8th edition & Harrison, 18th ed.*

Explanation:

- The anemia in H.pylori infection is due to **chronic blood loss** due to **Gastritis** or **Gastric ulcer.**
- Chronic blood loss typically causes **Iron deficiency anemia**, which presents with **microcytic** & **hypochromic** anemia

14. Sequestration crisis of sickle cell anemia is characterized by all *except:*

A. Severe abdominal pain
B. Reduced reticulocyte count
C. Sudden hypovolemia
D. Increased splenomegaly

Ans: B. Reduced reticulocyte count

Ref: *Robbins Pathologic Basis of Disease, 8th edition*

Explanation:

Sequestration crisis of sickle cell anemia

- Sequestration crises results from trapping of large amounts of red cells in the spleen and sometimes in the liver.
- Acute splenic sequestration is one of the important causes of early mortality in Sickle cell disease.
- In **homozygos (HbSS) patients** the **life time prevalence** of acute splenic sequestration is **7%-30%.**
- It may be seen as early as **8 weeks of age** although usually an **initial event** is seen in **toddlers.**
- In **HbSC and HbS/thalassaemia** patients the initial event tends to occur later in life (even into adulthood).
- During a crisis the sequestered sickle cells cause the **spleen** to become **grossly enlarged**.
  This is more **common in infancy** as repeated sequestration and infarction of the spleen during childhood gradually results in an **auto-splenectomy**.
- There is marked **pallor** with **cardiovascular collapse** due to **loss of effective circulating volume (Hypovolemia).**
- A patient with a sequestration crisis is usually severely anaemic (**2-3 g/100 ml**), but the **reticulocyte count will be high** (in contrast to the aplastic crisis where the **reticulocyte** count is low or **zero**).
- Sequestration crises also occur in **pregnant women**.
- Immediate management of sequestration crises is aimed at **correcting hypovolaemia** with **emergency blood transfusion**.
- The subsequent management depends on the recurrence rate of splenic sequestration and may include observation, **chronic transfusion** and **splenectomy**

Note:

- Sequestration crises **recur**
- **Splenectomy** is **curative** - and is recommended after **two episodes**
- Similar **sequestration episodes** may occur in the **liver in adults**.

15. All-trans retinoic acid (ATRA) is used in the treatment of:

A. APL
B. CML
C. ALL
D. CLL

Ans: A. APL

Ref: *Robbins Pathologic Basis of Disease, 8th edition*

Explanation:

"The t(15;17) not only has pathogenic significance, but also guides therapy, since tumors with this translocation respond to pharmacologic doses of all-trans retinoic acid (ATRA)"

Acute promyelocytic leukemia (APL)

- Subtype of AML with characteristic translocation t(15;17)
- The t(15;17) creates fusion gene that encodes a part of the **retinoic acid receptor-α (RARα)** fused to a portion of a protein called PML
- **PML-RARα fusion** protein interacts instead with transcriptional repressors, which results in an inhibition of granulocytic maturation
- AMLs with the t(15;17) also have frequent activating mutations **in FLT3**, a receptor tyrosine kinase that transmits signals that increase cellular proliferation and survival.
- The combination of **PML-RARα** and **activated FLT3** is a potent inducer of **AML**.
- The t(15;17) not only has pathogenic significance, but also guides therapy, since tumors with this translocation **respond** to pharmacologic doses of **all-trans retinoic acid (ATRA)**.

- **ATRA** binds to the **PML-RARα fusion protein** and **antagonizes** its inhibitory effect on the transcription of target genes.
- Remarkably, the resulting activation of transcription overcomes the block in differentiation, and within **1 to 2 days** the **neoplastic promyelocytes** begin to **differentiate** into **neutrophils**, which rapidly die.
- The response to ATRA proves that the major effect of PML-RARα is to block differentiation, and stands as one of the most successful uses of a targeted therapy in a human cancer.

16. Earliest lesion seen in atherosclerosis is:

A. Fatty streaks **B.** Intimal thickening
C. Fibrinoid necrosis **D.** Plaque

Ans: A. Fatty streaks

Ref: *Robbins Pathologic Basis of Disease, 8th edition.*

Explanation:

*"**Fatty streaks** are the **earliest lesions** in **atherosclerosis**" Ref: Robbins*

Morphology of Atherosclerosis

Fatty Streaks

- These are the **earliest lesions** in atherosclerosis.
- They are composed of **lipid-filled foamy macrophages**.
- Beginning as multiple minute flat yellow spots, they eventually coalesce into elongated streaks 1 cm or more in length.
- These lesions are not significantly raised and do not cause any flow disturbance
- Aortas of infants **less than 1 year old** can exhibit fatty streaks, and such lesions are seen in virtually all children older than 10 years, regardless of geography, race, sex, or environment.
- The relationship of fatty streaks to atherosclerotic plaques is uncertain
- They may evolve into precursors of plaques, not all fatty streaks are destined to become advanced lesions.

Atherosclerotic Plaque

- The key processes in atherosclerosis are **intimal thickening** and **lipid accumulation**
- Atheromatous plaques **impinge** on the **lumen of the artery** and grossly appear white to yellow; **superimposed thrombus** over ulcerated plaques is **red-brown**.
- Plaques vary from **0.3 to 1.5 cm** in diameter but can coalesce to form larger masses
- Atherosclerotic lesions are **patchy**, on cross-section, the lesions appear "**eccentric**"
- **Local flow disturbances** (e.g., turbulence at branch points) leads to increased susceptibility to plaque formation.
- In **descending order**, the most extensively involved vessels are the
  - **Lower abdominal aorta (MC)**
  - **The coronary arteries (Second MC)**
  - The popliteal arteries
  - The internal carotid arteries
  - Vessels of the circle of Willis
- Vessels of the upper extremities are usually spared, as are the mesenteric and renal arteries, except at their ostia.

Atherosclerotic plaques have three principal components:

(1) Cells, including smooth muscle cells, macrophages, and T cells
(2) ECM, including collagen, elastic fibers, and proteoglycans
(3) Intracellular and extracellular lipid

- **Superficial fibrous cap** composed of **smooth muscle cells** and **dense collagen**.
- Beneath and to the side of the cap (the "**shoulder**") is a **more cellular area** containing **macrophages, T cells, and smooth muscle cells**.
- Deep to the fibrous cap is a **necrotic core**, containing **lipid** (primarily cholesterol and cholesterol esters), **debris from dead cells**, **foam cells** (lipid-laden macrophages and smooth muscle cells), **fibrin**, variably **organized thrombus**, and other **plasma proteins** and **cholesterol**
- The **periphery** of the lesions show **neovascularization** (proliferating small blood vessels;
- Plaques generally continue to **change** and **progressively enlarge** due to **cell death** and **degeneration**, synthesis and **degradation** (remodeling) of ECM, and organization of **thrombus**.
- Atheromas often undergo **calcification**

Atherosclerotic plaques are susceptible to the following clinically important changes

- **Rupture, ulceration, or erosion** of the intimal surface of atheromatous plaques exposes the blood to highly thrombogenic substances and induces **thrombosis**.
- Such thrombosis can partially or completely occlude the lumen and lead to downstream ischemia.
- If the patient survives the initial thrombotic occlusion, the clot may become organized and incorporated into the growing plaque.

• **Hemorrhage into a plaque**. Rupture of the overlying fibrous cap, or of the thin-walled vessels in the areas of neovascularization, can cause intra-plaque hemorrhage; a contained hematoma may expand the plaque or induce plaque rupture.
• **Atheroembolism**. Plaque rupture can discharge atherosclerotic debris into the bloodstream, producing microemboli
• **Aneurysm formation**. Atherosclerosis-induced pressure or ischemic atrophy of the underlying media, with loss of elastic tissue, causes weakness resulting in aneurysmal dilation and potential rupture.

17. Askin tumor:

A. Primitive neuroectodermal tumor in chest
B. Cholangiocarcinoma arising from bifurcation of bile duct
C. Lung adenocarcinoma involving apical region
D. Enterochromaffin cell tumor

Ans: A. PNET in chest

Ref: *Benbrahim Z et al. Askin's tumor: a case report and literature review. World J Surg Oncol. 2013; 11: 10.*

Explanation:

Askin tumors (PNET of Chest wall)

- **Primitive neuroectodermal tumors (PNET)** arising from the **chest wall.**
- Ewing sarcoma and peripheral primitive neuroectodermal tumor (previously called peripheral neuroepithelioma) were originally described in the early 1900s as distinct clinicopathologic entities.
- They are rare **malignant small round cell tumors** that arise from the **primitive nerve cells** of the nervous system, but they can also occur outside the central nervous system in the chest wall, pelvis and extremities.
- **Askin's tumor** is a **PNET** of the **thoracopulmonary** region
- It develops from the **soft tissues** of the **chest wall**, particularly in the **paravertebral region**.
- Askin's tumor occurs in **young Caucasian adults** and is associated with **poor prognosis**.
- Cholangiocarcinoma arising from bifurcation of bile duct - **Klatsin tumor**
- Lung adenocarcinoma involving apical region - **Pancoast tumor**

Other named Tumors:

- **Buschke–Löwenstein tumor**- Giant condyloma acuminatum
- **Ackerman tumor** - Subtype of Verrucous Carcinoma (Carcinoma cuniculatum)
- **Grawitz tumor -** Renal cell carcinoma
- **Krukenberg tumor** - Metastatic secondaries in GIT from an ovarian primary
- **Kuttner's stumor -** Sialadenitis (sialoadenitis) - Inflammation of a salivary gland
- **Potts puffy tumor** - Frontal osteomyelitis with subperiosteal abscess
- **Wilms tumor** - Nephroblastoma affecting children

18. Most common site of Ca stomach? (Repeat)

A. Lesser curvature **B.** Greater curvature
C. Antrum **D.** Fundus

Ans: C. Antrum

Ref: *Robbins Pathologic Basis of Disease, 8th edition.*

Explanation:

"Most gastric adenocarcinomas involve the gastric antrum; the lesser curvature is involved more often than the greater curvature" (Ref: Robbins)

Gastric Adenocarcinoma

- Adenocarcinoma is the most common malignancy of the stomach, comprising over 90% of all gastric cancers.
- Early symptoms are non-specific and resemble those of chronic gastritis, including **dyspepsia**, **dysphagia**, and **nausea**.
- Weight loss, anorexia, altered bowel habits, anemia, and hemorrhage manifests in advanced stages
- As a result, these tumors are often discovered at advanced stages

Morphology

- Most gastric adenocarcinomas involve the gastric antrum
- The lesser curvature is involved more often than the greater curvature
- Gastric tumors are divided into two major types based on morphology
  - Intestinal type
  - Diffusive infiltrative type
- Tumors with **intestinal morphology** tend to form **bulky tumors** composed of **glandular structures** while cancers with a **diffuse infiltrative** growth pattern are more often composed of **signet-ring cells**
- ***Intestinal-type adenocarcinomas*** typically grow along broad cohesive fronts to form either an **exophytic mass** or an **ulcerated tumor**.
- The neoplastic cells often contain **apical mucin vacuoles**, and **abundant mucin** may be present in gland lumens.

- **Diffuse gastric cancer** is generally composed of **discohesive cells** that **do not form glands** but instead have **large mucin vacuoles** that **expand the cytoplasm** and push the **nucleus to the periphery**, creating **signet-ring cell** morphology.
- **Extracellular mucin release** in either type of gastric cancer can result in formation of large **mucin lakes** that dissect tissue planes.
- A mass may be difficult to appreciate in diffuse gastric cancer, but these infiltrative tumors often evoke a **desmoplastic** reaction that stiffens the gastric wall.
- When there are large areas of infitration, diffuse rugal flattening and a rigid, thickened wall may impart a **leather bottle** appearance termed **linitis plastica.**.
- **Breast** and **lung cancers** that **metastasize** to the **stomach** may also create a **linitis plastica–like appearance.**

Clinical characteristics

- *The* ***depth of invasion*** *and the* ***extent of nodal*** *and* ***distant metastasis at the time of diagnosis*** *remain the* ***most powerful prognostic indicators*** *for gastric cancer.*
- In advanced cases gastric carcinoma may first be detected as metastases to the supraclavicular sentinel lymph node, also called ***Virchow's node***.
- Gastric tumors can also metastasize to the periumbilical region to form a **subcutaneous nodule**, termed a ***Sister Mary Joseph nodule***.
- Local invasion into the duodenum, pancreas, and retroperitoneum is also characteristic.

19. **Ig A deposition in glomeruli is seen in:**
A. SLE nephritis **B.** PSGN
C. MPGN **D.** HSP nephritis

Ans: D. HSP nephritis

Ref: *Robbins Pathologic Basis of Disease, 8th edition.*

Explanation:

"Whereas ***IgA nephropathy*** *is typically an* ***isolated renal disease****, similar* ***IgA deposits*** *are present in a systemic disorder of children,* ***Henoch-Schönlein purpura****, which has many* ***overlapping features*** *with IgA nephropathy" Ref: Robbins.*

"IgA is deposited in the glomerular mesangium in a distribution similar to that of IgA nephropathy. This has led to the concept that ***IgA nephropathy*** *and* ***Henoch-Schönlein purpura*** *are* ***manifestations*** *of the* ***same disease****" Ref: Robbins. (See Table 11)*

Table 11 : Summary of Glomerular Findings in Major Primary Glomerulonephritides

Disease	*Light Microscopy*	*Fluorescence Microscopy*	*Electron Microscopy*
IgA nephropathy	Focal mesangial proliferative glomerulonephritis; mesangial widening	**IgA**±IgG, IgM, and C3 in mesangium	Mesangial and paramesangial dense deposits
HSP Nephritis	Mesangial proliferation capillary to crescentic glomerulonephritis	**IgA**±IgG and C3 in mesangium	Mesangial deposits
Postinfectious glomerulonephritis	Diffuse endocapillary proliferation; leukocytic infiltration	**Granular** IgG and C3 in GBM and mesangium	**Subepithelial** humps
Goodpasture syndrome	Extracapillary proliferation with crescents; necrosis	**Linear IgG** and C3; fibrin in crescents	No deposits; GBM disruptions; fibrin
Chronic glomerulonephritis	Hyalinized glomeruli	Granular or negative	
Membranous glomerulopathy	Diffuse capillary wall thickening	Granular IgG and C3; diffuse	**Subepithelial deposits**
Minimal-change disease	**Normal**; lipid in tubules	**Negative**	**Loss of foot processes**; no deposits
Focal segmental glomerulosclerosis	Focal and segmental sclerosis and hyalinosis	Focal; IgM + C3	Loss of foot processes; epithelial denudation
Membranoproliferative glomerulonephritis (MPGN) type I		IgG + C3; C1q + C4	**Subendothelial deposits**
Dense-deposit disease (MPGN type II)	Mesangial and endocapillary proliferation; GBM thickening; splitting	C3±IgG; no C1q or C4	**Dense deposits**

20. **Which cell doesn't take part in atherogenesis?**
A. Neutrophil **B.** Platelet
C. Monocyte **D.** Smooth muscle

Ans: A. Neutrophil

Ref: *Robbins Pathologic Basis of Disease, 8th edition*

Explanation:

PATHOGENESIS OF ATHEROSCLEROSIS

There are two dominant hypotheses:

- Intimal cellular proliferation
- The repetitive formation and organization of thrombi.
- The contemporary view of atherogenesis incorporates elements of both theories and also the risk factors (***Response-to-injury hypothesis***)
- *Atherosclerosis is a chronic inflammatory and healing response of the arterial wall to endothelial injury.*
- *Lesion progression occurs through the interaction of **modified lipoproteins, monocyte-derived macrophages,** and **T lymphocytes** with the **normal cellular** constituents of the **arterial wall***

Atherosclerosis is produced by the following pathogenic events:

- ***Endothelial injury***, which causes (among other things) increased vascular permeability, leukocyte adhesion, and thrombosis.
- ***Accumulation of lipoproteins*** (mainly LDL and its oxidized forms) in the vessel wall.
- ***Monocyte adhesion*** *to the endothelium*, followed by migration into the intima and transformation into ***macrophages*** and ***foam cells.***
- ***Platelet adhesion.***
- *Factor release* from activated platelets, macrophages, and vascular wall cells, inducing ***smooth muscle cell recruitment***, either from the media or from circulating precursors.
- ***Smooth muscle cell proliferation** and **ECM production.***
- ***Lipid accumulation*** both **extracellularly** and within cells (**macrophages** and **smooth muscle cells).**

21. **Amyloid deposits are seen in which thyroid malignancy?**
A. Medullary Ca **B.** Papillary Ca
C. Anaplastic Ca **D.** Follicular Ca

Ans: A. Medullary Ca

Ref: *Robbins Pathologic Basis of Disease, 8th edition.*

Explanation:

*"**Acellular amyloid deposits**, derived from altered **calcitonin polypeptides**, are present in the adjacent **stroma** in many cases of **Medullary carcinoma of thyroid**" Ref: Robbins*

Medullary Carcinoma of Thyroid

- These are **neuroendocrine neoplasms** derived from the **parafollicular cells,** or **C cells.**
- Accounts for approximately **5%** of thyroid neoplasms.
- Medullary carcinomas, similar to normal C cells, **secrete calcitonin**, the measurement of which plays an important role in the diagnosis and postoperative follow-up of patients.
- May also secrete other polypeptide hormones, such as **serotonin**, **ACTH**, and **vasoactive intestinal peptide (VIP)**.
- About **70%** of tumors arise sporadically.
- The remainder occurs in the setting of **MEN syndrome 2A or 2B** or as familial tumors without an associated MEN syndrome.
- Activating point mutations in the **RET protooncogene (chr 10)** - both familial and sporadic medullary carcinomas.
- Cases associated with MEN types 2A or 2B occur in **younger** patients.
- Familial medullary carcinomas arises in **4th - 5th** decade.

Morphology

- Sporadic medullary thyroid carcinomas present as a **solitary nodule.**
- In contrast, **bilaterality** and **multicentricity** are common in **familial cases**.
- Larger lesions often contain areas of **necrosis** and **hemorrhage** and may extend through the capsule of the thyroid.
- The tumor tissue is firm, pale gray to tan, and infiltrative.
- Microscopically, medullary carcinomas are composed of **polygonal to spindle-shaped cells**, which may form **nests, trabeculae**, and even **follicles**.
- Small, more anaplastic cells are present in some tumors and may be the predominant cell type. **Acellular amyloid deposits** derived from **calcitonin polypeptides** are present in adjacent stroma.
- **Calcitonin** is readily demonstrable within the **cytoplasm** of the tumor cells and in **stromal amyloid** by **immunohistochemical methods**.
- One of the peculiar features of **familial medullary cancers** is the presence of

multicentric C-cell hyperplasia in the surrounding thyroid parenchyma, a feature that is usually **absent in sporadic lesions**.

- **Foci of C-cell hyperplasia** are believed to represent the **precursor lesions** from which **medullary carcinomas arise.**

Clinical Course

- **Sporadic cases** presents with mass in the **neck** and **dysphagia** or **hoarseness**.
- **Paraneoplastic syndrome** can occur, caused by the secretion of a peptide hormone (e.g., **diarrhea** due to the secretion of **VIP**, or **Cushing syndrome** due to **ACTH**).
- Notably, **hypocalcemia** is **NOT** a prominent feature, **despite** the **presence** of **raised calcitonin** levels.
- Secretion of **carcinoembryonic antigen (CEA)** by the neoplastic cells is a useful biomarker.

22. Osmotic fragility of RBCs are increased in:

A. Hereditary Spherocytosis
B. Sickle cell anemia
C. Thalessemia
D. PNH

Ans: A. Hereditary Spherocytosis

Ref: *Robbins Pathologic Basis of Disease, 8th edition*

Explanation:

*"In two thirds of the patients with **Hereditary Spherocytosis**, the red cells are **abnormally sensitive to osmotic lysis** when incubated in **hypotonic salt solutions**, which causes the influx of water into spherocytes with little margin for expansion"*

Ref: Robbins.

Hereditary Spherocytosis (HS)

- This inherited disorder is caused by intrinsic defects in the red cell membrane skeleton.
- Red blood cells are spheroid, less deformable, and vulnerable to splenic sequestration and destruction.
- Majority of cases are **autosomal dominant** (75%).

Pathogenesis

- The remarkable elasticity and durability of the normal red cell are attributable to the physicochemical properties of its specialized membrane skeleton which lies closely apposed to the internal surface of the plasma membrane.
- Its chief protein component, **spectrin**, consists of two polypeptide chains, α and β, which form intertwined **(helical) flexible heterodimers**.
- The "**head**" regions of spectrin dimers self-associate to form **tetramers**, while the "**tails**" associate with **actin oligomers**.
- Each actin oligomer can bind multiple spectrin tetramers, thus creating a two-dimensional spectrin-actin skeleton that is connected to the cell membrane by two distinct interactions.
- The first, involving the proteins **ankyrin** and **band 4.2**, binds **spectrin** to the transmembrane ion transporter, **band 3**.
- The second, involving protein 4.1, binds the "tail" of **spectrin** to another transmembrane protein, **glycophorin A**.
- HS is caused by diverse mutations that lead to an insufficiency of membrane skeletal components.
- The life span of the affected red cells is **decreased on average to 10 to 20 days** (Normal -120 days)
- The pathogenic mutations most commonly affect **ankyrin**, **band 3**, **spectrin**, or **band 4.2**.
- Young HS red cells are normal in shape, but the deficiency of membrane skeleton reduces the stability of the lipid bilayer, leading to the loss of **membrane fragments as red cells age** in the circulation.
- The loss of membrane relative to cytoplasm "forces" the cells to assume the **smallest possible diameter for a given volume**, namely, a **sphere**.
- The invariably beneficial effects of **splenectomy** prove that the spleen has a **cardinal role** in the premature demise of **spherocytes**.
- Normal red cells must undergo extreme deformation to leave the cords of Billroth and enter the sinusoids.
- Because of their spheroidal shape and reduced deformability, the hapless spherocytes are trapped in the splenic cords, where they provide a happy meal for phagocytes.
- **After splenectomy** the **spherocytes persist,** but the **anemia is corrected**

Morphology

- The most specific morphologic finding is **spherocytosis**, apparent on smears as abnormally small, dark-staining (hyperchromic) red cells lacking the central zone of pallor.
- **Spherocytosis** is **distinctive** but **not pathognomonic**, since other forms of membrane loss, such as in autoimmune hemolytic anemias, also cause the formation of spherocytes.
- Other features are common to all hemolytic anemias.

- These include:
  - **Reticulocytosis**
  - **Marrow erythroid hyperplasia**
  - **Hemosiderosis**
  - Mild jaundice.
  - **Cholelithiasis** (pigment stones - 40% to 50% cases)
  - Moderate splenic enlargement
- Splenomegaly results from congestion of the cords of Billroth and increased numbers of phagocytes needed to clear the spherocytes.

Clinical Features

- The diagnosis is based on **family history, hematologic findings**, and **laboratory evidence**.
- In two thirds of the patients the red cells are abnormally **sensitive to osmotic lysis** when incubated in **hypotonic salt solutions**, which causes the influx of water into spherocytes with little margin for expansion.
- HS red cells also have an **increased mean cell hemoglobin concentration**, due to **dehydration** caused by the **loss of K+ and H2O**.
- The characteristic clinical features are **anemia, splenomegaly**, and **jaundice**.
- The generally stable clinical course is sometimes punctuated by **aplastic crises**, usually triggered by an **acute parvovirus** infection.
- **Parvovirus** infects and **kills red cell progenitors**, causing red cell production to cease until an effective immune response commences, generally in **1 to 2 weeks**.
- Because of the reduced life span of HS red cells, cessation of erythropoiesis for even short time periods leads to sudden worsening of the **anemia**.
- Transfusions may be necessary to support the patient until the immune response clears the infection.
- Hemolytic crises are produced by intercurrent events leading to increased splenic destruction of red cells (e.g., infectious mononucleosis); these are clinically less significant than aplastic crises.
- **Gallstones**, found in many patients, can also produce symptoms.
- **Splenectomy** treats the anemia and its complications, but brings with it the **risk of sepsis**. *(See the following Figure)*

23. Which of the following conditions exhibit allelic heterogenicity?

A. Beta thalassemia
B. Sickle cell disease
C. HOCM
D. Duchenne musclar dystrophy

Ans: A. Beta thalassemia

Ref: *Robbins Pathologic Basis of Disease, 8th edition & Thompson & Thompson. Genetics in Medicine.*

Explanation:

- A **single mutant gene** may lead to many end effects, termed ***pleiotropism***
- **Mutations at several genetic loci** may produce the same trait ***(genetic heterogeneity)***.
- **Sickle cell anemia** is an example of **pleiotropism**.

Allelic heterogeneity means that **different mutations within a single gene locus** (forming multiple alleles of that gene) cause the same phenotypic expression. There are over 1000 known mutant alleles of the **CFTR gene** that cause **cystic fibrosis** (Classic example) *(See Table 12 on the next page)*

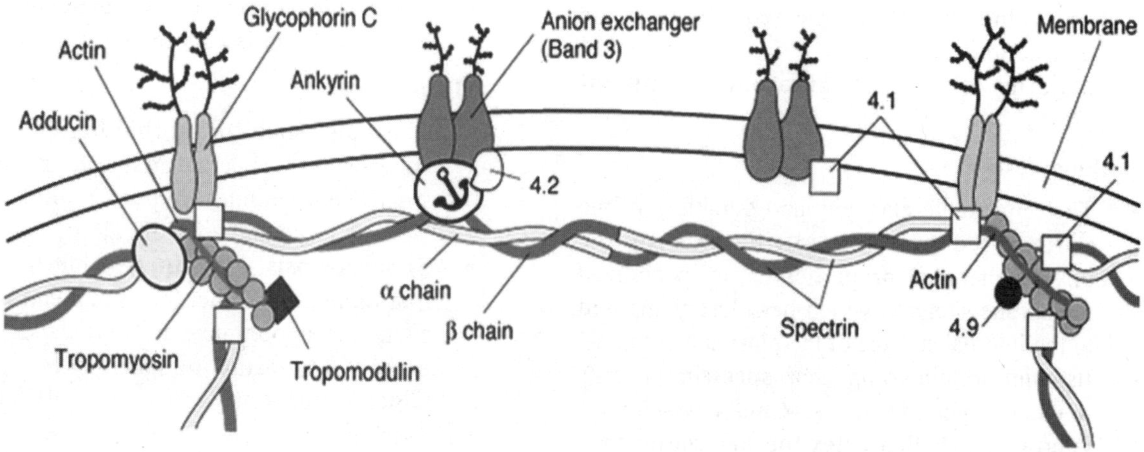

Table 12
The Various Types of Heterogeneity Associated with Genetic Disease

Type of Heterogeneity	Definition	Examples
Genetic beterogeneity		
Allelic heterogeneity	The occurrence of more than one allele at a locus	β-Thalassemia mutations in β-globin Phenylalanine hydroxylase mutations in PKU Perinatal lethal osteogenesis imperfecta (type II), from mutations in the α1 collagen gene
Locus heterogeneity	The association of more than one locus with a specific clinical phenotype	Biopterin metabolism defects causing by perphenylalaninemia
Clinical or phenotypic beterogeneity	The association of more than one phenotype with mutations at a single locus	Phenylalanine hydroxylase mutations causing PKU, variant PKU, or non-PKU hyperphenylalaninemia α-L-Iduronidase mutations causing Hurler syndrome or Scheie syndrome

MICROBIOLOGY

1. **Gas gangrene is caused by:**
   A. Clostridium botulium
   B. Clostridium perfringens
   C. Clostridium difficile
   D. Clostridium tetani

Ans. B. Clostridium perfringens

Ref: *Ananthnarayan R, Paniker CKJ. Textbook of Microbiology. 8th Edition. Hyderabad: Universities Press; 2009. Pg. 251*

Explanation:

Gas gangrene

Caused by

- *Cl. perfringens*
- *Cl. septicum*
- *Cl. odematieuns*
- *Cl. sporogenes*
- *Cl histolyticum* (Aerotolerant anaerobe)

Virulence factors

- ***Exotoxins*** – hemolytic, lethal and necrotic effects, help in spreading of the infection
- ***Alpha toxin (lecithinase)*** –splits lecithin
- ***Collagenase (Kappa)***
- ***Hyaluronidase*** – breaks down hyaluronic acid in muscles cells
- ***Theta toxin haemolysin***
- ***Leucocidin*** – kills leucocytes
- Gamma, delta, theta, lambda, mu & eta toxin

Food poisoning

- Gastroenteritis – *Cl. perfringens* (type A)
- Necrotising enterocolitis – *Cl. perfringens* (type C)
- Botulism – *Cl. botulinum*

Acute colitis (Antibiotic associated diarrhoea) – *Cl. difficile*

2. **Non motile clostridia is:**
   A. Clostridium tetanomorphum
   B. Clostridium histolyticum
   C. Clostridium septicum
   D. Clostridium perfringens

Ans. D. Clostridium perfringens

Ref: *Ananthnarayan R, Paniker CKJ. Textbook of Microbiology. 8th Edition. Hyderabad: Universities Press; 2009. Pg. 249*

Explanation:

- Most Clostridia are **motile** with **peritrichate flagella**.
- The motility is slow and has been described as 'stately'.
- Only ***Cl perfringens*** and ***Cl tetani*** **Type VI** are **nonmotile**.

3. **False regarding brucellosis is:**
   A. Transmitted my milk ingestion
   B. Cephalosporins is the drug of choice
   C. Causes gastroenteritis
   D. Causes spinal spondylosis

Ans. B. Cephalosporins is the drug of choice

Ref: *Ananthnarayan R, Paniker CKJ. Textbook of Microbiology. 8th Edition. Hyderabad: Universities Press; 2009. Pg. 345*
Jawetz, Melnick, & Adelberg's. Text book of Medical Microbiology, 25th Edition. 2010.

Explanation:

Brucellosis

- It is a **zoonotic disease**
- All three major species of brucellae are pathogenic to human beings.
- **Br melitensis** is the most pathogenic, **Br abortus** and **Br suis** being of intermediate pathogenicity.
- Slow-growing **Gram-negative coccobacilli**
- Primarily occurs through **occupational exposure** (e.g. exposure to cattle, sheep, pigs), but also by consumption of **unpasteurised milk products**
- It causes **Malta Fever** or **Undulant Fever**

Clinical features

- The incubation period is **1–6 weeks**.
- The onset is insidious, with malaise, fever, weakness, aches, and sweats.
- The fever usually rises in the afternoon; its fall during the night is accompanied by drenching sweat.
- There may be gastrointestinal and nervous symptoms.
- Lymph nodes enlarge, and the spleen becomes palpable. Hepatitis may be accompanied by jaundice.
- Deep pain and disturbances of motion, particularly in vertebral bodies, suggest **osteomyelitis**.
- Chronic stage is characterized by weakness, aches and pains, low-grade fever, nervousness, and other nonspecific manifestations compatible with **psychoneurotic symptoms**.

Diagnosis

- Blood culture technique
- Serological method
  - Standard Agglutination Test
  - ELISA
  - RIA
- Diagnosis of infected milk - **Milk ring test** (Abs against Brucella is detected).

Treatment

The usual regimen is a combination of **doxycycline** for 45 days with **streptomycin** 1M daily for the first 2 weeks in adults, and in children **cotrimoxazole** along with **rifampicin** or **gentamycin**.

4. **Other name of Cachetin is:**

A. TNF - alpha **B.** IL -2
C. IL -12 **D.** IFN -gamma

Ans. A. TNF - alpha

Ref: *Ananthnarayan R, Paniker CKJ. Textbook of Microbiology. 8th Edition. Hyderabad: Universities Press; 2009. Pg. 149*

Explanation:

Tumour necrosis factor (TNF)

- It occurs as two **types**, **alpha** and **beta**.
- A serum factor found to induce **hemorrhagic necrosis** in certain tumours was named the tumour necrosis factor.
- The same substance was independently described as **cachectin**, a serum factor causing the wasting syndrome (cachexia) during chronic infections.
- This has been renamed **TNFα**.
- It is formed principally by **activated macrophages and monocytes**.
- It resembles **IL 1** in possessing a very wide spectrum of biological activities such as participation in the manifestations of endotoxic shock. It exerts immunomodulatory influence on other cytokines.
- **TNFβ**, formerly known as **lymphotoxin**, is produced principally by **T helper cells**. Its effects are similar to those of **TNFα**.

5. **Which of these is sporicidal?**

A. Alcohol **B.** Phenol
C. Chlorine **D.** Glutaraldehyde

Ans. D. Glutaraldehyde

Ref: *Ananthnarayan R, Paniker CKJ. Textbook of Microbiology. 8th Edition. Hyderabad: Universities Press; 2009. Pg. 35-8.*

Explanation: *(See Table 13)*

Table 13

Disinfectant	Effective against	Characteristic
Alcohols Compounds (Ethanol, methanol, isopropyl alcohol)	Active against bacteria. Methanol is active against fungal spores	Good general use disinfectant
Aldehydes (Formaldehyde, Glutaraldehyde)	Active against bacteria and virus and spores	Good activity against bacteria , virus and spores
Chlorine	Good disinfectant for blood and body fluid spills	Active against bacteria, virus and moderate action against spores

6. **Which of the following specimen is not refrigerated prior to inoculation? (Repeat)**

A. Blood B. CSF
C. Urine D. Urine

Ans. B. CSF

Ref: *Ananthnarayan R, Paniker CKJ. Textbook of Microbiology. 8th Edition. Hyderabad: Universities Press; 2009. Pg. 332*

Explanation:

- **Haemophilus influenzae** is an important cause of **meningitis.**
- The disease is more common in children between **two months and three years** of age. Infections are caused by the **capsulated strains**, type B accounting for most cases.
- **CSF specimen** from suspected children should be plated promptly on a suitable medium such as **blood agar or chocolate agar** and incubated in an environment **of 5-10 per cent CO_2** and **high humidity.**
- As this bacillus is **very sensitive to low temperatures**, CSF specimens **should never be refrigerated** before inoculation.

7. **Toxic shock syndrome caused by Staphylococcus is due to:**

A. Hemolysins B. Super antigens
C. Coagulase D. Hyaluronidase

Ans. B. Super antigens

Ref: *Ananthnarayan R, Paniker CKJ. Textbook of Microbiology. 8th Edition. Hyderabad: Universities Press; 2009. Pg. 198-9.*

Explanation:

Microbial super antigens such as **Streptococcal protein A** and **Staphylococcal enterotoxin** can stimulate the broad range T & B cells irrespective of their antigenic specificity.

Toxic Shock Syndrome

- TSST is the cause of toxic shock syndrome (TSS). TSST is a **superantigen.**
- Superantigens **stimulate T cells non-specifically without normal antigenic recognition**
- Up to one in five T cells be activated, whereas only 1 in 10,000 are stimulated during a usual antigen presentation.
- Cytokines are released in large amounts, causing the symptoms of **TSS.**
- Superantigens bind directly to **class II major histocompatibility** complexes of antigen-presenting cells outside the conventional antigen-binding grove.

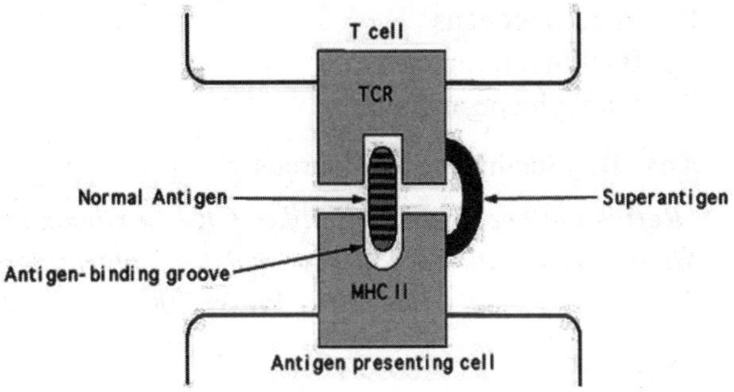

8. **Which is the largest pathogenic bacillus ?**

A. Bacillus cereus
B. Bacillus subtilis
C. Bacillus megaterium
D. Bacillius anthracis

Ans. D. Bacillius anthracis

Ref: *Ananthnarayan R, Paniker CKJ. Textbook of Microbiology. 8th Edition. Hyderabad: Universities Press; 2009. Pg. 242*

Explanation:

Bacillus anthracis

Considerable historical interest is attached to the anthrax bacillus.

- ***First pathogenic bacterium*** to be observed under the **microscope**
- ***First communicable disease*** shown to be **transmitted** by **inoculation** of infected blood
- ***First bacillus*** to be **isolated in pure culture** and shown to possess **spores**
- ***First bacterium*** used for the **preparation** of an **attenuated vaccine**
- The anthrax bacillus is the **largest of pathogenic bacteria**, measuring 3-10 μm x 1-1.6 μm.

Characteristics of Bacillus anthracis

- ***Bamboo stick appearance***
- Polypeptide capsule - ***M'Fadyeans reaction*** (stain with Polychrome Methylene blue)
- Edge of colony under dissecting Microscope shows "***Medusa Head appearance***"
- Nutrient agar –***Frosted glass appearance***
- Blood Agar – No or Minimal Hemolysis
- Selective Medium – ***PLET medium*** (Polymyxin, Lysozyme, EDTA, thallous acetate)
- Gelatin Stab Culture – ***Inverted Fir Tree appearance***
- "***String of Pearls***" – media with .05 - .5 U PenG/ml

9. **Ritter's disease is caused by:**
A. Pseudomonas aeruginosa
B. Pneumococcus
C. Bacillus antrhracis
D. Staphylococcus aureus

Ans. D. Staphylococcus aureus

Ref: *Ananthnarayan R, Paniker CKJ. Textbook of Microbiology. 8th Edition. Hyderabad: Universities Press; 2009. Pg. 199*

Explanation:

Staphylococcal scalded skin syndrome:

- **Exfoliative (epidermolytic) toxin**, also known as **ET** or **'exfoliatin'**, is responsible for the 'staphylococcal scalded skin syndrome' (SSSS)
- It is an exfoliative skin disease in which the outer layer of the **epidermis** gets separated from the underlying tissues.
- The severe form of **SSSS** is known as **Ritter's disease** in the **newborn** and **toxic epidermal necrolysis in older patients**.
- Milder forms are **pemphigus neonatorum** and **bullous impetigo**.

10. **Basophilic inclusion bodies seen in:**
A. Polio virus **B.** Adenovirus
C. Measles virus **D.** Herpes virus

Ans. B. Adenovirus

Ref: *Ananthnarayan R, Paniker CKJ. Textbook of Microbiology. 8th Edition. Hyderabad: Universities Press; 2009. Pg. 444.*
Jawetz, Melnick, & Adelberg's. Text book of Medical Microbiology, 25th Edition. 2010.

Explanation:

- **Inclusion bodies** are nuclear or cytoplasmic **aggregates** of **stainable substances**, usually **proteins**. They typically represent **sites** of **viral multiplication** and usually consist of **viral capsid proteins**.

Types of inclusion bodies:

- **Location**
  - ***Cytoplasm*** - Eg: Poxvirus
  - ***Nucleus*** - Eg: Herpesvirus
  - ***Both*** - Eg: Measles
- **Staining property**
  - ***Eosinophilic (Pink)***. Most viral infections. Eg: Negri bodies (Rabies), Molluscum contagiosum
  - ***Basophilic (Blue)***. Eg: Adenovirus
- **Size**
  - Small, multiple inclusion - Eg: Guarneri bodies (Vaccinia)
  - Large inclusions - Eg: Bollinger bodies (Fowlpox)
  - Very large inclusions - Eg: Molluscum bodies
- **Intranuclear**
  - ***Cowdry type A*** - Variable size & granular. Eg: Herpes, Yellow fever (HAY)
  - ***Cowdry type B*** - Well circumscribed & multiple. Eg: Adenovirus, Polio (BAP)

11. **The cyclic trend seen with influenza is due to:**
A. Antigenic drift **B.** Antigenic shift
C. Endemicity **D.** Virulence

Ans. A. Antigenic drift

Ref: *Ananthnarayan R, Paniker CKJ. Textbook of Microbiology. 8th Edition. Hyderabad: Universities Press; 2009. Pg. 496*
Jawetz, Melnick, & Adelberg's. Text book of Medical Microbiology, 25th Edition. 2010

Explanation:

- A unique feature of the **influenza virus** is its ability to undergo **antigenic variation.**
- Antigenic variability is highest in **influenza virus type A** and **less in type B**, while it has **not been demonstrated in type C.**
- Antigenic variation is of two type-s: **antigenic drift** or **antigenic shift**.
- **Antigenic drift**
  - The gradual sequential change in antigenic structure occurring **regularly at frequent intervals** is known as antigenic drift. Here, the new antigens, though different from the previous antigens, are yet **related to them,** so that they react with antisera to the predecessor virus strains, to varying degrees.
  - Antigenic drift is due to mutation and selection, the process being influenced by the presence of antibodies to the predecessor strains in the host population.
  - Antigenic drift accounts for the periodical epidemics of influenza. Influenza outbreaks occur in waves, which depends on the interplay between extent of antigenic drift of the predominant virus and waning immunity in the population.
- **Antigenic shift**
  - Antigenic shift is an **abrupt, drastic, discontinuous variation** in the antigenic structure, resulting in a **novel virus strain**

unrelated antigenically to predecessor strains.
- Such changes may involve hemagglutinin, neuraminidase or both.
- Antibodies to predecessor viruses do not neutralise the new variants and can, therefore, spread widely in the population causing major epidemics or pandemics.
- The changes involved in antigenic shift are due to **genetic re-assortment**

12. Quadrivalent HPV vaccine protects against:

A. HPV 6,11,16,18
B. HPV 6, 11, 31, 32
C. HPV 16, 18, 31, 35
D. HPV 11, 16, 30, 33

Ans. A. HPV 6,11,16,18

Ref: *Jawetz, Melnick, & Adelberg's. Text book of Medical Microbiology, 25th Edition. 2010.*

Explanation:

Quadrivalent HPV vaccine

- It is a **noninfectious recombinant vaccine** produced in yeast and containing virus-like particles composed of **HPV L1** proteins.
- The vaccine contains particles derived from **HPV types 6, 11, 16, and 18.**
- The vaccine is effective at preventing persistent infections by the four HPV types and the development of HPV-related genital precancerous lesions.
- It is **not effective** against **established HPV disease.**
- **Adolescent** and **young adult females** make up the initial target population for vaccination.
- It is **not known how long vaccine-induced immunity lasts.**

13. Thick walled fungal resting spores formed by condensation of hyphal elements is:

A. Basidiospore **B.** Arthrospore
C. Chlamydospores **D.** Blastospore

Ans. C. Chlamydospores

Ref: *Ananthnarayan R, Paniker CKJ. Textbook of Microbiology. 8th Edition. Hyderabad: Universities Press; 2009. Pg. 601*

Explanation:

- **Arthrospore**: A spore formed by segmentation and fragmentation of vegetative hyphae, usually but not always in a chain. Commonly seen in **Trichosporon, Geotrichum, Coccidioides.**
- **Blastospore**: A spore formed through a **budding process** as seen in **yeast**.
- **Chlamydospore**: A thick-walled resting spore formed within a **hyphal** segment. It is formed by condensation from an **intercalary or terminal hyphal cell** and contains stored food and is capable functioning as a resting spore. Seen in **Candida**.

FORENSIC MEDICINE

1. Metabolic acidosis and visual damage occurs in poisoning due to:

A. Methanol **B.** Ethanol
C. Cocaine **D.** Opium

Ans: A. Methanol

Ref: *The Essentials of Forensic Medicine and Toxicology by KS Narayan Reddy. 29th edition. 2010. Pg: 521*

Explanation:

Methyl alchohol (Methanol) Poisoning

- Methanol has a high toxicity in humans.
- The median lethal dose is typically 100 mL
- Methanol is toxic by two mechanisms.
  - Methanolcan be fatal due to its **CNS depressant properties** in the same manner as ethanol poisoning.
  - In a process of **toxication**, it is metabolized to formic acid (which is present as the formate ion) via formaldehyde in a process initiated by the enzyme alcohol dehydrogenase in the liver.
- Methanol is converted to **formaldehyde** via alcohol dehydrogenase **(ADH)** and **formaldehyde** is converted to **formic acid** (formate) via aldehyde dehydrogenase **(ALDH)**.
- **Formate** is **toxic** because it inhibits **mitochondrial cytochrome c oxidase**, causing the symptoms of **hypoxia** at the cellular level, and **metabolic acidosis.**
- Methanol poisoning can be treated with the antidotes **ethanol or fomepizole**
- Both drugs act to **reduce the action** of **alcohol dehydrogenase** on methanol by means of **competitive inhibition,** so it is excreted by the kidneys rather than being transformed into toxic metabolites.
- Further treatment may include giving sodium bicarbonate for metabolic acidosis, and **hemodialysis** or **hemodiafiltration** can be used to remove methanol and formate from the blood.

- **Folinic acid** or **folic acid** is also administered to enhance the metabolism of formate.
- The initial symptoms of methanol intoxication include:
  - Central nervous system depression
  - Headache
  - Dizziness
  - Nausea
  - lack of coordination
  - Confusion
- Unconsciousness and death (with large doses)
- Death due to respiratory failure.
- Physical examination may show Tachypnea
- Ophthalmologic examination may show **dilated pupils** with hyperemia of the optic disc and retinal edema.

2. All are feature of cocaine intake *except:*

A. Hemorrhagic stroke **B.** Seizures
C. Alcoholism **D.** Priapism

Ans: D. Priapism

Ref: *The Essentials of Forensic Medicine and Toxicology by KS Narayan Reddy. 29th edition. 2010. Pg: 544*

Explanation:

Acute Cocaine intoxication

Two clinical stages

A. Stage of excitement
- Hyperthermia (Cocaine fever)
- Intracranial bleed
- Paraesthesia

B. Stage of Depression
- Arrthytmias
- Respiratory failure
- Cardiac failure

Complications
- Convulsions
- Headache
- Ischaemic /Hemorrhagic stroke
- Subarachnoid hemorrhage

Cocaine Addiction / Chronic poisoning / Cocainism

- Blackening of tongue and teeth
- Ulceration and perforation of nasal septum
- Magnan symptoms/ formication/ Cocaine bugs: Feeling of bugs/ small insects creeping under the skin- a form of tactile hallucination
- Euphoria followed by depression
- Alcohol dependance
- Hyperactivity
- Loss of libido
- Impotence in males
- Gynecomastia

3. Colour of urine in phenol poisoning: (Repeat)

A. Red **B.** Green
C. Yellow **D.** Blue

Ans: B. Green

Ref: *The Essentials of Forensic Medicine and Toxicology by KS Narayan Reddy. 29th edition. 2010. Pg:*

Explanation:

Refer 2011 Forensic medicine question explanation

4. Sample of spinal cord preseved in: (Repeat)

A. Strychnine poisoning
B. Arsenic poisoning
C. Yellow Oleander poisoning
D. Nerve gas poisoning

Ans: A. Strychnine poisoning

Ref: *The Essentials of Forensic Medicine and Toxicology by KS Narayan Reddy. 29th edition. 2010. Pg:*

Explanation:

Refer 2011 Forensic medicine question explanation

5. A doctor leaves a swab in abdomen during surgery. Under which doctrine will a criminal suit be filed against him?

A. Criminal negligence **B.** Civil negligence
C. Res ispa loquitor **D.** Vicarious liability

Ans: A. Criminal negligence

Ref: *The Essentials of Forensic Medicine and Toxicology by KS Narayan Reddy. 29th edition. 2010. Pg:33*

Explanation:

Criminal negligence: When a doctor shows gross absence of skill and care during treatment resulting in death of patient

Medical Negligence is considered to be criminal negligence if:

a. When a doctor shows gross absence of skill or care during treatment resulting in serious injury to or death of a patient
b. When a doctor performs an illegal act
c. When an assaulted person dies, the defence may attribute the death to the negligence or undue interference in the treatment of the deceased by the doctor.

Section 304-A IPC deals with Criminal Negligence *"Whosoever causes the death of any person by doing any rash or negligent act not amounting to culpable homicide shll be punished with imprisonment upto 2 years or with fine or with both". (See Table 14)*

Table 14 : Difference between Civil and Criminal Negligence

Trait	Civil Negligence	Criminal Negligence
Offence	No specific or clear violation of law needs to be proved	Must have specifically violated a particular criminal law in question
Negligence	Simple absence of care & skill	Gross negligence, inattention or lack of competency
Conduct of Physician	It is compared to a generally accepted simple standard of professional conduct	Not compared to a single test
Consent for act	Good defence; cannot recover damages	Not a defence; can be prosecuted
Trial by	Civil Court	Criminal Court
Evidence	Strong evidence is sufficient	Guilt should be proved beyond doubt
Punishment	Liable to pay damages	Imprisonment

Resispa loquitor - 'the thing or fact speaks for itself'

In this situation, the patient need not prove negligence of the physician because it is obvious.

The rule is applied when:

a. that in the absence of negligence the injury would not have occured ordinarily.
b. the doctor had exclusive control over the injury producing instrument or treatment.
c. patient was not guilty of contributory negligence
   - These enables the lawyer to prove the case without medical evidence.

Vicarious liability (Liability for act of another)

An employer is responsible not only for his own negligence, but also for the negligence of his employees, by the principle ***"respondeat superior" (Let the master answer).***

In practice, the principal doctor becomes responsible for any negligence of his assistant.

6. A criminal negligence suit against a doctor must be filed within:

A. 6 months **B.** 1 year
C. 2 years **D.** 4 year

Ans: C. 2 years

Ref: *The Essentials of Forensic Medicine and Toxicology by KS Narayan Reddy. 29th edition. 2010.*

Explanation:

- Time limitation to sue for criminal negligence against a doctor is **2 years**

Refer explanation to the previous question.

7. Incised looking lacerated wounds are seen in:

A. Hand **B.** Thorax
C. Abdomen **D.** Forehead

Ans: D. Forehead

Ref: *The Essentials of Forensic Medicine and Toxicology by KS Narayan Reddy. 29th edition. 2010. Pg: 171*

Explanation:

Incised- like or Incised- looking wounds

- Lacerations produced without excessive skin crushing may have relatively sharp margins
- Blunt force on areas where the skin is close to bone, and the subcutaneous tissues are scanty
- Produces a wound which by linear splitting of the tissues, may look like a incised wound
- The sites are:
  - Scalp & Forehead
  - Eyebrows
  - Cheek bones
  - Lower jaw
  - Iliac crest
  - Perineum
  - Shin

8. 'Hatter's shakes' are see in poisoning due to:

A. Mercury **B.** Arsenic
C. Lead **D.** Copper

Ans: A. Mercury

Ref: *The Essentials of Forensic Medicine and Toxicology by KS Narayan Reddy. 29th edition. 2010.*

Explanation:

Symptoms of Mercury Poisoning:

Acid metallic taste, hoarse voice, greyish white coating of tongue, blood-stained stool, circulatory collapse, necrosis of jaw, membranous, colitis, proximal renal tubular necrosis.

Acrodynia (Acro-Limbs Odynia-Pain) is seen in mercury poisoning (aka Pink's Disease).

It is characterized by Pain, swelling and parasthesia of Limbs.

Mimimata disease—Contamination of fish with mercury, at a place called Minimate Bay in Japan.

Chronic Poisoning (Hydrar gyrism)

- The symptoms are salivation, sore mouth and throat, fine tremors of the tongue, hands, arms, anemia.
- **Shaking palsy** is associated with Hg poisoning. Mercurial tremors are also called **hatter's shakes or glass blower's shake or Danbury Tremors.**
- **Mercurial erethism** is seen in persons working with mercury in mirror manufacturing firms. Erethism is characterized by shyness, timidity, irritability, loss of confidence, mental depression, loss of memory and insomnia. (Psychological symptoms).
- **Mercuria lentis** is a peculiar eye change due to brownish deposit of mercury through the cornea on the anterior lens capsule (Brown-Malt Reflex). It is bilateral and has no effect on visual acuity

9. **Acrodynia is a feature of:**
   A. Iron deficiency anemia
   B. Mercury poisoning
   C. Copper poisoning
   D. Zinc poisoning

Ans: B. Mercury poisoning

Ref: *The Essentials of Forensic Medicine and Toxicology by KS Narayan Reddy. 29th edition. 2010.*

Explanation:

Symptoms of Mercury Poisoning:

Acid metallic taste, hoarse voice, greyish white coating of tongue, blood-stained stool, circulatory collapse, necrosis of jaw, membranous, colitis, proximal renal tubular necrosis.

Acrodynia (Acro-Limbs Odynia-Pain) is seen in mercury poisoning (aka Pink's Disease).

It is characterized by Pain, swelling and parasthesia of Limbs.

Mimimata disease—Contamination of fish with mercury, at a place called Minimate Bay in Japan.

Chronic Poisoning (Hydrar gyrism)

- The symptoms are salivation, sore mouth and throat, fine tremors of the tongue, hands, arms, anemia.
- **Shaking palsy** is associated with Hg poisoning. Mercurial tremors are also called **hatter's shakes or glass blower's shake or Danbury Tremors.**
- **Mercurial erethism** is seen in persons working with mercury in mirror manufacturing firms. Erethism is characterized by shyness, timidity, irritability, loss of confidence, mental depression, loss of memory and insomnia (Psychological symptoms).
- **Mercuria lentis** is a peculiar eye change due to brownish deposit of mercury through the cornea on the anterior lens capsule (**Brown-Malt Reflex**). It is bilateral and has no effect on visual acuity.

PSM

1. **What is true about case fatality rate?**
   A. It is a ratio
   B. It is not useful for acute disease
   C. Related to virulence
   D. Not useful in chronic diseases

Ans: C. Related to virulence

Ref: *Park's Preventive and Social Medicine, 22nd edition. Pg 55*

Explanation:

Case Fatality Rate

- **Number of death due to the case × 100 / Number of cases**
- It is **proportion**, as numerator is part of denominator
- It is definitely useful in **acute diseases**
- Usefulness is **limited in chronic** diseases, but surely useful to some extent
- As **virulence** increases, **CFR** increases

2. **Confounding factor can be eliminated by:**
   A. Matching **B.** Correlation
   C. Standardization **D.** Randomization

Ans: A. Matching

Ref: *Park's Preventive and Social Medicine, 22nd edition. Pg 69.*

Explanation:

Confounding

- It is the factor which **confuses** the **association** between **two variables.**
- It is defined as one which is associated both with exposure an disease, and is distributed unequally in study and control groups.
- Control of confounding can be done at design stage and at analysis stage.

- At design stage, **restriction** (appropriate inclusion and exclusion criteria), **matching** cases and **control** can avoid confounding.
- At analysis stage, **stratification, regression analysis** can control confounding.
- **Correlation** is a statistical method of testing association.
- **Randomization** is done for balance of prognosis.

3. **Which is done even after control of disease?**
 A. Surveillance
 B. Vaccination
 C. Chemoprophylaxis
 D. Prolonged treatment

 Ans: A. Surveillance

 Ref: *Park's Preventive and Social Medicine, 22nd edition. Pg 118*

 Explanation:
 - **Surveillance** is **continuous scrutiny** of occurrence of disease or health related events to take action.
 - So, even after control of disease, one needs to keep an eye on the occurrence of disease, so that it is identified in time to take action.
 - All other options are distracters.

4. **Primary and secondary prevention of a disease is done for:**
 A. Control
 B. Eradication
 C. Elimination
 D. Surveillance

 Ans: A. Control

 Ref: *Park's Preventive and Social Medicine, 22nd edition. Pg 41-2*

 Explanation:
 - Both primary and secondary prevention are essential for **control**, though **secondary prevention** is the key.
 - Most of **national programs** are aimed at **secondary prevention for control**.
 - Surveillance is just a distracter.
 - **Public health surveillance** is the ongoing **systematic collection, analysis,** and **interpretation of data,** closely integrated with the timely dissemination of these data to those responsible for preventing and controlling disease and injury.
 - For **eradication and elimination**, it is only **primary prevention** which is essential, like **vaccination, life style modification, standard of living** etc.
 - Thus here answer is control of disease.

5. **A vaccine's efficacy is calculated to be 95 %. It literally means:**
 A. 5 out of 100 children can get infection even after vaccination
 B. 95% of children will not get the disease
 C. 95% are no longer susceptible to infection following vaccination
 D. 95 percentile of the population is protected

 Ans: B. 95% of children will not get the disease

 Ref: *Park's Preventive and Social Medicine, 22nd edition.*

 Explanation:
 - **Vaccine efficacy:** Reduction in incidence of a disease among people who have received vaccine compared to the incidence in unvaccinated people.
 Study design – RCT
 VE=(ARU-ARV)*100/ARU
 - **Vaccine effectiveness:** real world situation, how much reduction of disease it causes in population.
 Study design: Retrospective Case Control Study, quasi cohort/retrospective cohort, case cohort, Proportion of people getting infection despite vaccination

6. **Most sensitive parameter in monitoring iodine deficiency control programme is:**
 A. Goitre
 B. Urine T3, T4
 C. Growth retardation
 D. Neonatal hypothyroidism

 Ans: D. Neonatal hypothyroidism

 Ref: *Park's Preventive and Social Medicine, 22nd edition. Pg 579*

 Explanation:
 - **Iodine level in salt** at **consumption** level **15 ppm.**
 - Iodine level in salt at **production** level **30 ppm**
 - Iodine **oil injection** will **provide protection** for **4 years.**
 - Sensitive indicator for consumption of appropriate level of iodine is **urine level of iodine.**
 - Any area is said to be endemic to **IDD**, if prevalence of goiter is **>10%** among general population or **>5%** among school going children or median iodine excretion is **<100µg/l.**
 - RDA- **150 µ gram.**
 - **Most sensitive parameter in** monitoring **iodine deficiency control programme is – Neonatal hypothyroidism.**

7. **Which of the following is a killed vaccine? (Repeat)**
A. Japenese encephalitis
B. Measles
C. BCG
D. Yellow fever

Ans: A. Japenese encephalitis

Ref: *Park's Preventive and Social Medicine, 22nd edition. & Ananthanarayan, Paniker CJ. Textbook of Microbiology. 8th Edition. London: John Wiley & Sons; 2009. Pg. 88, 451*

Explanation:

Types of vaccines

Live attenuated vaccine	Killed vaccine	Subunit vaccine	Toxoid
Oral Polio Vaccine (Sabin)	Injectable Polio Vaccine (Salk)	Hepatitis B vaccine (HbSAg)	Tetanus toxoid
Yellow Fever	Rabies	Typhim-Vi (Typhoid Vi antigen)	Diphtheria toxoid
Varicella	Japanese encephalitis		
Measles	Cholera		
Mumps			
Rubella			
BCG			
Typhoral (mutant S. typhi strain Ty2 1a)			

8. **Most common cause of death in the under five age group in developing countries is:**
A. Malnutrition
B. Respiratory diseases
C. Diarrhea
D. Road traffic accidents

Ans: A. Respiratory diseases

Ref: *Park's Preventive and Social Medicine, 22nd edition. Million Death Study Collaborators, Bassani DG et al. Causes of neonatal and child mortality in India: a nationally representative mortality survey. Lancet. 2010 Nov 27;376(9755):1853-60.*

Explanation:

Indian Data (Ref: Lancet Article)

Top 2 causes of Under-5 mortality (Accounts for >78% of total Under-5 deaths).
1. Pneumonia
2. Diarrhoeal diseases

Top 3 causes of neontal mortality (Accounts for >78% of total neonatal deaths)
1. Prematurity and low birthweight
2. Neonatal infections
3. Birth asphyxia and birth trauma

9. **Which respiratory illness is more common in a paper mill worker?**
A. Anthracosis **B.** Byssinosis
C. Bagassosis **D.** Asbestosis

Ans: C. Bagassosis

Ref: *Park's Preventive and Social Medicine, 22nd edition*

Explanation:

*"**Byssinosis**, also called "**brown lung disease**" or "**Monday fever**", is an occupational lung disease caused by exposure to **cotton dust** in inadequately ventilated working environments"*

Pneumoconiosis

- It is a group of occupational lung disease and a restrictive lung disease caused by the inhalation of various particles specific to workplace
- It is classified depending upon the **type of dust**
  - **Coalworker's pneumoconiosis** (Miner's lung, black lung or anthracosis)-Coal, Carbon
  - **Asbestosis** - Asbestos
  - **Silicosis** ("grinder's disease" or Potter's rot) - Silica
  - **Bauxite fibrosis** - Bauxite
  - **Berylliosis** - Beryllium
  - **Siderosis** - Iron
  - **Byssinosis** - Cotton
  - **Silicosiderosis** - Mixed dust containing silica and iron
  - **Labrador lung** (found in miners in Labrador, Canada) - Mixed dust containing Iron, Silica and Anthophyllite, a type of asbestos

10. **RNTCP target level:**
A. 70 % detection 85 % cure
B. 70 % detection 85 % cure
C. 80 % detection 75 % cure
D. 80 % detection 75 % cure

Ans: A. 70 % detection 85 % cure

Ref: *Park's Preventive and Social Medicine, 22nd edition. & http://www.health.mp.gov.in/tb.htm (RNTCP document) 2012 revised*

Explanation:

The goal of RNTCP is to cure ***at least 85% of new smear-positive cases*** *of tuberculosis and to* ***detect at least 70% of such patients****, after the desired cure rate has been achieved.*

11. The number of live births/no of females 15-45 in the population denotes: (Repeat)

A. General fertility rate
B. Total fertility rate
C. Gross reproduction rate
D. Age specific fertility rate

Ans: A. General fertility rate

Ref: *Park's Preventive and Social Medicine, 22nd edition. & http://censusindia.gov.in/vital_statistics/Vital_Rates/Vital_rates.aspx*

Explanation:

General fertility rate (GFR):
The number of births in a year divided by the number of women aged 15–44, times 1000. It focuses on the potential mothers only, and takes the age distribution into account.

Gross reproduction rate (GRR)

- It is the average number of daughters that would be born to a woman (or a group of women) if she survived at least to the age of 45 and conformed to the age-specific fertility rate of a given year. It is often regarded as the extent to which the generation of daughters replaces the preceding generation of females.
- This rate is **similar** to the **net reproduction rate** but it ignores the fact that **some women** will **die before completing** their childbearing years
- The GRR is particularly relevant where **sex ratios** are significantly affected by the **use of reproductive technologies.**

Total fertility rate (TFR)

- Also called as fertility rate, period total fertility rate (PTFR) or total period fertility rate (TPFR) It is the average number of children that would be born to a woman over her lifetime if:
  - She were to experience the exact current age-specific fertility rates (ASFRs) through her lifetime.
  - She were to survive from birth through the end of her reproductive life.
- It is obtained by summing the single-year age-specific rates at a given time.

Net reproduction rate (NRR)

- It is defined as the number of *daughters* a woman would have in her lifetime if she were subject to prevailing age-specific fertility *and mortality* rates in the given year.
- When the NRR is exactly **one**, then each generation of women is exactly reproducing itself.
- NRR is particularly relevant where the number of male babies born is very high
- This is a significant factor in world population, due to the high level of gender imbalance in the very populous nations of China and India.
- The gross reproduction rate (GRR), is the same as the NRR, except that—like the TFR—it ignores life expectancy.

Latest Indian Data (Census 2011)

Crude birth rate	24.8
General Fertility rate	95.3
Total Fertility rate	3
Gross reproduction rate	1.4

ENT

1. Type of deafness seen in early stages of Meniere's disease:

A. Low frequency conductive hearing loss
B. Low frequency sensorineural hearing loss
C. High frequency conductive hearing loss
D. High frequency sensorineural hearing loss

Ans: B. Low frequency sensorineural hearing loss

Ref: *Diseases of the Ear Nose and Throat by PL Dhingra 5th edn .2010.Page 113*

Explanation:

- **Hearing loss in Meniere's disease** is **sensorineural type** and is **fluctuating.**
- It is associated with **episodic vertigo, tinnitus** and **sensation** of fullness of ear.
- **Early** Meniere's has **low frequency loss** and the **PTA** curve is **rising type.**
- **Later** on the **higher frequencies** are **affected** and the **PTA curve becomes flat** and finally it becomes **sloping type.**

2. Most common cause of acute otitis media in children:

A. E coli
B. H influenzae
C. Pneumococcus
D. Staph aureus

Ans : C. Pneumococcus

Ref: *Diseases of the Ear Nose and Throat by PL Dhingra 5th edn .2010.Page 69*

Explanation:

Most Common organisms ASOM in **infants and children** is

- ***Streptococcus pneumoniae*** – 30%
- ***Haemophilus influenzae*** – 20%
- ***Moraxella catarrahalis*** – 12%
- Other organisms are like ***Streptococcus pyogenes***, ***Staphylococcus aureus***

3. **Characteristic feature of TB otitis media: (Repeat)**
   A. Multiple perforations in TM
   B. Mastoiditis
   C. Middle ear effusion
   D. Ear discharge

Ans: A. Multiple perforations in TM

Ref: *Diseases of the Ear Nose and Throat by PL Dhingra 5th edn .2010.Page 83*

Explanation:

- **TB otitis media** is mostly **secondary** to **pulmonary TB.**
- More common in **children** and **young adults**
- Patients have **painless ear discharge** which may be **foul smelling** and **severe conductive hearing loss** which is out of proportion to symptoms.
- On examination **multiple perforations** are seen on the tympanic membrane, **pale granulation tissue** in the middle ear and there maybe **facial nerve palsy**
- Investigations include culture of the discharge, Histopathological examination of the granulation tissues and chest X-ray for ruling out pulmonary TB.
- Treatment is with Anti tubercular drugs.

4. **Most common site of fracture mandible:**
   A. Ramus
   B. Angle of mandible
   C. Neck of the condyle
   D. Coronoid process

Ans: C. Neck of the condyle

Ref: *Diseases of the Ear Nose and Throat by PL Dhingra .5th edn .2010.Page 199, Apley's System of Orthopedics and fractures, 9th ed & Anyanechi C E, Saheeb B D. Mandibular Sites Prone to Fracture: Analysis of 174 Cases in a Nigerian Tertiary Hospital. Ghana Med J. 2011 September; 45(3): 111–114.*

Explanation:

- Most common site of fracture mandible is the **Condyle > Angle & Body > Symphisis.**
- Fracture of the **ramus, coronoid** and **alveolar process** are rare.
- Clinical features are that of **pain** and **trismus.**
- On examination, there may be **deviation of the jaw** to the **opposite side, echymosis** of the oral mucosa , **malocclusion of teeth,** step deformity and crepitus.
- Investigations include X-rays left and right oblique view of the mandible, Orthopantomogram and PA view of the skull for the condyle.
- Treatment is with either open or closed reduction and fixation.

The most commonly fractured sites in Mandible are: *(Ref: Apley)*

- Body (29%)
- Condyle (26%)
- Angle (25%)
- Symphysis (17%)
- Ramus (4%)
- Coracoid (1%)

Other Locations of fracture in mandible

- Alveolar
- Coronoid
- Ramus
- Parasymphysis

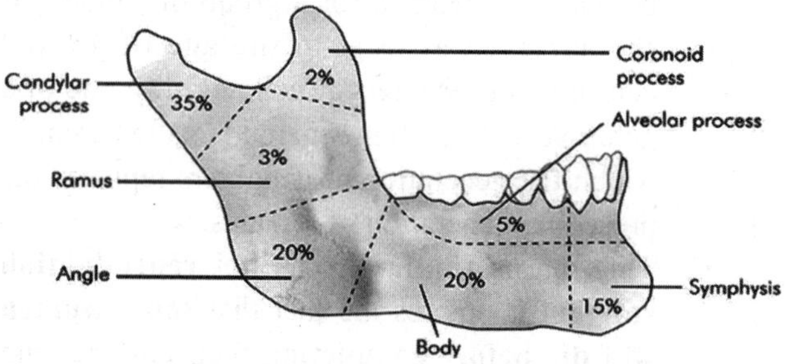

5. **Perilymph communicates with subarachnoid space through:**
   A. Ductus reunions
   B. Helicotrema
   C. Utriculosaccular duct
   D. Cochlear aqueduct

Ans: D. Cochlear aqueduct

Ref: *Diseases of the Ear Nose and Throat by PL Dhingra 5th edn .2010.Page 12*

Explanation:

- **Perilymph**
  - Composition is like extracellular fluid
  - Lies between the bony and membranous labyrinth
  - Rich in Na+ ions

- **Endolymph**
  - Fills the membranous labyrinth.
  - It is rich in K^+ ions.
  - Composition is like intracellular fluid.
  - Secreted by the **stria vascularis** of the crista and dark cells which are seen in the utricle and the ampullary ends of the semi circular canals.

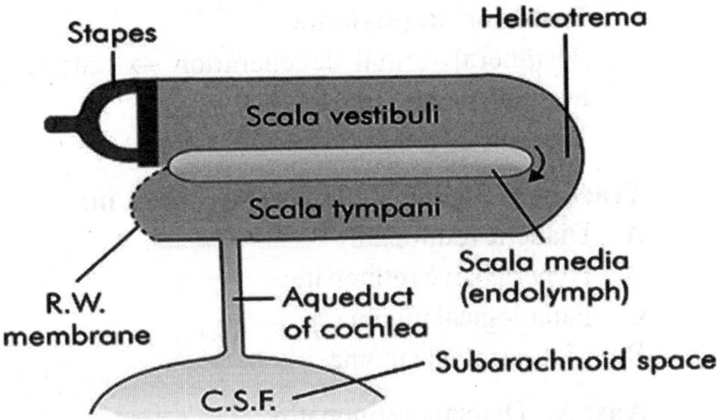

6. **Level of tracheostomy is by which of the following anatomical landmark? (Repeat)**
   A. Cricoid cartilage
   B. Isthmus of thyroid
   C. 2nd tracheal ring
   D. 3rd tracheal ring

   Ans: B. Isthmus of the thyroid

Ref: *Diseases of the Ear Nose and Throat by PL Dhingra 5th edn .2010.Page 337*

Explanation:

Types of tracheostomy based on position

- **High tracheostomy** – Above the thyroid isthmus through the first tracheal ring
  - Increased risk of sub glottic edema and stenosis
- **Mid tracheostomy** - At the level of thyroid isthmus, through the 2nd or 3rd tracheal ring
  - Isthmus is divided or retracted
  - Most commonly done
- **Low tracheostomy** – Below the isthmus
  - Increased risk of injury to great vessels in the neck

7. **Depolarization of cochlea due to:**
   A. Potassium influx
   B. Potassium efflux
   C. Sodium influx
   D. Sodium efflux

   Ans: A. Potassium influx

Ref: *Diseases of the Ear Nose and Throat by PL Dhingra 5th edn.2010.Page13 and 19*

Explanation:

- There exists a potential **difference approx (125mv)** between the **K^+ rich endolymph (+80mv)** and the **inner hair cells (-45mv).**
- When the **ion channels** of the hair cells open, K^+ is driven **into the hair cells** because of this potential difference and causes depolarization.
- This mechanism helps covert the mechanical energy of sound into electrical impulses.
- This gradient and energy for transduction is provided by the **Na^+/K^+ ATPase pump** in the **stria vascularis.**

OPHTHALMOLOGY

1. **The changes seen in accommodation during near reflex are all *except:***
   A. Increase in curvature of lens
   B. Contraction of ciliary muscle
   C. Convergence of visual axis
   D. Dilatation of the pupil

   Ans: D. Dilatation of the pupil

Ref: *Kanski Clinical Ophthalmology 6th edition pg no: 803; Parson's Diseases of the eye 22nd edition pg no 58.*

Explanation:

Near reflex is a **synkinesis** which is activated when the gaze is changed from a distant to a near target.

- It comprises
  - Accommodation
  - Convergence
  - Miosis
- During accommodation, the circular ciliary muscle contracts→the zonules relax → the capsule is relieved of tension àthe curvature of the anterior lens capsule increases → the converging effect of the lens is increased → the near object is focused on the retina. The radius of curvature of the anterior lens capsule is decreased from 10 to 6 mm.

Near reflex pathway:

- Impulses from the medial recti muscles while converging → third cranial nerve → mesencephalic nucleus of the trigeminal nerve → presumptive convergence centre in the pretectal or tectal region → **Edinger Westphal nucleus** a → Third nerve → spincter muscle of the iris.

2. **Most common malignant intraorbital tumor in childhood:**
   A. Malignant melanoma
   B. Retinoblastoma

C. Rhabdomyosarcoma
D. Neuroblastoma

Ans: C. Rhabdomyosarcoma

Ref: *Kanski Clinical Ophthalmology 6th edition pg no:200-201*

Explanation:

"The most common primary orbital malignancy of childhood is rhabdomyosarcoma (embryonal sarcoma)"

RHABDOMYOSARCOMA

- Derived from the undifferentiated **mesenchymal** cell rests which have the potential to differentiate into the **striated muscle.**
- HISTOLOGY: **Tadpole** or **TENNIS –RACKET rhabdomyoblasts.**
- The most common **secondary intraorbital tumour** is **neuroblastoma.**
- The most common **intraocular tumour** is **retinoblastoma.**

3. **False about pathological myopia is:**
A. Vitreous opacities
B. Retinal degenaration
C. Myopic crescents
D. Shallow ant chamber

Ans: D. Shallow anterior chamber

Ref: *Parson's Diseases of the Eye 22nd edition pg no 73; Kanski Clinical Ophthalmology 6th edition pg no 654 -655*

Explanation:

Pathological myopia:

- **Refractive error > -6 D** or the **axial length of the globe > 26 mm.**
- Hereditary
- **Females** are more commonly involved.
- Starts at the age of **5 years** & continues to increase till **25 years** of age.
- Pathogenesis: Disturbance of growth + degeneration of the of the coats of the eye (mainly the posterior half of the globe) → progressive & excessive anteroposterior elongation of the globe

Ocular features:

- Prominent eyes
- Pupil dilated
- Anterior chamber deep
- **Myopic chorioretinal degeneration** usually starts in the 5th decade.
  - **Pale large disc** with temporal crescent
  - **Supertraction crescent** on the nasal side of the disc
  - **Choroidal degeneration** in the central fundus
  - **Foster Fuch's spot** in the fovea due to choroidal thrombosis
  - **Lacquer cracks** – linear breaks in the **Bruch's membrane**
  - **Posterior staphyloma**
  - Peripheral retinal degeneration → Lattice & cystoids degenerations
  - Vitreous degeneration → Floaters

4. **Tractional retinal detachment is seen in:**
A. Diabetic retinopathy
B. Hypertensive retinopathy
C. Pathological myopia
D. Malignant melanoma

Ans: A. Diabetic retinopathy

Ref: *Parson's Diseases of the Eye 22nd edition pg no 323; Kanski Clinical Ophthalmology 6th edition pg no 654 - 655; Basak Diseases of the Eye 5th edition, pg no 324*

Explanation:

RETINAL DETACHMENT (RD)

- The separation of the neurosensory retina from the pigment epithelium.
- Embryologically, the neurosensory retina develops from the inner layer of the optic vesicle and the pigmented epithelium develops from the outer layer.
- There is a potential space called **subretinal space** in between them.

Classification of RD

- Rhegmatogenous – Rhegma means break.
- Non rhegmatogenous – Tractional & exudative

Tractional RD

- The sensory retina is pulled from the RPE by the vitreo retinal traction membranes

Symptoms

- Slow & progressive loss of field.
- No H/O floaters or flashes of light.

Signs

- RD configuration is concave.
- The highest elevation of retina occurs at the site vitreorteinal traction.
- Mobility of the detached retina is severely reduced.

Causes

- Retinopathy of prematurity
- Diabetic retinopathy
- Eales disease
- CRVO
- Persistent hyperplastic primary vitreous
- Plastic cyclitis
- Parsplanitis
- PENETRATING INJURY

5. **Topical glucocorticoids in eyes causes:**
   A. Glaucoma
   B. Optic atrophy
   C. Retinal detachment
   D. Corneal ulcer

Ans: A. Glaucoma

Ref: *Parson's Diseases of the Eye Pg:358; Basak Diseases of the Eye 5th edition, pg no 50*

Explanation:

STEROIDS

- Systemic and topical steroids – causes, **Posterior subcapsular cataract**
- Topical steroids – causes, **Open angle glaucoma**
- There is **no safe dosage**
- Who is **Steroid responder**?
  After 6 weeks of topical steroids, if the IOP
  - >30mmHg – high responders
  - 22-30mmHg – moderate responders
  - No change - non responders
- Strong steroids [dexamethasone, betamethasone, prednisolone] →more potent in increasing the IOP
  - **Fluoromethalone →** lesser propensity to increase IOP
  - **Difluprednate →** strong steroid but least potent to increase IOP

Other Local Side Effects:

- Increased risk of super infection
- Delayed wound healing
- Corneal melting

Indications of steroids in eye:

- ***Sterile ocular inflammation***
  - Disciform keratitis
  - Episcleritis
  - Scleritis
  - Uveitis
  - Optic neuritis
- *Allergic problems*
  - Phlycten
  - Vernal catarrah
  - Allergic blepharo conjunctivitis
- ***Post operative***
  - Following cataract surgery
  - Keratoplasty
  - Vitrectomy
  - Trabeculectomy

6. **The characteristic feature of diabetic papillopathy:**
   A. Bulging optic disc with telengiectatic vessels
   B. Multiple hemorrhagic spots
   C. Optic disc pallor
   D. Cupping of optic disc

Ans: A. Bulging optic disc with telengiectatic vessels

Ref: *Kanski Clinical Ophthalmology 6th edition pg no 796*

Explanation:

DIABETIC PAPILLOPATHY

- ***Transient visual dysfunction*** associated with optic disc swelling.
- Pathogenesis: Unclear; may be due to small vessel disease.
- Signs:
  - Defective vision **6/12**.
  - Unilateral or bilateral **disc swelling & hyperemia.**
  - Disc surface **telangiectasia.**

MEDICINE

1. **All are features of rabies encephalitis *except:***
   A. Tonic spasm of the body
   B. Hypersalivation
   C. Sound Phobia
   D. Hypotonic paralysis

Ans: C. Sound Phobia

Ref: *Harrison's Principles of Internal Medicine, 18th ed.*

Explanation:

Rabies Encephalitis

- Two acute neurologic forms of rabies are seen in humans:
  - **Encephalitic** (furious) in 80%
  - **Paralytic** in 20%.
- The Common features include **fever, confusion, hallucinations, combativeness,** and **seizures.**
- **Autonomic dysfunction** is common and may result in **hypersalivation, gooseflesh, cardiac arrhythmia,** and **priapism.**

Encephalitic rabies

- Episodes of **hyperexcitability** are typically followed by periods of **complete lucidity** that become **shorter** as the disease progresses.
- Rabies encephalitis is distinguished by **early brainstem involvement**, which results in the classic features of **hydrophobia** (involuntary, painful contraction of the diaphragm and accessory respiratory, laryngeal, and pharyngeal muscles in response to swallowing liquids) and **aerophobia** (the same features caused by stimulation from a draft of air).
- These symptoms are probably due to **dysfunction of infected brainstem neurons** that normally inhibit inspiratory neurons near the **nucleus ambiguus**, resulting in **exaggerated defense reflexes** that protect the respiratory tract.
- The combination of **hypersalivation** and **pharyngeal dysfunction** is also responsible for the classic appearance of "**foaming at the mouth**"
- Brainstem dysfunction progresses rapidly, and **coma** followed within days by **death** is the rule unless the course is prolonged by supportive measures.
- With such measures, late complications can include **cardiac and/or respiratory** failure, disturbances of **water balance (SIADHor diabetes insipidus)**, **noncardiogenic pulmonary edema (ARDS)**, and **gastrointestinal hemorrhage**.
- **Cardiac arrhythmias** may be due to dysfunction affecting vital centers in the brainstem or to myocarditis.
- **Multiple-organ failure** is common in patients treated aggressively in critical care units.

Paralytic Rabies

- About **20%** of patients have **paralytic rabies** in which muscle **weakness** predominates
- Cardinal features of encephalitic rabies (hyperexcitability, hydrophobia, and aerophobia) are lacking.
- There is early and prominent **flaccid muscle weakness**, often beginning in the **bitten extremity** and spreading to produce **quadriparesis** and **facial weakness**.
- **Sphincter involvement** is common, **sensory involvement** is usually **mild**, and these cases are commonly **misdiagnosed as Guillain-Barré syndrome.**
- Patients with paralytic rabies generally **survive a few days longer** than those with encephalitic rabies, but **multiple-organ failure** nevertheless ensues.

2. Oochronosis occurs in: (Repeat)

A. Alkaptonuria **B.** Isovaleric aciduria
C. Phenyl ketonuria **D.** Tyrosinemia

Ans: A. Alkaptonuria

Ref: *Harrison's Principles of Internal Medicine, 18th ed.*

Explanation:

Alkaptonuria

- Autosomal Recessive
- Due to **deficiency** of ***homogentisic acid oxidase***
- **Clinical features**
  - Oochronosis
  - Arthritis
  - Cardiac valve involvement
  - Coronary artery calcification
  - Pigmented heart valves, sclera, joint, skin & renal calculi
  - Urine darkens on standing
- **Nitisinone** used to reduce urinary excretion of homogentisic acid

3. Which of the following is not seen in Non-ketotic hyperosmolar coma?

A. Insidious onset
B. Kussmaul's breathing
C. Seen in elderly
D. Seen in type 2 DM

Ans: B. Kussmaul's breathing

Ref: *Harrison's Principles of Internal Medicine, 18th & Nelson Textbook of Pediatrics, 19th ed.*

Explanation:

"Notably absent are symptoms of nausea, vomiting, and abdominal pain and the Kussmaul respirations characteristic of DKA." Ref: Harrison

Nonketotic Hyperosmolar Coma

- Aka **Hyperglycemic Hyperosmolar State**
- This syndrome is characterized by
  - Severe hyperglycemia (blood glucose >800 mg/dL)
  - Absence of or only slight ketosis
  - Nonketotic acidosis
  - Severe dehydration
  - Depressed sensorium or frank coma
  - Neurologic signs that may include grand mal seizures, hyperthermia, hemiparesis, and positive Babinski signs.

Clinical Features

- Classically, elderly **individual** with **type 2 DM**, with a **several-week history** of **polyuria, weight loss**, and **diminished oral intake** that culminates in **mental confusion, lethargy**, or **coma**.
- The physical examination reflects **profound dehydration** and **hyperosmolality** and **reveals hypotension, tachycardia**, and **altered mental status**.
- **Nausea, vomiting, abdominal pain** and **Kussmaul respirations** (characteristic of DKA) are **ABSENT**
- Precipitated by a serious, concurrent illness such as **myocardial infarction, stroke** or **Sepsis**.

Pathophysiology

- **Relative insulin deficiency** and **inadequate fluid intake** are the underlying causes of HHS.
- Insulin deficiency **increases hepatic glucose production** (through **glycogenolysis** and **gluconeogenesis**) and impairs glucose utilization in skeletal muscle.
- **Hyperglycemia** induces an **osmotic diuresis** that leads to **intravascular volume depletion**, which is exacerbated by **inadequate fluid replacement**.
- The **absence of ketosis** in HHS is **not well understood**.
- Presumably, the **insulin deficiency** is only **relative** and **less severe** than in **DKA**.
- **Lower levels of counterregulatory** hormones and free fatty acids have been found in HHS than in DKA.
- Liver is less capable of ketone body synthesis or that the insulin/glucagon ratio does not favor ketogenesis.

Laboratory Abnormalities and Diagnosis

- Most notable are the:
  - **Marked hyperglycemia** [plasma glucose may be >55.5 mmol/L (1000 mg/dL)],
  - **Hyperosmolality** (>350 mosmol/L), and
  - **Prerenal azotemia**.
- The measured serum sodium may be normal or slightly low despite the marked hyperglycemia.
- The corrected serum sodium is usually increased [add 1.6 meq to measured sodium for each 5.6-mmol/L (100 mg/dL) rise in the serum glucose].
- In contrast to DKA, acidosis and ketonemia are absent or mild.
- A small anion-gap metabolic acidosis may be present secondary to increased lactic acid.
- Moderate ketonuria, if present, is secondary to starvation.

Treatment:

- Volume depletion and hyperglycemia are prominent features of both HHS and DKA.
- In both disorders, careful monitoring of the patient's fluid status, laboratory values, and insulin infusion rate is crucial.
- Underlying or precipitating problems should be aggressively sought and treated.
- In HHS, **fluid losses** and **dehydration** are usually more pronounced than in DKA
- The patient with HHS is usually **older**, more likely to have **mental status changes**, and more likely to have a **life-threatening precipitating event** with accompanying comorbidities.
- Even with proper treatment, HHS has a substantially **higher mortality rate** than DKA (up to **15%**).
- Fluid replacement should initially stabilize the hemodynamic status of the patient (1–3 L of 0.9% normal saline over the first 2–3 h).
- Because the fluid deficit in HHS is accumulated over a period of days to weeks, the **rapidity of reversal** of the hyperosmolar state must **balance** the **need for free water repletion** with the risk that too rapid a reversal may worsen neurologic function.
- If the serum sodium > 150 mmol/L (150 meq/L), 0.45% saline should be used.
- After hemodynamic stability is achieved, the IV fluid administration is directed at reversing the free water deficit using hypotonic fluids (0.45% saline initially, then 5% dextrose in water, D5W). The calculated free water deficit (which averages 9–10 L) should be reversed over the next 1–2 days (infusion rates of 200–300 mL/h of hypotonic solution).
- **Hypophosphatemia** may occur during therapy and can be improved by using KPO4 and beginning nutrition.
- A reasonable regimen for HHS begins with an **IV insulin bolus** of 0.1 units/kg followed by IV insulin at a constant **infusion** rate of 0.1 units/kg per hour.
- The insulin infusion should be continued until the patient has resumed eating and can be transferred to a **SC insulin regimen.**

4. **A 30 year old female presents with amenorrhea, galactorrhea and bitemporal heminanopia. What is the most probable diagnosis?**

A. Pituitary macroadenoma
B. Craniopharygioma
C. Meningioma
D. Pinealoma

Ans: A. Pituitary Macroadenoma

Ref: *Harrison's Principles of Internal Medicine, 18th ed.*

Explanation:

*"More symmetric compression of the optic chiasm by a **pituitary adenoma**, **meningioma**, **craniopharyngioma**, **glioma**, or aneurysm results in a **bitemporal hemianopia**" Ref: Harrison*

Pituitary adenomas

- They are the most common cause of pituitary hormone hypersecretion and hyposecretion syndromes in adults.
- They account for >15% of all intracranial neoplasms.
- At autopsy, up to 25% of all pituitary glands harbor an unsuspected **microadenoma (<10 mm** diameter). *(See Table 15)*

PROLACTINOMAS (Pitiuitary adenoma involving Lactotroph)

- Most common type of hyperfunctioning pituitary adenoma (Accounts for 30% of all cases)
- These lesions range from **small microadenomas** to **large, expansile tumors** associated with substantial mass effect. Microscopically, **weakly acidophilic** or **chromophobic** cells are present ***(sparsely granulated prolactinoma)***;
- **Rarely** prolactinomas are strongly **acidophilic** ***(densely granulated prolactinoma).***
- Prolactin can be demonstrated within the cytoplasmic secretory granules by immunohistochemical stains.
- Can undergo **dystrophic calcification**, ranging from isolated **psammoma bodies** to extensive calcification of virtually the entire tumor mass ("**pituitary stone**").
- **Increased Prolactin secretion** (even microadenomas secrete sufficient prolactin to cause hyperprolactinemia).
- **Prolactinemia**, cause **amenorrhea**, **galactorrhea**, **loss of libido**, and **infertility**.
- The diagnosis of an adenoma is made more readily in women than in men, especially between the ages of **20 and 40 years**, presumably because of the sensitivity of menses to disruption by **hyperprolactinemia.**
- **Prolactinoma** underlies almost a **quarter of cases** of **amenorrhea.**
- In contrast, in men and older women, the hormonal manifestations may be subtle, allowing the tumors to reach considerable size (**macroadenomas**) before being detected clinically.

Meningiomas

- They are found **incidentally** following **neuroimaging** for unrelated reasons.
- They can also present with **headaches, seizures,** or **focal neurologic deficits.**
- On imaging studies, appear as a **partially calcified**, densely enhancing **extraaxial tumor** arising from the **dura**
- Occasionally they may have a **dural tail**, consisting of **thickened**, enhanced **dura** extending like a **tail** from the **mass.**

Table 15 : Classification of Pituitary Adenomas

Pituitary Cell Type	Hormone	Tumor Type	Associated Syndrome[*]
Corticotroph	ACTH and other POMC-derived peptides	ACTH cell (corticotroph) adenoma	Cushing syndrome Nelson syndrome
Somatotroph	GH	GH cell (somatotroph) adenoma	Gigantism (children) Acromegaly (adults)
Lactotroph	Prolactin	Prolactin cell (lactotroph) adenoma	Galactorrhea and amenorrhea (in females) Sexual dysfunction, infertility
Mammosomatotroph	Prolactin, GH	Mammosomatotroph	Combined features of GH and prolactin excess
Thyrotroph	TSH	TSH cell (thyrotroph) adenoma	Hyperthyroidism
Gonadotroph	FSH, LH	Gonadotroph, "null cell," oncocytic adenomas	Hypogonadism, mass effects, and hypopituitarism

Craniopharyngiomas

- Craniopharyngiomas are **rare**, usually **suprasellar**, partially **calcified**, solid, or mixed solid-cystic benign tumors that arise from **remnants of Rathke's pouch**.
- They have a **bimodal** distribution, occurring predominantly in **children** but also between the **ages of 55 and 65 years.**
- They present with **headaches**, **visual impairment**, and **impaired growth** in children and **hypopituitarism** in **adults**. Treatment involves **surgery**, **radiotherapy**, or the combination of the two.

5. Dorsal column lesions are associated with loss of:

A. Ankle jerk
B. Knee jerk
C. Proprioception
D. Superficial abdominal reflexes

Ans: C. Proprioception

Ref: *Harrison's Principles of Internal Medicine, 18th ed.*

Explanation:

The posterior column (dorsal column)

- It refers to the area of white matter in the dorsomedial side of the spinal cord.
- It is made up of the **fasciculus gracilis** and **fasciculus cuneatus**
- It is part of an **ascending pathway** that is important for **well-localized fine touch** and conscious **proprioception** called the **posterior column-medial lemniscus** pathway.
- **Joint capsules, tactile** and **pressure receptors** send a signal through the **dorsal root ganglia** up through the **fasciculus gracilis** for **lower body** sensory impulses and the **fasciculus cuneatus** for **upper body impulses.**
- Once the fasciculus gracilis reaches the nucleus gracilis and the fasciculus cuneatus reaches the nucleus cuneatus in the **lower** medulla, they begin to **cross over** the medulla as the **internal arcuate** fibers.
- When they reach the **contralateral side**, they become the **medial lemniscus**, which is the **second part** of the **posterior column-medial lemniscus** pathway.
- Lesions in this pathway can diminish or completely abolish **tactile sensations** and **movement** or **position sense** below the lesion.

Tests of sensation

Modality	Pathway
Light touch	Large fast-conducting axons Dorsal columns Medial lemniscus
Proprioception	
Vibration	
Two-point discrimination	
Pinprick (superficial pain)	Smaller slower-conducting axons Spinothalamic tracts
Deep pain	
Temperature	
Stereognosis	Parietal cortex (only valid if peripheral sensory function intact)
Graphaesthesia	
Two-point discrimination	

6. Decreased erythropoietin levels are seen in:

A. End stage renal disease
B. Heart failure
C. Polycytic kidney disease
D. Advanced Liver failure

Ans: A. End stage renal disease

Ref: *Harrison's Principles of Internal Medicine, 18th ed.*

Explanation:

End-stage renal disease is replaced by the term ***stage 5 CKD*** (Chronic kidney disease).

*"The primary cause in patients with **CKD** is insufficient production of erythropoietin (EPO) by the diseased kidneys" Ref: Harrison.*

Causes of Anemia in CKD

- Relative deficiency of erythropoietin
- Diminished red blood cell survival
- Bleeding diathesis
- Iron deficiency
- Hyperparathyroidism/bone marrow fibrosis
- Chronic inflammation
- Folate or vitamin B12 deficiency
- Hemoglobinopathy
- Comorbid disease

7. Not a complication of major blood transfusion : (Repeat)

A. Hypercalemia **B.** Hyperkalemia
C. Volume overload **D.** Hypocalcemia

Ans: A. Hypercalcemia

Ref: *Harrison's Principles of Internal Medicine, 18th ed.*

Explanation:

Complications of Blood Transfusion

Early

- Haemolytic reactions

- Immediate
- Delayed

- Non-haemolytic febrile reactions
- Allergic reactions to proteins, IgA
- Transfusion-related acute lung injury
- Reactions secondary to bacterial contamination
- Circulatory overload (Volume overload)
- Air embolism
- Thrombophlebitis
- ***Hyperkalaemia***
- Citrate toxicity
- ***Hypocalcemia***
- Hypothermia
- Clotting abnormalities (after massive transfusion)

Late

- Transmission of infection
  - **Viral (hepatitis A, B, C, HIV, CMV)**
  - **Bacterial (Treponeum pallidum, Salmonella)**
  - **Parasites (malaria, toxoplasma)**
- Graft-vs-host disease
- Iron overload (after chronic transfusions)
- Immune sensitization (Rhesus D antigen)
  - RBC leakage during storage increases the concentration of potassium in the unit. Neonates and patients in renal failure are at risk for ***hyperkalemia***.
  - Preventive measures, such as using fresh or washed RBCs, are warranted for neonatal transfusions because this complication can be fatal.
  - Citrate, commonly used to anticoagulate blood components, chelates calcium and thereby inhibits the coagulation cascade.
  - ***Hypocalcemia***, manifested by circumoral numbness and tingling sensation of the fingers and toes, may result from multiple rapid transfusions.
  - Because citrate is quickly metabolized to bicarbonate, calcium infusion is seldom required in this setting.

8. **Episodic hypertension is characteristic of:**

A. Carcinoid tumor
B. Insulinoma
C. Pheochromocytoma
D. Zollinger Ellison syndrome

Ans: C. Pheochromocytoma

Ref: *Harrison's Principles of Internal Medicine, 18th ed.*

Explanation:

"Classically, ***pheochromocytoma*** *patients have* ***episodic hypertension****, but sustained hypertension is also common" Ref: Harrison.*

Other three options do not cause hypertension commonly.

PHEOCHROMOCYTOMA

Pheochromocytomas are neoplasms composed of **chromaffin** cells, which synthesize and release **catecholamines** and in some instances **peptide** hormones.

Traditionally, pheochromocytomas have been associated with a **"rule of 10s"**.

- 10% of pheochromocytomas are **extra-adrenal**, occurring in sites such as the organs of **Zuckerkandl** and the **carotid** body. Pheochromocytomas that develop in extra-adrenal **paraganglia** are designated **paragangliomas.**
- 10% of sporadic adrenal pheochromocytomas are **bilateral**; this figure may rise to as high as **50%** in cases that are associated with **familial** syndromes
- 10% of adrenal pheochromocytomas are biologically **malignant**, defined by the presence of metastatic disease.
- 10% of adrenal pheochromocytomas are **not associated with hypertension**. Of the 90% that present with hypertension, approximately two thirds have **"paroxysmal" episodes** associated with sudden rise in blood pressure and palpitations.

Familial conditions assc with Pheochromocytoma

- Multiple endocrine neoplasia, type 2A (MEN-2a)
- Multiple endocrine neoplasia, type 2B (MEN-2b)
- Neurofibromatosis, type 1 (NF1)
- Von Hippel-Lindau (VHL)
- Familial paraganglioma 1, 2, 3 & 4
  - The tumors are composed of **polygonal to spindle-shaped chromaffin cells** or **chief cells**, clustered with the **sustentacular cells** into **small nests or alveoli** (**zellballen pattern**) by a rich vascular network.

9. **Not true regarding POEMS syndrome: (Repeat)**

A. Osteolytic lesions
B. Hypertrichosis
C. Papilledema
D. Amenorrhea

Ans: A. Osteolytic lesions

Ref: *Harrison's 18th edn, pg 3080*

Explanation:

POEMS syndrome

- ***P**olyneuropathy*, ***o**rganomegaly*, ***e**ndocrinopathy*, ***m**ultiple myeloma*, and ***s**kin changes*.
- It is associated with **osteosclerotic myeloma, Waldenstorm's macroglobulinemia, MGUS** but not the classical osteolytic multiple myeloma
- Elevations in **IL-1α, IL-6, TNF-β & VGEF** implicated
- **Polyneuropathy:** Sensory & motor deficits characterised by distal, symmetrical weakness spreading proximally
- Hepatomegaly and lymphadenopathy occur in about two-thirds of patients, and splenomegaly is seen in one-third.
- **Endocrine**:
  - ***Amenorrhea*** in women
  - **Impotence** and gynecomastia in men
  - Hyperprolactinemia
  - Papilledema
  - Type 2 diabetes mellitus
  - Hypothyroidism
  - Adrenal insufficiency
- **Skin changes:**
  - ***Hyperpigmentation***
  - ***Hypertrichosis***
  - Skin ***thickening***
  - ***Digital clubbing***
- **Others**
  - Peripheral edema
  - Ascites
  - Pleural effusions
  - Fever
  - Thrombocytosis.
- Not all the components of POEMS syndrome may be present initially.
- Treatment: Like myeloma. **Plasmapheresis does not appear** to be of benefit in POEMS syndrome.

10. Hypercalcemia is caused by all *except:*

A. Hyperparathyroidism
B. Thyrotoxicosis
C. Phenytoin
D. Lytic skeletal metastasis

Ans: C. Phenytoin

Ref: *Harrison's Principles of Internal Medicine, 18th ed.*

Explanation:

Phenytoin causes hypocalcemia

"Mild hypercalcemia occurs in up to 20% of thyrotoxicosis patients, but hypercalciuria is more common" Ref: Harrison.

Causes of Hypercalcemia

I. Parathyroid-related

- Primary hyperparathyroidism Adenoma(s) Multiple endocrine neoplasia Carcinoma
- Lithium therapy
- Familial hypocalciuric hypercalcemia

II. Malignancy-related

- Solid tumor with metastases (breast)
- Solid tumor with humoral mediation of hypercalcemia (lung, kidney)
- Hematologic malignancies (multiple myeloma, lymphoma, leukemia)

III. Vitamin D—related

- Vitamin D intoxication
- 1,25 (OH)2D; sarcoidosis and other granulomatous diseases
- Idiopathic hypercalcemia of infancy

IV. Associated with high bone turnover

- Hyperthyroidism
- Immobilization
- Thiazides
- Vitamin A intoxication

V. Associated with renal failure

- Severe secondary hyperparathyroidism
- Aluminum intoxication
- Milk-alkali syndrome

11. Wernicke hemianopic pupil is seen in lesion of

A. Optic radiation
B. Optic tract
C. Optic chiasma
D. Afferent tract

Ans: B. Optic tract

Ref: *Harrison's Principles of Internal Medicine, 18th ed.*

Explanation:

Wernicke's Hemianopic Pupil

- It indicates that the lesion is in **optic tract.**
- Here, the light reflex is absent when light is thrown on the temporal half of the retina of the affected side and nasal half of the retina of the opposite side.
- Light reflex is present when the light is thrown on the nasal half of the affected side and temporal half of the opposite side.
- The patient also has **homonymous hemianopia** as the lesion is in **optic tract.**

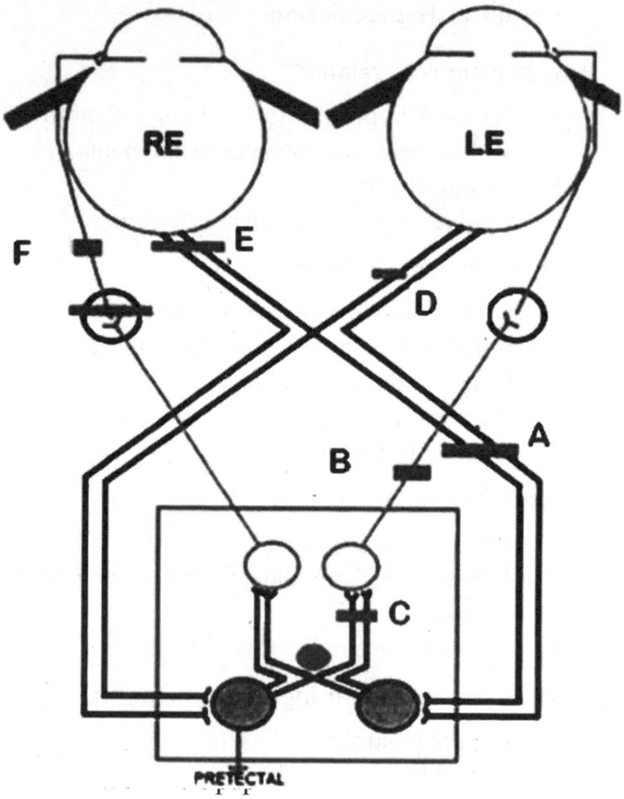

B- Pseudo Argyll Robertson Pupil
C- Argyll Robertson Pupil
D- **Marcus** Gunn Pupil
E- Amaurotic pupil
F- Adie's Pupil

12. **Not seen in hypervitaminosis A:**
    A. Alopecia
    B. Polyuria
    C. Pseudotumor cerebri
    D. Hyperlipidemia

Ans: B. Polyuria

Ref: *Harrison's Principles of Internal Medicine, 18th ed.*

Explanation:

- **Polyuria** is characteristically seen in chronic **Hypervitaminosis D**
- Seen in **normal adults** who ingest **15 mg/d** and **children** who ingest **6 mg/d** of vitamin A over a period of **several months.**

Effects of Hypervitaminosis A

- Angular cheilitis
- Glossitis
- Vomiting
- Bone demineralization
- Pain
- Hypercalcemia
- Lymph node enlargement
- **Hyperlipidemia**
- Amenorrhea
- **Pseudotumor cerebri** with increased intracranial pressure and papilledema.
- Liver fibrosis with portal hypertension Coarse bone growths
- Excessive skin dryness/peeling (desquamation)
- **Alopecia**
- Intracranial hypertension
- Liver problems
- Premature epiphyseal closure
- Reduced bone mineral density that may result in osteoporosis
- Skin discoloration

Note: When vitamin A is provided in excess to **pregnant women, congenital malformations (teratogenic effect)** have included **spontaneous abortions, craniofacial abnormalities,** and **valvular heart disease.**

13. **ECG change seen in hypocalcemia: (Repeat 2011)**
    A. QT prolongation
    B. Prolonged PR interval
    C. Shortened PR interval
    D. QT Shortening

Ans: A. QT prolongation

Ref: *Harrison's Principles of Internal Medicine, 18ed.*

Explanation:

Clinical Manifestations of Hypocalcemia

- Patients with hypocalcemia may be **asymptomatic** if the decreases in serum calcium are relatively mild and chronic.
- Moderate to severe hypocalcemia is associated with **paresthesias**, usually of the **fingers, toes,** and **circumoral** regions due to **increased neuromuscular irritability.**
- **Chvostek's sign** (twitching of the circumoral muscles in response to gentle tapping of the facial nerve just anterior to the ear) may be elicited.
- **Carpal spasm** may be induced by inflation of a blood pressure cuff to 20 mmHg above the patient's systolic blood pressure for 3 min (**Trousseau's sign**).
- Severe hypocalcemia can induce **seizures, carpopedal** spasm, **bronchospasm, laryngospasm,** and
- **ECG: Prolongation of the QT interval.**

Clinical Manifestations of Hypercalcemia

Mild hypercalcemia (up to 11–11.5 mg/dL)

- It is usually asymptomatic
- Recognized only on routine calcium measurements.
- Vague **neuropsychiatric** symptoms, like trouble concentrating, personality changes, or depression
- Assc with **peptic ulcer disease** or **nephrolithiasis**, and increased **fracture risk**.

More severe hypercalcemia (>12–13 mg/dL)

- **CNS** symptoms: Lethargy, stupor, or coma
- **Gastrointestinal** symptoms (nausea, anorexia, constipation, or pancreatitis).
- Decreased **renal concentrating ability**, causing **polyuria** and **polydipsia**.
- **Bone pain** or pathologic **fractures** (in long-standing hyperparathyroidism).
- ECG changes: **Bradycardia**, **AV block**, and **Short QT interval**

14. All except are features plummer vinson syndrome: (Repeat)

A. Hypertrophy of oral mucosa
B. Dysphagia
C. Glossitis
D. Iron deficiency anemia

Ans: A. Hypertrophy of oral mucosa

Ref: *Harrison's Principles of Internal Medicine, 18ed.*

Explanation:

Plummer–Vinson syndrome (PVS)

- Also called **Paterson–Brown–Kelly syndrome** or **sideropenic dysphagia**
- **It is Premalignant**
- Presents as a triad of
  - Dysphagia
  - Esophageal webs
  - Iron deficiency anemia
- It most usually occurs in postmenopausal women.

Clinical features

- Burning sensation with the tongue and oral mucosa
- **Atrophy of lingual papillae** produces a smooth, shiny, red dorsum of the tongue.
- Dysphagia
- Pain
- Weakness
- Odynophagia
- **Atrophic glossitis**
- Angular stomatitis
- The condition is associated with **koilonychia**, **glossitis**, **cheilitis**, and **splenomegaly**.
- Hemogram – **Microcytic hypochromic** anemia suggestive of Iron deficiency
- Increased risk of **squamous cell carcinoma of Esophagus**

15. Which is not a disease with mitochondrial inheritance? (Repeat)

A. Leber's hereditary neuropathy
B. Myotonia congenita
C. Kayre searns disease
D. MELAS

Ans: B. Myotonia congenita

Ref: *Harrison's Principles of Internal Medicine, 18ed.*

Explanation:

- **Myotonia congenita** is a **chloride channelopathy**

Common mitochondrial inheritance diseases include

- **Mitochondrial myopathy (eg:** Kayre searns disease, MELAS, MERRF, CPEO)
- **Kayre searns disease**
  - Retitinitis pigmentosa
  - AV block
  - Cerebellar ataxia
  - Hearing loss
- **Diabetes mellitus and deafness (DAD)**
  - This combination at an early age can be due to mitochondrial disease
  - Diabetes mellitus and deafness can also be found together for other reasons
- **Leber's hereditary optic neuropathy (LHON)**
  - Visual loss beginning in young adulthood
  - Eye disorder characterized by progressive loss of central vision due to degeneration of the optic nerves and retina
  - Wolff-Parkinson-White syndrome
  - Multiple sclerosis-type disease
- **Leigh syndrome, subacute sclerosing encephalopathy**
  - After normal development the disease usually begins late in the first year of life, although onset may occur in adulthood
  - A rapid decline in function occurs and is marked by seizures, altered states of consciousness, dementia, ventilatory failure
- **Neuropathy, ataxia, retinitis pigmentosa, and ptosis (NARP)**
  - Progressive symptoms as described in the acronym
  - Dementia

- **Myoneurogenic gastrointestinal encephalopathy (MNGIE)**
  - Gastrointestinal pseudo-obstruction
  - Neuropathy
- **Myoclonic Epilepsy with Ragged Red Fibers (MERRF)**
  - Progressive myoclonic epilepsy
  - "Ragged Red Fibers" – clumps of diseased mitochondria accumulate in the — subsarcolemmal region of the muscle fiber and appear as "Ragged Red Fibers" when muscle is stained with modified **Gömöri trichrome** stain
  - Short stature
  - Hearing loss
  - Lactic acidosis
  - Exercise intolerance
- **Mitochondrial myopathy, encephalomyopathy, lactic acidosis, stroke-like symptoms (MELAS)**
- **Chronic progressive external ophthalmoplegia (CPEO)**

16. **Reiter's disease is associated with: (Repeat)**
   A. Psedomanas auerignosa
   B. Shigella flexneri
   C. Streptococcus pyogenes
   D. Pneumococcus

Ans: B. Shigella flexneri

Ref: *Harrison's Principles of Internal Medicine, 18th ed.*

Explanation:

Causes of Reiter's syndrome (Reactive arthritis)

- Reactive arthritis is associated with the HLA-B27 gene on chromosome 6 and by the presence of enthesitis as the basic pathologic lesionand is triggered by a preceding infection.
  - **Shigella flexneri** (MC, both epidemic & sporadic)
  - **Shigella sonnei**
  - **Shigella dysenteriae**
  - **Salmonella** spp
  - **Yersinia enterocolitica**
  - Y. pseudotuberculosis
  - **Campylobacter** jejuni
  - **Chlamydia** trachomatis
  - **Ureaplasma** urealyticum

17. **Kartagener's syndrome includes all *except*: (Repeat)**
   A. Situs inversus **B.** Bronchiectasis
   C. Lobar emphysema **D.** Sinusitis

Ans: A. Lobar emphysema

Ref: *Harrison's Principles of Internal Medicine, 18th ed. & Medscape*

Explanation:

Kartagener's syndrome

- Triad of Situs inversus, Chronic sinusitis, and Bronchiectasis
- Associated with **Primary ciliary dyskinesia**
- Patients present with **chronic upper** and **lower respiratory tract disease** resulting from **ineffective mucociliary clearance**.
- A typical presentation is that of **rhinorrhea** and **mucopurulent discharge** since **birth**.
- **Immotile spermatozoa** result in **male sterility**.
- **Nasal polyps** are seen in 30% cases
- **Recurrent chronic sinusitis**
- **Recurrent otitis media**
- Recurrent LRIs by **Pseudomonas & Hemophilus influenzae**

18. **Reverse splitting of S2 seen in:**
   A. VSD **B.** Severe AS
   C. RBBB **D.** ASD

Ans: B. Severe AS

Ref: *Hutchison's Clinical Methods, 22nd ed.*

Explanation:

Causes of Reverse splitting (Second heart sound A2 occuring after P2)

- Complete LBBB
- Aortic stenosis
- Right ventricular ectopics
- Left ventricular outflow tract obstruction
- Chronic severe Hypertension
- Ischemic heart disease
- WPW syndrome

(See Figure on the next page)

19. **Dicrotic pulse is seen in: (Repeat)**
   A. AS with AR
   B. HOCM
   C. Dilated cardiomyopathy
   D. Aortic dissection

Ans: C. Dilated cardiomyopathy

Ref: *Harrison's Principles of Internal Medicine, 18th ed.*

Explanation:

Abnormal Pulses

Anacrotic Pulse

- This is slow rising pulse of smaller amplitude seen in conditions like aortic stenosis

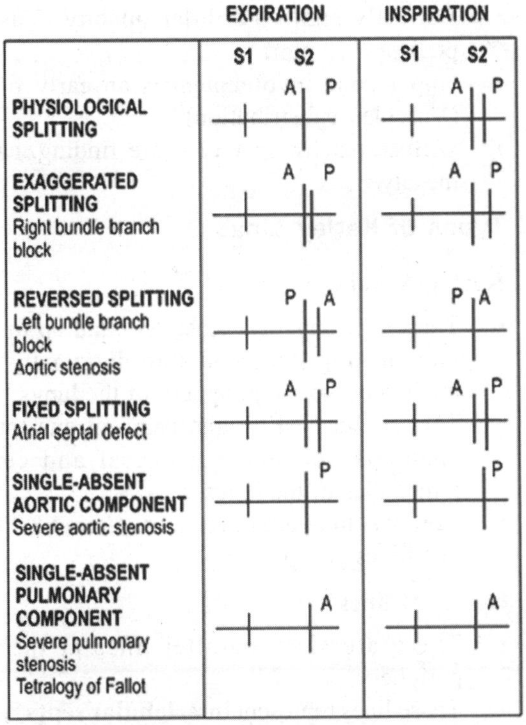

- Anacrotic means upbeating; refers to exaggerated anacrotic notch seenin AS

Double beating Pulses

- Occurs when there are two palpable arterial pulses per cardiac cycle

A. Bisferiens Pulse

- Two positive peaks during systole
- Felt best in carotid arteries
- Seen in Severe AR, Combined AR and AS, HOCM & in high output states

B. Bifid Pulse

- Commonly recorded than palpated
- The initial spike is followed by a mid systolic pulse collapse and then by late systolic impulse
- Seen in Hypertrophic cardiomyopathy

C. Dicrotic Pulse

- Second palpable component is a diastolic reflection wave.
- The detectable delay between two palpable peaks is much longer than in bisferiens pulse
- Seen in Dilated & Restricted Cardiomyo-pathy or Severe LV dysfunction, Aortic regurgitation, Typhoid fever, Cardiac tamponade

Pulsus Alternans

- Strong and weak beat occuring alternatively
- Seen in left ventricular dysfunction

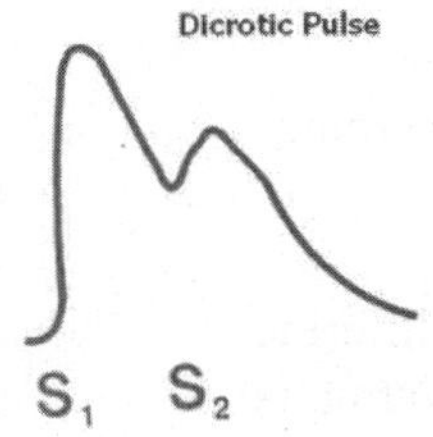

20. Photosensitivity is seen in:

A. SLE
B. Kawasaki disease
C. Rheumatoid arthritis
D. Polyarteritis nodosa

Ans: A. SLE

Ref: *Harrison's Principles of Internal Medicine, 18th ed.*

Explanation:

Conditions associated with Photosensitivity

Type	Disease
Genetic	Erythropoietic porphyria Erythropoietic protoporphyria Porphyria cutanea tarda—familial Variegate porphyria Hepatoerythropoietic porphyria **Albinism** **Xeroderma pigmentosum** Rothmund-Thomson syndrome **Bloom syndrome** Cockayne's disease Kindler syndrome **Phenylketonuria**
Metabolic	**Porphyria cutanea tarda**—sporadic **Hartnup disease** Kwashiorkor **Pellagra** **Carcinoid syndrome**
Immediate Delayed	Solar urticaria Drug photoallergy Persistent light reaction/chronic actinic dermatitis
Neoplastic and degenerative	Photoaging **Actinic keratosis** **Melanoma** and nonmelanoma skin cancer
Idiopathic	Polymorphous light eruption Hydroa aestivale Actinic prurigo
Photoaggravated	**Lupus erythematosus** Systemic Subacutecutaneous Discoid **Dermatomyositis** **Herpes simplex** **Lichen planus** actinicus Acnevulgaris (aestivale)

Other Miscellaneous conditions assc with photosensitivity

- Sjögren's syndrome
- Psoriasis
- Atopic eczema
- Erythema multiforme
- Seborrhoeic dermatitis
- Autoimmune bullous diseases
- Mycosis fungoides
- Smith–Lemli–Opitz syndrome
- Sinear Usher syndrome
- Rosacea
- Darier's disease
- Kindler-Weary syndrome

21. **Kerley B lines are seen in: (Repeat)**
A. Pulmonary edema
B. Pulonary embolism
C. Pleural effusion
D. HOCM

Ans: A. Pulmonary edema

Ref: *Harrison's Principles of Internal Medicine, 18th ed. & Arun Babu T et al. Pulmonary edema, Recent Advances in Pediatrics, Spl Vol-24, Edited by Suraj Gupte.*

Explanation:

Cardiogenic Pulmonary edema

Chest radiography

- Cardiomegaly
- Kerley-B lines – Thickening of interlobar septa
- Basilar edema
- Absence of air bronchograms
- Presence of pleural effusion (particularly bilateral)

Echocardiogram

Echocardiography is useful to evaluate left ventricular function, valvular function and pericardial disease.

Pulmonary capillary wedge pressure (PCWP)

PCWP can be measured with a pulmonary arterial catheter. This method helps in differentiating CPE from NCPE. In CPE, PCWP is elevated and large V waves and rapid Y descent may be seen.

Non-Cardiogenic Pulmonary edema (ARDS)

Chest radiography

- Hemodynamic — Peribronchial and Perivascular cuffing, diffuse streakiness - indicated interlobular fluid and distended lymphatics
- Septal lines - Kerley A & B
- Butterfly sign - Perihilar opacity (Vascular pedicle > 70 mm)
- Upper zone involvement is an early finding (Vascular re distribution)
- Diffuse patchy opacity - late finding, cardiomegaly.

Types of Kerley Lines

Kerley A lines

- These are longer (at least 2cm and up to 6cm) unbranching lines coursing diagonally from the hila out to the periphery of the lungs.
- They are caused by distension of anastomotic channels between peripheral and central lymphatics of the lungs.
- Kerley A lines are never seen without Kerley B or C lines also present.

Kerley B lines

- These are short parallel lines at the lung periphery.
- These lines represent **interlobular septa**, which are usually **less than 1 cm** in length and parallel to one another at **right angles to the pleura**.
- They are located **peripherally in contact with the pleura** near the lung bases
- These seen in **Congestive Heart Failure** (CHF) and **Interstitial Lung Diseases** (ILd).

Kerley C lines

- These are the **least commonly** seen of the Kerley lines.
- They are **short, fine lines** throughout the lungs, with a **reticular** appearance.
- They represent **thickening of anastomotic lymphatics**

22. **Skip lesions are seen in: (Repeat)**
A. Crohn's disease
B. Ulcerative colitis
C. Ischemic bowel disease
D. Typhoid colitis

Ans: A. Crohn's disease

Ref: *Harrison's Principles of Internal Medicine, 18ed.*

Explanation:

Crohn's disease

- MC site-***terminal ileum*** with ***rectal sparing***, ***skip areas*** +
- It is ***transmural***, hence more of fistula formation
- More of systemic symptoms, pain, abdominal mass
- ***Toxic megacolon***→ Perforation
- Intraabdominal abscess, fallopian tube scarring → infertility

- Intestinal obstruction, massive hemorrhage, malabsorption, severe perianal disease
- ***Cobblestoning on endoscope***
- Responds to antibiotics, recurs after surgery
- ***ASCA-positive***
- Treatment – Antibiotics, corticosteroids, sulfasalazine, mercaptopurine, azathioprine, methotrexate, cyclosporine, tacrolimus
- **Anti-TNF**: Infliximab, adalimumab, certolizumab pegol
- **Anti-integrin**: Natalizumab
- Risk of Ca increases with duration & severity of the disease

23. All are true regarding rheumatic chorea *except:* (Repeat)

A. Absent in sleep
B. May cause Neurologic sequelae
C. Lasts for 4 to 10 wks
D. Common in girls

Ans: B. May cause Neurologic sequle

Ref: *Harrison's Principles of Internal Medicine, 18ed &Nelson's Textbook of Pediatrics. 19th Edition*

Explanation:

CHOREA

- Occurs in **10-15%** of patients
- Presents as an **isolated, subtle, neurologic behavior** disorder
- Symptoms include
  - Emotional lability
  - Incoordination
  - Poor school performance
  - Uncontrollable movements
  - Facial grimacing
  - Symptoms exacerbated by **stress** and **disappearing with sleep**
- The latent period from acute GAS infection to chorea is usually longer than for arthritis or carditis and can be months.
- Commonly **occurs** in the **absence of other manifestations**
- **Prolonged latent period** after group A streptococcal infection
- Found mainly in **females.**
- Onset can be **insidious**, with symptoms being present for several months before recognition.
- Clinical maneuvers to elicit features of chorea include:
  - Demonstration of **milkmaid's grip** (irregular contractions of the muscles of the hands while squeezing the examiner's fingers).
  - ***Spooning and pronation*** of the hands when the patient's arms are extended.
  - ***Wormian darting movements*** of the ***tongue*** upon ***protrusion.***
  - Examination of ***handwriting*** to evaluate ***fine motor*** movements.
- Chorea **does not cause** permanent neurologic sequelae.
- Chorea eventually resolves completely, usually **within 6 weeks.**

24. Tall 'T' waves are seen in: (Repeat)

A. Hyperkalemia
B. Hypocalcemia
C. Hypercalcemia
D. Hypokalemia

Ans: A. Hyperkalemia

Ref: *Harrison's Principles of Internal Medicine, 18ed.*

Explanation:

ECG changes in Hyperkalaemia

- Tall T waves (Earliest sign)
- Prolonged PR interval
- Widened QRS interval
- Flattened P waves
- Arrythmias including bradycardia, ventricular tachycardia or fibrillation
- Sinus arrest or nodal rhythm with possible asystole

ECG changes in Hypokalaemia

- Flattened T waves
- ST segment depression
- Prolonged QT interval
- Tall U waves
- Atrial arrythmias
- Ventricular tachycardia or ventricular fibrillation

25. True statement regarding pulse oximetry in Methemoglobinemia:

A. No effect
B. Falsely high value in mild cases
C. Falsely low values in severe cases
D. Falsely high values in severe cases

Ans: D. Falsely high values in severe cases

Ref: *Harrison's Principles of Internal Medicine, 18th ed. & Emedicine Medscape*

Explanation:

Pulse oximetry in Methhemoglobinemia

- Findings of bedside pulse oximetry in the presence of methemoglobinemia may be misleading. Pulse oximetry measurements with **low-levels of methemoglobinemia** often result in **falsely low values** for oxygen saturation and are often **falsely high** in those with **high-level methemoglobinemia.**

- The pulse oximeter only measures the relative absorbance of **2 wavelengths of light (660 nm** and **940 nm)** to differentiate oxyhemoglobin from deoxyhemoglobin.
- The ratio of absorption of light at each of these wavelengths is converted into oxygen saturation by using calibration curves.
- Methemoglobin **increases absorption of light** at **both wavelengths** (more **at 940 nm**) and therefore offers **optical interference** to pulse oximetry by **falsely absorbing light.**
- As a result, oxygen saturations by pulse oximetry in methemoglobinemia plateau at about **85%**; therefore, a patient with a methemoglobin level of **5%** and a patient with a level **of 40%** have approximately the same saturation values on pulse oximetry (~**85%**).
- The severity of the cyanosis does not correspond to the pulse oximetry reading: a patient may appear **extremely cyanotic** but still have a pulse oximetry reading in the high **80s**.
- However, newer **multiwavelength pulse oximeters** have been developed that can detect methemoglobinemia with an accuracy comparable to that achievable with co-oximeters.

26. Neutropenia is seen in all *except:*

A. Scurvy
B. Aplastic anemia
C. Typhoid fever
D. Chloramphenicol

Ans: A. Scurvy

Ref: *Harrison's Principles of Internal Medicine, 18 ed.*

Explanation:

Severity of neutropenia based on the absolute neutrophil count (ANC) measured in cells per microliter of blood:

- **Mild neutropenia** (1000 ≤ ANC < 1500) — minimal risk of infection
- **Moderate neutropenia** (500 ≤ ANC < 1000) — moderate risk of infection
- **Severe neutropenia** (ANC < 500) — severe risk of infection.

Causes of Neutropenia

- Causes can be divided into the following groups:

Decreased production in the bone marrow due to:

- Aplastic anemia
- Arsenic poisoning
- Cancer, particularly blood cancers
- Hereditary disorders (e.g. Congenital neutropenia, cyclic neutropenia)
- Radiation
- Vitamin B 12, Folate or copper deficiency.

Increased destruction:

- Autoimmune neutropenia.
- Chemotherapy treatments, such as for cancer and autoimmune diseases

Marginalisation and sequestration:

- Hemodialysis

Medications:

- Chloramphenicol
- Phenytoin
- Indomethacin
- Propylthiouracil
- Carbimazole
- Chlorpromazine
- Trimethoprim/sulfamethoxazole
- Clozapine
- Ticlodipine

Infections

- Tuberculosis
- Typhoid fever
- Brucellosis
- Tularemia
- Measles
- Infectious mononucleosis
- Malaria
- Viral hepatitis
- AIDS

27. All of the following are seen in cardiac tamponade *except:* (Repeat)

A. Pulsus paradoxus
B. Warm periphery
C. Feeble heart sounds
D. Less urine output

Ans: B. Warm periphery

Ref: *Harrison's Principles of Internal Medicine, 18th ed.*

Explanation:

Cardiac Tamponade

- The accumulation of **fluid** in the **pericardial space** in a quantity sufficient to cause serious

obstruction to the inflow of blood to the ventricles results in cardiac tamponade.

- The most common causes of tamponade are
  - Neoplastic disease
  - Idiopathic pericarditis
  - Renal failure
  - Tuberculosis (Developing countries)
- Tamponade may also result from bleeding into the pericardial space after cardiac operations, trauma, and treatment of patients with acute pericarditis with anticoagulants.
- The three principal features of **tamponade (Beck's triad)** are
  - Hypotension
  - Soft or absent heart sounds
  - Jugular venous distention with a prominent x descent but an absent y descent.
- There are both **limitation of ventricular filling** and **reduction of cardiac output**.
- Tamponade may also develop more slowly, and in these circumstances the clinical manifestations may resemble those of **heart failure**, including **dyspnea**, **orthopnea**, **hepatic engorgement** and **decreased urine output.**
- There may be **reduction in amplitude of the QRS complexes**, and **electrical alternans** of the **P, QRS, or T waves.**
- **Paradoxical Pulse:** Greater than normal (>**10 mmHg**) inspiratory decline in systolic arterial pressure.

Diagnosis

- When pericardial effusion causes tamponade, **Doppler ultrasound** shows that tricuspid and pulmonic valve flow velocities increase markedly during inspiration, whereas pulmonic vein, mitral, and aortic flow velocities diminish.
- Often the **right ventricular cavity** is **reduced** in diameter, and there is late **diastolic inward motion (collapse)** of the **right ventricular free wall** and the **right atrium**.
- Transesophageal echocardiography may be necessary to diagnose a loculated or hemorrhagic effusion responsible for cardiac tamponade.

Pericardiocentesis

- If manifestations of **tamponade** appear, **echocardiographically** or **fluoroscopically** guided **pericardiocentesis** must be carried out
- **Intravenous saline** may be administered as the patient is being readied for the procedure, but the pericardiocentesis must not be delayed.

SURGERY

1. **Least recurrence rate with incisional hernia repair is seen in:**

   A. Laparoscopic herniorrhaphy
   B. On lay mesh repair
   C. In lay mesh repair
   D. Component separation technique

   Ans: A. Laparoscopic herniorrhaphy

Ref: Kingsnorth A. The management of incisional hernia. Ann R Coll Surg Engl. 2006 May;88(3):252-60.

Explanation:

Operative Management of Incisional hernias

a. **The laparoscopic approach** (Recurrence rate 2.9 – 9.3%)
b. **Open prosthetic mesh techniques**
   - The inlay technique (Recurrence rate – 44%)
   - The onlay technique (Recurrence rate – 15%)
   - The sublay technique (Recurrence rate – 33%)
c. **Components separation techniques** (Recurrence rate – 32%)

2. **Charcot's triad:**

   A. Abdominal Pain, fever, jaundice
   B. Fever, jaundice, abdominal distention
   C. Fever, Vomiting, Jaundice
   D. Jaundice, Fever, Diarrhea

   Ans: A. Adbominal Pain, Fever, Jaundice

Ref: Bailey and Love's Short Practice of Surgery 25th Edition, Robbins Pathology 8th ed, Nelson Pediatrics 19th ed, Harrison Principles of internal medicine, 18th ed.

Explanation:

Charcot's Triad

- Seen in cholangitis
- Pain
- Jaundice
- Fever

Few important triads in medicine

Saint's Triad

- Diverticulosis
- Gall stones
- Hiatus hernia

Whipple's triad

Seen in **Insulinoma** (most common functioning tumor of the endocrine pancreas)

- Fasting-induced neuroglyopenic symptoms of hypoglycemia (diaphoresis, shaking, mental confusion, obtundation, and seizures)
- Low blood glucose levels (40 to 50 mg/dl)
- Relief of symptoms after the administration of glucose.

Beck's Triad

- Seen in Cardiac Tamponade
- Hypotension
- Soft or absent heart sounds
- Jugular venous distention (increased JVP)

Murphy's Triad

- Seen in Acute appendicitis
- Pain
- Fever
- Vomiting

Mackler's triad

- Seen in Boerhaave's syndrome
- Pain
- Vomiting and
- Subcutaneous emphysema

Sandbolm's triad

- Seen in Hemobilia
- Pain
- Jaundice
- Hematemesis

Chiari triad

- Seen in Aorto enteric fistula
- Midthoracic pain
- Sentinel arterial hemorrahage
- Exsanguination

Virchow's triad

- Abnormalities that lead to thrombus formation
- Endothelial injury
- Stasis or turbulent blood flow
- Hypercoagulability of the blood

Currarino triad

- Anorectal malformations (ectopic anus, anal stenosis, imperforate anus)
- Sacral bone anomalies (hypoplasia, poor segmentation)
- Presacral anomaly (anterior meningoceles, teratoma, cyst)

Female athlete triad

- Disordered eating
- Amenorrhea
- Osteoporosis

Kartagener triad

- Situs inversus totalis
- Chronic sinusitis
- Bronchiectasis

Samter triad

- Nasal polyps
- Aspirin sensitivity
- Asthma

Carney triad

- Gastric GIST
- Paraganglioma
- Pulmonary chondroma

Classical triad of features in Diseases

Felty syndrome – Triad of Rheumatoid arthritis, Splenomegaly, and Neutropenia

Whipple disease - Triad of Diarrhea, Weight loss, and Malabsorption.

Reiter syndrome - Triad of Arthritis, Urethritis, and Conjunctivitis

Wegener granulomatosis - Triad of

- Acute necrotizing granulomas of the upper & lower respiratory tract
- Necrotizing or granulomatous vasculitis affecting small to medium-sized vessels
- Glomerulonephritis

Plummer-Vinson syndrome- Triad of Esophageal webs, Microcytic hypochromic anemia & atrophic glossitis

Achalasia cardia - Triad of incomplete LES relaxation, increased LES tone, esophageal aperistalsis

Solitary rectal ulcer - Triad of rectal bleeding, mucus discharge, and an inflammatory lesion of the anterior rectal wall.

Spasmus nutans - Triad of nystagmus, head tilt, and head nodding

Hepatopulmonary syndrome (HPS) - Triad of chronic liver disease, hypoxemia, and intra-pulmonary vascular dilations (IVPD)

Hemochromatosis – Triad of pigment cirrhosis with hepatomegaly, skin pigmentation, and diabetes mellitus

Anhidrotic ectodermal dysplasia – Triad of absence of sweat glands, anomalous dentition, and hypotrichosis

DRESS syndrome – Triad of Fever, rash and hepatitis

Gradenigo syndrome - Triad of suppurative OM, paralysis of the external rectus muscle, and pain in the ipsilateral orbit.

Infantile glaucoma – Triad of epiphora (tearing), photophobia (sensitivity to light), and blepharospasm (eyelid squeezing)

Kearns-Sayre syndrome - Triad of progressive external ophthalmoplegia, pigmentary degeneration of the retina, and onset before age 20 yr.

Andersen-Tawil syndrome - Triad of periodic paralysis, potentially fatal cardiac ventricular ectopy

Hemolytic uremic syndrome – Triad of Microangiopathic hemolytic anemia, thrombocytopenia, and renal insufficiency

Prune-belly syndrome, also called **triad syndrome** or **Eagle-Barrett syndrome**

MacCune Albright Syndrome - Triad of Polyostotic disease, Precocious puberty, and Cutaneous pigmentation

Botulism – Triad of acute onset of a symmetric flaccid descending paralysis with clear sensorium, no fever, and no paresthesias

Klippel-Feil syndrome - Triad of short neck, low hairline, and restriction of neck motion

3. **Most common tumor arising from appendix is:**
   A. Melanoma
   B. Carcinoid tumor
   C. Adenocarcinoma
   D. Mucinous carcinoma

Ans: B. Carcinoid tumor

Ref: Robbins Pathologic basis of Disease, 8th ed.

Explanation:

Tumors of the Appendix

- The most common tumor of the appendix is the **carcinoid**.
- It is usually discovered incidentally at the time of surgery or examination of a resected appendix.
- This neoplasm most frequently involves the **distal tip** of the appendix, where it produces a **solid bulbous swelling** up to **2 to 3 cm** in diameter.
- Although **intramural** and **transmural extension** may be evident, nodal metastases are very infrequent, and distant spread is exceptionally rare.
- Conventional adenomas or non-mucin-producing adenocarcinomas also occur in the appendix and may cause obstruction and enlargement that mimics acute appendicitis.
- **Mucocele**, a dilated appendix filled with **mucin**, may simply represent an obstructed appendix containing **inspissated mucin** or be a consequence of **mucinous cystadenoma** or **mucinous cystadenocarcinoma**.
- In the latter instance, invasion through the appendiceal wall can lead to intraperitoneal seeding and spread. In women the resulting peritoneal implants may be mistaken for mucinous ovarian tumors.
- In the most advanced cases the abdomen fills with tenacious, semisolid mucin, a condition called **pseudomyxoma peritoneii**
- This disseminated intraperitoneal disease may be held in check for years by repeated debulking but, in most instances, follows an inexorably fatal course

4. **Acute emphysematous cholecystitis is caused by: (Repeat)**

A. E coli	**B.** Staph aureus
C. Pseudomonas	**D.** Strep pyogenes

Ans: A. E coli

Ref: Schwartz's Principles of Surgery, 9th Edition. & Medscape online

Explanation:

Emphysematous cholecystitis

- Aka **clostridial cholecystitis,**
- Emphysematous cholecystitis is a rare form of acute, usually gangrenous, cholecystitis, associated with the presence of gas in the gallbladder
- Pathogenesis is related to acute inflammation of the gallbladder, which often begins aseptically, complicated by a secondary infection with gas-forming bacilli.
- **Cholelithiasis** is also present in half the patients, who are frequently diabetic.
- It is an acute infection of the gallbladder wall caused by gas-forming organisms (e.g.)
  – **Clostridium**
  – **Escherichia coli**
  – **Klebsiella**
- This condition is a surgical emergency.
- An infrequent, insidious, and rapidly progressive form of acute cholecystitis, emphysematous cholecystitis is characterized by early gangrene, perforation of the gallbladder and high mortality.

- Emphysematous cholecystitis is associated with much higher rates of gangrene and perforation of the gallbladder and significantly increased rates of mortality **(15-25%).**
- **X-ray:** ***Gas bubbles*** in the surface of gall bladder (Ref: Schwartz)
- The diagnosis is usually made on the basis of radiographs that show a **globular, gas-filled shadow** in the region of the **gallbladder**.
- Later, **intramural** or **submucosal** gas may appear, and gas may also appear in the **pericholecystic** area, denoting extension of the pathologic process outside the confines of the gallbladder.
- The treatment of choice is **early surgery**, since % of perforation is **40 to 60 %.**
- **Cholecystectomy** is indicated, but if it is not feasible, **cholecystostomy** should be performed.
- If **choledocholithiasis** is present, and exploration of the common duct may be required.
- The mortality rate is significantly greater than that for nonemphysematous cholecystitis.

5. **True about Superior mesentric artery syndrome is all *except:***

A. Long mesentery
B. Compression of duodenum
C. Common after Scoliosis surgery
D. Narrow aortomesenteric angle

Ans: A. Long mesentery

Ref: *Robbins Pathologic basis of Disease, 8th ed.*

Explanation:

Superior mesenteric artery (SMA syndrome or Wilkie syndrome

- It is an uncommon but well recognized clinical entity characterized by **compression** of the **third, or transverse, portion** of the **duodenum** between the **aorta and the superior mesenteric artery.**
- This results in **chronic**, **intermittent**, or **acute complete** or **partial duodenal obstruction**.

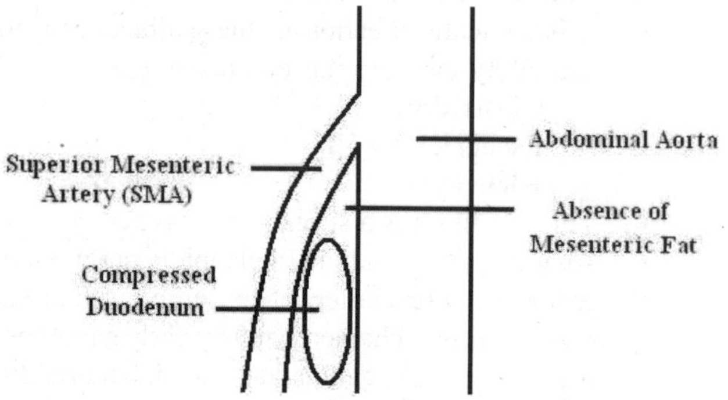

- The **superior mesenteric artery** usually forms an angle of approximately **45°** with the **abdominal aorta**, and the **third part of the duodenum crosses caudal** to the origin
- Any factor that sharply narrows the aortomesenteric angle to approximately **6-25°** can cause entrapment and compression of the third part of the duodenum
- The patient often presents with **chronic upper abdominal symptoms** such as epigastric pain, nausea, eructation, voluminous vomiting (bilious or partially digested food, postprandial discomfort, early satiety, and sometimes, subacute small bowel obstruction.
- Symptoms of superior mesenteric artery (SMA) syndrome often develop from **6-12 days after scoliosis** surgery.
- The symptoms are typically **relieved** when the patient is in the **left lateral decubitus**, **prone**, or **knee-to-chest position**, and they are often **aggravated** when the patient is in the **supine** position. These maneuvers are thought to **reduce the small bowel mesenteric tension** at the **aortomesenteric angle.**
- An **asthenic habitus** is noted in about 80% of cases.
- Abdominal examination may reveal a **succussion splash**.
- **Peptic ulcer** disease has been noted in **25-45%** of the patients, and **hyperchlorhydria** has been noted in **50%**.
- Patients can present with signs of **subacute small bowel obstruction**.

6. **All are causes of dynamic intestinal obstruction *except:***

A. Gall stones
B. Bands
C. Intussusception
D. Mesenteric vascular occlusion

Ans: D. Mesenteric vascular occlusion

Ref: *The Washington Manual of Surgery, 6th edition, Bailey and Love's Short Practice of Surgery 25th Edition & Schwartz's Principles of Surgery, 9th Edition*

Explanation:

Intestinal obstruction

- **Defn**: Lack of transit of intestinal contents
- Classification according to pathology

Dynamic: Where peristalsis is working against a mechanical obstruction
Adynamic: Where there is absence of peristalsis without obstruction

- Absent peristalsis (eg: Paralytic ileus)
- Non-propulsive form (eg: Mesenteric vascular occlusion, Pseudo-obstruction)

Causes of Dynamic intestinal obstruction

Intraluminal Causes

- Impacted stools
- Foreign bodies
- Bezoars
- Gall stones
- Ascariasis
- Meconium ileus

Intramural causes

- Atresia
- Inflammatory stricture – TB, Crohn's disease
- Malignant stricture – Ca Colon, GIST

Extramural causes

- Intraperitoneal bands and adhesions
- Hernia
- Volvulus
- Intussusception

7. **All are indications for surgery in bronchiectasis *except:***

A. Refractory foul smelling copious sputum
B. Hemoptysis
C. Bilateral disease
D. Bleeding

Ans: C. Bilateral disease

Ref: *Schwartz's Principles of Surgery, 9th Edition*

Explanation:

"Patients with diffuse bilateral disease, of which cystic fibrosis is the best example, rarely benefit from resection and should be considered for lung transplantation as they approach end-stage disease." (Ref: Schwartz)

Treatment of Bronchiectasis

- The majority of patients with bronchiectasis **do not require operative treatment**.
- **Postural drainage** and **chest physical therapy** minimize retention of purulent sputum, and antibiotic treatment of all episodes of pneumonitis should be pursued indefinitely.
- When **debilitating effects** of **chronic infection** become prominent and surgery is contemplated, the anatomy should be defined carefully with CT scan before resection is planned.
- When **extensive saccular disease** is confined to **one lobe** or **segment** in a sufficiently **symptomatic** patient, **resection** is a **clear choice**.
- In children, **interference with growth** is often the **sign of debility**.
- **Frequent hemoptysis** associated with localized disease deserves operation.
- Patients with **diffuse bilateral disease**, of which **cystic fibrosis** is the best example, **rarely benefit from resection** and should be considered for **lung transplan**tation as they approach end-stage disease.
- The operative strategy is to **remove as little normal lung as possible** without entering the central focus of infection.
- This usually requires **segmentectomy** or **lobectomy** and depends on an accurate preoperative assessment of the diseased segments.
- **Pneumonectomy** is **rarely indicated** in this disease.

8. **All are complications of gall stones *except:***

A. Diverticulosis
B. Acute cholangitis
C. Mucocele
D. Empyema of Gallbladder

Ans: A. Diverticulosis

Ref: *Bailey and Love's Short Practice of Surgery 25th Edition & Schwartz's Principles of Surgery, 9th Edition*

Explanation:

Complications of Gall Stones

- Acute and Chronic cholecystitis
- Jaundice
- Mucocele of GB
- Empyema of GB
- Gangrene of GB
- Sepsis
- Ca Gall Bladder
- Cholangitis
- Pancreatitis
- ***Mirrizi syndrome***: Biliary duct obstruction secondary to stone impaction in hartman's pouch of GB
- Gallstone ileus

9. **Klatskin tumor is:**

A. Common hepatic duct tumor
B. Merkel Cell Ca of Skin
C. Adenocarcinoma of Anal canal
D. Primitive neuroectodermal tumor of chest wall

Ans: A. Common hepatic duct tumor

Ref: Robbins Pathologic basis of Disease. 8th ed.

Explanation:

Klatskin tumor (or hilar cholangiocarcinoma)

- It is a **cholangiocarcinoma** (cancer of the biliary tree) occurring at the **confluence of the right and left hepatic bile ducts**.
- Cancer of the bile duct, cholangiocarcinoma, can occur anywhere along the biliary tract from the ampulla of Vater to the intrahepatic biliary radicals.
- The **hepatic duct bifurcation** is the **most frequently involved site** accounting for approximately **60–80%** of cholangiocarcinomas.
- **Primary sclerosing cholangitis**, an idiopathic inflammatory condition of the biliary tree, has been clearly associated with the development of cholangiocarcinoma in up to **40%** of patients.
- **Congenital biliary cystic disease**, such as **choledochal** cysts or **Caroli's disease**, has also been associated with malignant transformation in up to **25%** of cases.
- Chronic biliary tract parasitic infection, seen commonly in Southeast Asia due to **Clonorchis sinensis** and **Opisthorchis viverrini**, has also been identified as a risk factor.
- Although gallstones and cholecystectomy are not thought to be associated with an increased incidence of cholangiocarcinoma, hepatolithiasis and choledocholithiasis may predispose to malignant change.
- Finally, industrial exposure to **asbestos** and **nitrosamines**, and the use of the radiologic contrast agent, **Thorotrast** (thorium dioxide), are considered to be risk factors for the development of **cholangiocarcinoma**.

10. Most common esophageal motility disorder is:

A. Nut cracker esophagus
B. Esophageal web
C. Diffuse esophageal spasm
D. Achalasia cardia

Ans: D. Achalasia cardia

Ref: Robbins Pathologic basis of disease, 8th ed.

Explanation:

ACHALASIA CARDIA

- Increased tone of the lower esophageal sphincter (LES), as a result of **impaired smooth muscle relaxation**, is an important cause of **esophageal obstruction**.
- Release of nitric oxide and vasoactive intestinal polypeptide from inhibitory neurons, along with interruption of normal cholinergic signaling, allows the LES to relax during swallowing.
- Achalasia is characterized by the **triad** of:
  - **Incomplete LES relaxation**
  - **Increased LES tone**
  - **Aperistalsis of the esophagus**
- Primary achalasia is caused by failure of distal esophageal inhibitory neurons and is, by definition, idiopathic.
- Degenerative changes in neural innervation, either intrinsic to the esophagus or within the extraesophageal vagus nerve or the dorsal motor nucleus of the vagus, may also occur.
- Secondary achalasia may arise in **Chagas disease**, in which **Trypanosoma cruzi** infection causes destruction of the myenteric plexus, failure of peristalsis, and esophageal dilatation. **Duodenal**, **colonic**, and **ureteric myenteric plexi** can also be affected in Chagas disease.
- **Achalasia-like disease** may be caused by
  - Diabetic autonomic neuropathy
  - Infiltrative disorders such as malignancy
  - Amyloidosis
  - Sarcoidosis
  - Lesions of dorsal motor nuclei
  - Polio
  - Surgical ablation.
- X-ray: **Absence of Gastric fundus shadow**
- Barium Swallow findings
  - **Bird's beak or rat tail appearance**
  - **Dilatation of proximal esophagus**
  - **Air fluid level** in esophagus
- Treatment options for **primary** and **secondary achalasia** include **laparoscopic myotomy** and **pneumatic balloon dilatation.**
- Heller's Pyloromyotomy
- Pneumatic dilatation
- **Botulinum neurotoxin (Botox) injection**, to **inhibit LES cholinergic neurons**, can also be effective.
- **Calcium channel blockers and nitrates.**

11. A 1 cm coin lesion is seen on chest X-ray in the right upper lobe. FNAC shows adenocarcinoma. Appropriate management is:

A. Excision and observation
B. Excision and chemotherapy
C. Neoadjuvant chemotherapy followed by excision
D. Excision and Chemoradiation

Ans: A. Excision and observation

Ref: Schwartz's Principles of Surgery, 9th Edition & Sabiston Textbook of Surgery, 19th Edition

Explanation:

"Early stage lung cancer (Stages I and II) may successfully be treated with surgery alone and, in most patients, yields long-term survival rates." (Ref: Sabiston)

Principles of Management of Lung Adenocarcinoma

- Treatment options include
- Surgery for localized disease
- Chemotherapy for metastatic disease
- Radiation therapy for local control in patients whose condition is not amenable to surgery.
- Radiation therapy and chemotherapy together are better than chemotherapy or radiation therapy alone for primary treatment of advanced stage lung cancer.

Solitary Pulmonary Nodule

- Among patients with lung cancer, the best survival can be expected in cases presenting with asymptomatic solitary peripheral pulmonary nodule on chest x-ray **(coin lesions)**
- The solitary pulmonary nodule (SPN) - **abnormal density up to 4 cm** in **diameter, rounded** or **ovoid** in appearance surrounded by a **zone of lung tissue** by x-ray, and **free of cavitation** or associated **lung infiltrates.**
- **Eccentric flecks** of **calcium** may be present
- Recent analyses suggest that approximately **80 percent** of all coin lesions were malignant in patients over 50 years of age.
- The differential diagnosis of an SPN includes many entities
  - Malignant tumors
  - Benign tumors
  - Pulmonary hamartoma
  - Granuloma
  - Pulmonary arteriovenous fistula
  - Pulmonary infarction
- Surgery is rarely indicated for the nonmalignant lesions if diagnosis is confirmed.
- Where calcification is present, **CT** is useful in selecting the rare patient who can be observed safely.
- CT scans have the capacity to measure **absorption coefficients**, which indicate **tissue density.**
- For many years there has been a difference of opinion regarding the management of patients with SPNs, with some groups **advocating early thoracotomy** with resection of the lesion for all patients above 35 years of age and others urging a more **conservative approach** with greater emphasis on diagnostic studies and observation.
- Although the resection policy did result in **a 50 percent frequency** of removal of benign lesions, **excellent cure rates** could be expected if primary malignancies were found.
- **Serial radiographs** provide the data for calculation of growth rate, and it usually is possible to detect that a lesion is growing within a few weeks.
- The doubling time of malignant nodules is usually between **37 and 465 days.**
- If the lesion is growing **more slowly** or **more rapidly** than this, the evidence is in favor of **benignity.**
- With the advent of **video-assisted thoracoscopic techniques, resection** of **nodules** in the **periphery of the lung** result in **minimal morbidity** and **virtually no mortality.**

12. **Regarding treatment of meningioma: (Repeat)**
    A. Surgery and observation
    B. Preop chemo and surgery
    C. Surgery and postop radiotherapy
    D. Removal of duramater

Ans: D. Removal of duramater

Ref: Robbins Pathologic Basis of Disease, 8th edition & Schwartz's Principles of Surgery, 9th Edition

Explanation:

Refer 2011 Pathology question explanation

Principles of Management – Meningioma

- *Currently, surgery alone is the mainstay of therapy.*
- *Radiotherapy can be tried form grade 1 meningiomas after resection.*
- *There is no role for only chemotherapy or only radiotherapy or combined surgery + radiotherapy.*

"Radiation therapy is often considered for WHO grade I meningiomas after subtotal (incomplete) tumor resections. The clinical decision to irradiate after a subtotal resection is somewhat controversial and not recommended" (Ref: Schwartz)

MENINGIOMAS

- Benign tumors of adults
- Arise from the meningothelial cell of the arachnoid & is often attached to the dura

- Found along any of the external surfaces of the brain & within the ventricular system arising from the stromal arachnoid cells of the choroid plexus.
- Prior radiation therapy, typically decades earlier, is a risk factor

Morphology

- Meningiomas are usually **rounded masses** with **well-defined dural bases** that compress underlying brain but are easily separated from it
- Extension into the **overlying bone** may be present.
- The surface of the mass is usually encapsulated with thin, fibrous tissue and may have a bosselated or polypoid appearance.
- They may also grow en plaque, in which the tumor spreads in a **sheetlike** fashion along the surface of the dura.
- This form is commonly associated with **hyperostotic reactive changes** in the overlying **bone**.
- The lesions range from firm and fibrous to finely gritty
- Lesions may contain numerous calcified ***psammoma bodies***.
- Gross evidence of necrosis or extensive hemorrhage is not present.

Histological Grades

- Most meningiomas have a relatively low risk of recurrence or aggressive growth, and so are considered **WHO grade I/IV.** Various histologic patterns are observed, with no prognostic significance.

These include

- **Syncytial ("meningothelial")**: Whorled clusters of cells without visible cell membranes
- **Fibroblastic:** Elongated cells with abundant collagen deposition between them
- **Transitional**: Shares features of the syncytial and fibroblastic types
- **Psammomatous**: Conatins ***psammoma bodies***, formed from calcification of the syncytial nests of meningothelial cells
- **Secretory**: Conatins PAS-positive intracytoplasmic droplets and intracellular lumens by electron microscopy
- **Microcystic**: Has loose, spongy appearance.

- **Xanthomatous** degeneration, **osseous metaplasia**, and moderate nuclear **pleomorphism** are common in meningiomas.
- **Atypical meningiomas (WHO grade II/IV)**
  - These lesions have higher rate of recurrence and more aggressive local growth, and may require radiation therapy in addition to surgery.
  - They are distinguished from lower grade meningiomas by the presence of either a **mitotic index** of four or more mitoses per 10 high power fields or at least three atypical features (increased cellularity, small cells with a high nuclear-to-cytoplasmic ratio, prominent nucleoli, patternless growth, or necrosis).
  - Certain histologic patterns **(Clear cell and chordoid)** are also considered to be grade II/IV because of their more aggressive behavior.
- **Anaplastic (malignant) meningioma** (**WHO grade III/IV**)
  - It is a highly aggressive tumor with the appearance of a high-grade sarcoma, but retaining some histologic evidence of meningothelial origin.
  - **Mitotic rates** are often extremely high (**>20 mitoses per 10 high power fields**).
  - **Papillary meningioma** (with pleomorphic cells arranged around fibrovascular cores) and **rhabdoid meningioma** (with sheets of tumor cells with hyaline eosinophilic cytoplasm containing intermediate filaments) both have such a high propensity to recur that they are also considered to be WHO grade III/IV tumors.
- Meningiomas are commonly ***immunoreactive*** for epithelial membrane antigen.
- ***Keratin*** is restricted to lesions with the secretory pattern, and these tumors are also positive for ***carcinoembryonic antigen***.

Molecular Genetics

- The most common cytogenetic abnormality is **loss** of **long arm of chromosome 22 (22q).**
- The deletions include the region that harbors the **NF2 gene**, which encodes the protein **Merlin**

Clinical Features

- Meningiomas are slow-growing lesions that present either with vague nonlocalizing symptoms or with focal findings referable to compression of underlying brain.
- Common sites of involvement are
  - **Parasagittal aspect of the brain convexity** (MC site)

- Dura over the lateral convexity
- Wing of the sphenoid
- Olfactory groove
- Sella turcica
- Foramen magnum

- They are uncommon in children & shows **female predominance (3 : 2)**
- Sex ratio (Female: Male) is **10 : 1** for **spinal meningiomas**
- Most meningiomas **(90%)** are categorized as **benign tumors**, with the remaining **10%** being **atypical or malignant**.
- Lesions are usually solitary, but when present at multiple sites, especially in association with acoustic neuromas or glial tumors, a diagnosis of NF2 should be considered.
- It expresses ***progesterone receptors*** and may ***grow more rapidly*** during ***pregnancy***.

Treament

- Combined Surgery and Radiotherapy and not Radiotherpy alone
- Prognosis is good if the entire tumor is surgically removed.
- However, this is not always possible due to the location of the tumor.

The constant principles in meningioma resection are the following:

- If possible, all involved or **hyperostotic bone** should be removed.
- The dura involved by the tumor as well as a dural rim that is free from tumor should be resected (**duraplasty** is performed).
- **Dural tails** that are apparent on MRI are best **removed**, even though some may not be involved with the tumor.
- Provision for harvesting a suitable dural substitute (pericranium or fascia lata) is done
- The surgeon also can use **commercially** available **dural substitutes**.

Simpson Grade	Completeness of Resection	10-year Recurrence
Grade I	Complete removal including resection of underlying bone and associated dura	9%
Grade II	Complete removal + coagulation of dural attachment	19%
Grade III	Complete removal w/o resection of dura or coagulation	29%
Grade IV	Subtotal resection	40%

13. Secondary brain injury seen in:

A. Concussion
B. Diffuse axonal surgery
C. Seizures
D. Intracrebral hematoma

Ans: C. Seizures

Ref: *J. Claude Hemphill. Multimodal Monitoring and Neurocritical Care Bioinformatics: Secondary Brain Injury. Medscape education.*

Explanation:

- When patients have an acute neurological catastrophe such as **traumatic brain injury (TBI)** or stroke, damage to the brain can occur at the time of the initial event.
- This damage is termed **primary brain injury**, and the underlying mechanisms include:
  - ***Intraparenchymal or extra-axial traumatic or spontaneous hemorrhage***
  - ***Diffuse axonal injury*** (in TBI)
  - ***Focal or global ischemia*** from acute ischemic stroke or global cerebral ischemia during cardiac arrest.
- Although interventions (eg: surgical hematoma evacuation) can be undertaken to limit or reverse primary brain injury, much of the primary damage may be **irreversible**.
- This primary brain injury initiates a cascade of biochemical events that are **reversible**. This process is termed **secondary brain injury**
- **Secondary brain injury** can generally be considered as two related concepts:
  - ***Cellular injury cascades***
  - ***Secondary brain insults*** (SBIs).
- An example of the cellular injury cascade is the ischemic cascade in which events such as excitotoxicity, intracellular calcium influx, and free radical membrane damage are ongoing.
- Hence, ultra-early ischemic stroke treatment via **revascularization** of an occluded intracranial artery with thrombolytic agents is intended to restore perfusion before permanent cell death, thereby reversing this secondary brain injury.
- In addition to initiating ischemic and apoptotic cell injury cascades, primary brain injuries make injured, but salvageable, brain tissue vulnerable to SBIs.
- **Hypotension**, **hypoxia** and **hypoglycemia** are all examples of SBIs in which decreased substrate delivery to an injured brain further worsens injury.
- On the other hand, **fever**, **seizures** and **hyperglycemia** are examples of SBIs in which

increased metabolic demand may outstrip compensatory mechanisms and result in further injury.

Examples of primary and secondary brain injury in TBI

Primary	Secondary
• Intracerebral hemorrhage • Subdural hemorrhage • Subarachnoid hemorrhage • Epidural hemorrhage • Cerebral contusion • Cerebral laceration • Axonal stretch injury	• Edema • Impaired metabolism • Altered cerebral blood flow • Free radical formation • Excitotoxicity • Increased intracranial tension • Seizures

14. **Migratory thrombophlebitis seen in: (Repeat)**

A. Pancreatic Ca
B. Breast Ca
C. Bronchogenic Ca
D. Prostate Ca

Ans: A & D

Ref: *Robbins and Cotran Pathologic Basis of Disease: 8th edition*

Explanation:

*"Migratory thrombophlebitis, known as the **Trousseau sign**, occurs in about **10% of Adenocarcinoma of pancreas** patients and is attributable to the elaboration of platelet-aggregating factors and procoagulants from the carcinoma or its necrotic products" Ref: Robbins*

Migratory Thrombophlebitis (Trousseau Syndrome)

- It is associated with a significant risk of underlying **malignancy**, esp **Pancreas, Lung,** and **Prostate.**
- The **veins** of the **neck, chest, abdomen,** and **lower extremities** are involved either sequentially or simultaneously.
- The **hypercoagulable state** associated with cancer is **multifactorial** in origin, and may be induced by **inflammatory cytokines, acute-phase reactants, circulating tissue factor,** and **cancer microparticles.**

15. **True regarding Warthin's tumor: (Repeat)**

A. Shows hot spot on tc 99 scan
B. Most common tumor of minor salivary glands
C. Most malignant tumor
D. Common in females

Ans: A. Shows hot spot on tc99 scan

Ref: *Robbins Pathologic basis of Disease, 8th edition & Sabiston Textbook of Surgery, 19th Edition*

Explanation:

*"The only neoplasms of salivary glands known to consistently concentrate **Tc-99m** pertechnetate (Hot spot) are **Warthin's tumor** and **oncocytoma**" Ref: Sabiston*

WARTHIN TUMOR (PAPILLARY CYSTADENOMALYMPHOMATOSUM)

- This curious **benign** neoplasm with its intimidating histologic name is the **second most** common **salivary gland neoplasm.**
- It arises almost ***exclusively in the parotid gland*** (the only tumor virtually restricted to the parotid. and occurs more commonly in **males** than in females, usually in the **fifth to seventh decades of life.**
- About **10% are multifocal** and **10% bilateral.**
- **Smokers** have eight times the risk of non-smokers for developing these tumors.
- The tumor is **slow growing, painless,** and usually appears in the **tail of the parotid gland** near the angle of the mandible

Morphology:

- Most Warthin tumors are round to oval, encapsulated masses, 2 to 5 cm in diameter, usually arising in the superficial parotid gland, where they are readily palpable.
- Transection reveals a pale gray surface punctuated by narrow cystic or **cleftlike spaces** filled with a **mucinous** or **serous secretion.**
- On microscopic examination these spaces are lined by a **double layer of neoplastic epithelial cells** resting on a dense lymphoid stroma sometimes bearing germinal centers.
- The spaces are frequently narrowed by **polypoid projections** of the lymphoepithelial elements.
- The double layer of lining cells is distinctive; it consists of a surface palisade of columnar cells having an abundant, finely granular, eosinophilic cytoplasm, that imparts an oncocytic appearance, which rests on a layer of cuboidal to polygonal cells.
- **Oncocytes** are epithelial cells stuffed with **mitochondria,** which impart the granular appearance to the cytoplasm.
- Secretory cells are dispersed in the columnar cell layer, accounting for the secretions within the cystically dilated lumens.
- On occasion, there are foci of **squamous metaplasia.**
- The occasional finding of small salivary gland rests in lymph nodes in the neck suggests that

these tumors arise from the aberrant incorporation of similar inclusion-bearing lymphoid tissue in the parotids.
- Rarely, **Warthin tumors** have arisen within **cervical lymph nodes**, a finding that should not be mistaken for metastases.
- These neoplasms are **benign**, with recurrence rates of only **2%** after **resection**

16. Most common cause of pseudopancreatic cyst: (Repeat)

A. Acute pancreatitis
B. Abdomen trauma
C. Post pancreatic surgery
D. Pancreatic Carcinoma

Ans: A. Acute Pancreatitis

Ref: *Sabiston Textbook of Surgery, 19th Edition. Pg 1524-25 & Schwartz's Principles of Surgery, 9th Edition*

Explanation:

"Pancreatic pseudocysts occur usually as a complication of pancreatitis, although some occur after trauma" (Ref: Schwartz).

Pancreatic Pseudocysts

- Pancreatic pseudocysts occur in 5% to 15% of patients who have peripancreatic fluid collections after Acute Pancreatitis.
- By definition, the capsule of a pseudocyst is composed of collagen and granulation tissue and it is not lined by epithelium.
- The fibrotic reaction typically requires at least 4 to 8 weeks to develop.

Clinical features

Upto 50% develop symptoms
- Abdominal pain
- Early satiety
- Nausea
- Weight loss

Diagnosis

- Elevated pancreatic enzyme levels in plasma is suggestive
- CT or MRI can confirms the diagnosis
- EUS with FNA is indicated for patients in whom the diagnosis is not clear
- Cyst Fluid analysis
  - High amylase
  - Absence of mucin
  - Low carcinoem-bryonic antigen (CEa) levels

Management

Asympomatic patients

Only observation is indicated because spontaneous regression has been documented in up to 70% of asymptomatic patients .

Factors favoring spontaneous regression

- Pseudocysts smaller than 4 cm in diameter
- Located in the tail
- No evidence of pancreatic duct obstruction or communication with the main pancreatic duct.

Symptomatic Patients

Management options are

Endoscopic Management

- Transgastric / transduodenal endoscopic drainage – for pseudocysts in close contact (defined as <1 cm) with the stomach and duodenum.
- Transpapillary drainage can be attempted in pancreatic pseudocysts communicating with the main pancreatic duct.
- For pancreatic duct stricture is associated with a pancreatic pseudocyst, endoscopic dilation and stent placement are indicated

Surgery

- Indicated for patients with pancreatic pseudocysts that cannot be treated with endoscopic techniques and patients who fail endoscopic treatment
- Depends on the location of the cyst.
- Pancreatic pseudocysts closely attached to the stomach should be treated with a cyst-gastrostomy.
- Pancreatic pseudocysts located in the head of the pancreas that are in close contact with the duodenum are treated with a cystoduodenostomy
- For pseudocysts are not in contact with the stomach or duodenum the surgical treatment is a roux-en-y cystojejunostomy.

Percutaneous drainage

- Percutaneous drainage is only indicated for septic patients secondary to pseudocyst infection
- High incidence of external fistula

Complications of Pseudocyst

- Bleeding
- Pancreaticopleural fistula
- Bile duct obstruction
- Duodenal obstruction
- Rupture into the abdominal cavity
- Infection

17. **Treatment of choice of squamous cell cancer of anal canal not involving deep structures: (Repeat)**

A. Abdominoperineal resection
B. Wide excision with chemotherapy
C. Chemoradiation
D. Wide excision with radiotherapy

Ans: C. Chemoradiation

Ref: *Bailey & Love's Short Practice of Surgery, 25th Edition 1269 & Sabiston Textbook of Surgery, 19th Edition 1405-6*

Explanation:

SQUAMOUS CELL CARCINOMA OF ANAL CANAL

Risk factors

- HPV (especially subtypes 16, 18, 31 or 33)
- HIV
- Transplant recipients

Clinical features

- Pain and bleeding- most common
- Can also present with discharge, mass or pruritus
- Advanced tumours may cause faecal incontinence
- Spreads to inguinal lymph nodes

Diagnosis- By Biopsy

Management

Concurrent Chemoradiation (Nigro Protocol) is the treatment of choice

- External-beam radiation therapy combined with 5-fluorouracil (5-FU) and Mitomycin C based chemotherapy

Role of surgery

- **Abdomino Perinael resection(APR)** is indicated in:
  1. patients who are already in need of a stoma for fecal incontinence.
  2. when chemotherapy or radiation therapy is contraindicated.
  3. residual disease after radiation therapy plus chemotherapy.
- Wide local excision may be considered for small lesions, but Chemoradiation is the treatment of choice.

Note:

1. It is **concurrent chemoradiotherapy** i.e chemotherapy and radio therapy offered simultaneously, the current treatment of choice
2. **Cisplatin** is used in metastatic anal cancer.

ORTHOPEDICS

1. **Clergyman's knee is due to involvement of: (Repeat)**

A. Infrapatellar bursa
B. Suprapatellar bursa
C. Prepatellar bursa
D. Semimembranous bursa

Ans: A. Infrapatellar bursa

Ref: *Apley's Orthopedics, 9th ed.*

Explanation:

Infrapatellar bursitis (clergyman's knee)

- It is the inflammation of the infrapatellar bursa, which is located just below the patella.
- It is often called "clergyman's knee" due to its historical frequency amongst clergyman, who injured the bursa by kneeling on hard surfaces during prayer.

Prepatellar bursitis

- Also known as **beat knee**, **carpet layer's knee**, **coal miner's knee**, **housemaid's knee**, **rug cutter's knee**, or **nun's knee**
- It is an inflammation of the prepatellar bursa at the anterior to patella.
- It is marked by swelling at the knee, which can be tender to the touch but which does not restrict the knee's range of motion.
- It is most commonly caused by trauma to the knee by chronic trauma over a period of time.
- As such, prepatellar bursitis commonly occurs among individuals whose professions require frequent kneeling.

2. **Mosaic pattern of lamellar bone is classically seen in: (Repeat)**

A. Paget's disease **B.** Osteomalacia
C. Osteopetrosis **D.** Osteomyelitis

Ans: A. Paget's disease

Ref: *Robbins Pathologic Basis of Disease, 8th ed.*

Explanation:

Paget Disease (Osteitis Deformans)

- This unique skeletal disease can be divided into three phases:
- An initial osteolytic stage.
- A mixed osteoclastic-osteoblastic stage, which ends with a predominance of osteoblastic activity.

- A burnt-out quiescent osteosclerotic stage.
- The net effect is a **gain in bone mass**; however, the newly formed bone is **disordered** and **architecturally unsound**
- Paget disease usually begins in late adulthood (average age at diagnosis, 70 years) and becomes progressively more common thereafter.

Pathogenesis

- The cause of Paget disease remains uncertain, and current evidence suggests both environmental and genetic factors.
- Autosomal dominant pattern of inheritance (15% to 40%)
- Mutations in the ***SQSTM1*** gene are present in **40% to 50%** of cases of **familial Paget disease**, and in 5% to 10% of patients without a family history.
- The ***SQSTM*** mutations enhance **NF-κB activation** by **RANK signaling**, leading to **increased osteoclast activity**

Morphology

- Shows remarkable histologic variation over time and from site to site.
- The hallmark is the **mosaic pattern** of lamellar bone.
- This pattern, which is likened to a **jigsaw puzzle**, is produced by **prominent cement lines** that **anneal haphazardly oriented units of lamellar bone.**
- In the **initial lytic phase** there are waves of **osteoclastic activity** and numerous **resorption pits**.
- The **osteoclasts** are **abnormally large** and have many more than the **normal 10 to 12 nuclei;** sometimes **100 nuclei** are present.
- Osteoclasts persist in the **mixed phase**, but now many of the bone surfaces are lined by **prominent osteoblasts**.
- The **newly formed bone** may be **woven or lamellar**, but eventually all of it is remodeled into **lamellar bone.**
- As the **mosaic pattern unfolds** and the **cell activity decreases**, the **periosseous fibrovascular tissue recedes** and is replaced by **normal marrow**.
- Bone is larger than normal and composed of coarsely thickened trabeculae and cortices that are soft and porous and lack structural stability. These aspects make the bone vulnerable to deformation under stress; consequently, it fractures easily.

Clinical Course

- Paget disease is monostotic in about **15%** of cases and polyostotic in the remainder.
- The **axial skeleton or proximal femur** is involved in up to **80%** of cases.
- Even though no bone is immune, involvement of the **ribs, fibula, and small bones of the hands and feet** is **unusual.**
- ***Pain*** localized to the affected bone is common.
- It is caused by **microfractures** or by **bone overgrowth** that compresses spinal and cranial nerve roots.
- Enlargement of the **craniofacial skeleton** may produce ***leontiasis ossea*** and a cranium so heavy that is difficult for the person to hold the head erect.
- The weakened pagetic bone may lead to **invagination of the skull base *(platybasiA.*** and compression of the posterior fossa structures.
- Weight bearing causes **anterior bowing of the femurs** and **tibiae** and **distorts the femoral heads**, resulting in the development of ***severe secondary osteoarthritis.***
- ***Chalkstick-type*** **fractures** occur in the long bones of the lower extremities.
- **Compression fractures** of the **spine** result in **spinal cord injury** and the development of **kyphoses**.
- The hypervascularity of pagetic bone warms the overlying skin, and in severe polyostotic disease the increased blood flow acts like an **arteriovenous shunt**, leading to **high-output heart failure** or exacerbation of underlying cardiac disease.
- A variety of **tumor and tumor-like conditions** develop in pagetic bone.
- The benign lesions include giant-cell tumor, giant-cell reparative granuloma, and extra-osseous masses of hematopoiesis. The most dreaded complication is **sarcoma**, which occurs in **0.7% to 0.9%** of all individuals with Paget disease, and in **5% to 10%** of those with **severe polyostotic disease**.
- The **sarcomas** are usually **osteosarcoma** or **fibrosarcoma**, and they arise in Paget lesions in the long **bones, pelvis, skull, and spine**.
- The diagnosis can frequently be made from the **radiographic findings**.
- Pagetic bone is typically enlarged with **thick, coarsened cortices** and **cancellous bone**

- Active disease has a **wedge-shaped lytic leading edge** that may progress along the length of the bone at a rate of **1 cm per year**
- Many affected individuals have elevated **serum alkaline phosphatase levels** and **increased urinary excretion of hydroxyproline.**

3. **Disc prolapse involving L4 nerve root typically presents with: (Repeat)**
   A. Weakness of hip flexion
   B. Absent ankle jerk
   C. Weakness of hip extension
   D. Absent knee jerk

   Ans: D. Absent ankle jerk

Ref: *Harrison's Principles of Internal Medicine, 18th ed.*

Explanation:

Lumbosacral Radiculopathy—Neurologic Features *(See Table 16)*

Neurologic Examination

Deep Tendon Reflexes

- L4 Nerve Root (L3-4 disc): Patellar Reflex or Knee jerk
- S1 Nerve Root (L5-S1 disc): Achilles Reflex or Ankle jerk

Motor Exam

- L4 Nerve Root (L3-4 disc): Ankle dorsiflexion
- L5 Nerve Root (L4-5 disc): Great toe dorsiflexion (extensor hallucis longus)
- S1 Nerve Root (L5-S1 disc): Ankle plantar flexion (gastrocnemius-soleus complex)

Sensory Exam

- L4 Nerve Root (L3-4 disc): Medial malleolus
- L5 Nerve Root (L4-5 disc): Dorsal third metatarsophalangeal joint
- S1 Nerve Root (L5-S1 disc): Lateral heel

Radicular patterns by disc herniation type

Central DIsk herniation

- Nerve root affected is ABOVE the disc
- Example: Central L3 disc herniation causes findings above the L2-3 Nerve root

Paracentral disk herniation

- Nerve root affected is AT the disc
- Example: Paracentral L3 disc herniation causes findings at the L2-3 Nerve root

Lateral disk herniation

- Nerve root affected is BELOW the disc (foraminal effects)

Table 16

	Examination Findings			
Lumbosacral Nerve Roots	**Reflex Absent**	**Sensory**	**Motor**	**Pain Distribution**
L2	—	Upper anterior thigh	Psoas (hip flexion)	Anterior thigh
L3	—	Lower anterior thigh Anterior knee	Psoas (hip flexion) Quadriceps (knee extension) Thigh adduction	Anterior thigh, knee
L4	**Quadriceps (Knee reflex)**	Medial calf	Quadriceps (knee extension) Thigh adduction Tibialis anterior (foot dorsiflexion)	Knee, medial calf Anterolateral thigh
L5	—	Dorsal surface—foot Lateral calf	Peroneii (foot eversion) Tibialis anterior (foot dorsiflexion) Gluteus medius (hip abduction) Toe dorsiflexors	Lateral calf, dorsal foot, posterolateral thigh, buttocks
S1	**Gastrocnemius/soleus (Ankle reflex)**	Plantar surface—foot Lateral aspect—foot	Gastrocnemius/soleus (foot plantar flexion)Abductor hallucis (toe flexors) Gluteus maximus (hip extension)	Bottom foot, posterior calf, posterior thigh, buttocks

- Example: Lateral L3 disc herniation causes findings at the L3-4 Nerve root

4. **All are true about Rotator cuff syndrome *except:***

A. Fracture	**B.** Weakness
C. Tendinitis	**D.** Rupture

Ans: A. Fracture

***Ref:** Apley's System of Orthopedics and Fractures, 9th ed, pg 341.*

Explanation:

The most common cause of pain around the shoulder is a disorder of the rotator cuff.

This is sometimes referred to rather loosely as **'rotator cuff syndrome'**

It comprises at least four conditions with distinct clinical features and natural history:

- Supraspinatus impingement syndrome and tendinitis
- Tears of the rotator cuff
- Acute calcific tendinitis
- Biceps tendinitis and/or rupture.

Clinical Features

Three patterns are encountered:

- **Subacute tendinitis** – the ***'painful arc syndrome'***, due to vascular congestion, microscopic haemorrhage and oedema.
- **Chronic tendinitis** – Recurrent shoulder pain due to tendinitis and fibrosis.
- **Cuff disruption** – Recurrent pain, weakness and loss of movement due to tears in the rotator cuff.

5. **All the following causes osteopenia:**

A. Rickets	**B.** Osteopetrosis
C. Osteomalacia	**D.** Osteonecrosis

Ans: B. Osteopetrosis

***Ref:** Harrison's Principles of Internal Medicine, 18th ed & Nelson Textbook of Pediatrics*

Explanation:

Osteopenia

- It is a condition where bone mineral density is lower than normal.
- It is considered to be a precursor to osteoporosis.
- However, not every person diagnosed with osteopenia will develop osteoporosis.
- Technically, Osteopenia is defined as a **bone mineral density T-score** between **-1.0 and -2.5.**

What is T-score?

- The T-score is the relevant measure when screening for osteoporosis.
- It is the bone mineral density (BM**D.** at the site when compared to the young normal reference mean.
- It is a comparison of a patient's BMD to that of a healthy thirty-year-old.
- The criteria of the World Health Organization are:
  - **Normal** is a T-score of -1.0 or higher
  - **Osteopenia** is defined as between **-1.0 and -2.5**
  - **Osteoporosis** is defined as **-2.5 or lower,** meaning a bone density that is two and a half standard deviations below the mean of a thirty-year-old man/woman.

Causes of Osteopenia

- Rickets
- Metabolic bone disease
- Osteoporosis esp Postmenopausal women
- Osteomalacia
- Rheumatoid arthritis
- Ankylosing spondylitis
- Osteomyelitis
- Osteonecrosis
- Multiple myeloma
- Coeliac disease

6. **Position of lower limb in post polio deformity of hip: (Repeat)**

A. Extension, Adduction, Internal rotation
B. Extension, Abduction, Internal rotation
C. Flexion, Abduction, External rotation
D. Flexion, Adduction, External rotation

Ans: C. FABER

***Ref:** Turek's Orthopaedics –Principles and Their Applications, 4th edition, p 529*

Explanation:

Post polio paralysis

- During the acute and convalescent phases of poliomyelitis the patient lies supine in the so called **'frog-legged'position** with hips flexed **(F)**, abducted **(AB)** and externally rotated **(ER)**; the knees flexed and the feet in equinovarus position.
- Initially this position may be assumed because of the muscle spasm in these muscles.
- Later contractures involving the fascia and intermuscular septum occur.
- Contracture of the muscles contribute at a later stage.

- With the advent of growth these deformities get worse and adaptive bony changes make correction more difficult.

7. **Bone to bone metastasis is commonly seen in:**
   A. Osteosarcoma
   B. Ewing's sarcoma
   C. Chondrosarcoma
   D. Reticulum cell carcinoma

Ans: ?? A or B

***Ref:** Apley's System of Orthopedics and Fractures, 9th ed, pg 216.*

Explanation:

I couldn't find answer in any textbook. But an internet source (without reference/citation) mentioned that Ewings sarcoma and osteosarcoma can cause bony secondaries.

Secondaries in Bone

- The skeleton is one of the commonest sites of secondary cancer;
- In patients over 50 years bone metastases are seen more frequently than all primary malignant bone tumours together.
- The commonest source is carcinoma of the **breast**; next in frequency are carcinomas of the **prostate, kidney, lung, thyroid, bladder** and **gastrointestinal tract.**
- In 10% cases - No primary tumour is found
- The commonest sites for bone metastases are the **vertebrae, pelvis**, the prox**imal half of the femur** and the **humerus**. Spread is usually via the **blood stream.**

8. **Diaphyseal tumor among the following is:**
   A. Chondromyxofibroma
   B. Giant cell tumor
   C. Chondroblastoma
   D. Primitive neuroectodermal bone tumor

Ans: D. Primitive neuroectodermal bone tumor

***Ref:** Robbins Pathologic Basis of Disease, 8th ed. Multiple sources*

Explanation:

Primitive neuroectodermal group of tumor affecting bone is Ewing's sarcoma

Bone tumors according to the site of origin within the bone

Epiphysis

- Chondroblastoma
- Giant cell tumor
- Subchondral bone cyst

Metaphysis

- Non Ossifying Fibroma
- Simple bone cyst
- Chondromyxoid fibroma
- Osteosarcoma
- Chondrosarcoma
- Enchondroma
- Fibrosarcoma
- Osteoblastoma
- Osteoid osteoma
- Aneurysmal bone cyst
- Fibrous dysplasia
- Fibrous cortical defect

Diaphysis

- Ewing's sarcoma,
- Simple bone cyst
- Aneurysmal bone cyst
- Enchondroma
- Fibrous dysplasia
- Osteoblastoma.
- Multiple myeloma
- Eosinophilic granuloma (Langerhans cell histiocytosis)
- Osteoid osteoma
- Adamantinoma

9. **All are true regarding CTEV *except:***
   A. Hindfoot varus
   B. Cavus
   C. Increased dorsiflexion
   D. Forefoot adduction

Ans: C. Increased dorsiflexion

***Ref:** Nelson's Textbook of Pediatrics, 19th ed.*

Explanation:

Plantar flexion (cavus) is seen in CTEV, not increased dorsiflexion

Congenital Talipes Equinovarus (Clubfoot) CTEV

- Deformity involving malalignment of the **calcaneotalar-navicular** complex.
- Components of this deformity - mnemonic **CAVE (cavus, adductus, varus, equinus).**
- **Plantar flexion (cavus)** of the 1st ray and **adduction** of the **forefoot/midfoot** on the **hindfoot**. The **hindfoot** is in **varus** and **equinus**)
- Clubfoot is extremely common in patients with **myelodysplasia** and **arthrogryposis.**
- Congenital clubfoot is seen in approximately 1/1,000 births.
- Etiology is **multifactorial** environmental factors in a genetically susceptible host.

- The risk is approximately 1 in 4 when both a parent and one sibling have clubfeet.
- It occurs more commonly in males **(2:1)**
- Bilateral in **50%** of cases.
- The pathoanatomy involves both **abnormal tarsal morphology (plantar** and **medial deviation** of the **head** and **neck** of the **talus)** and abnormal relationships between the tarsal bones in all three planes.

Clinical Manifestations

- The spine should be inspected for signs of **occult dysraphism**.
- Examination of the infant clubfoot demonstrates **forefoot cavus** and **adductus** and **hindfoot varus** and **equinus.**
- All patients exhibit **calf atrophy**.
- Both **internal tibial torsion** and **leg-length discrepancy** (shortening of the ipsilateral extremity) may be present.

Radiographic Evaluation

- Anteroposterior and lateral radiographs are recommended, often with the foot held in the maximally corrected position.
- The **navicular** bone does not ossify until **3-6 yr** of age
- A common radiographic finding is "**parallelism**" between lines drawn through the axis of the **talus** and the **calcaneus** on the lateral radiograph, indicating **hindfoot varus.**
- Many clinicians believe that **radiographs are not required** in the evaluation and treatment

Treatment

- **Nonoperative treatment** is initiated in **all infants** and should be started **as soon as possible following birth.**
- Techniques have included **taping** and **strapping**, **manipulation** and **serial casting**, and **functional treatment**.
- Historically, a significant percentage of patients treated by manipulation and casting required a surgical release, which was usually performed between 3 and 12 mo of age. Although many feet remain well aligned after surgical releases, a significant percentage of patients have required additional surgery for recurrent or residual deformities.
- **Stiffness** remains a concern at long-term follow-up.
- The **Ponseti method** of clubfoot treatment involves a specific technique for **manipulation** and **serial casting** and may be best described as minimally invasive rather than nonoperative.
- The order of correction follows the mnemonic CAVE. Weekly cast changes are performed, and 5 to 10 casts are typically required.
- The most difficult deformity to correct is the **hindfoot equinus**, for which ~90% of patients require an outpatient **percutaneous tenotomy** of the heel cord.
- Following the tenotomy, a long leg cast with the foot in **maximal abduction (70 degrees)** and **dorsiflexion** is worn for **3 wk**; the patient then begins a **bracing program**.
- An **abduction brace** is worn full time for **3 mo** and then at **nighttime** for **3-5 yr**.
- A subset of patients require transfer of the **tibialis anterior tendon** to the middle cuneiform for **recurrence**. Although most patients require some form of surgery, the procedures are minimal in comparison with a surgical release, which requires **capsulotomy** of the major joints (and lengthening of the muscles) to reposition the joints in space.
- **Functional treatment**, or the **French method**, involves daily manipulations (supervised by a physical therapist) and splinting with elastic tape, as well as continuous passive motion (machine required) while the baby sleeps.
- **Surgical realignment** has a definite role in the management of clubfeet, especially in the minority of congenital clubfeet that have failed nonoperative or minimally invasive methods, and for the neuromuscular and syndromic clubfeet that are characteristically rigid.
- Common surgical approaches include a **release of the involved joints** (realign the tarsal bones), a lengthening of the shortened posteromedial musculotendinous units, and usually pinning of the foot in the corrected position.
- **Triple arthrodesis** is **reserved** as salvage for **painful, deformed feet** in **adolescents** and **adults.**

10. A 60 yrs diabetic presents with swelling and pain in the ankle joint and foot. X-ray shows soft tissue swelling, loose bodies and bony sclerosis. Most probable diagnosis is:

A. Osteoarthritis
B. Neuropathic joint
C. Gouty arthritis
D. Septic arthritis

Ans: B. Neuropathic joint

Ref: *Harrison's Principles of Internal Medicine, 18th ed.*

Explanation:

Neuropathic Joint Disease

- Neuropathic joint disease (Charcot's joint) is a progressive destructive arthritis associated with **loss of pain sensation & proprioception.**
- Normal muscular reflexes that modulate joint movement are decreased.
- Without these protective mechanisms, joints are subjected to repeated trauma, resulting in progressive cartilage and bone damage.
- **Diabetes mellitus** is the **most frequent** cause of neuropathic joint disease.

Causes

- Diabetes mellitus (Most common)
- Tabes dorsalis
- Leprosy
- Yaws
- Syringomyelia
- Meningomyelocele
- Congenital indifference to pain
- Peroneal muscular atrophy (Charcot-Marie-Tooth disease)
- Amyloidosis.

- **Tabes dorsalis**, - Knees, hips, and ankles are most commonly affected
- **Syringomyelia** - Glenohumeral joint, elbow, and wrist
- **Diabetes Mellitus** - ***Tarsal*** and ***tarsometatarsal*** joints are most commonly affected.

Pathology

- There is fragmentation and eventual loss of articular cartilage with eburnation of the underlying bone.
- **Osteophytes** are found at the joint margins.
- **Erosions** are present on the joint surface.
- Fractures, devitalized bone, intraarticular loose bodies, and microscopic fragments of cartilage and bone may be present.

Clinical Manifestations

- Usually begins in a **single joint** and then becomes apparent in other **joints**
- The involved joint progressively enlarges due to **bony overgrowth** and **synovial effusion**.
- **Loose bodies** may be palpated in the joint cavity.
- **Joint instability**, **subluxation**, and **crepitus** occur as the disease progresses.
- Most commonly seen in **diabetes mellitus** (Incidence -0.5%)
- The **tarsal** and **tarsometatarsal** joints are most often affected, followed by the **metatarso-phalangeal** and **talotibial** joints.
- Downward collapse of the tarsal bones leads to convexity of the sole, referred to as a "**rocker foot**".
- **Large osteophytes** may protrude from the top of the foot.
- **Calluses** frequently form over the **metatarsal heads** and may lead to **infected ulcers** and **osteomyelitis**.
- Radiographs may show **resorption** and **tapering** of the **distal metatarsal bones**.
- The term **Lisfranc fracture-dislocation** is sometimes used to describe the destructive changes at the **tarsometatarsal** joints.

11. Fracture of 1st metacarpal bone: (Repeat)

A. Barton's fracture
B. Bennett's fracture
C. Chauffer's fracture
D. Boxer's fracture

Ans: B. Bennett's fracture

Ref: *Apley's Orthopedics, 9th ed. & Internet Sources*

Explanation:

Fracture	Description
Aviator fracture	Fracture of neck of **Talus**
Bankart's fracture	Fracture of **anterior glenoid** associated with **anterior shoulder dislocation**
Barton's fracture	**Distal radius fracture** involving the articular surface with dislocation of the radiocarpal joint
Bennett's fracture	Intra-articular fracture of **base** of **Thumb metacarpal**
Bosworth fracture	Fracture of **distal fibula** with posterior dislocation of the proximal fibula behind the tibia
Boxer's fracture	Fracture of **neck of little metacarpal**
Bumper fracture **tibial plateau**	Compression **fracture of lateral**
Chance fracture	**Horizontal** fracture of **vertebral body**
Chauffeur's fracture	**Intra-articular** fracture of **radial styloid**
Chopart's fracture-dislocation	**Foot dislocation** through **talonavicular and calcaneocuboid** joints with associated **fractures**, usually after ankle twisting.treated in a non weight bearing cast for 6–8 weeks
Clay shoveller's fracture	**Spinous process** fracture of **C6, C7 or T1**
Colles' fracture	**Distal radius fracture** with dorsal angulation, impaction and radial drift
Duverney fracture	Isolated fracture of the **iliac wing**
Essex-Lopresti fracture	Comminuted **radial head** fracture with interosseous membrane disruption and distal radioulnar joint subluxation

Contd.

Contd.

Galeazzi fracture	**Radius shaft** fracture with dislocation of distal radioulnar joint
Gosselin fracture	V-shaped **distal tibia** fracture extending into the tibial plafond
Hangman's fracture	Fracture of **both pedicles of C2**
Hill-Sachs fracture	Impacted **posterior humeral head** fracture occurring during anterior shoulder dislocation
Holstein-Lewis fracture	Fracture of the **distal third of the humerus** resulting in entrapment of the radial nerve
Holdsworth fracture	**Unstable spinal** fracture-dislocation at the thoracolumbar junction
Hume fracture	**Olecranon** fracture with anterior dislocation of radial head
Jefferson fracture	Fracture of **first cervical vertebra**
Jones fracture	Fracture of **base of 5th metatarsal** extending into intermetatarsal joint
Le Fort fractures	Series of **facial fractures**
Le Fort's fracture the ankle	Vertical fracture of **distal fibula** with of avulsion of medial malleolus
Lisfranc fracture	Fracture dislocation of **midfoot**
Maisonneuve fracture	Spiral fracture of **proximal fibula**
Malgaigne's fracture	Vertical **pelvic** fracture through both pubic rami and the ilium orsacroiliac joint with vertical displacement
March fracture	Stress fracture of a **metatarsal** shaft
Monteggia fracture	Proximal **ulna** fracture with dislocation of radial head
Moore's fracture	Distal **radius** fracture with ulnar dislocation and entrapment of styloid process under annular ligament
Pipkin fracture-dislocation	Posterior dislocation of hip with avulsion fracture of fragment of **femoral head** by the ligamentum teres
Pott's fracture	**Bimalleolar** fracture of the ankle
Rolando fracture	Comminuted fracture of **base of first metacarpal**
Runner's fracture	Stress fracture of distal fibula 3–8 cm above the lateral malleolus
Salter–Harris fracture	Fractures involving a growth plate
Segond fracture	Lateral **tibial** plateau avulsion fracture with anterior cruciate ligament tear
Shepherd's fracture	Fracture of the lateral tubercle of the posterior process of the **talus**
Smith's fracture	**Distal radius** fracture with volar displacement
Stieda fracture	Avulsion fracture of the **medial femoral condyle** at the origin of the medial collateral ligament
Tillaux fracture	Salter–Harris III fracture of the **tibia**
Toddler's fracture	Undisplaced spiral fracture of **distal tibia** in children under 8 years old

12. Least common joint to be affected in ankylosing spondylitis is:

A. Sacroiliac joint
B. Temporomandibular joint
C. Costovertebral joint
D. Hip joint

Ans: B. Temporomandibular joint

Ref: *Harrison's Principles of Internal Medicine, 18th ed.*

Explanation:

"Sacroiliitis is often the earliest manifestations of AS"

AS primarily affects the **axial skeleton** and **peripheral joints**

- Common sites include the:
  - Sacroiliac joint
  - Costosternal junctions
  - Spinous processes
  - Iliac crests
  - Greater trochanters
  - Ischial tuberosities
  - Tibial tubercles
  - Heels
  - **Arthritis** in the **hips** and **shoulders** ("root" joints) occurs in **25–35%** of patients.
  - Severe isolated hip arthritis or bony chest pain may be the presenting complaint.

OBS AND GYNE

1. Magnesium sulphate is contraindicated in:

A. Placenta previa **B.** Preeclampsia
C. Epilepsy **D.** Myasthenia gravis

Ans: D. Myasthenia gravis

Ref: *Dutta: Textbook of Obstetrics 7th ed pg 508,509,234*

Explanation:

MAGNESIUM SULPHATE

- Acts by **competitive inhibition of calcium ion** either at **motor end plate.**
- At **cell membrane**: It decreases **calcium influx, decreases Ach release** and its sensitivity at motor end plate.
- It acts as a **direct depressant on uterine muscle** causes **vasodilation** and **increases cerebral**, uterine and **renal blood flow**.
- It **decreases intracranial edema.**
- **Pritchard regimen**—4gm 20% soln given slow I.V. over 15 to 20 min and 4 gm i.m. in each buttock {loading dose}. Further 4gm given i.m. in alternate buttocks every 4 hours till 24 hours

- Therapeutic level of mgso4 4 to 7 meq/l

Side effect

  - Flushing
  - Perspiration
  - Headache
  - Muscle weakness
  - Pulmonary edema.
- In **neonate** it causes **lethargy**, ***hypotonia*** and ***respiratory depression.***
- **Contraindications—myasthenia gravis, impaired renal function.**
- **Antidote**—Inj. **calcium gluconate** 10% 10ml I.V.

2. **Pseudomyxoma peritonei occurs due to:**
A. Mucinous cystadenoca ovary
B. Ca colon
C. Adenoma stomach
D. Pancreatic adenocarcinoma

Ans: A. Mucinous cystadenoca ovary

Ref: *Shaws Textbook of Gynecology 15th ed pg 375*

Explanation:

MUCINOUS TUMOURS OF OVARY

- Multiloculated cyst lined by **columnar epithelium**
- Cut surface shows multilocular and **honey comb appearance**
- Can grow to large size **5 to 10 kgs, pedunculated.**
- Usually unilateral (Bilateral in 5% cases)
- Usually Benign (5 to 10% malignant).
- Bilateral — metastasis from GI tract, mucocele of appendix, primary adenoca appendix.
- In women **30 to 60** years.
- Has a **glistening** surface.
- If tumor ruptures it may lead to formation of **pseudomyxoma peritonei** and viscera show extensive adhesions.
- **Appendicectomy** prevents this condition as mucocele of appendix often causes this complication.

3. **Most ideal site for sterilisation by tubectomy is:**
A. Ampulla **B.** Isthumus
C. Fimbriated extremity **D.** Interstitial portion

Ans: B. Isthumus

Ref: *Dutta Textbook of Gynecology 7th ed pg 554*

Explanation:

- Most ideal site for tubectomy consists mainly of **isthumus** and **ampullary part of tube** [proximal and middle 3rd].

METHODS OF STERILISATION

- **Pomeroy Tubal Ligation** — In this method of tubal ligation, a loop of tube is "strangled" with a suture. Usually, the loop is cut and the ends cauterized or "burned".
- **Uchida technique**—Proximal end of resected tube is buried into the serous coat along the antimesentric border.
- **Irving procedure**—The proximal ends of the tube are buried into the posterior surface of uterus.
- **Madlener technique**—Loop of the tube is crushed with artery forceps and tied with black silk.
- **Kroener method** of fimbriectomy.
- **laparoscopic method** using **rings, clips** and **electrocoagulation.**

4. **Most common site of fertilisation is:**
A. Interstitium
B. Isthumus
C. Ampulla
D. Infundibulum

Ans: C. Ampulla

Ref: *Dutta: Textbook of Obstetrics 7th ed pg 21, 22*

Explanation:

FERTILISATION

- Process of fusion of sperm with ovum forming zygote.
- Fertilisation occurs in the ampullary end of the tube.

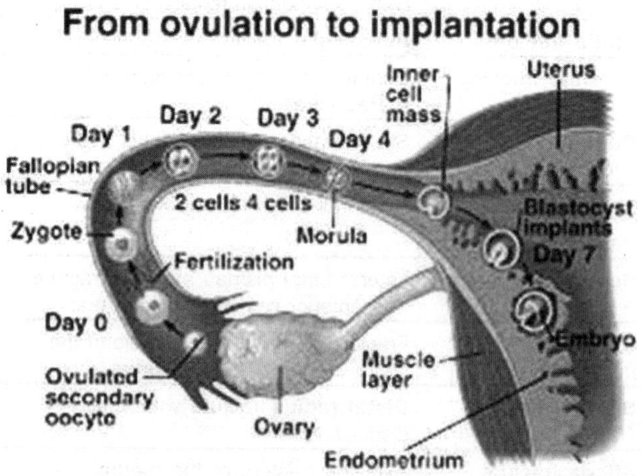

- Complete dissolution of **corona radiata** occurs by chemical action of **hyaluronidase** liberated from **acrosomal cap** of hundreds of **sperm** present at the site.

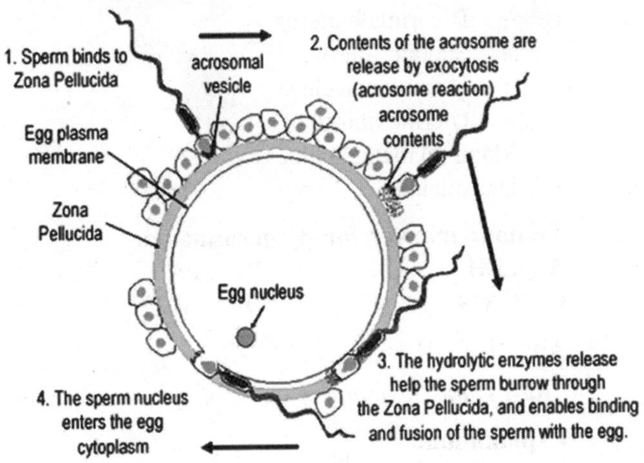

5. **How will you prevent bleeding after IUCD insertion?**
   A. Aspirin
   B. Progesterone only pill
   C. Combined oral pills
   D. Tranexamic acid

Ans: D. Tranexamic acid

Ref: *Dutta: Textbook of Obstetrics, 7th ed pg 540*

Explanation:

– The excessive bleeding after IUCD insertion involves increased menstrual blood loss, prolongation of duration of periods, intermenstrual bleeding.
– Tranexamic acid may be given for short term relief.

Adverse Effects or Complications from IUDs

- Cramping
- Displaced threads
- Ectopic pregnancy
- Embedment or fragmentation of IUD
- Expulsion
- Infertility
- Pelvic infections
- Septicemia during pregnancy
- Tubo-ovarian damage
- Uterine or cervical perforation
- Vaginal bleeding, with or without anemia
- Vasovagal reaction (on insertion)

6. **Not an epithelial tumor: (Repeat)**
   A. Hilus cell tumor
   B. Clear cell carcinoma
   C. Transitional cell tumor
   D. Endometrioid ca

Ans: A. Hilus cell tumor

Ref: *Shaws Textbook of Gynecology 15th ed pg 367*

Explanation:

- **Hilus cell (similar to leydig cells) tumor** is a **virilising mesenchymoma.**
- Clear cell ca is otherwise mesonephroid tumor of epithelial origin.
- **Transitional cell Ca** includes **benign and malignant brenner tumor.**

WHO classification of ovarian tumours

I	**Common epithelial tumours:**
	• Serous tumours • Mucinous tumours • Endometrioid tumours • Clear cell (mesonephroid tumours) • Brenner tumours • Mixed epithelial tumours • Undifferentiated carcinoma • Unclassified epithelial tumours
II	**Sex cord (gonadal stromal) tumours:**
	• Granulosa-stromal cell tumours, theca cell tumours • Androblastomas: Sertoli-Leydig cell tumours • Gynandroblastomas • Unclassified
III	**Lipid (lipoid) cell tumours**
IV	**Germ cell tumours:**
	• Dysgerminoma • Endodermal sinus tumour (Yolk sac tumor) • Embryonal carcinoma • Polyembryoma • Choriocarcinoma • Teratoma • Mixed forms
V	**Gonadoblastoma:**
	• Pure • Mixed with dysgerminoma or other germ cell tumours
VI	**Soft tissue tumours not specific to ovary**
VII	**Unclassified tumours**
VIII	**Secondary (metastatic) tumours**
IX	**Tumour-like conditions**

7. **Which is the most common ovarian tumor in pregnancy?**
   A. Serous cystadenoma
   B. Mucinous cystadenoma
   C. Dermoid tumor
   D. Solid teratoma

Ans: C. Dermoid tumor

Ref: Dutta: Textbook of Obstetrics 7th ed pg 310

Explanation:

OVARIAN TUMOR IN PREGNANCY

- Incidence—1 in 2000
- Incidence of **dermoid cyst** increased two folds in pregnancy
- **Effects of tumor:**
  - Retention of urine
  - Malpresentation
  - Mechanical distress
  - Non engagement of head
- **Effects on tumor:**
  - Torsion
  - Hemorrhage
  - Rupture
  - Infection
- Diagnosis—abdominal examination to detect swelling
- Vaginal examination-**Hingorani Sign**—a groove felt in between uterus and tumor
- Investigations-**USG**
- Treatment—Surgery best **14 to 16 weeks** if uncomplicated.
- If complicated, surgery is performed irrespective of gestation

8. **Most common cause of spontaneous abortion in first trimester:**
A. Chromosomal anomalies
B. Uterine anomalies
C. Antiphospholipid antibody syndrome
D. Hypothyroidism

Ans: A. Chromosomal anomalies

Ref: Dutta: Textbook of Obstetrics 7th ed pg 160

Explanation:

COMMON CAUSES OF MISCARRIAGE

First Trimester

- Genetic factors [50%]
- Endocrine [LPD, Thyroid abnormalities, Diabetes]
- Immunological disorders [Autoimmune, Alloimmune]
- Infection
- Unexplained

Second Trimester

- Anatomic
  - Cervical incompetence
  - Bicornuate uterus
  - Septate uterus
  - Uterine synechiae
  - Uterine fibroid
- Maternal medical illness
- Unexplained

9. **Tumour marker for dysgerminoma:**
A. LDH **B.** CEA
C. CA19 **D.** CA125

Ans: A. LDH

Ref: Dutta Textbook of Gynecology 5th ed pg 367

Explanation:

DYSGERMINOMA

- Most common **malignant germ cell tumour**
- Arises from undifferentiated form of germ cells
- Majority occurs before 30 years
- **HCG** assays are **positive**
- 20 to 30 % occurs in pregnancy
- May be associated with **endodermal sinus tumour** or **choriocarcinoma**
- **5 to 15** cm diameter
- Micro—**Uniform large round cells**
- Treatment—Laparotomy, surgical staging and unilateral salpingooopherectomy [for stage 1] with chemotherapy
- Chemotherapy—Carboplatin, BEP,VBP,VAC regimens[bleomycin, etoposide, cisplatin, vinblastine, actinomycin D, cyclophosphamide]
- Combination chemotherapy for recurrent disease—POMB-ACE [Vincristine, Bleomycin, Methotrexate, Cisplatin, Etoposide, Actinomycin D, Cyclophosphamide]
- Tumour markers—**HCG, AFP, LDH**

10. **Vasectomy leads to all *except:* (Repeat)**
A. Decreased libido
B. Sperm granuloma
C. Antisperm antibody
D. Infection

Ans: A. Decreased libido

Reference: *Bailey and Love's Short Practice of Surgery 25th Edition*

Explanation:

Complications of Vasectomy

Short-term complications include:

- Temporary bruising,
- Genito urinary infection (2.5%)
- Fistula

- Bleeding/ Hematoma

The primary long-term complications are

- Vasectomy failure (0.2%)
- ***Chronic pain (Orchalgia)*** conditions or syndromes that can affect any of the scrotal, pelvic and/or lower-abdominal regions, known as ***post-vasectomy pain syndrome***.
- After a vasectomy, the natural duct for sperm, the vas deferens, is closed off. The testicles continue to produce sperm at a rate of about 50,000 cells per minute. These sperm cells build up pressure in the delicate epididymis portion of the testicles, which eventually ruptures from the pressure. This can occur spontaneously or often when there is stress in the area, such as when a man is ejaculating. These ruptures can lead to what many men have described as an ***ice pick-in-the-testicle-like sensation.***
- Long-term post-vasectomy pain (2% -33%)
- ***Antisperm antibodies***

Post-vasectomy pain syndrome (PVPS)

- It is chronic and debilitating condition that may develop immediately or several years after vasectomy.
- The pain can be constant orchialgia or epididymal pain, or it can be pain that occurs only at particular times such as with intercourse, ejaculation, or physical exertion.

11. Most common cause of vesicovaginal fistula is: (Repeat)

A. Laparoscopy
B. Abdominal hysterctomy
C. Obstructed labour
D. Cystoscopy

Ans: C. Obstructed labour

Ref: *DC Dutta's Textbook of Gynaecology 6th edition pg 401*

Explanation:

VESICOVAGINAL FISTULA

- **MC type** of genito urinary fistula
- **Causes**

A. Obstetrical :

- Accounts for **80 % cases of VVF in developing countries**
- 5 - 15 % cases in developed countries
- VVF may result from
  - **Ischaemia**
    - o Obstructed labour : Ischaemic necrosis of the bladder base following prolonged compression of the bladder base between fetal head and pubic symphysis – infection – sloughing – fistula
    - o **Take 3-5 days following delivery to roduce ischaemic fistula**
    - o MC in developing countries
  - **Traumatic**
    - o Instrumental vaginal delivery
      - ·· Forceps – specially with **Kielland's** forceps
      - ·· Destructive operations
      - ·· Instruments used for **Craniotomy** procedure – perforators and cranioclasts
      - ·· Injury may be inflicted by bony spicule of fetal skull
    - o Abdominal surgeries
      - ·· Hysterectomy for rupture uterus
      - ·· LSCS
  - **Traumatic injuries manifests soon after delivery**

B. Gynaecological causes:

- Accounts for **80 % fistulas in developed countries**
- **MC type** of VVF in **developed** countries
- **Causes**
  - Operative injury – anterior colporrhaphy, TAH
  - **Traumatic** – illegal abortions, pelvic fractures
  - Advanced **malignancies** of genital tract organs
  - **Radiation therapy** for Ca cervix
    - o Due to end **arteritis obliterans**
    - o Takes long time to develop – 1-2 yrs
  - Infective – vaginal TB, LGV, Schistosomiasis, Actinomycosis
  - **Uretero vaginal fistula**
    - o **2nd common cause** of urinary fistula
    - o MC site of injury to **ureter**
      - ·· In hysterectomies - Ureteric tunnel in Mackenrodt's ligament
      - ·· In radical surgery for Ca cervix - Near crossing of pubocervical ligament

12. Clue cells are seen in: (REPEAT 2013)

A. Bacterial vaginosis
B. Moniliasis

C. Trichomoniasis
D. Gardenella vaginalis

Ans: A. Bacterial vaginosis

***Ref:** Shaw's Textbook of Gynecology 15th edition pg.131*

Explanation:

GARDNERELLA VAGINOSIS

- Alteration in normal vaginal flora
- **Decrease in number of lactobacilli in vaginal discharge** - lactobacilli reduce pH and release hydrogen peroxide toxic to other bacteria
- 100 fold increase in anerobic bacteria
- **Hemophilus vaginalis, Gardnerella, Mobiluncus and Mycoplasma hominis**—cause
- Vaginal discharge without discharge
- White, milky non-viscous discharge, **pH** of discharge more than **4.5**
- **Whiff Test - Fishy odour** when vaginal discharge is mixed with 10% KOH - due to release of amino metabolites from various organisms
- Presence of **Clue Cells** - epithelial cells with granular cytoplasm caused by gram negative bacilli adhering on the surface
- Wet smear, gram stain and culture are investigations

Treatment:

- Metronidazole 500mg bd for 7 days
- Ampicillin 500mg or cephalosporin 500mg bd for 7 days
- Tetracycline 500mg 4 times a day
- Doxycycline 100mg bd
- Sulphafurazole 1g 4 times daily for 10-14 days
- Clindamycin 300mg daily for 7 days
- Clindamycin 2%cream locally
- Ornidazole 500mg vaginal tablet for 7 days
- **Lacteal** is protein free acidifying lactate gel neutralises vaginal ph 5ml applied for 7 days

AMSEL CRITERIA for diagnosing Bacterial Vagninosis

- Thin, white, yellow, homogeneous discharge
- Clue cells on microscopy
- pH of vaginal fluid >4.5
- Release of a fishy odor on adding alkali—10% potassium hydroxide (KOH) solution.
- **At least three of the four criteria** should be present for a confirmed diagnosis.

13. Which is not a complication specific to monochorionic twins?

A. Malpresentation
B. Conjoint twins
C. Twin to twin transfusion
D. Growth retardation of one fetus

Ans: A. Malpresentation

***Ref:** Dutta: Textbook of Obstetrics 5th ed pg 307*

Explanation:

Problems specific to Monochorionic Twins

- Twin to twin transfusion syndrome
- Twin reverse arterial perfusion (TRAP) or Acardiac twin
- Monoamnionicity – High mortality due to cord problems
- Dead fetus syndrome
- Conjoint twins
- Discordant twins

14. Ca cervix with involvment of upper 1/3rd vagina but not the parametrium is: (Repeat)

A. Stage IIA **B.** Stage IIIA
C. Stage IIB **D.** Stage IIIB

Ans: A. Stage IIA

***Ref:** Shaw's Textbook of Gynecolgy pg 412*

Explanation:

CARCINOMA CERVIX STAGING

Stage I

- Stage I is carcinoma strictly confined to the cervix;
- The diagnosis of both Stages IA1 and IA2 should be based on microscopic examination of removed tissue, preferably a cone, which must include the entire lesion.
  - **Stage IA**: Invasive cancer identified only microscopically. Invasion is limited to measured stromal invasion with a maximum depth of 5 mm and no wider than 7 mm.
    - **Stage IA1**: Stage IA1: Measured invasion of the stroma no greater than 3 mm in depth and no wider than 7 mm diameter.
    - **Stage IA2**: Stage IA2: Measured invasion of stroma greater than 3 mm but no greater than 5 mm in depth and no wider than 7 mm in diameter.
  - **Stage IB**: Stage IB: Clinical lesions confined to the cervix or preclinical lesions greater than Stage Ia. All gross lesions even with superficial invasion are Stage IB cancers.
    - **Stage IB1**: Stage IB1: Clinical lesions no greater than 4 cm in size.

- o **Stage IB2**: Stage IB2: Clinical lesions greater than 4 cm in size.

Stage II

- Stage II is carcinoma that extends beyond the cervix, but does not extend into the pelvic wall.
- The carcinoma involves the vagina, but not as far as the lower third.
  - **Stage IIA**: No obvious parametrial involvement. Involvement of up to the upper two-thirds of the vagina.
  - **Stage IAB**: Obvious parametrial involvement, but not into the pelvic sidewall.

Stage III

- Stage III is carcinoma that has extended into the pelvic sidewall.
- On rectal examination, there is no cancer-free space between the tumour and the pelvic sidewall.
- The tumour involves the lower third of the vagina.
- All cases with ***hydronephrosis*** or a non-functioning kidney are Stage III cancers.
  - **Stage IIIA**: No extension into the pelvic sidewall but involvement of the lower third of the vagina.
  - **Stage IIIB**: Extension into the pelvic sidewall or hydronephrosis or non-functioning kidney.

Stage IV

- Stage IV is carcinoma that has extended beyond the true pelvis or has clinically involved the mucosa of the bladder and/or rectum.
  - **Stage IVA**: Spread of the tumour into adjacent pelvic organs.
  - **Stage IVB**: Spread to distant organs.

15. Schiller duval bodies seen in: (REPEAT 2013)

A. Endodermal sinus tumour
B. Embryonal carcinoma
C. Dermoid cyst
D. Brenner tumour

Ans: A. Endodermal sinus tumour

***Ref:** Dutta Textbook of Gynecology 5th edition pg.368*

Explanation:

- **Schiller duval bodies** are characteristic histological feature of **endodermal sinus tumour**.
- They are tuft of vascular tissue inside cystic spaces lined by flattened epithelium.

ENDODERMAL SINUS TUMOUR

- Originate from **multipotential embryonal tissue** as a result of selective differentiation of yolk sac structures
- Peak - 15 to 20 years of age
- Second most common malignant germ cell tumour of ovary
- Unilateral, solid, >10 cms diameter
- **Micro-schiller duval bodies**, eosinophilic hyaline bodies containing alphaprotein
- Associated with **dysgerminoma**
- Treatment- surgical staging and unilateral salpingo oopherectomy
- **Combination chemotherapy - POMB-ACE regimen** (cyclophosphamide, vincristine, methotrexate, bleomycin, actinomycin D, cisplatin, etoposide) **VAC regimen, VBP regimen**
- Tumor marker- **alphafetoprotein >20 microgm/ml**, Elevated **alpha 1 antitrypsin**
- Respond well to chemotherapy and good survival rate

16. Least common tumor in vagina among the following is: (Repeat)

A. Metastasis from cervix
B. Metastasis from endometrium
C. Metastasis from choriocarcinoma
D. Primary vaginal carcinoma

Ans: D. Primary vaginal carcinoma

***Ref:** Dutta Textbook of Gynecology 5th ed pg 325*

Explanation:

PRIMARY VAGINAL CARCINOMA

- Incidence very rare 0.6 per 100000 women [**1%** of genital malignancies]
- Etiology:
  - HPV
  - **VAIN** [vaginal intraepithelial neoplasia]
  - Diethyl stilboesterol
  - Irradiation
  - Pessary usage
  - White race
- **Upper 3rd** of vaginal **posterior** wall
- **MC - Squamous cell ca 90%,** adenoca, melanoma, sarcoma
- Spread- lymphatic, direct and blood borne
- C/f—abnormal vaginal bleeding, foul smelling discharge
- Investigations—cytolgy, colposcopy, biopsy
- Treatment—surgery and radiotherapy

SECONDARY VAGINAL CA

- Follows ca of cervix, vulva, urethra by direct spread

- Metastasis in **lower 3rd vagina** or **vault** occurs in choriocarcinoma or endometrial ca
- Commoner than primary ca

17. OC pills prevent all *except:* (Repeat)

A. Ca colon
B. Ca endometrium
C. Ca breast
D. Ca cervix

Ans: D. Ca cervix

Ref: *Shaw's Textbook of Gynaecology 15th Edition Pg: 232.*

Explanation:

Infact, OCPs are associated with increased risk of Endocervical cancer.

OCPS & Malignancy

- **Combined OC pills** reduce the incidence of **ovarian cancer** by **40%** and **uterine cancer** by 50% if taken for 1 year.
- Risk of **Colonic** and **anorectal** cancer is reduced by **30-40%.**
- Regarding **breast cancer**, the role of combined pills is still **controversial**. Some studies reported that women who took combined pills for more than 4 years are at risk of breast cancer. But the risk disappears after 10 years of stopping the drug. But, lately evidence based data fail to prove the adverse role of pills on breast cancer.
- Regarding cervical cancer, risk of **endocervical cancer** is **increased** has been reported in women who used combined pills for more than 5 years.
- OCPs are also associated with Hepatocellular Carcinoma.

Benefits of combined OC pills:

- Menorrhagia
- Polymenorrhea
- Dysmenorrhea
- Premenstrual tension
- Benign breast neoplasia
- Functional ovarian cysts
- PID
- Rheumatoid arthritis
- Acne
- PCOD
- Endometriosis
- Ovarian cancer
- Endometrial cancer
- Anorectal cancer
- Colon cancer

18. Primary amenorrhoea is seen in all *except:* (Repeat)

A. Kallman syndrome
B. Rokitansky syndrome
C. Ashermann syndrome
D. Turner's syndrome

Ans: C. Ashermann syndrome

Ref: *Dutta's Gynecology pg 433*

Explanation:

(See Table 17 and Figure on the next page)

Asherman's syndrome or Fritsch syndrome

- It is characterized by **adhesions** and **fibrosis** of the **endometrium.**
- Most often associated with **dilation** and **curettage** of the **intrauterine cavity**.
- Patients present with **secondary amenorrhea.**

Table 17 : Causes of Primary Amenorrhea

Outflow tract Anomalies/ obstruction	Gonadal/end-organ disorders	Pituitary and hypothalamic
Uterine: ▪ Mullerian agenesis (2nd MC cause) Vaginal: ▪ Vaginal atresia, ▪ Cryptomenorrhoea ▪ Imperforate hymen.	▪ **Gonadal dysgenesis**, including Turner syndrome, is the most common cause ▪ **Androgen insensitivity** syndrome (Testicular feminization syndrome) ▪ **Receptor abnormalities for hormones FSH and LH** ▪ Specific forms of **congenital adrenal hyperplasia** ▪ **Swyer syndrome** ▪ **Galactosaemia** ▪ **Aromatase deficiency** ▪ **Prader-Willi syndrome** ▪ **Male pseudo-hermaphroditism**	Hypothalamic: **Kallmann syndrome**

Approach to Primary Amenorrhea

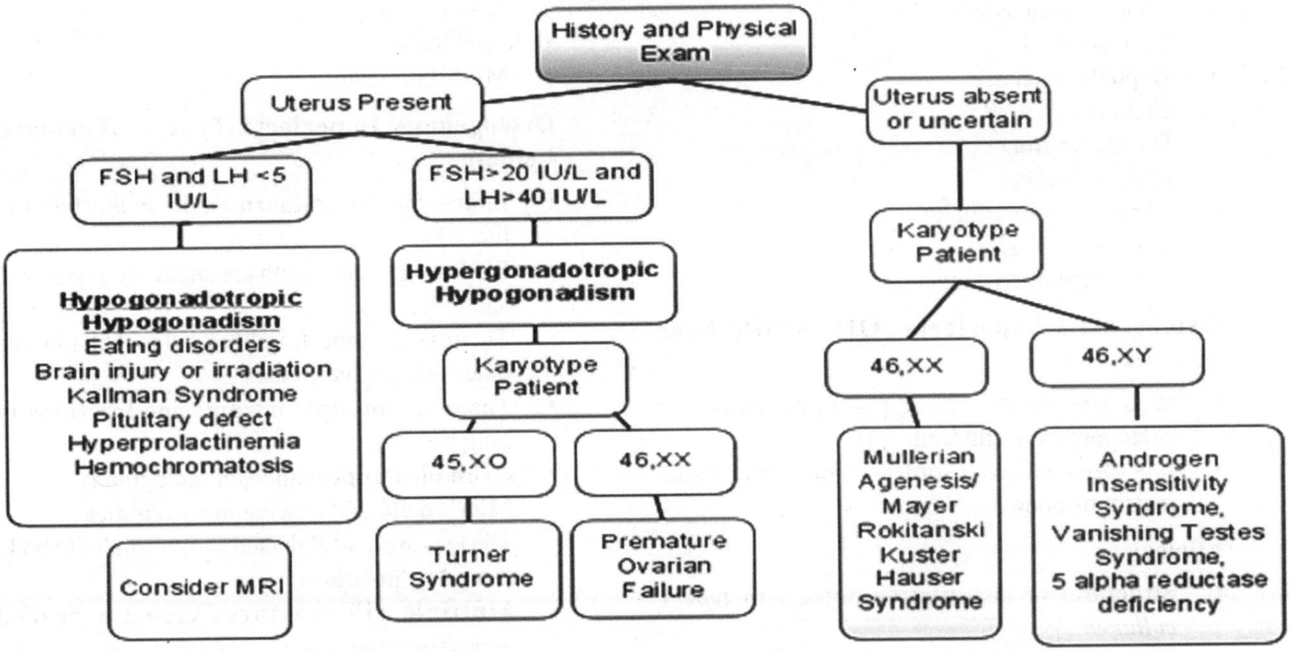

PEDIATRICS

1. **Most common cause of Acute otitis media in children is:**
   - **A.** Strep pneumoniae
   - **B.** Strep pyogenes
   - **C.** Staph aureus
   - **D.** Pseudomonas

Ans: A. Strep pneumoniae

Ref: *Nelson's Textbook of Pediatrics. 19th Edition*

Explanation:

Three pathogens predominate in Acute Otitis Media (AOM)

- *Streptococcus pneumoniae* (MC Organism)
- Nontypeable *Haemophilus influenzae*
- *Moraxella catarrhalis.*

Less common causes

- Group A streptococcus
- *Staphylococcus aureus*
- Gram-negative organisms.
- *Alloiococcus otitidis.*
- Rhinovirus
- Respiratory syncytial virus (RSV)

→ "*In countries where widespread use of conjugate pneumococcal vaccine is employed, nontypeable H. influenzae has overtaken S. pneumoniae as the most common pathogen; found in 40-50% of cases"(Ref: Neslon)*

Organisms causing Chronic suppurative otitis media (CSOM) in children

- *Pseudomonas aeruginosa (MC Organism)*
- *Staph aureus*
- *Streptococcus pneumoniae*
- *Nontypeable Haemophilus influenzae*
- *Moraxella catarrhalis.*

2. **Child with recurrent fractures and wormian bones is most likely to have:**
   - **A.** Osteogenesis imperfecta
   - **B.** Rickets
   - **C.** Battered baby syndrome
   - **D.** Shaken baby syndrome

Ans: A. Osteogenesis imperfecta

Ref: *Nelson's Textbook of Pediatrics. 19th Edition*

Explanation:

- **Soft areas (craniotabes)** are occasionally found in the **parietal bones** at the vertex near the sagittal suture; they are more common in **premature infants** and in infants who have been exposed to **uterine compression.** Though such soft areas are usually insignificant.
- Soft areas in the **occipital region** suggest the irregular calcification and **wormian bone formation.**

Conditions associated with Wormian bones

- Osteogenesis imperfecta
- Cleidocranial dysostosis
- Lacunar skull
- Hypophosphatasia
- Cretinism
- Down syndrome.
- Healing Rickets
- Chronic hydrocephalus
- Pyknodysostosis
- Pachydermoperiostosis

Osteogenesis imperfecta (OI) (brittle bone disease)

- It is the most common genetic cause of osteoporosis in children.
- It is a generalized disorder of connective tissue matrix of bone.

Etiology

- Structural or quantitative defects in ***type I collagen***.
- Type I collagen is the primary component of the extracellular matrix of bone and skin.
- Other cases are caused by recessive null mutations in a collagen-modifying enzyme, ***prolyl 3-hydroxylase 1*** (coded by the *LEPRE1* gene on chromosome 1p34.1) or its associated protein, ***CRTAP.***

Pathology

- The bone matrix contains ***abnormal type I collagen fibrils.***
- Relatively ***increased*** levels of ***types III and V collagen***.
- Several noncollagenous proteins of bone matrix are also reduced.
- The ***hydroxyapatite crystals*** deposited on matrix are poorly aligned with the long axis of fibrils.

Clinical Manifestations

OI has the triad of

- Fragile bones
- Blue sclerae
- Early deafness.

The ***Sillence classification*** divides OI into four types based on clinical and radiographic criteria.

Osteogenesis Imperfecta Type I (Mild)

- Mild disease
- Families have blue sclerae
- Recurrent fractures in childhood, and
- Presenile hearing loss (30-60%).
- **Dentinogenesis imperfecta**.
- Easy bruising
- Joint laxity
- Mild short stature

Osteogenesis Imperfecta Type II (Perinatal Lethal)

- Infants may be **stillborn or die** in the 1st yr of life.
- Birthweight and length are small for gestational age.
- There is extreme fragility of the skeleton and other connective tissues.
- There are **multiple intrauterine fractures** of long bones
- **Crumpled appearance** on radiographs
- **Micromelia** and bowing of extremities
- The legs are held abducted at right angles to body **(frog-leg position)**
- **Multiple rib fractures** create a beaded appearance, and the
- **Small thorax** leading to respiratory insufficiency.
- The skull is large for body size, with enlarged anterior and posterior fontanels.
- **Sclerae are dark blue-gray**.

Osteogenesis Imperfecta Type III (Progressive Deforming)

- Most severe nonlethal form of OI
- Results in significant physical disability.
- Birthweight and length are often low normal.
- Fractures usually occur in utero.
- Relative **macrocephaly** and **triangular facies**
- Fractures occur from inconsequential trauma and heal with deformity.
- Disorganization of the bone matrix results in a **"popcorn" appearance** at the **metaphyses**
- Basal Flaring of rib cage has & Pectal deformity.
- **Scoliosis** and **vertebral compression**.
- **Extreme short stature**.
- Scleral hue ranges from white to blue.

Osteogenesis Imperfecta Type IV (Moderately Severe)

- In utero fractures & congenital bowing of lower long bones.
- Recurrent fractures after ambulation.
- Fracture rates decrease after puberty.
- X-ray: osteoporosis; metaphyseal flaring and vertebral compressions
- Moderate short stature.

- Scleral hue may be blue or white.

Osteogenesis Imperfecta Type V (Hyperplastic Callus) and Type VI (Mineralization Defect)

- Have distinct findings on bone histology.
- Hyperplastic callus
- Calcification of the interosseous membrane of the forearm
- Radiodense metaphyseal band.
- The genetic etiology is unknown. (No collagen defect)
- They constitute <5% of OI populations.

Osteogenesis Imperfecta Types VII and VIII (Recessive Form)

- Types VII and VIII patients have null mutations in ***P3H1*** and ***CRTAP***, respectively.
- Clinically they **overlap types II and III OI**
- Distinct features including
- **White sclerae**
- **Rhizomelia**
- Small to normal head circumference
- Surviving children have **severe osteochondrodysplasia**
- Extreme short stature
- Dual energy X-ray absorptiometry (DEXa) L1-L2 z-score in the -6 to -7 range

3. **Cleft lip is repaired at: (Repeat)**
   A. 2 - 4month **B.** 1 - 4 weeks
   C. 6 - 12 months **D.** 12 - 18 months

   Ans: A. 2 – 4 months

   Ref: *Nelson's Textbook of Pediatrics. 19th Edition*

   Explanation:

   "Surgical closure of a ***cleft lip*** *is usually performed by* ***3 mo of age****, when the infant has shown satisfactory weight gain and is free of any oral, respiratory, or systemic infection." Ref: Nelson*

   "In an otherwise healthy child, ***closure of the palate*** *is usually done* ***before 1 yr of age*** *to enhance normal speech development." Ref: Nelson*

   - Modification of the **Millard rotation-advancement technique** is the most commonly used technique; a staggered suture line minimizes notching of the lip from retraction of scar tissue.
   - The initial repair may be revised at **4 or 5 yr** of age.
   - **Corrective surgery** on the nose may be **delayed until adolescence.**
   - Nasal surgery can also be performed at the time of the lip repair.
   - Cosmetic results depend on the extent of the original deformity, healing potential of the individual patient, absence of infection, and the skill of the surgeon.

4. **Parkland formula is: (Repeat)**
   A. %of burn area*body wt*4
   B. %of burn area*body wt / 4
   C. %of burn area*body surface area*4
   D. %of burn area*body surface area / 4

   Ans: A. % of burn area*body wt*4

   Ref: *Nelson's Textbook of Pediatrics. 19th Edition*

   Explanation:

   Parkland's Formula

   Total percentage body surface area × weight (kg) × 4 = volume (ml)
   Half this volume is given in the first 8 hours, and the second half is given in the next 16 hours

5. **Surfactant is produced by: (Repeat)**
   A. Type 2 pneumocytes
   B. Type 1 Pneumocytes
   C. Clara cells
   D. Endothelium

   Ans: A. Type 2 pneumocytes

   Ref: *Nelson's Textbook of Pediatrics. 19th Edition*

   Explanation:

   - **Surfactant** is produced by **Type 2 pneumocytes**

6. **First sinus to develop in a growing fetus:**
   A. Maxillary **B.** Frontal
   C. Ethmoidal **D.** Sphenoidal

   Ans: A. Maxillary

   Ref: *Nelson's Textbook of Pediatrics. 19th Edition*

   Explanation:

   - Ethmoid sinus is significantly developed at birth

   (See Table 18 on the next page)

7. **Maintenance IV fluids per day for child weighing 10 kg: (Repeat)**
   A. 400 ml **B.** 500 ml
   C. 800 ml **D.** 1000 ml

   Ans: A. 1000 ml/day

   Ref: *Nelson's Textbook of Pediatrics. 19th Edition.*

   Explanation:

   The Holliday-Segar Method:

   - In the Holliday-Segar Method, fluid and electrolyte requirements are empirically based

Table 18 : Radiological appearance of Different sinuses

Maxillary	Status at birth	Growth	First radiological evidence
	Present	Rapid growth from birth to 3 years and 7-12 years. Reaches adult size by 15 years	4-5 months after birth
Ethmoid	Present	Reaches adult size by 12 years	1 year
Frontal	Absent	Invades frontal bone by age of 4 years and increases till teens	6 years
Sphenoid	Absent	Reaches sella turcica by age of 7 years, dorsum sellae by late teens and basisphenoid by adult age and reaches full size between 15 years to adult age.	4 years

on the caloric needs of the average hospital patient.

- The same formula is used for calculating **calorie requirement** as well as **fluid requirement**

Relation of Body Weight to Maintenance fluids	
For each kilogram in this range	Daily fluid requirement per kilogram
First 1-10 kg	100 ml/kg/day
Next 11-20 kg	50 ml/kg/day
For >20 kg	20 ml/kg/day

- For **10 kg** child, Maintanence fluid for 24 hours = **10** × 100 = **1000 ml/day**
- For **15 kg** child, Maintanence fluid for 24 hours = **10** × 100 + **5**× 50 = **1250 ml/day**
- For **25 kg** child, Maintanence fluid for 24 hours = **10** × 100 + **10**× 50 + **5**× 20 = **1600 ml/day**

8. Pincer grasp is seen at: (Repeat)

A. 5-6 months **B.** 7-8 months
C. 9-11 months **D.** >12 months

Ans: C. 9 - 12 months

Ref: *Nelson's Textbook of Pediatrics. 19th Edition.*

Explanation:

Fine Motor Milestones

Fine motor milestone	Median age of attainment in months
Grasps rattle	3.5
Reaches for objects	4
Palmar grasp gone	4
Transfers object hand to hand	5.5
Bidextrous grasp	5
Palmar grasp	7
Pincer grasp	9
Thumb-finger grasp	8
Turns pages of book	12
Scribbles	13
Builds tower of 2 cubes	15
Builds tower of 6 cubes	22

9. Most common complication of mumps in children:

A. Orchitis **B.** Aseptic meningits
C. Myocarditis **D.** Pancreatitis

Ans: B. Aseptic meningitis

Ref: *Nelson's Textbook of Pediatrics. 19th Edition*

Explanation:

"The most common complications of mumps are ***meningitis, with or without encephalitis,*** *and* ***gonadal involvement.****"*

Common complications

- Aseptic meningitis
- Encephalitis
- Orchitis
- Myocarditis
- Arthritis

Uncommon complications include

- Conjunctivitis
- Optic neuritis
- Pneumonia
- Nephritis
- Pancreatitis
- Thrombocytopenia.
- Thyroiditis

Complications of Mumps

Maternal infection with mumps during the 1st trimester of pregnancy results in increased fetal wastage.

Meningitis and Meningoencephalitis

- Mumps virus is neurotropic and is thought to enter the CNS via the choroid plexus and
- Infect the choroidal epithelium and ependymal cells
- Symptomatic CNS involvement occurs in 10-30% of infected individuals
- CSF pleocytosis has been found in 40-60% of patients with mumps parotitis.

- The meningoencephalitis ***may occur before, along with, or following the parotitis.***
- It most commonly manifests ***5 days after the parotitis.***
- Clinical findings vary with age. Infants and young children have fever, malaise, and lethargy, whereas older children, adolescents, and adults complain of headache and demonstrate meningeal signs.
- CSF in mumps meningitis has a **white blood cell pleocytosis** of 200-600/mm^3 with a predominance of lymphocytes.
- The **CSF glucose** content is **normal** in most patients, but a moderate hypoglycorrhachia (glucose content 20-40 mg/dL) may be seen in 10-20% of patients.
- The CSF **protein** content is **normal or mildly elevated.**
- Less common CNS complications of mumps include transverse myelitis, aqueductal stenosis, and facial palsy.
- Sensorineural hearing loss is rare but has been estimated to occur in 0.5-5.0/100,000 cases of mumps.

Orchitis and Oophoritis

- In adolescent and adult males, **orchitis** is **2nd only to parotitis** as a common finding in mumps.
- Involvement in **prepubescent boys is extremely rare**
- **After puberty, orchitis** occurs in **30-40%** of males.
- It begins within days following onset of parotitis
- Moderate to high fever, chills, and exquisite pain and swelling of the testes.
- In d"**30%** of cases the orchitis is **bilateral**.
- **Atrophy** of the **testes** may occur
- **Sterility is rare** even with bilateral involvement.
- **Oophoritis is uncommon** in postpubertal females but may cause severe pain and may be confused with appendicitis when located on the right side.
- **Mumps Myocarditis** Has been linked to later development of **endocardial fibroelastosis.**

10. Max limit of cardiothoracic ratio in chidren below 2 years:

A. 0.40 **B.** 0.45
C. 0.50 **D.** 0.55

Ans: C. 0.50

Ref: *Nelson's Textbook of Pediatrics. 19th Edition & Park's Pediatric Cardiology for Practitioners*

Explanation:

- Measurement of the cardiothoracic (CT) ratio is by far the simplest way to estimate the heart size in older children.
- The CT ratio is obtained by relating the
- Largest transverse diameter of the heart to the widest internal diameter of the chest:
- **CT ratio = (A + B) ÷ C**
- where A and B are maximal cardiac dimensions to the right and left of the midline, respectively, and C is the widest internal diameter of the chest.
- A CT ratio of more than **0.5** indicates cardiomegaly.
- The CT ratio cannot be used with accuracy in **newborns** and **small infants,** in whom a good inspiratory chest film is rarely obtained.
- In this situation, the degree of **inadequate inspiration** should be taken into consideration.
- Also, an estimation of the cardiac volume should be made by inspecting the **posteroanterior** and **lateral views instead of the CT ratio**

11. False about hartnup's disease:

A. Defect in neutral aminoacid transport
B. Mental retardation is the common presentation
C. Most children are asymptomatic
D. Photosenitivity

Ans: B. Mental retardation is the common presentation

Ref: *Nelson's Textbook of Pediatrics. 19th Edition*

Explanation:

Hartnup disease

- It is a rare inborn error of metabolism with **autosomal recessive** inheritance.
- Neutral amino acids, including **tryptophan,** are not transported across the brush border epithelium of the intestine and kidneys,
- This results in deficiency of synthesis of **nicotinamide**
- It causes a **photo-induced pellagra-like syndrome.**
- Increased urinary **monoamine monocarboxylic amino acids.**
- **Cutaneous signs** precede neurologic manifestations
- Eczematous, occasionally vesiculobullous eruption noted on the face and extremities in a **glove-and-stocking photodistribution.**
- **Hyperpigmentation** and **hyperkeratosis** may supervene and are intensified by further exposure to sunlight.

- Episodic flares may be precipitated by febrile illness, sun exposure, emotional stress, and poor nutrition.
- Emotional instability and **episodic cerebellar ataxia**.
- Neurologic symptoms are fully **reversible**.
- Administration of **nicotinamide** and protection from sunlight improves both cutaneous and neurologic manifestations.

12. Hyaline membrane deposition is seen in: (Repeat)

A. ARDS
B. RDS
C. Pumonary hemorrhage
D. Interstitial lung disease

Ans: B. RDS

Ref: *Nelson's Textbook of Pediatrics. 19th Edition*

Explanation:

- **Hyaline membrane disease (HMd)** is the old terminology for **RDS (Respiratory distress syndrome)**

13. Patient with VSD develops pulmonary hypertension. Which of the following will present?

A. Cyanosis
B. Initial resolution of symptoms
C. Clubbing
D. Ejection systolic murmur in pulmonary area

Ans: D. Ejection systolic murmur in pulmonary area

Ref: *Nelson's Textbook of Pediatrics. 19th Edition*

Explanation:

Pulmonary hypertension

- Loud P2
- Palpalbel P2 (Diastolic shock)
- Ejection systolic murmur in pulmonary area
- When the ratio of pulmonary to systemic resistance approaches **1 : 1**, the shunt becomes **bidirectional, signs of heart failure abate**, and the patient begins to show **signs of cyanosis**
- **Cyanosis, resolution of symptoms** and **clubbing** occurs when there is **reversal of shunt (Eisenmenger syndrome)**

14. In which of the following tubercular infection steroid is used? (Repeat)

A. TB Lymphadenitis
B. TB Osteomylitis
C. Endobronchial TB
D. Neurotuberculosis

Ans: D. Neurotuberculosis

Ref: *Harrison's Principles of Internal Medicine, 18ed. & Nelson textbook of Pediatrics, 19ed.*

Explanation:

Indications for Steroids in TB

- TB meningitis (Definite evidence of decreasing neurologic sequelae)
- TB Pericarditis
- Pleural TB
- Miliary disease

Doubtful benefit in

- Endobronchial TB
- TB peritonitis
- TB osteomyelitis
- Laryngeal TB
- TB Lymphadenitis
- Genitourinary TB

15. Most common cause of congenital hypothyroidism: (Repeat)

A. Thyroid dysgenesis
B. Maternal antibodies
C. Inborn errors of thyroid hormone defects
D. Maternal iodine deficiency

Ans: A. Thyroid dysgenesis

Ref: *Nelson's Textbook of Pediatrics. 19th Edition. Pg.1895*

Explanation:

"Most cases of congenital hypothyroidism results from thyroid dysgenesis"(Ref:Nelson)

Refer 2013 Pediatrics Question Explanation.

DERMATOLOGY

1. Fishnet appearance in immunoflorescence is seen in:

A. Pemphigus vulgaris
B. Bullous pemphigoid
C. Dermatitis herpetiformis
D. Darier disease

Ans: A. Pemphigus vulgaris

Ref: *Vesiculobullous Disorders. In: Thappa DM, editor. Essentials in Dermatology, 2nd ed., Jaypee 2009;114-26).*

Explanation:

- Pemphigus is an autoimmune blistering disorder characterized by ***autoantibody formation*** against the intercellular cementing substance called ***desmogleins.***
- The mechanism of cell separation is called ***acantholysis***- loss of intercellular substance

causing separation of the epidermal keratinocytes which become rounded→result in intraepidermal blister.

- These large rounded keratinocytes with large nucleus, perinuclear halo and peripheral condensation of cytoplasm are called the ***acantholytic cells*** – seen in Tzanck smear.

Types of pemphigus:

- Pemphigus vulgaris (variant-pemphigus vegetans)- most common type
- Pemphigus foliaceus (variant-pemphigus erythematosus; endemic pemphigus or fogoselvagem)
- Paraneoplastic pemphigus
- Drug induced pemphigus
- IgA pemphigus
- Neonatal pemphigus

Clinical features:

- Fluid filled bullae → rupture → painful erosions with no tendency to spontaneous healing.
- Painful mucosal erosions- oral (most common; almost in all cases in pemphigus vulgaris); genital mucosa, pharynx, larynx,conjunctiva, urethra
- ***Bulla spread sign/ Asboe Hansen sign- positive.***
- ***Nikosky sign***- peeling of skin leaving behind erosions when tangential pressure applied over areas of normal looking skin or over bony prominences (other conditions- staphylococcal scalded skin syndrome, toxic epidermal necrolysis).

Diagnosis:

- Tzanck smear- acantholytic cells; histopathology; direct and indirect immunofloresence.

Treatment:

- ***Systemic steroids*** are mainstay of treatment.
- Adjuvants- cyclophosphamide, azathioprine, methotrexate, mycophenolate mofetil, dapsone, plasmapheresis, iv immunoglobulins; biological agent- Rituximab (anti CD20).
  (See Table 19 on next Page)

2. **A 22 year old sexually active male presents with painful, foul smelling genital ulcer which bleeds easily to touch and has excessive granulation tissue. What is the most probable diagnosis? (Repeat)**

A. Chancroid **B.** Herpes
C. Syphilis **D.** Donovaniosis

Ans: A. Chancroid

Ref: *Thappa DM, editor. Essentials in Dermatology, 2nd ed., Jaypee 2009.*

Explanation:

Repeat: Refer 2013 Dermat question explanation

CHANCROID

- Aka **Soft sore, Soft Chancre, Ulcus molle**
- Causative agent: **Hemophilus ducrei**
- Incubation period: 3 days – 2 weeks (1-5 days average)
- Extremely **painful**
- **Suppurative ulcers** of genital mucosa
- Soft **friable, non-indurated**, ragged undermined edges
- **Foul smelling** yellow grey **exudate**
- Suppurative inguinal lymph nodes (Bubo)
- **Ito-Reenstierna test** - Intradermal test
- **Pyogenic Ulceration**

Treatment

- **Azithromycin** 1g single oral dose (or)
- Ceftriaxone 250 mg im single dose (or)
- Ciprofloxacin 500 mg bd for 3 days.

3. **Vitilgo is most commonly associated with:**

A. Diabetes mellitus **B.** Addisons disease
C. Hypothyroidism **D.** Diabetes insipidus

Ans: B. Addisons disease

Ref: *Rook's Dermatology, 8th ed*

Explanation:

VITILIGO

- Characterized by well circumscribed, milky white cutaneous macules devoid of identifiable melanocytes.

Pathogenesis

- Loss of Melanocytes
- Multiple mechanisms causing the pathology
  - Autoimmune
  - Autocytotoxic
  - Neural
  - Biochemical
  - Intrinsic (Genetic) Theory

Clinical features

- Diagnostic lesion is the vitiligo macule, which is of variable size, shape, has milky white color and scalloped margins.
- May appear at any age . Peak onset 5 -30 years
- ***Vitiligo fuminans / Galloping Vitiligo***: Rapid worsening seen in vitiligo.

Table 19 : Characteristics of Various Pemphigus Disorders (High yield table)

Features	Pemphigus vulgaris	Pemphigus foliaceus	Bullous pemphigoid	Dermatitis herpetiformis
Antigen	Desmoglein 3	Desmoglein 1	BP 180, BP 230	Unknown
Level of split	Intraepidermal - suprabasal	Intraepidermal- subcorneal	Subepidermal	Subepidermal
Mechanism of blister	Acantholysis	Acantholysis	Basement membrane zone disruption	Basement membrane zone disruption
Age	40-60 years	40-50 years	>60 years	20-55 years
Symptoms	Pain	Pain (less severe)	Pruritus	Intensely pruritic
Type of blister	Flaccid bullae on normal or erythematous skin	Transient blisters	Tense bullae on normal or erythematous or urticated skin	Grouped erythematous papules and papulovesicles; vesicles excoriated
Nature of erosion	Painful erosions with no tendency to spontaneous healing	Crusted moist scaly erosions	Erosions heal spontaneously	-
Distribution	Scalp, face, trunk, axilla, groins, pressure sites	Seborrheic distribution	Flexural aspect of limbs, lower abdomen, groin, axilla	Extensor aspect of limbs (elbows, knees), buttock, nasal cleft, shoulder, upper back, face, scalp
Bulla spread sign	+	Transient vesicles	+/-	Vesicles not seen as excoriated
Nikolsky sign	+	+	-	-
Mucosal involvement	Almost in all patients; may be presenting or the only feature (80-90%)	Uncommon	Rare; never presenting feature; desquamative gingivitis (40%)	Common but asymptomatic
Tzanck smear	Acantholytic cells	Acantholytic cells	Eosinophils	Neutrophils
HPE	Suprabasal cleft with row of tomb stone appearance	Subcorneal split	Subepidermal blister with eosinophils	Neutrophilic microabscess at tips of dermal papillae
DIF	Intercellular **IgG** deposists throughout the *epidermis* in fish net pattern	Intercellular **IgG** deposists in upper *epidermis*	Linear **IgG** and **C3**deposists in *basement membrane zone*	Granular **IgA** deposists in *dermal papilla*
IIF	Antibody titres correlate with disease severity	Antibody titres correlate with disease severity	Antibody titres do not correlate with disease severity	Negative or anti basement membrane zone or dermal autoantibodies. Antithyroid or antigliadin antibodies present
Associations	Thymoma, myasthenia gravis, lymphoma, bronchogenic carcinoma	-	Gastric carcinoma, diabetes, rheumatoid arthritis, psoriasis	Gluten sensitive enteropathy
Main stay of treatment	Steroids+adjuvants	Steroids+adjuvants	Steroids+adjuvants	Dapsone Gluten free diet

- ***Leukotrichia*** - depigmentation of hair; may occur in vitiligo.

Classification

Localized:

a. Focal
b. Segmental
c. Mucosal

Generalised:

a. Acrofacial vitiligo
b. Vitiligo Vulgaris
c. Lip-tip vitiligo
d. Mixed
e. Universal vitiligo

Special signs in Vitiligo

- **Trichrome sign:** Also known as ***'vitiligo gradata'***. It is presence of coloured zone (intermediate color) between the normal skin and depigmented macules
- **Quadrichrome vitiligo** implies presence of additional 4th colour.
- **Koebner's phenomenon:** Development of new vitiligo lesions along the lines of trauma.

Association with other diseases

- Autoimmune thyroid disease
- Addison's disease
- Pernicious anemia
- Diabetes mellitus

Association with dermatological conditions

- Alopecia areata
- Scleroderma
- Psoriasis
- Collagen vascular disorders

Vogt koyanagi Harada syndrome - Characterised by

- Vitiligo
- Poliosis
- Uveitis
- Dysacousia
- Alopecia

Medical Treatment

A. Systemic:

- Psoralen
- Corticosteroids
- Immunomodulators
- Khellin
- Phenylalanine
- Antioxidants

B. Topical:

- Topical PUVA
- Topcial potent steroids
- Human placental extract
- Calcipotriol
- Topical psudocatalase+ calcicum + UVB
- Cosmetic camouflage
- Depigmentation with 20% monobenzyl ether

Surgical Management:

Indications: Stable Vitiligo - i.e no new lesions for last two years
Refractory to medical treatment

Modalities

- Punch grafting
- Split skin thickness graft
- Blister grafting
- Melanocyte culture & transplantation
- Tatooing

4. PUVA treatment is not used in:

A. Melasma
B. Vitiligo
C. Psoriasis
D. Cutaneous T cell lymphoma

Ans: A. Melasma

Ref: *Rook's Dermatology, 8th ed*

Explanation:

PUVA Therapy

Psoralens + UV-A radiation

Three Psoralens are used clinically

- 8 methoxypsoralen (8 MOP)
- 5 methoxypsoralen (5 MOP)
- Trimethyl psoralen (TMP)

- They are active only when combined with UVA radiation.
- It interferes with DNA synthesis and blocks epidermal cell proliferation.
- Also has immunomodulatory and immunosuppressive effects.
- Induced epidermal thickening and melanogenesis.

Dosage

- Oral 8-MOP given in a dose of 0.6 -0.8 mg/kg/ weight/day.
- Two hours later, patient is exposed to UV-A radiation at a dose of 1 Joule/square cm
- UV-A dose gradually increased depending on skin type and onset of erythema
- Therapy given 2 -3 times per week

- Number of exposures required for control: 15 - 25

Indications

- Psoriasis
- Vitiligo
- Photodermatoses
- Cutaneous T-cell lymphoma

Side effects

- Nausea and Vomiting
- Cutaneous:
  - Acute sunburn
  - Irreversible pigmentation
  - PUVA Lentigenes
  - Actinic keratoses
  - Premature aging of skin
- Ocular – Cataract (Prevented by using sunglasses during treatment)
- Carcinogenesis

5. **Leukonychia is seen in:**
   A. Hypoalbuminemia
   B. Onycomycosis
   C. Lead Poisoning
   D. Psoriasis

Ans: A. Hypoalbuminemia

Ref: *Rook's Dermatology, 8th ed*

Explanation:

- **Leukonychia is** white e discolouration of nails attributable to nail matrix dysfunction.
- It is seen in ***hypoalbuminaemia*** of ***chronic liver disease.***
  (See table 20 on the next page)

6. **All are seen in dermatomyositis *except:***
   A. Calcinosis cutis
   B. Heliotropic rash
   C. Shawl sign
   D. Gottron's rash

Ans: A. Calcinosis cutis

Ref: *Connective tissue disorders. In: Thappa DM, editor. Essentials in Dermatology, 2nd ed., Jaypee 2009;134-47.*

Explanation:

- **Calcinosis cutis** is characteristically seen in **CREST syndrome**

Dermatomyositis

Connective tissue disorder characterized by inflammatory myositis presenting with proximal muscle weakness and cutaneous manifestations in the form of:

Pathognomonic features:

- **Gottron's papules** – violaceous flat topped **papules** on IP joints and knuckles; also knee, elbow, medial malleoli.
- **Gottron's sign**- violaceous erythematous **macules** with or without edema at the above mentioned sites.

Characteristic features:

- **Heliotrope rash**- periorbital violaceous erythema with edema.
- **Shawl sign** - erythema and scaling with or without poikiloderma over shoulder region.
- Periungual telangiectasia and dystrophic cuticles.
- Mechanic's hands-hyperkeratosis, scaling, fissuring and hyper pigmentation over fingertips, sides of thumbs and fingers.

Compatible features:

- **Calcinosis cutis**
- Poikilodermaa trophicans vasculare

CREST SYNDROME

- **Limited** form of **systemic scleroderma.**
- **Anti centromere antibody** (remember as centromere is the central small part so anti centromere antibody in limited type in comparison to progressive systemic sclerosis where anti-scl 70 refers to diffuse sclerosis).

  C-Calcinosis cutis
  R-Raynaud's phenomenon
  E-Esophageal dysmotility
  S-Sclerodactyly
  T-Telangiectasia

- Progressive systemic sclerosis- cutaneous + internal organ fibrosis
- American Rheumatism Association criteria (ARA criteria 1980) for systemic sclerosis
- 97% sensitivity; 98% specificity
- One major+two or more minor

Major:

- Scleroderma proximal to digits affecting limbs, face, neck, trunk

Minor:

- Sclerodactyly
- Digital pitted scarring
- Bilateral basal pulmonary fibrosis

Table 20 : Other Nail Abnormalities

Nail abnormality	Description	Causes
Koilonychia	Reverse curvature in the longtitudinal and transverse axis	Iron deficiency anemia
Macronychia / Micronychia	Too small or large nails	—
Onycholysis	Distal or lateral seperation of the nail from nail bed	Psoriasis Onychomycosis
Pterygium	Central fibrotic tongue like band from proximal nail fold joins the nail bed dividing the nail proximally into two.	Lichen Planus
Subungual hyperkeratosis	Excessive collection of squamous debris under the free edge of nail	Psoriasis Onychomycosis
Onychogryphosis	Nail get thickened and grows upwards in a spiral manner	Chronic trauma
Pachynychia congenital	Hypertrophy of nails associated with nail bed and hyponychial hyperkeratosis	—
Beau's lines	Transverse grooves on nails	Temporary cessation of nail formation Chemotherapy Hypocalcemia Nail infection Coronary occlusion Malnutrition
Terry's nail	Nail is white proximally but normal distally	Congestive cardiac failure Cirrhosis Diabetes mellitus
Pitting	Punctate erosions on nail surface	Psoriasis Alopecia areata
Red Lunulae	Nails shows erythema of lunula	Psoriasis (Dotted red lunula) Congestive cardiac failure Cirrhosis SLE
Splinter hemorrhages	Longitudinal hemorrhages in nail bed	Psoriasis Dermatitis Fungal Infections Infective endocarditis SLE Mycosis fungoides Rheumatoid arthritis
Mees lines	Whitening or discoloration of the nail in bands or "stria" that run parallel the lunula (nail base)	Cirrhosis Chemotherapy Heavy metal poisoning (Arsenic, Thallium) Trauma
Muehrcke's nails	White lines (leukonychia) that extend all the way across the nail and lie parallel to the lunula (half moon)	Nonspecific Assc with decreased protein synthesis Hypoalbuminemia Nephrotic syndrome

ANESTHESIOLOGY

1. **Plasma potassium concentration is increased with:**

   A. Succinyl choline **B.** Atracurium
   C. Pancuronium **D.** Propofol

   Ans: A. Succinyl choline

Ref: *Ajay Yadav, Short textbook of Pediatrics 1st edition Pg 86 & Miller Textbook of Anaesthesia. 6th edition*

Explanation:

Systemic Effects of Succinyl choline

- **Cardiovascular system -** Profound Bradycardia
- **Hyperkalemia** – due to excessive muscle fasciculations
- **CNS** – Increases intracranial tension
- **Eye** – Increases intraocular tension
- **GIT** – Increases intragastric pressure, increases salivation, gastric secretions & peristalsis
- **Muscle pains** – due to excessive muscle contractions
- **Malignant hyperthermia** – SCh is the most common drug causing this
- **Anaphylaxis**
- **Masseter spasm**

2. **Drug used to prevent nausea and vomiting:**

   A. Propofol
   B. Fentanyl
   C. Nitrous oxide
   D. Sevoflurane

   Ans: A. Propofol

Ref: *Ajay Yadav, Short textbook of Pediatrics 1st edition Pg 73 & Miller Textbook of Anaesthesia. 6th edition*

Explanation:

Propofol has antiemetic property and has the least incidence of nausea and vomiting.

PROPOFOL

- Comercial prepartions is **Oil based** and contains Soyabean oil, **Egg Lecithin & Glycerol**
- Causes **pain during injection**, avoided by prior injection by lignocaine
- Can **support the growth of bacteria**, to be used within 6 hrs of opening the vial
- **Drug of choice for day care surgery**

Anesthetic properties

- Induction is achieved in 15 seconds (Arm brain circulation time)
- Consciousness is regained in 5 – 10 minutes (due to redistribution)
- Elimination half life – 2-4 hours
- No analgesic property
- Not a muscle relaxant

Metabolism

- Metabolised by liver and excreted by kidneys
- Clearance rate is 20 times more rapid than Thiopentone

Systemic Effects

- Major CVS effect is **hypotension and vagal bradycardia**
- **Better blunting of airway reflexes** compared to thiopentone
- **Respiratory depression is more severe** than Thiopentone
- **Has Cerebral protection effect** (Similar to thiopentone)
- Can cause **muscle twitchings or myoclonus**
- Has **antiemetic property**
- **Antipruritic property**
- **Decreases intraocular pressure**

Uses

- Agent of choice for **Day care anesthesia**
- Agent of choice for **total intravenous anesthesia (TIVA)** in combination with **Fentanyl**
- Used to produce **sedation** in ICU
- Agent of choice in patients susceptible to **Malignant hyperthermia**

3. **Drug producing haematological side effect is:**

   A. Nitrous oxide **B.** Halothane
   C. Ketamine **D.** Sevoflurane

   Ans: A. Nitrous oxide

Ref: *Ajay Yadav, Short Textbook of Anesthesia, 1st edition, pg 59.*

Explanation:

Nitrous oxide *produces* ***Aplastic anemia*** and ***Megaloblastic anemia***

NITROUS OXIDE (LAUGHING GAS)

- Stored as liquid in ***blue*** color cylinder
- **1.5** times more heavier than ***air***
- **35** times more soluble than ***nitrogen***

Anesthetic properties

- It is not a complete anesthetic.
- It is used as a ***carrier gas*** to other anesthetics
- MAC is ***104%*** (It is not possible to deliver, so not a complete anesthetic).
- Maximum concentration which can be given is ***66%.***

- A minimum of 33% of Oxygen has to be given (Otherwise can cause severe hypoxia)
- It is usually given as N20 66% and O2 33% mixture
- Blood gas coefficient *is 0.47* making it agent with faster induction and recovery
- ***Good analgesic***
- ***Not a muscle relaxant***
- When given with other inhalational agent, it increases the concentration of that agent ***(Second gas effect***) and also its own concentration (***Concentration effect***)
- Sudden stoppage can lead to ***Diffusion Hypoxia***(Should always be tapered slowly by giving 100% oxygen)

Metabolism

- It is ***not metabolized*** in human body.
- It is excreted unchanged in lungs
- Small amount is excreted via skin (Percutaneous excretion)
- Impurities in N2O cylinder can cause severe laryngospasm, methhemoglobinemia and Pulmonary edema

Systemic Actions

- **CVS:** It does not depress the myocardium in vivo, so it can be safely used in patients with cardiac disease and shock
- **CNS:** It increases cerebral metabolic rate and raises intra cranial tension
- **RS:** It causes tachypnea and decrease tidal volume, maintaining minute volume
- Ventilatory response to hypoxia is blunted
- No significant effect on Liver and Kidneys

Side Effects

- **Hematological:** It inactivates vitamin B12 (If used for >6 hours) → defective folate metabolism → Bone marrow depression → ***Aplastic anemia*** and ***Megaloblastic anemia***
- **CNS:** Vitamin B12 deficiency can cause Demyelination of spinal cord (Subacute degeneration of spinal cord) especially involving posterior columns and lateral spinothalamic tracts
- **Closed Gas Spaces:** Compliant spaces like gut, penumoperitoneum, pneumothorax and non-compliant spaces like middle ear cavity, pneumoencephalum can develop very high pressure following nitrous oxide inhalation.
- This happens because for 1 mole of nitrogen removed, 35 moles of nitrous oxide enter (35 times more soluble than nitrogen.
- Therefore, Nitrous oxide is **contraindicated** in
  - Pneumothorax
  - Pneumoperitoneum
  - Pneumoencephalum
  - Middle ear surgery
  - Posterior fossa surgery
  - Laproscopic surgery
  - Acute intestinal obstruction and volvulus of gut
  - Eye surgeries

Uses in Anesthesia

- As a supplement to anesthesia (not a complete anesthetic)
- As a carrier gas for inhalational agents
- As analgesic in obstetrics, dental pain, burn dressing and acute trauma

4. **Best treatment for relieving pain during intra-partum period is:**

A. Neuraxial block
B. Epidural anesthesisa
C. IV ketamine
D. General Anesthesia

Ans: B. Epidural anesthesia

Ref: *Ajay Yadav, Short Textbook of Anesthesia, 1st edition, pg 123*

Explanation:

Epidural (Extradural) anesthesia

- The epidural space is a potential space.
- It contains connective tissue, venous plexuses, and adipose tissue.
- It is found between the connective tissue covering the vertebrae and the **ligamentum flavum** posteriorly and the **dura mater** anteriorly.
- Laterally it is bound by the **pedicles** and the **intervertebral foramina**.
- It extends from the **foramen magnum**, where the dura is fused to the base of the skull, to the **sacral hiatus**.
- The plica mediana dorsalis is a connective tissue band that may extend from the dura mater to the ligamentum flavum, which divides the posterior epidural space into right and left compartments.
- Clinically, this is significant because it may affect the spread of epidurally injected medications.

Indications

- All surgeries which can be performed under spinal anesthesia can be performed under epidural block

- Plus upper abdominal surgeries, thoracic surgeries and even neck surgeries can be performed under cervical epidural block
- Mainly used for controlling postoperative pain
- For painless labour
- To control chronic pain due to cancer and chronic pain conditions
- Acute occlusive vascular conditions
- Blood patch for postspinal headache

Site of action of drug

- Anterior and posterior nerve roots
- Mixed spinal nerves
- Drug diffuses through dura and arachnoid and inhibits descending pathways in spinal cord

Complications

- Inadequate patch block
- **Hypotension**
- **Apnea** (higher blocks)
- **Total spinal:** Accidental injection into subarachnoid space – presents with marked hypotension, bradycardia, apnea, dilated pupils and coma
- **Dural puncture**
- Invascular injection
- Local anesthetic toxicity
- **Horner's syndrome** (Cervical block)
- Epidural hematoma
- Epidural abscess
- Anterior spinal artery syndrome
- Needle injury to spinal cord
- Epiduro-cuteaneous fistula
- Trigeminal nerve palsy
- Intraocular hemorrhage

Other methods tried in Obstetric analgesia - Regional nerve blocks

- Subarachnoid (Spinal) anesthesia
- Pudendal nerve block

5. **Drugs used in advanced life support include all *except:***

A. Calcium	**B.** Amiodarone
C. Vasopressin	**D.** Adrenaline

Ans: A. Calcium

Ref: *ALS Protocol guidelines 2010. Pdf & American Heart Association. 2005 American Heart Association (AHA) guidelines for cardiopul-monary resuscitation (CPR) and emergency cardiovascular care (ECC) of pediatric and neonatal patients: pediatric basic life support. Pediatrics. 2006 May; 117(5):e 989-1004.*

Explanation:

Advanced Life Support (ALS) is a set of life-saving protocols and skills that extend Basic Life Support to further support the circulation and provide an open airway and adequate ventilation (breathing).

AHA 2010 guidelines : Drugs used are:

- Epinephrine
- Vasopressin
- Amiodarone

(Atropine has been removed in the new 2010 guidelines)

RADIOLOGY & RADIOTHERAPY

1. **Gamma knife contains**

A. Cs 127	**B.** Co 60
C. Iridium 92	**D.** Tc99

Ans: B. Cobalt 60

Reference: *Emedicine Medscape*

Explanation:

Gamma Knife

- The Gamma Knife is used to treat brain tumors by administering high-**intensity cobalt radiation** therapy in a manner that concentrates the radiation over a **small volume**.
- A Gamma Knife typically contains **201 cobalt-60** sources of approximately **30 curies (1.1 TBq)**, each placed in a circular array in a heavily shielded assembly.
- The device aims gamma radiation through a **target point** in the **patient's brain**.
- The patient wears a specialized helmet that is surgically fixed to the skull, so that the brain tumor remains stationary at the target point of the gamma rays.
- An ablative dose of radiation is thereby sent through the tumor in one treatment session, while surrounding brain tissues are relatively spared.
- **Gamma Knife therapy**, like all radiosurgery, uses doses of radiation to kill cancer cells and shrink tumors, delivered precisely to avoid damaging surrounding healthy brain tissue.

- Gamma Knife radiosurgery is able to accurately focus many beams of **gamma radiation** to converge on one or more tumors.
- Each individual beam is of relatively low intensity, so the radiation has little effect on intervening brain tissue and is concentrated only at the tumor itself.
- Gamma Knife radiosurgery has proven effective for patients with **benign or malignant brain tumors up to 4 centimeters** in size, vascular malformations such as an **arteriovenous malformation** (AVM), **pain** or other functional problems.
- For treatment of **trigeminal neuralgia**, the procedure may be used repeatedly on patients.

2. Gold standard test for pulmonary embolism: (Repeat)

A. CT Angiography **B.** MRI
C. PET **D.** Echocardiography

Ans: A. CT Angiography

Ref: *Harrison's Principles of Internal Medicine, 18ed. Chapter 262. Deep Venous Thrombosis and Pulmonary Thromboembolism*

Explanation:

- **Tests**:
  - D-Dimer assay- sensitive 'rule out' test
  - False positive inMI, pneumonia, sepsis, cancer, pregnancy, post-op state
  - ABG- low pO2 & pCO2, high A-a gradient
  - S.troponin, heart- type fatty acid binding protein, BNP, NT-pro BNP} due to RV microinfarction
- **ECG:**
  - Sinus tachycardia
  - Acute right axis deviation
  - RBBB
  - S1Q3TS sign
  - T-wave inversion in V1-V4
- **CXR:**
  - **Hampton's sign**-peripheral wedge shaped density above diaphragm
  - **Westermark's sign** – focal oligemia
  - **Palla's sign**- enlarged right pulmonary artery
- **ECHO- Mc-Connel's sign**- Hypokinesia of RV free wall, normal RV apex
- **Multidetector**-row spiral CT- Very sensitive, non invasive test
- **Pulmonary angiography with CT — Gold standard** Test (Most specific)

3. Which isotope use to assess myocardial function?

A. 99m Tc MDP
B. 99mTc Sestamibi
C. 99m Tc Exametazime
D. 99m Tc Pyrophosphate

Ans: B. 99m Tc Sestamibi

Ref: *Emedicine Medscape*

Explanation:

Rubidium-82 (1.26 min): Convenient **PET agent** in **myocardial perfusion** imaging.

Technetium (99mTc) sestamibi

- It is a pharmaceutical agent used in nuclear medicine imaging. The drug is a coordination complex consisting of the radioisotope technetium-99m bound to six **methoxyisobutylisonitrile (MIBI) ligands**.
- The scan of a patient using MIBI is commonly known as a "**MIBI scan.**"
- It is mainly used to image the **myocardium (heart muscle)**.
- **Technetium (99mTc) sestamibi** is a lipophilic cation which, when injected intravenously into a patient, **distributes in the myocardium** proportionally to the **myocardial blood flow.**
- Single photon emission computed tomography (**SPECT**) imaging of the heart is performed using a gamma camera to detect the gamma rays emitted by the technetium-99m as it decays.
- **Two sets** of images are acquired.
- For one set, 99mTc MIBI is injected while the patient is at **rest** and then the myocardium is imaged.
- In the second set, the patient is **stressed** either by **exercising** on a **treadmill** or pharmacologically.
- The drug is injected at peak stress and then imaging is performed.
- The resulting two sets of images are compared with each other to distinguish **ischemic from infarcted areas** of the **myocardium.**
- It is also used in the work-up of **primary hyperparathyroidism** to identify **parathyroid adenomas**, for **radioguided surgery** of the **parathyroid** and in the work-up of **possible breast cancer.**

Note: Before introduction of Technetium isotopes, **Thallium-201** was used to assess myocardial function. It is obsolete now since it required large doses, has long half life and yielded poor quality images.

4. **Spider leg appearence is seen in:**
A. Adult polycystic kidney disease
B. Wilm's Tumor
C. Horse shoe kidney
D. Vesicoureteral reflux

Ans: A. Adult polycystic kidney disease

***Ref:** Harrison's online. 18th ed.*

Explanation:

Some important features in Contrast Radiographs

- **Spider leg** appearance — **Polycystic** kidney
- **Cobra head** appearance — **Ureterocele**
- **Flower vase** appearance of ureters — **Horse shoe** kidney
- **Sandy** patches — **Schistosomiasis** of bladder
- **Soap bubble** appearance — **Hydronephrosis**
- **Apple core** lesion on barium — **Ca colon**
- **Claw appearance** on barium enema — **Intussusception**
- **Saw tooth** appearance — **Diverticula** of colon
- **Birds beak** appearance of esophagus on barium meal — **Achalasia**
- **Cork screw** appearance of esophagus on barium meal — **Diffuse esophageal spasm**
- ***String sign of kantor***— **Crohn's** dissease
- **Thumb printing** sign — **Ischemic colitis**
- **EGG SHELL CALCIFICATION — Silicosis, Sarcoidosis, Scleroderma, Histoplasmosis, Amyloidosis, lymphoma** following radiotherapy

5. **String sign of Kantor is seen in:**
A. Crohn's disease **B.** Ulcerative colitis
C. Ca Colon **D.** Typhoid colitis

Ans: A. Crohn's disease

***Ref:** http://www.learningradiology.com*

Explanation:

String Sign of Kantor

- Seen in **Crohn's disease**
- Finding seen on contrast studies using primarily **barium**
- It is caused by **severe spasm secondary to irritability of the loop** producing the appearance of a **frayed cotton string**
- At first, **edema** and **spasm narrow the loop** but the narrowing is at least **partially distensible**
- Eventually the wall of the ileum may become **fibrotic** and the **lumen fixed** in diameter.

Imaging Findings

- Persistently **narrowed** but potentially distensible **terminal ileum**
- First sign of Crohn's ileitis is usually **shallow aphthous ulcers**
- **Short, linear ulcers** along the **mesenteric border** may also be seen with Crohn's ileitis
- Induration of the surrounding fat may cause the loop to be separated from the other small bowel loops (**Proud loop**)

PSYCHIATRY

1. **True regarding delirium: (Repeat)**
A. Irreversible
B. Insidious onset
C. Behavioral change due to alteration in cerebral metabolism
D. Clear consciousness

Ans: C. Behavioral change due to alteration in cerebral metabolism

***Ref:** Synopsis of Psychiatry, Kaplan & Sadock, 10th edition*

Explanation:

Delirium

It is a condition basically characterized by ***"alteration in consciousness"***.
It is **abrupt** (within 2 days) or **acute** (less than 2 weeks) in onset.
Synonyms - Acute organic brain syndrome, Acute organic psychosis, ICU psychosis.

It is characterized by the following set of symptoms:

1. **Clouding of consciousness**
2. **Disorientation** (*to time, place and person in that order of appearance*)
3. **Psychotic symptoms** (hallucinations-visual / auditory, delusions - persecutory) which are *fleeting & often ill-formed*
4. **Irrelevant talk** and / or **behaviour**
5. **Altered sleep-wake cycle**.

- All the symptoms are ***fluctuating in nature*** (i.e., their presence, severity vary from time to time in a given 24hrs) and usually worsen in night time (**sun downing**).
- It is usually **reversible**.
- But the mortality rate is high -10%.

The causes are many: anything which affects the brain structure / function (metabolism) result in delirium. The following table is highly useful in practice.

PRIMARY FOCAL LESIONS	PRIMARY DIFFUSE LESIONS
- Infarction - Tumor - Abscess	- Hemorrhage - Concussion injury - Meningitis
SECONDARY FOCAL LESIONS - Metastasis - Abscess	**SECONDARY DIFFUSE LESIONS** - Failure of other organs (heart, lungs, kidneys) - Sepsis

Depending upon the psychomotor activity, delirium is divided into types viz.

1. Hypoactive
2. Hyperactive (alcohol, benzodiazepine withdrawal)
3. Mixed.

Management:

1. Treat the causes
2. Low dose typical (first generation) antipsychotics like haloperidol
3. Benzodiazepines in case of alcohol withdrawal (**Lorazapam** is the drug of choice in case of decompensated liver state, commonly seen in these group, since it has no secondary active metabolites)
4. Reorientation, Restraint & Resuscitation (food & fluid balance)

2. Wernicke's encephalopathy occurs due to the deficiency of:

A. Thiamine
B. Riboflavin
C. Folate
D. Vitamin B12

Ans: A. Thiamine

Ref: *Synopsis of Psychiatry, Kaplan & Sadock, 10th edition.p.400.*

Explanation:

Wernicke's encephalopathy

- It is a condition which is **acute in onset** (cf. Korsakoff psychosis is **insidious**),
- It is characterized by the triad:
  1. **Confusion** (delirium tremens)
  2. **Ataxia** (in-coordination of movements)
  3. **Nystagmus** (due to **opthalmoplegia** and / or vestibular dysfunction). [CAN- the Mnemonic]
- Chronic alcohol intake depletes **thiamine** (Vitamin B1) by various mechanisms.
- During acute intoxication, such deficiency results in degeneration of paraventricular regions of brain (**mammillary bodies, thalamus** and **hypothalamus**).
- The treatment is **'THIAMINE'** IV **250-500mg/** day as slow infusion for first five days, followed by oral route (100mg tds) for at least 15days.
- It is **reversible** if treated early.
- Otherwise, the condition progresses into **"Korsakoff's psychosis"**, which is characterized by **amnesia** (both **anterograde & retrograde**) [declarative memory deficit], **confabulation** (to fill up the gaps in memory), **apathy & lack of insight**.
- Less than 20% only respond to thiamine and often need as long as two years to show moderate improvement.

Other neuropsychiatric disorders due to alcohol are:

- Cerebellar degeneration,
- Central Pontine Myelinosis &
- Corpus callosum demyelination (Marchiafava-Bignami disease).

Riboflavin deficiency:

- Mucositis (Chelitis, Stomatitis, Glossitis)
- Dermatitis (Seborrheic)
- Normochromic, normocytic anemia.

Folate deficiency - Depression.

Vitamin B12:

- Depression & Psychosis (both folate and Vit.B12 cause mental disorders either directly or by increasing homocysteine levels in brain).

3. All the following are used in the treatment of bipolar disorder *except:*

A. Gabapentin **B.** Valproate
C. Lithium **D.** Carbamazepine

Ans: A. Gabapentin

Ref: *Synopsis of Psychiatry, Kaplan & Sadock, 10th edition*

Expanation:

- **Bipolar disorder (BPAd)** is a psychiatric disorder characterized by the occurrence of one or more episodes of mania with (usually) or without (rarely) depressive episodes.
- Both poles of mood disturbance occur in the same patient.
- It is characterized by two phases- **illness phase & remission phase.**

- In the illness phase patient may have either mania or depression or a mixed picture.
- The genetic component of this illness is high compared to unipolar depression (*Note- there is no* ***unipolar mania,*** *since even a single episode is construed as bipolar disorder*).
- There are many subtypes like **Bipolar** I (mania + depression), **Bipolar** II (hypomania + depression) etc.
- The primary drugs for BPAD are "Mood Stabilizers".
- **Lithium, Valproate, Carbamazapine** are the first line drugs
- **Oxcarbazapine, Lamotrigine, Levitracetam** are second-line drugs.
- Some atypical anti-psychotics like ***Olanzapine, Quetiapine*** too have mood stabilizing property and often used alone in some cases.

Lithium

- It is the first MS studied and one of the two drugs (the other one is Clozapine) proved to **prevent suicide** effectively.
- It is neither protein bound nor metabolized in the body & excreted unchanged in urine.
- The mechanism of action is inhibition **of GSK3ß & inositol phosphatase** enzymes.
- Side effects are **diabetes insipidus, hypothyroidsm, seizures, Ebstein's anomaly (teratogenic)**.
- Useful in **seborrheic dermatitis & leucopenia.**
  - Prophylactic blood level – 0.4-0.8 Meq/L
  - Therapeutic blood level – 0.6-1.2 Meq/L
  - Toxic level – ≥ 1.2 Meq/L (the commonest first symptom of toxicity is coarse tremors & level above 1.8 Meq/L is the indication for hemodialysis)
- ***Valproate*** is a rapidly acting MS, (DOC for rapid cyclers - ≥ 4 episodes per year) with multiple mechanisms (blockade of voltage-gated sodium channels, inhibition of GABA transaminase). It causes hemorrhagic **pancreatitis, hepatic necrosis, hyperammonemia**, midline defects **(teratogenic)**.
- ***Carbamazapine*** is known to cause **agranulocytosis, Steven-Johnson's** syndrome, **SIADH** and often aggravates **absence seizures & juvenile myoclonic epilepsy**.
- ***Gabapentin*** is useful in "pain syndromes" & adjuvant to treat anxiety disorders.

4. Drug used in Alzheimer's disease *except:*

A. Rivastigmine **B.** Memantine
C. Donapezil **D.** Clonidine

Ans: D. Clonidine

Ref: *Synopsis of Psychiatry, Kaplan & Sadock, 10th edition.p.343.*

Expanation:

- **Alzheimer's disease / dementia** is the most common type of dementia across the globe (In India, **Vascular dementia is MC**).
- Dementia is a chronic, progressive condition characterized by:
  1. Decline in memory (Short term)
  2. Executive dysfunction (Agnosia, Aphasia and Apraxia).
- While many are irreversible, some have reversible causes- alcohol, head injury, deficiency states, metabolic and endocrinopathies.
- Alzheimer's dementia is due to progressive loss of neurons starting from basal nucleus (of Meynert) which in turn due to accumulation of neurofibrillary tangles (intracellular tau proteins) & amyloid plaques (**extracellular ßamyloid)** deposition.
- Since basal nucleus is the main place in brain where acetylcholine is synthesized (Ach is responsible for transferring immediate memory into short term memory), decline of memory is seen.
- *Recently,* ***aluminum*** *has been implicated for* ***Alzheimer's disease****.*

Cortical dementia	Sub-cortical dementia
Memory loss is early Aphasia is pronounced e.g., Alzheimer's dementia	Mood & motor symptoms first Memory disturbance is late e.g., Parkinson, Lewy body disease

The aim of treatment of Alzheimer's disease is preservation of existing cholinergic neurons (or at least Ach by preventing its degradation - which in turn done by inhibition of Ach-estrase).

The drugs used:

1. **Ach precursors**- Choline, Lecithine
2. **AchE inhibitors**- Donapezil, Rivastigmine, Galantamine (DRG)
3. **Antiglutamates** - Memantine
4. **New drugs** – Selegeline (MAOI-B type), Ondensetron, Estrogen, NSAIDs.

Clonidine is a **central sympatholytic (α)**, used to treat **essential hypertension, diabetic neuropathy, Opioid withdrawal, menopausal symptoms (hot flushes)**.

5. **True about explicit memory:**
A. Consciously present
B. Form of working memory
C. Type of sensory memory
D. Stored in striatum

Ans: A. Consciously present

Ref: Synopsis of Psychiatry, Kaplan & Sadock, 10th edition

Expanation:

- Memory are based on *long-term potentiation* (LTP) of cells, well developed in neurons.
- Human brain memory systems are classified in various ways
  1. Based on the time gap between storage and retrieval - immediate, recent, remote
  2. Based on the duration and capacity of storage- short term & long term
     Conversion of short (living) term memory into long term occurs at Hippocampus.
  3. Long term memory in turn- declarative (explicit) & non-declarative (implicit)
     Declarative memory needs conscious effort for retrieval of information
  4. Declarative memory is of two types- Episodic & Semantic
     - **Episodic memory** denotes information about self and personal events (one's age). It is also known as "auto-biographical memory". Stored in Entorhinal cortex & Thalamus (mammillary body).
     - **Semantic memory** denotes general information and knowledge (time-independent, like how many continents on the earth?). Stored in medial temporal lobes. May get affected alone as in herpes simplex infection (leaving episodic memory intact!)
  5. **Non-declarative memory** (procedural memory) is the type of memory used to store information related to skills (writing, driving) & stored in cerebellum. Priming is an important component and it is stored in Striatum.
     - Sensory memory is an ultra-short-acting memory of nerve endings at sense organs. Working memory is a type of memory important for executive functioning (Prefrontal cortex is essential for it). Emotional memory is stored in Amygdala.

The steps of memory process are:
1. Reception
2. Registration
3. Retention
4. Rehearsal
5. Retrieval

6. **All are true regarding cocaine toxicity *except:***
A. Seizures
B. Myocardial infarction
C. Amantidine is the drug of choice
D. Mania symptoms

Ans: C. Amantidine is the drug of choice

Ref: Synopsis of Psychiatry, Kaplan & Sadock, 10th edition

Expanation:

Cocaine

- It is an alkaloid (from ***Erythroxylon coca).***
- It is has high dependence potential.
- The routes of use are many:
  1. **Inhalation** of cocaine powder- *snorting* (MC method**).**
  2. **Smoking** – *free basing* (cocaine in crack jam) [least dangerous method]
  3. **Ingestion**- *rush* as an aphrodisiac (cocaine + Opioid=speed balls)
  4. **Intravenous** injection- most dangerous method (risk of Hepatitis & HIV due to needle sharing , local gangrene due to additives)
- It **causes**
  - *Perforation of nasal septum*
  - COPD
  - Sepsis
  - *Endocarditis*
  - Hypertension
  - Myocardial infarction
  - Stroke
  - Autonomic over activity
  - Seizures
  - Mania-like picture
  - Post-intoxication depression (*crash*).
- Treatment of **intoxication- Amylnirite**
- Treatment of **withdrawal - Imipramine / Amitryptaline**.

7. **True regarding anxiety is all *except:* (Repeat)**
A. Adaptive response
B. Alert signal
C. Autonomic hyperactivity
D. Always pathological

Ans: D. Always pathological

Ref: Synopsis of Psychiatry, Kaplan & Sadock, 10th edition

Explanation:

- Anxiety is a state of mind characterized by **alertness**, in response to any **threatening stimulus** and it is an **adaptive response**.
- It has **cognitive symptoms (inattention → forgetfulness)**
- **Emotional symptoms** (feeling on the edge)
- **Autonomic symptoms** (hyper-sympathetic state)
- **Physical symptoms** (muscle tension).
- While anxiety is due to an internal, vague, distant stimuli, fear is a response to a stimulus which is external, well-defined and immediate.
  - Also Refer Psychiatry question explanation in 2011 paper.

JIPMER–2009

ANATOMY

1. **'Milky spots' present in the greater omentum consists of:**
A. Macrophages B. Neutrophils
C. Lymphocytes D. Langerhans cells

Ans: A. Macrophages

Ref: *Gray's Anatomy, 39th edition, 2008, Page 1132*

Explanation:

'Milky spots'

- These are dense, oval or round visible spots in the **greater omentum** (policeman of abdomen).
- 'Milky spots' contains numerous fixed **macrophages**.
- These macrophages are easily mobilized.

* Other areas where 'Milky spots' present: **Pleura.**

2. **Skin over the angle of mandible and parotid area is supplied by:**
A. Auriculotemporal nerve
B. Posterior auricular nerve
C. Great auricular nerve
D. Facial nerve

Ans: C. Great auricular nerve

Ref: *Gray's Anatomy, 39th edition, 2008, Page 515*

Explanation:

- **Great auricular nerve** is a branch from **cervical plexus.**
- Root value – **ventral rami of C2 and C3**.
- Important relation or location present in the post-triangle of neck, from the middle of post-border of sternomastoid muscle it crosses obliquely and reach angle of mandible.
- Area supplied:
  – **Skin over the angle of mandible**
  – **Lower part of auricle of the ear**
  – **Skin over the parotid gland**

3. **The following are present in seminiferous tubules *except*:**
A. Sertoli cells B. Leydig cells
C. Spermatid D. Spermatogonia

Ans: B. Leydig cells

Ref: *Wheater's Functional Histology: A Text and Colour Atlas, 5th edition, 2007, Pages 348 & 349*

Explanation:

Seminiferous tubules contain:

- **Germ cells in various stages**, i.e. Spermatogonia dark and light type A, type B spermatogonia, primary spermatocytes, secondary spermatocytes, spermatid and spermatozoa.
- **Sertoli cells**: non–germ cells, which support and nourish the developing spermatozoa.

Note:

- **Leydig cells**: They are endocrine cells present outside the seminiferous tubules, i.e. in the interstitial spaces between tubules.

4. **Abductor of vocal cord is (Repeat):**
A. Posterior cricoarytenoid
B. Lateral cricoarytenoid
C. Cricothyroid
D. Oblique arytenoids

Ans: A. Posterior cricoarytenoid

Ref: *Gray's Anatomy, 40th edition, pg. 580*

Explanation:

Muscles of Vocal Cords

Action	Intrinsic muscle
Abductor	Posterior cricoarythenoid
Adductor "TILAC"	Thyroarythenoid Inter arythenoid Lateral cricoarythenoid
Tensor of vocal cord	Cricothyroid Thyroarythenoid
Openers of laryngeal inlet	Thyroepiglottic
Closers of laryngeal inlet	Inter arythenoid Aryepiglottic

Nerve supply of larynx:

Motor

- All intrinsic muscles of the laryngx are supplied by recurrent laryngeal nerve except for cricothyroid which is supplied by external laryngeal nerve.

Sensory

- Upto to the level of vocal fold is supplied by internal laryngeal nerve.
- Below the level of vocal cord is supplied by recurrent laryngeal nerve.

5. **Vestibular anus is classified under which of the following anorectal anomalies?**

A. Imperforate anus
B. High anorectal
C. Low anorectal
D. Mid anorectal

Ans: B. High anorectal

Ref: *Keith L Moore and T.V.N. Persaud The developing human clinically oriented embryology, 8th edition,2008, Page 240*

Explanation:

High anorectal anomalies (Rectum ends superior to puborectalis muscle).

- Most common type of anorectal anomaly (**2/3 of anorectal anomaly**).
- Rectum **ends blindly superior to puborectalis muscle**.
- There is a **fistula to the bladder (rectovesical fistula**) or **urethra (rectourethral fistula**) in males or to the vagina (**rectovaginal fistula**) or to the vestibule of the vagina (**rectovestibular fistula**).
- In this case it is rectovestibular fistula – vestibular anus (not anus but rectum opens into vestibule of vagina).
- Diagnosis: Presence of **meconium** in the **vestibule of vagina.**
- Embryological cause: Incomplete separation of the cloaca by the urorectal septum.

6. **Which organ develops from both ectoderm and mesoderm?**

A. Adrenal **B.** Pancreas
C. Kidney **D.** Spleen

Ans: A. Adrenal

Ref: *Langman's embryology, 11th ed.*

Explanation:

Adrenal gland

- The adrenal gland develops from 2 components:
  a. A **mesodermal** portion, which forms the **cortex.**
  b. An **ectodermal** portion, which forms the **medulla.**

Pituitary gland

- The pituitary gland develops from two separate sources:
  a. **Rathke's pouch,** which is an ectodermal outpocketing of the stomodeum immediately in front of the buccopharyngeal membrane.
  b. A **downward extension** from the **floor of the diencephalon.**
- The **Rathke's pouch** gives rise to the **pars anterior,** pars intermedia and the pars tuberalis.
- The cavity of the pouch may persist as the intraglandular cleft.
- The **diverticulum** from the **diencephalon** gives rise to the **posterior lobe** and the **infundibulum;** its cavity persists as the **infundibular recess.**

Kidney

- The definitive human kidney arises from two distinct sources:
  a. The **excretory tubules or nephrons** are derived from the **metanephric mesoderm** also called the **metanephric blastema.**
  b. The **collecting part** is derived from a **diverticulum** of the **mesonephric duct** called the **ureteric bud.**

Pancreas

- The pancreas develops from **dorsal and ventral buds**, from a part of the gut that later forms the **2nd part of the duodenum.**
- The **dorsal bud** arises from the **dorsal aspect of the gut** and grows into the **mesogastrium** and the **mesoduodenum.**
- The ventral bud arises from the **ventral aspect of the gut** at the junction of the **foregut** and midgut, in the inferior angle between the **hepatic bud and the duodenum.**

Spleen

- The spleen is developed from **mesoderm** within the **dorsal mesogastrium.**
- A number of lobules appear which fuse to form a single mass, which projects under the cover of the left leaf of the dorsal mesogastrium.
- The appearance of the spleen in the dorsal mesogastrium divides it into the gastrosplenic ligament in front and the lienorenal ligament behind.

- The primordium of the splenic tissue differentiates into branching trabecular cords and numerous free cells which differentiate into blood forming cells.

7. **Morrison pouch is:**
   A. Right subphrenic space
   B. Right subhepatic space
   C. Right infracolic space
   D. Right extraperitoneal space

Ans: B. Right subhepatic space

Ref: *Gray's Anatomy, 39th edition, 2008, Page 1135*

Explanation:

Right subhepatic space or hepatorenal recess or pouch of Morrison:

Situation: lies between right lobe of liver and kidney.

Boundaries:

Superior – inferior layer of coronary ligament
Laterally – right lateral abdominal wall.
Medially – second part of duodenum, hepatic flexure of colon and pancreas.
Posteriorly – anterior surface of right kidney.

Clinical significance:

In supine position it is more dependent than right paracolic gutter.
So postoperative infected fluid collections are more common.

8. **All the following organs are developed from endoderm *except:* (Repeat)**
   A. Liver
   B. Kidney
   C. Pancreas
   D. Urinary bladder

Ans: B. Kidney

Ref: *Keith L Moore and T.V.N. Persaud, The Developing Human Clinically Oriented Embryology, 8th edition,2008, Pages 219,244-252 and 257*

Explanation:

Development of Kidney

- **From 2 sources:**
  a. **Collecting part from – Ureteric bud,** which is developed from nephrogenic cord (intermediate mesoderm).
  b. **Excretory part** – from metanephric blastema, which is developed from metanephric masss of mesenchyme (intermediate mesoderm).

Also Note

- **Pancreas and liver**: Developed from endoderm of foregut.
- **Urinary bladder**: Developed from endoderm of vesical part of urogenital sinus (ventral part of endodermal cloaca).

9. **Hassal corpuscles are seen in: (Repeat)**
   A. Thymus **B.** Thyroid
   C. Parathyroid **D.** Spleen

Ans: A. Thymus

Ref: *Gray's Anatomy, 40th Ed, Pg 939*

Explanation:

Hassal's corpuscles

- These are **whorls** of **flattened, concentrically** layered **medullary epithelial cells,** and are characteristic features of the **thymic medulla.**
- They start to form before birth and their numbers increase throughout life.
- Their **function** is **not clear**, although they may represent a **site for removal of dying, apoptotic thymocytes**, because their centres are eosinophilic, partly keratinized and often contain cellular debris.

10. **All the following develops from Wolffian duct *except:* (Repeat)**
    A. Eoophoron **B.** Paraoophoron
    C. Gartner duct **D.** Bartholin duct

Ans: D. Bartholin duct

Ref: *Gray's Anatomy 40th Ed, Pg 1305*

Explanation:

Derivatives of Mesonephric duct (Wolffian duct)

1. Kidney-collecting tubules, pelves and calyces
2. Ureter
3. Trigone of the bladder
4. Prostatic urethera
5. Epididymis
6. Vas deferens
7. Seminal vesicle
8. Ejaculatory duct
9. Part of prostate
10. Appendix of testis

Derivative of Paramesonephric Duct (Mullerian duct)

1. Uterus
2. Fallopian tube
3. Part of vagina

Note:

- Scrotum develops from genital swelling.
- Testis and ovary develops from genital ridge.

11. **Red nucleus is present in:**
   A. Upper pons
   B. Lower pons
   C. Midbrain
   D. Medulla

Ans: C. Midbrain

Ref: *Gray's Anatomy, 40th edition, pg. 280*

Explanation:

Red Nucleus

- The red nucleus is a pink, ovoid mass, approximately 5 mm in diameter and lying **dorsomedial** to the **substantia nigra**.
- The tint appears only in fresh material and is caused by a **ferric iron pigment** in **its multipolar** neurons.
- Small multipolar neurons occur in all parts of the nucleus.
- The magnocellular element is considered phylogenetically old, which accords with the parvocellular predominance in primates.
- Rostrally, the red nucleus is poorly demarcated, and it blends into the reticular formation and caudal pole of the interstitial nucleus.
- It is traversed and surrounded by fascicles of nerve fibres, including many from the **oculomotor** nucleus.

12. **All the following are true about trochlear nerve** ***except:***
   A. Purely motor
   B. Only nerve emerging from ventral aspect of brain stem
   C. Originates from midbrain at level of inferior colliculus
   D. Supplies only the superior oblique muscle

Ans: B. Only nerve emerging from ventral aspect of brain stem

Ref: *Gray's Anatomy:Anatomical basis of clinical practice by Susan Standring,Churchill Livingstone: 40th edition, 2008, Pg. 666*

Explanation:

Trochelar Nerve

- The trochlear nerve is the **fourth** cranial nerve and innervates **superior oblique exclusively**.
- It is the **only cranial nerve** to emerge from the **dorsal surface** of the brain stem, passing from the midbrain onto the lateral surface of the crus of the cerebral peduncle.
- It runs through the lateral dural wall of the cavernous sinus and then crosses the oculomotor nerve to enter the orbit through the **superior orbital fissure**, above the common tendinous ring and levator palpebrae superioris, and medial to the frontal and lacrimal nerves.
- The trochlear nerve travels but a short distance to enter the superior (orbital) surface of superior oblique.

13. **One of the following is supplied by median nerve:**
   A. 1st and 2nd lumbricals
   B. Hypothenar muscles
   C. Palmar interossei
   D. Dorsal interossei

Ans: A. 1st and 2nd lumbricals

Ref: *Gray's Anatomy:Anatomical basis of clinical practice by Susan Standring,Churchill Livingstone, 40th edition, 2008, Pg. 895*

Explanation:

Brachial plexus branch	Origin	Spinal segment	Function
Median nerve	Medial and lateral cords	**C5 to T1**	**Motor:** • All muscles in anterior compartment of forearm (except flexor carpi ulnaris and medial half of flexor digitorum profundus) • Three thenar muscles • Two lateral lumbrical muslces **Sensory**: Skin over the palmar surface of the lateral three and one half digits and lateral side of palm and middle of wrist

14. **The following muscles are supplied by radial nerve below the spiral groove** ***except:***
   A. Brachialis
   B. Brachioradialis
   C. Extensor carpi radialis longus
   D. Anconeus

Ans: D. Anconeus

Ref: *Gray's Anatomy:Anatomical basis of clinical practice by Susan Standring, Churchill Livingstone, 40th edition, 2008, Pg. 829,837*

Explanation:

Radial Nerve ($C_{5678}T_1$)	
Above elbow	**Below elbow**
• **Above spiral groove :** - Triceps (long, medial head) - Posterior cutaneous nerve of arm • **In spiral groove : Sensory** - Posterior cutaneous nerve of forearm - Lateral cutaneous nerve of arm • **Anconeus** - Triceps (medial and lateral heads) • **Between spiral groove and lateral epicondyle** - Brachialis - Brachioradialis - Extensor carpi radialis longus	• Posterior interosseous nerve supply remaining Ms. i.e. - Abductor pollicis longus - Extensor pollicis longus and brevis - Extensor indicis Supinator - Extensor digitorum - Extensor digit, minimi - Extensor carpi ulnaris - Extensor carpi radialis brevis

PHYSIOLOGY

1. **Carotid body baroreceptor is most sensitive to: (Repeat)**
   A. Mean blood pressure
   B. Diastolic blood pressure
   C. Systolic blood pressure
   D. Pulse pressure

Ans: D. Pulse pressure

Ref: *1. Pal GK, Blood Pressure and Its Regulation, In: Textbook of Medical Physiology, Ahuja Publishing House, 2007; 80: 646-49*

2. WF Ganong, Cardiovascular Regulatory Mechanisms, In: Review of Medical Physiology, 24th ed, California: McGraw-Hill Companies 2012, p593

Explanation:

Refer to 2013 Physiology question explanation:

- Baroreceptors regulate blood pressure in the pressure range of 50-200 mmHg.
- Baroreceptors are very sensitive to changes in pulse pressure.

2. **Inhibition of prolactin is caused by: (Repeat)**
   A. Dopamine
   B. Dobutamine
   C. TRH
   D. AT-II

Ans: A. Dopamine

Ref: *Pal GK, Pituitary Gland: The Anterior Pituitary. In: Textbook of Medical Physiology, Ahuja Publishing House, 2007; 44:332*

Explanation:

Regulation of Prolactin Secretion

- **Prolaction Increased by:**
  – PRF
  – Sleep, stress, breast feeding
  – Also released by **TRH** and hormones in the **glucagon family (secretin, glucagon, VIP and gastric inhibitory polypeptide [GIP])**
  – **AT-II**
  – Oxytocin
  – Dopamine antagonist (phenothiazine)
  – Adrenergic blockers
  – Serotonin agonists
- **Prolactin Decreased by:**
  – Dopamine
  – Somatostatin
  – Prolactin
  – GABA

3. **Waves on EEG during stage 4–NREM period of sleep is: (Repeat)**
   A. Alpha **B.** Beta
   C. Delta **D.** Theta

Ans: C. Delta

Ref: *Pal GK, Reticular Formation, EEG and Sleep, In: Textbook of Medical Physiology, Ahuja Publishing House 2007; 119:895*

Explanation:

Non - REM Sleep (Slow Wave Sleep)

- **Stage 1**
  – Beta to alpha rhythm
- **Stage 2**
  – Amplitude increases
  – **Sleep spindle** (12-14Hz; 50μV; for about 2 Seconds) and **K complexes** (high amplitude)
- **Stage 3**
  – High amplitude; low frequency

- **Stage 4**
  - Delta rhythm
- **Autonomic and visceral changes**
  - ↓ heart rate and BP
  - ↓ body temperature
  - Slow regular respiration
  - ↑ GI activity
  - ↓ muscle tone
  - No rapid eye movement

4. **Action potential is transmitted in myofibrils via:**

A. Terminal cisterns
B. T- Tubules
C. Longitudinal
D. Sarcomere

Ans: B. T- Tubules

Ref: *Pal GK, Muscle, In: Textbook of Medical Physiology, Ahuja Publishing House 2007; 20:177*

Explanation:

- **T-Tubules** are **tubular extensions** of **sarcolemma**, that penetrate to the center at the junctions of A and I bands. It is involved in conduction of **action potential** from **NMJ** to the **triad** formed by **terminal cisternae and L tubules** (part **of sarcotubular system**).
- **Terminal cisternae** – dilated region at both ends of elongated tubules (L-tubules), a part of Sarcoplasmic reticulum - involved in calcium release.

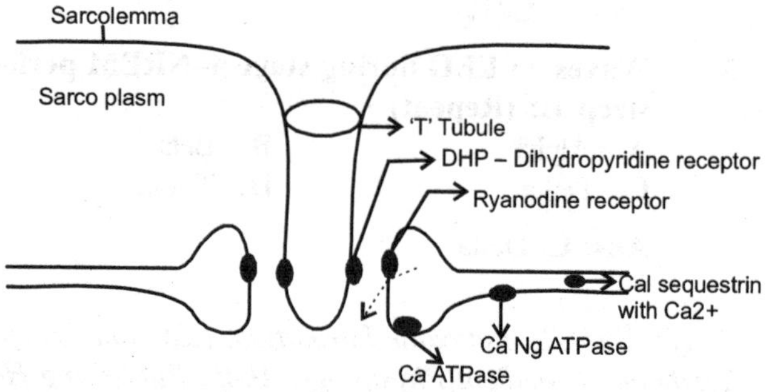

Sarco-Tubular System

- **Sarcomere** – structural functional unit of myofibril; portion of myofibril between two successive Z lines.

5. **Following is true of hormone leptin** ***except:***

A. It is found in increased levels in obese
B. Site of action is hypothalamus
C. It is produced by adipose all
D. It increases appetite

Ans: D. It increases appetite

Ref: *Pal GK, Functions of Hypothalamus, In: Textbook of Medical Physiology, Ahuja Publishing House, 118:889*

Explanation:

Leptin

- Protein of 167 amino acids
- Manufactured primarily in the **adipocytes**
- High leptin level occurs in **obesity** - ↑ **sympathetic** activity; ↓ **food intake**
- Low leptin level occurs in **starvation** - ↑ **para-sympathetic** activity; ↑ **food intake**
- Acts on **hypothalamus, arcuate nucleus** identifies plasma **leptin** concentration.
- Regulates onset of **puberty**
- **Stimulates thyroid** function
- **Controls glucocorticoid secretion**

6. **Function of brown fat is: (Repeat)**

A. Glycogenosis
B. Gluconeogenesis
C. Glycogenolysis
D. Thermogenesis

Ans: D. Thermogenesis

Ref: *WF Ganong, Excitable Tissue: Nerve, In: Review of Medical Physiology, 21st ed, California: McGraw-Hill Companies 2012, p27*

Explanation:

Brown Fat

- More abundant in **infants** but is present in **adults** as well (between the **scapulas**, at the **nape of the neck**, along the **great vessels** in the **thorax** and **abdomen**, and in other scattered locations in the body).
- Have an extensive **sympathetic innervation** (fat cells and its blood vessels); also contain many **mitochondria.**
- In these mitochondria, there is a **second proton conductance** that **does not generate ATP,** depends on a **32-kDa uncoupling protein (UCP1)**; involved in **heat production.**

7. **Which of the following hormones increase during sleep?**

A. Insulin　　**B.** ACTH
C. GH　　**D.** Glucocorticoid

Ans: C. GH

Ref: *Pal GK, Pituitary Gland: The Anterior Pituitary, In: Textbook of Medical Physiology, Ahuja Publishing House 2007; 44:328,336*

Explanation:

- **70%** of total 24 hours GH secretion occurs during **sleep**. **Adequte sleep** promotes **growth.**
- **ACTH** – **75%** of daily secretion occurs in **early morning.**
- **Insulin secretion** is mainly decided by **glucose uptake** and its **plasma concentration.**
- **Glucocorticoid** secretion follows the **ACTH pattern.**

8. **Which of the following has least half-life?**
   A. Norepinephrine **B.** Insulin
   C. Calcitonin **D.** PTH

Ans: A. Norepinephrine

Ref: *1. The Adrenal Medulla 48:380*
2. Endocrine Pancreas 49:389
3. Parathyroid Gland 50:411, 414
In: Pal GK, Textbook of Medical Physiology Ahuja Publishing House, 2007

Explanation:

Half life of Hormones

- **Catecholamines** – **1-3 minutes**
- **Insulin** – **5-8 minutes**
- **Calcitonin** – **5-10 minutes**
- **PTH** – about **10 minutes**

9. **Which of the following will not decrease Glomerular filtration rate (GFR)? (Repeat)**
   A. Increased hydrostatic pressure in tubule
   B. Increased capillary oncotic pressure
   C. Hypoproteinemia
   D. Mesangial cell contraction

Ans: C. Hypoproteinemia

Ref: *Pal GK. Glomerular Filtration, In: Textbook of Medical Physiology, 2nd ed, Ahuja Publishing House 2011; 61: 522*

Explanation:

GFR – Glomerular Filtration Rate

Amount of filtrate formed by glomerular filtering membrane of both kidneys in a unit time.
Normal GFR – 125 ml/min

Factors Affecting Glomerular Filtration Rate

- Changes in renal blood flow
  - Increase in renal blood flow, promotes filtration
- Changes in glomerular capillary hydrostatic pressure
  - Increases glomerular filtration
- Changes in systemic blood pressure
- Afferent or efferent arteriolar constriction
- Changes in hydrostatic pressure in Bowman's capsule
- Ureteral obstruction
- Edema of kidney inside tight renal capsule
- Changes in concentration of plasma proteins: dehydration, hypoproteinemia
- Changes in Kf
- Changes in glomerular capillary permeability
- Changes in effective filtration surface area

10. **Receptor for stretch reflex is:**
    A. Muscle spindle
    B. Golgi tendon organ
    C. Proprioceptors
    D. Paccinian corpuscle

Ans: A. Muscle spindle

Ref: *Pal GK, The Spinal Reflexes. In: Textbook of Medical Physiology, 2nd ed, Ahuja Publishing House 2011; 112: 839*

Explanation:

- **Stretch reflex** – Reflex contraction of the muscle to stretch when a skeletal muscle (with intact nerve supply) is stretched
- **Type**
  - Phasic stretch reflex
  - Tonic stretch reflex
- **Phasic stretch reflex**
  - Stimulus – sudden stretch
  - Receptor – muscle spindle
  - Afferent – Ia
  - Efferent – Motor neuron (reciprocal innervation – contraction of agonist, relaxation of antagonist)
  - Importance – immediate correction of spinal motor output in moment – to moment motor control
- **Tonic stretch reflex**
  - Stimulus – sustained stretch
  - Receptor – muscle spindle
  - Afferent – Ia, II
  - Efferent – Motor neuron (reciprocal innervation – contraction of agonist, relaxation of antagonist)
  - Importance – role in muscle tone, regulation of posture
- **Golgi Tendon organ** is involved in **inversed stretch reflex.**

11. **Type–2 skeletal muscle fibers are rich in:**
    A. Mitochondria **B.** ATPase activity
    C. Anaerobic glycolysis **D.** Oxidation

Ans: B and C. ATPase activity (Myosin ATPase) and Anaerobic glycolysis

***Ref:** Berne & Levy, Physiology, 6th Ed, Chapter 12, Skeletal Muscle Physiology, Page 243-244.*

Explanation:

- There are **2 types** of **Type II** skeletal muscle fibers (Type **II-A**, Type **II-B**).
- Even if we consider it as Type II - B skeletal fiber, it has more than one **answer**.
  - Skeletal muscle can be classified as either **fast-twitch** (also called type IIA and type IIB or **slow-twitch** (also called type I) muscle.
  - Type IIA, are found in mammals but are uncommon in humans. They have both high glycolytic and high oxidative capacity.

Basic Classification of Skeletal Muscle Fiber Types

	Type I Slow Oxidative (Red)	Type II-B Fast Glycolytic (White)	Type II-A Fast Oxidative (Red)
Myosin isoenzyme (ATPase rate)	Slow	***Fast***	Fast
Sarcoplasmic reticular Ca^{++} pumping capacity	Moderate	High	High
Diameter (diffusion distance)	Moderate	Large	Small
Oxidative capacity: Mitochondrial content, capillary density, myoglobin	High	Low	Very high
Glycolytic capacity	Moderate	***High***	High

12. Sertoli cells secrete:

A. FSH
B. Androgen binding protein
C. Testosterone
D. LH

Ans: B. Androgen binding protein

***Ref:** Rhoades Rodney A Bell, David R, Medical Physiology: Principles for Clinical Medicine, 3rd Edition. Chaper 36, Male Reproductive System. Page 674 (Picture Ref) & GK Pal, Textbook of Medical Physiology, Chapter 54, Male Reproductive System. Page 440*

Explanation:

Functions of Sertoli Cell

1. Germ cell development – Structural support
2. Nourishment and growth of spermatid
3. Phagocytosis (residual bodies during maturation)
4. Formation of tubular fluid
5. Support spermiation - secrete plasminogen activator
6. Endocrine function (Sertoli cell secretes)
   - **Inhibin, Follistatin** - ↓ FSH
   - **Activin** - ↑ FSH
   - **MIS** (Mullerian Inhibiting Substance)– 8th weak of IUL
   - **Estrogen** - From androgen by aromatase
7. It **has FSH, testosterone (receptors)** sensitivity. They do not secrete testosterone.
8. Secretory functions
   i. **Androgen Binding Protein (ABP)**- Binds with DHT, testosterone and transport to epididymis
   ii. H-Y antigen - development of gonads
   iii. Also produce plasminogen activator
9. Blood Testis Barrier (BTB)
10. Paracrine effect on leydig cell

13. 'A' wave of electroretinogram corresponds to activity in:

A. Rods and cones
B. Pigment epithelium
C. Ganglion cell layer
D. Nerve fiber layer

Ans: A. Rods and cones

***Ref:** Pal GK, Movements of the Eye, In: Textbook of Medical Physiology, Ahuja Publishing House, 2007 965*

Explanation:

Electroretinography

- It is the recording of retinal electrical activities
- **Negative 'a' wave** - from retinal photoreceptors (Rods, Cones)
- **Positive 'b' wave** - from bipolar cells
- **'c' wave** - pigment epithelium
- Used in diagnosing **retinal detachment, retinal dystrophy, vitamin A deficiency**

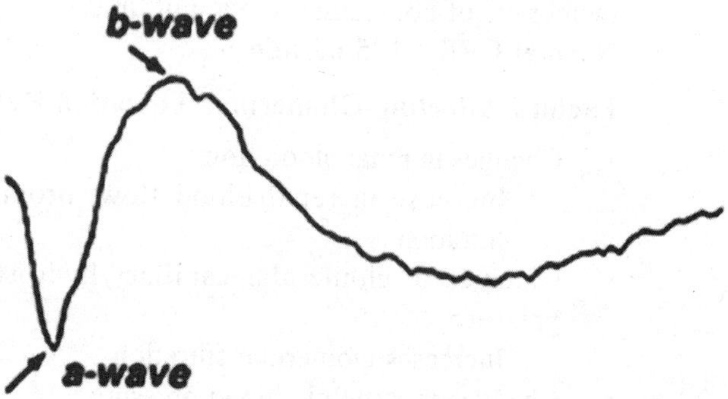

14. **Meissner's plexus are present in:**

A. Mucosa **B.** Submucosa
C. Muscularis layer **D.** Serosa

Ans: B. Submucosa

Ref: Ganong Medical Physiology, 21st ed.

Explanation:

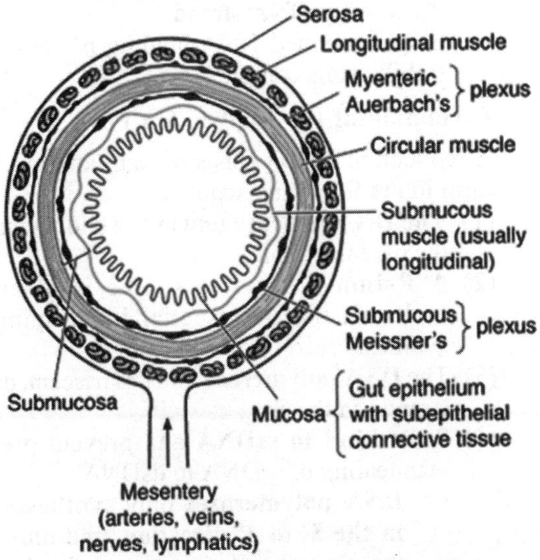

All segments of the GI tract are divided into four layers:

- The mucosa (epithelium, lamina propria, and muscular mucosae)
- The submucosa (**Meissner's plexus)**
- The muscularis propria (inner circular muscle layer, intermuscular space and outer longitudinal muscle layer) (**Myenteric Auerbach plexus** – between longitudinal and circular layers)
- The serosa

BIOCHEMISTRY

1. **Most stable amino acid at the physiological pH is:**

A. Histidine **B.** Lysine
C. Arginine **D.** Glycine

Ans: A. Histidine

Ref: 'Textbook of Medical Biochemistry' by Dinesh Puri, 3rd edn, Chapter 4, p49

Explanation:

- **Histidine** with an **imidazole ring** functions as **a general acid base catalyst**.
- **pKa range** of histidine is **6.5-7.4**, which **ionizes within the physiological pH range.**

2. **All are polyunsaturated fatty acids *except:***

A. Linoleic acid **B.** Linolenic acid
C. Palmitic acid **D.** Arachidonic acid

Ans: C. Palmitic acid

Ref: Harper's Illustrated Biochemistry, 29th edition, Pg142

Explanation:

- **Palmitic acid** is 16 carbon containing **saturated fatty acid**.
- All human cells can synthesize **palmitic acid** from **acetyl coA**.
- **Linoleic and linolenic acid** are the nutritionally essential fatty acids.
- **Arachidonic acid** is **semi-essential FA**, if we take enough of essential fatty acids arachidonic acid can be synthesized in our body, or else this also becomes essential.

1. **Arachidonic acid** is a **PUFA** but arachidic acid is saturated FA. Both contain 20 carbons.
2. Active fatty acid is called as **acyl coA** and active acetate is called as **acetyl coA.**
3. **Eicosonoids** are **20 carbon** containing physiologically active compounds synthesized from arachidonic acid.

3. **All the following causes non-ketotic hypoglycemia *except:***

A. Galactosemia
B. Fructose intolerance
C. Hyperinsulinemia
D. Alcohol intoxication

Ans: D. Alcohol intoxication

Ref: Harper's Illustrated Biochemistry, 29th edition

Explanation:

- **Ketosis** implies **ketonuria** and **ketonemia.**
- Increased production of ketone bodies (**Acetone, Acetoacetate, beta hydroxyl butyrate)** occurs due to low levels/absence of insulin accompanied by elevated counter regulatory hormones mainly, **glucagon, epinephrine** and **cortisol.**
- **Carnitine deficiency** is another cause for **non-ketotic hypoglycemia.**

Causes for Ketotic Hypoglycemia

- Alcohol intoxication
- Starvation

4. **7-Methyl guanosine cap is present in: (Repeat)**

A. mRNA **B.** tRNA
C. rRNA **D.** DNA

Ans: A. mRNA

Ref: Harper's Illustrated Biochemistry, 28th edition, Chapter 36, p-349

Explanation:

*"The 5' cap is found on the 5' end of an **mRNA** molecule and consists of a **guanine nucleotide** connected to the mRNA via an unusual **5' to 5' triphosphate** linkage.*

*This guanosine is methylated on the 7 position directly after capping in vivo by a methyl transferase. It is referred to as a **7-methylguanylate cap**, abbreviated **m^7G**"*

Capping - 5' end

- Addition of modified nucleotide
- 7-methylguanosine to 5' end
- Guanyl transferase and methyl transferase.

Functions

- mRNA recognition
- Promotion of 5' proximal intron excision.
- Prevention of degradation by exonucleases.
- Regulation of Nuclear Transport/Export
- Promotion of translation and stability

5. **During DNA replication, Okazaki fragments are seen in relation to:**

A. Leading strand **B.** Lagging strand
C. Both **D.** Helicase

Ans: B. Lagging strand

Ref: *Harper's Illustrated Biochemistry, 29th edition*

Explanation:

DNA SYNTHESIS and REPLICATION

Steps Involved in DNA Replication:

1. Identification of the origins of replication
2. Unwinding (denaturation) of dsDNA to provide an ssDNA template
3. Formation of the replication fork
4. Initiation of DNA synthesis and elongation
5. Formation of replication bubbles with ligation of the newly synthesized DNA segments
6. Reconstitution of chromatin structure

Classes of Proteins Involved in Replication

Protein	Function
DNA polymerases	Deoxynucleotide polymerization
Helicases	Processive unwinding of DNA
Topoisomerases	Relieve torsional strain that results from helicase-induced unwinding
DNA primase	Initiates synthesis of RNA primers
Single-strand binding proteins	Prevent premature reannealing of dsDNA
DNA ligase	Seals the single strand nick between the nascent chain and Okazaki fragments on lagging strand

The Origin of Replication

- At the origin of replication (ori), there is an association of sequence-specific dsDNA-binding proteins with a series of direct repeat DNA sequences.
- The interaction of proteins with ori defines the start site of replication and provides a short region of ssDNA essential for initiation of synthesis of the nascent DNA strand.
- Single-stranded DNA-binding proteins (SSBs) stabilize this complex.

Formation of the Replication Fork

A replication fork consists of four components that form in the following sequence:

(1) **The DNA helicase** unwinds a short segment of the parental duplex DNA
(2) A **Primase** initiates synthesis of an RNA molecule that is essential for priming DNA synthesis
(3) The **DNA polymerase** initiates nascent, daughter strand synthesis
(4) **SSBs bind to ssDNA** and prevent premature reannealing of ssDNA to dsDNA.
   - **DNA polymerases** only **synthesize DNA in the 5' to 3' direction**, and only one of the several different types of polymerases is involved at the replication fork.
   - Because the DNA strands are antiparallel, the polymerase functions asymmetrically.
   - On the leading (forward strand, the DNA is synthesized continuously.
   - On the lagging (retrograde) strand, the DNA is synthesized in short fragments, the so-called Okazaki fragments.
   - Several **Okazaki fragments** (upto 250) must be sequentially synthesized for each replication fork.
   - To ensure that this happens, the **helicase** acts on the **lagging strand** to unwind dsDNA in a 5' to 3' direction.
   - The helicase associates with the primase to afford the latter proper access to the template.
   - This allows the RNA primer to be made and, in turn, the polymerase to begin replicating the DNA.
   - This is an important reaction sequence since DNA polymerases cannot initiate DNA synthesis de novo. The mobile complex between helicase and primase has been called a primosome.
   - As the synthesis of an **Okazaki fragment** is completed and the polymerase is released, a new primer has been synthesized.
   - The same polymerase molecule remains associated with the replication fork and proceeds to synthesize the next Okazaki fragment.

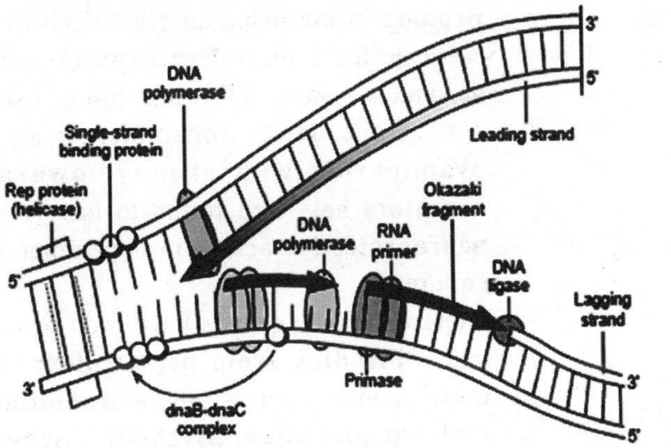

6. **All enzyme reactions are involved in substrate level phosphorylation *except:* (Repeat)**
   A. Phosphoglycerate kinase
   B. Succinate thiokinase
   C. Phosphofructokinase
   D. Pyruvate kinase

Ans: C. Phosphofructokinase

Ref: *Harper's Illustrated Biochemistry, 29th edition, Page 172 and 165*

Explanation:

- Usually **ATP** is produced when the **reducing equivalents** (NADH & FADH) reach **ETC**. Substrate level phosphorylation implies production of **ATP** when the **substrate** is converted to **product**, without involving Electron Transport Chain **(ETC)** in the inner mitochondrial membrane.
- Here the substrate is converted to product the extra energy in the substrate is utilized for the synthesis of ATP.
- Among the three options **Pyruvate kinase, Phosphoglycerate kinase and Succinate thiokinase** are involved in **substrate level phosphorylation**.
- **Phosphofructokinase** catalyses **rate limiting step in glycolysis** which **rather consumes one ATP.**

Examples for **substrate level phosphorylation**:

In Glycolysis:

1. Phosphoglycerate kinase
2. Pyruvate kinase

In Kreb's cycle (also known as TCA cycle, citric acid cycle)

1. Succinate thiokinase

7. **Lesh–Nyan syndrome is due to deficiency of: (Repeat)**
   A. HGPRTase **B.** CPS I
   C. CPS II **D.** PRPP synthetase

Ans: A. HGPRTase

Ref: *Harper's Illustrated Biochemistry, 29th edition, Page 335, 339 & 742*

Explanation:

Lesh-Nyhan Syndrome

This syndrome is characterized by:

- Hyperuricemia
- Urolithiasis
- Self mutilation
- CNS manifestations
- Extrapyramidal involvement (Choreathethosis, Dystonia, Ophisthotonus)

Enzyme Defect

- Hypoxanthine-guanine Phosphoribosyl Transferase (HGPRTase).
- This enzyme is involved in purine salvage it converts hypoxanthine to inosine mono phosphate (IMP).
- In absence of this enzyme intracellular PRPP levels will be elevated.
  Mutation in gene producing HGPRTase may be due to deletion, frame shift mutation, base substitutions or aberrent mRNA splicing.
  Note: Salvage reactions require less energy than the de novo synthesis.

8. **Pyridoxal phosphate is needed in: (Repeat)**
   A. Glucogenolysis
   B. Fatty acid oxidation
   C. Glycogenesis
   D. Gluconeogenesis

Ans: A. Glucogenolysis

Ref: *Harper's Illustrated Biochemistry,28th edition*

Explanation:

- Glycogenolysis is the breakdown of glycogen.
- **Glycogen Phosphorylase** catalyzes phosphorolytic cleavage of the? **(1→4)** glycosidic linkages of glycogen, releasing glucose-1-phosphate as reaction product.
- **Glycogen$_{(n\ residues)}$ + P_i → glycogen $_{(n-1\ residues)}$ + glucose-1-phosphate**
- **Pyridoxal phosphate** (PLP), a derivative of vitamin B_6, serves as prosthetic group for Glycogen Phosphorylase. Pyridoxal phosphate (PLP) is held at the active site with the e-amino group of a **lysine** residue.

PHARMACOLOGY

1. **All the following are beta-blockers *except:***

   A. Esmolol **B.** Sotalol
   C. Celiprolol **D.** Formoterol

   Ans: D. Formoterol

   Ref: *Goodman & Gilman's The Pharmacological Basis of Therapeutics, 12th ed, 2011, Pg 293, 313-315, 829*

   Explanation:

   - **Esmolol** is a **cardioselective beta blocker** with a **short half life of 9-10 min**. It belongs to **second generation** beta blockers.
   - **Sotalol** is a beta blocker with additional action of **prolonging action potential duration** through **potassium channel blockade**. Hence it is used as an **anti-arrhythmic drug**.
   - **Celiprolol** is a **beta 1 selective blocker** with **intrinsic sympathomimetic activity**. It is a **third generation** beta blocker with **vasodilating property**. In addition to **celiprolol**, **betaxolol** and **nebivolol** also belongs to third generation with **cardio selective beta blocking activity** as well as **vasodilating** property.
   - **Formoterol** is a **long acting beta 2 adrenergic receptor agonist**. Food and drug administration (FDA) has placed a **warning** on the labeling information for **salmeterol**, **formoterol** and **arformoterol** (all long acting beta 2 agonists). Expert panels have recommended the use of long acting beta 2 agonists for either initial therapy or if inhalational corticosteroid alone is not successful in controlling asthma.

2. **True statement regarding bromocriptine is:**

   A. It acts as agonist to dopamine receptors
   B. It can be used in active peptic ulceration
   C. It does not cause postural hypotension
   D. It has possible neuroprotective effect

   Ans: A. It acts as agonist to dopamine receptors

   Ref: *Basic and Clinical Pharmacology by Katzung, 2012, 12th ed, Pg 489*

   Explanation:

   - **Bromocriptine** is a **dopaminergic D2 agonist** used in the treatment of **parkinsonism** in the past. Now it has been replaced by more efficacious newer dopaminergic drugs namely **ropinirole** and **pramipexole**.
   - Dopaminergic agonists cause **postural hypotension** as an adverse effect especially in the beginning of therapy.
   - **Bromocriptine** being an ergot derivative can cause **painful digital vasospasm** in a dose dependent manner following chronic use.
   - Among the newer dopaminergic agonists, **pramipexole** with affinity **towards D3 receptors** has been found to have possible **neuroprotective action** in dopaminergic cell cultures.
   - **Dopaminergic agonists** have been reported to cause **bleeding from peptic ulcer**. Hence dopaminergic agonists are **contraindicated** in **active peptic ulcer, psychotic diseases** and **recent myocardial infarction**.

3. **Which of the following is contraindicated in early pregnancy?**

   A. Heparin **B.** Phenytoin
   C. Chloroquine **D.** Penicillin

   Ans: B. Phenytoin

   Ref: *Basic and Clinical Pharmacology by Katzung, 2012, 12th ed, Pg 424, 605, 609,920, 922-924, 1043, 1485*

   Explanation:

   Heparin

   - It has molecular weight in the range of **5000-30,000**, hence it **does not cross placenta**.
   - Thus it is used in pregnancy due to lack of teratogenic effects in contrast to **warfarin** which crosses placenta and causes hemorrhagic disorder in the fetus.
   - In addition warfarin can affect **gamma glutamate residues** found in the **fetal bones** may cause serious **birth defects**.

   Phenytoin

   - It is **contraindicated** in all trimesters as it can cause **fetal hydantoin syndrome**.
   - However in a pregnant woman with epilepsy though it is required to reduce exposure to anti-seizure drugs care also should be taken to control maternal seizures.

   Chloroquine

   - It is an antimalarial drug is a safe drug in pregnant women and children.
   - In addition, the antimalarial drugs: Quinine, quinidine and mefloquine are also considered safe during pregnancy.
   - However **primaquine** should be avoided during pregnancy as the **fetus is deficient of G6PD enzyme** and may develop **hemolysis**.

Penicillin

- It can be used in pregnant women without any complications to mother and fetus, provided the mother is not allergic to penicillin.
- However in pregnant women suffering from **syphilis, penicillin** is the drug of choice and hence even those pregnant women allergic to penicillin need to be desensitized and treated with penicillin.

4. **Insulin sensitivity increases with following treatment *except:***

A. Metformin	**B.** Acarbose
C. Exercise	**D.** Fasting

Ans: D. Fasting

Ref: *Goodman & Gilman's The Pharmacological Basis of Therapeutics, 12th ed, 2011, Pg 1246, 1258, 1264, 1270*

Explanation:

- **Insulin sensitivity** refers to the **amount of glucose that can be cleared from the blood with a given dose of insulin.** Insulin sensitivity may be altered by **age, body weight, exercise, diseases** and **drugs. Active persons** are found to be **more sensitive to insulin** compared to those with **sedentary life style.** Insulin sensitivity has been found to be **inversely related to age** with insulin resistance more common in the **elderly** due to **reduced physical activity.**
- In **hyperglycemic** state, **metformin** decreases blood glucose by **lowering hepatic glucose production** and **enhancing peripheral glucose uptake.** This is attributed to **increase in insulin sensitivity** and **reduction in insulin resistance.**
- **Acarbose** an **α-glucosidase inhibitor** by reducing **postprandial plasma glucose** increases the release of glucoregulatory hormone, **GLP-1.** As a result acarbose **increases insulin sensitivity** and **reduces blood glucose.**
- **Fasting** leads to **hypoglycemia** which is associated with **reduction of insulin secretion** and the release of counter regulatory hormones namely epinephrine, glucagon, glucocorticoids etc. Hence the answer to above question is fasting which does not increase insulin sensitivity.

5. **All the following are anticonvulsants *except:***

A. Lamotrigine	**B.** Methylphenidate
C. Vigabatrin	**D.** Topiramate

Ans: B. Methylphenidate

Ref: *Goodman & Gilman's The Pharmacological Basis of Therapeutics, 12th ed, 2011, Pg 299, 592, 601, 603*

Explanation:

Methylphenidate

- It is structurally similar to **amphetamine** is a **mild CNS stimulant.**
- It is used in the treatment of **narcolepsy** and **attention deficit / hyperactivity disorder.**
- However at high dose it can **cause CNS stimulation** resulting in **convulsions.**
- The other drugs mentioned in the options namely **lamotrigine, vigabatrin** and **topiramate** are **antiepileptic drugs.**

Lamotrigine

- It is a **broad spectrum antiepileptic** used in **monotherapy** and **add on therapy** of **partial** and **generalized tonic – clonic seizures** in **adults.**
- It is also used in the treatment of **Lennox – Gastaut syndrome** in both **adults** and **children.**
- The most common adverse effects:
  - Ataxia
  - Blurred vision
  - Dizziness
  - Nausea
  - Vomiting
  - Rash
- **Stevens-Johnson syndrome** and **disseminated intravascular coagulation** are also reported with lamotrigine.

Vigabatrin

- It is used as an **adjunctive** therapy for **refractory partial complex seizures** in **adults.**
- It is used in treatment of **infantile spasms** especially in **children** with **infantile spasms** due to **tuberous sclerosis.**

Topiramate

- It is approved as initial monotherapy in patients atleast 10 years old and as adjunctive therapy for patients of 2 years of age for partial onset or primary generalized tonic clonic seizures.
- It is also approved for **Lennox Gastaut syndrome** in patients of **age more than 2 years** and for **prophylaxis** of **migraine** in adults.

6. **Side effect of valvular heart disease is seen with:**

A. Pergolide	**B.** Methylphenidate
C. Amphetamine	**D.** Pramipexole

Ans: A. Pergolide

Ref: *Goodman & Gilman's The Pharmacological Basis of Therapeutics, 12th ed, 2011, Pg 297,298, 299, 617; Basic and Clinical Pharmacology by Katzung, 2012, 12th ed, Pg 489*

Explanation:

- **Pergolide**, a **dopaminergic D1 and D2 agonist** once used in the treatment of **Parkinsonism** has now been **withdraw** as it was found to cause **valvular heart disease**.
- **Pramipexole**, a **selective D2 agonist** causes **CNS side effects** including **hallucination** and **confusion**. It also causes **nausea**, **fatigue**, **somnolence** and **orthostatic hypotension.**
- **Methylphenidate** structurally similar to **amphetamine** is a mild CNS stimulant. It is used in the treatment of **narcolepsy** and **attention deficit / hyperactivity disorder**. However at high dose it can cause CNS stimulation resulting in **convulsions**. Methyl phenidate is association with CNS side effects and is **contraindicated** in **glaucoma**.
- The adverse effects of amphetamine includes CNS effects:
  - Restlessness
  - Tenseness
  - Irritability
  - Tremor
  - Talkativeness
  - Fever
  - Insomnia
  - Euphoria
- It also produces cardiovascular side effects
  - Flushing
  - Headache
  - Pallor
  - Palpitation
  - Arrhythmia
  - Angina
  - Hypo or hypertension.
- Toxic dose can cause **convulsion**, **coma** and **cerebral hemorrhages**.

7. **Side effect of acute pancreatitis is due to following anti-HIV drugs:**

A. Lamivudine **B.** Zidovudine
C. Didanosine **D.** Zalcitabine

Ans: C. Didanosine

Ref: *Goodman & Gilman's The Pharmacological Basis of Therapeutics, 12th ed, 2011, Pg 1632, 1635, 1639, 1640*

Explanation:

- **Lamivudine** is associated with least adverse effects:
  - Headache
  - Nausea
  - Neutropenia
  - Hepatitis
  - Pancreatitis has been found to occur in children
- The adverse effects caused by **zidovudine** include:
  - Fatigue
  - Nausea
  - Anorexia
  - Headache
  - Insomnia
  - Bone marrow suppression
  - Nail hyperpigmentation
  - Myopathy
  - Hepatotoxicity and lactic acidosis (rare)
- **Didanosine** causes serious adverse effects including:
  - Peripheral neuropathy
  - Acute pancreatitis.
- Both these adverse effects are attributed to **mitochondrial toxicity** caused by didanosine.
- As **stavudine**, another nucleoside reverse transcriptase inhibitor is also associated with the occurrence of **peripheral neuropathy** and **pancreatitis**, it **should not be combined** with didanosine.
- **Zalcitabine** is associated with **peripheral neuropathy** the reason for which it is not currently marketed.

  Hence the answer to the above question is didansosine.

8. **Short acting anti-histamine is:**

A. Cetirizine **B.** Promethazine
C. Hydroxyzine **D.** Acrivastine

Ans: B. Promethazine

Ref: *Goodman & Gilman's The Pharmacological Basis of Therapeutics, 12th ed, 2011, Pg 921-922.*

Explanation:

- **Hydroxyzine**, is a long acting first generation antihistamine used in the treatment of skin allergies. It acts for a duration of 6-24 hrs.
- **Cetirizine** a second generation antihistamine acts for 12 – 24 hrs.
- **Acrivastine** belongs to second generation antihistamine and acts for a duration of 6-8 hrs.

- **Promethazine**, a first generation antihistamine acts for a duration of 4-6 hrs.
- Among the first generation antihistamines longer acting drugs include doxepin (6-24 hrs), chlorpheniramine (24 hrs) and meclizine (12-24 hrs). Of the 2nd generation antihistamines longer acting drugs are cetirizine (12-24 hrs), levocetirizine (12-24 hrs), azelastine (12-24 hrs), loratadine (24 hrs), desloratadine (24 hrs), ebastine (24 hrs), mizolastine (24 hrs), and fexofenadine (12-24 hrs).

9. Sumatriptan is contraindicated in:

A. Asthma
B. DM
C. Sepsis
D. Peripheral vascular disease

Ans: D. Peripheral vascular disease

Ref: *Goodman & Gilman's The Pharmacological Basis of Therapeutics, 12th ed, 2011, Pg 346, 348*

Explanation:

Sumatriptan is a $5HT_{1B/1D}$ agonist used in treatment of migraine. All triptans are effective in the treatment of acute migraine.

The available triptans include sumatriptan, naratriptan, rizatriptan, frovatriptan, zolmitriptan and eletriptan.

- **All triptans are contraindicated in:**
  - Ischemic or vasospastic coronary artery disease
  - History of stroke or transient ischemic attacks
  - Cerebrovascular disease
  - Peripheral vascular disease
  - Hemiplegic / basilar migraines
  - Ischemic bowel diseases
  - Uncontrolled hypertension
  - Within 2 weeks of MOA inhibitor administration
- Hence the answer to the above question is peripheral vascular disease.
- In addition, **naratriptan** is contraindicated in **severe hepatic and renal impairment** while **eletriptan** is contraindicated in **hepatic disease.**
- **Ergot alkaloids which are also used in migraine as that of triptans are contraindicated in:**
  - Pregnancy
  - Peripheral vascular disease
  - Coronary artery disease
  - Hypertension
  - Impaired hepatic or renal function
  - Sepsis
  - Within 24 hrs of triptan administration

10. The following macrolides are used for toxoplasmosis *except:*

A. Erythromycin **B.** Clarithromycin
C. Azithromycin **D.** Spiramycin

Ans: A. Erythromycin

Ref: *Goodman & Gilman's The Pharmacological Basis of Therapeutics, 12th ed, 2011, Pg 1421; Basic and Clinical Pharmacology by Katzung 2012, 12th ed, Pg 813-814*

Explanation:

- **Erythromycin is effective against**
  - Pneumococci
  - Streptococci
  - Staphylococci
  - Corynebacteria
  - Mycoplasma pneumonia
  - Legionella pneumophila
  - Chlamydia trachomatis
  - Chlamydia psittaci
  - Chlamydia pneumonia
  - H. pylori
  - Listeria monocytogenes
  - Mycobacterium Kansasii
  - Mycobacterium scrofulaceum
  - Neisseria
  - Bordetella, Bartonella
  - Ricketssia
  - Treponema pallidum
  - Campylobacter
  - H. influenza
- **Clarithromycin is active against**
  - Mycobacterium avium complex
  - Mycobacterium leprae
  - Toxoplasma gondii
  - H.influenza
- **Azithromycin is active against**
  - Mycobacterium avium complex
  - Toxoplasma gondii
  - H. influenza
  - Chalmydia
- **Spiramycin** concentrates in placental tissue and hence used in the treatment of acute toxoplasmosis during pregnancy to prevent fetal transmission.

11. Following are third generation cephalosporins *except:*

A. Cefuroxime **B.** Ceftriaxone
C. Ceftazidime **D.** Cefotaxime

Ans: A. Cefuroxime

Ref: Goodman & Gilman's The Pharmacological Basis of Therapeutics, 12th ed, 2011, Pg 1496; Basic and Clinical Pharmacology by Katzung, 2012, 12th ed, Pg 800

Explanation:

- **First generation cephalosporin**
  - Cefazolin
  - Cephalexin
  - Cefadroxil
  - Cephradine

  First generation cephalosporins are effective against *Streptococci, Staphylococcus aureus*
- **Second generation cephalosporin**
  - Cefuroxime
  - Cefuroxime axetil
  - Cefprozil
  - Cefmetazole
  - Loracarbef
    - Second generation cephalosporins are effective against *E.coli, Klebsiella, Proteus, H. influenzae, Moroxella catarralis*
- **Third generation cephalosporin includes**
  - Cefotaxime
  - Ceftriaxone
  - Cefdinir
  - Cefditoren pivoxil
  - Ceftibuten
  - Cefpodoxime
  - Ceftizoxime
  - Cefoperazone
  - Ceftazidime

  Third generation cephalosporins are effective against *Enterobactericeae, Pseudomonas aeruginosa, Serratia, Neisseria gonorrhea; among the 3rd generation cephalosporins, cefoperazone and ceftazidime are effective against pseudomonas.*
- **Fourth generation cephalosporin**
  - Cefepime

  Action is similar to third generation with enhanced resistance to some beta lactamases.

  The spectrum of cephalosporins extends more towards gram negative organisms with declining action against gram positive organisms as the generation increases.

  Recently, **Ceftaroline fosamil** – a prodrug of **ceftaroline** which is an active metabolite, has been approved for **methicillin resistant Staphylococci.**

12. **The mechanism of action of cephalosporin is:**

A. Interferes with cell wall synthesis
B. Inhibition of DNA gyrase
C. Inhibition of protein synthesis
D. Inhibition of DNA polymerase

Ans: A. Interferes with cell wall synthesis

Ref: Goodman & Gilman's The Pharmacological Basis of Therapeutics, 12th ed, 2011, Pg 1479, 1493; Basic and Clinical Pharmacology by Katzung, 2012, 12th ed, Pg 792

Explanation:

- **Cephalosporin** inhibits **bacterial cell wall synthesis**.
- Its mechanism of action is similar to **penicillin** as both are beta lactams.
- **Bacterial cell wall** plays a major role in the **growth and development of bacteria**.
- **Peptidoglycan**, a component of bacterial cell wall owing to its cross-linked structure offers strength to the cell wall.
- **Peptidoglycan** is composed of **N-acetyl-glucosamine** and **N-acetylmuramic acid** with **cross–linking**.
- A five amino acid peptide known as **pentapeptide** is linked to N-acetylmuramic acid and this peptide terminates as **D-alanyl–D-alanine**.
- **Penicillin Binding Protein (PBP) removes** terminal **alanine** from **D-alanyl –D-alanine** and forms **cross link** with the adjacent peptide, thus enhancing **cell wall rigidity**.
- Beta lactam antibiotics are structurally similar **to D-alanyl –D-alanine,** and hence **covalently bind** to **PBP,** resulting in **inhibition of transpeptidation reaction** which is essential for the **removal of D-alanine from D-alanyl–D-alanine.**
- As peptidoglycan synthesis is inhibited by cephalosporins as any other beta lactams, the **bacterial cell dies**. However cell death is maximum when the cells are **actively growing and synthesizing cell wall.**

13. **Autoinduction of biotransformation and action as a hormone is seen in:**

A. Carbamazepine **B.** Cimetidine
C. Corticosteroid **D.** Thyroxine

Ans: D. Thyroxine

Ref: Basic and Clinical Pharmacology by Katzung, 2012, 12th ed, Pg 684-685

Explanation:

- In **hyperthyroidism**, the half lives of **T_3 and T_4** are **decreased** owing to their **enhanced metabolic clearance**.

- Similarly in **hypothyroidism**, the **half lives of T_3 and T_4** are **increased** due to **reduced metabolic clearance**. This clearly shows the **autoinduction feature of thyroid hormones.**
- In **hyperthyroidism**, the required dose of **digoxin increases** while in **hypothyroidism lower dose** is sufficient.
- **Sedation** and **respiratory depression** is more with **sedatives** and **opioids** respectively in patients with **hypothyroidism** while these effects are **less in hyperthyroidism**.

14. Selective decrease in IgA is seen with administration of:

A. Phenytoin **B.** Diazepam
C. Clonazepam **D.** Phenobarbitone

Ans. A. Phenytoin

Ref: *Goodman & Gillman's The Pharmacological Basis of Therapeutics, 2011, 12th Edition, McGraw Hill, Burton LL, P 593*

Explanation:

- **Phenytoin** can cause **lymphadenopathy** similar to **Hodgkin's disease** and **malignant lymphoma**. This is attributed to **decrease** in **IgA production.**

Other Adverse Effects of Phenytoin

Neurologic

- Horizontal gaze nystagmus
- Sedation
- Cerebellar ataxia
- Cerebellar atrophy
- Ophthalmoparesis
- Seizures

Hematologic

- Megaloblastic anemia
- Agranulocytosis
- Aplastic anemia
- Leukopenia
- Thrombocytopenia.

Teratogenicity

- Phenytoin is a known teratogen and causes "fetal hydantoin syndrome"
- The syndrome consists of **craniofacial anomalies (broad nasal bridge, cleft lip and palate, microcephaly)** and a mild form of **mental retardation** (average IQ=71)

Dermatologic

- Hypertrichosis
- Rash
- Exfoliative dermatitis
- Pruritis
- Hirsutism
- Coarsening of facial features
- SJS and TEN

Others

- Gingival hypertrophy (overgrowth of the gums) (can be decreased with folate supplementation)
- Induction of reversible IgA deficiency
- Drug-induced lupus.
- Hypocalcemia

15. Which of the following is prothrombotic?

A. Thrombomodulin **B.** PGI2
C. Heparin **D.** ADP

Ans. D. ADP

Ref: *Basic and Clinical Pharmacology, 2012, 12th Ed, Tata McGraw Hill, Katzung BG, Masters SB, Trevor AJ, P 602-604*

Explanation:

- **Platelet** releases **ADP, thromboxane A2** and **serotonin**. The tissue factor which is exposed when endothelium is damaged binds to factor VIIa. This will activate various clotting factors finally converting prothrombin to thrombin.
- **PGI2, heparin and thrombomodulin** have anticoagulant in nature along with **Antithrombin. Protein C and Protein S** by proteolysing clotting factor **Va and VIIIa.**

16. Which of the following is not an analeptic agent?

A. Doxapram **B.** Nikethamide
C. Doxacurium **D.** Propylbutamide

Ans. C. Doxacurium

Ref: *A Complete Textbook of Medical Pharmacology S.K. Srivasthava, Vol 1, Avanchal Publishing Company 764*

Explanation:

- **Doxapram, Nikethamide, Prethcamide** are the **analeptics**, stimulate the **medullary centre.**
- **Nikethamide** is now withdrawn due to the risk of convulsion.
- **Doxacurium** is a **competitive neuromuscular blocker** while other drugs are known **respiratory stimulants.**

17. The neurotransmitter secreted by postganglionic sympathetic fibers innervating sweat glands is: (Repeat)

A. Nor epinephrine **B.** Epinephrine
C. Acetylcholine **D.** Dopamine

Ans: C. Acetylcholine

Ref: Katzung, 10th ed

Explanation:

- NE is the neurotransmitter of all postganglionic sympathetic fibers except the ones innervating the sweat glands, where acetylcholine is the neurotransmitter.

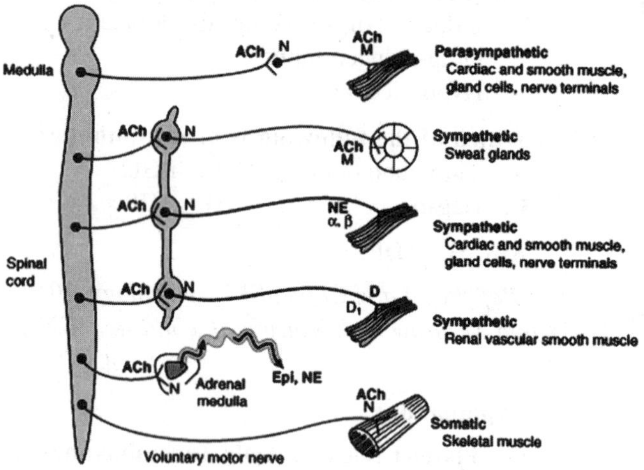

Fig: Schematic diagram comparing some anatomic and neurotransmitter features of autonomic and somatic motor nerves. (ACh, acetylcholine; D, dopamine; Epi, epinephrine; NE, norepinephrine; N, nicotinic receptors; M, muscarinic receptors)

- **Parasympathetic ganglia** are present near the **wall of the organ innervated.**
- Some **sympathetic postganglionic fibers** release **acetylcholine** or **dopamine rather** than **norepinephrine.**
- The **adrenal medulla,** a modified **sympathetic ganglion,** receives **sympathetic preganglionic fibers** and releases **epinephrine** and **norepinephrine** into the blood.
- The autonomic nervous system lends itself to division on anatomic grounds into two major portions: the **sympathetic (thoracolumbar)** division and the **parasympathetic (cranio-sacral)** division.
- The **sympathetic preganglionic fibers** leave the central nervous system through the **thoracic** and **lumbar spinal nerves.**
- The **parasympathetic preganglionic** fibers leave the central nervous system through the **cranial nerves** (especially the **third, seventh, ninth and tenth**) and the **third and fourth sacral spinal roots.**
- Most of the **sympathetic preganglionic fibers** terminate in **ganglia** located in the **paravertebral** chains that lie on either side of the spinal column.
- The remaining **sympathetic preganglionic fibers** terminate in **prevertebral ganglia,** which lie in front of the **vertebrae,** usually on the surface of the aorta.
- From the ganglia, postganglionic sympathetic fibers run to the tissues innervated. Some preganglionic parasympathetic fibers terminate in **parasympathetic ganglia** located outside the **organs** innervated: the **ciliary, pterygopalatine, submandibular, otic, and several pelvic ganglia.**
- The majority of **parasympathetic preganglionic fibers** terminate on **ganglion cells** distributed diffusely or in networks in the walls of the innervated organs.

18. Which of the following drugs is not used for the treatment of anaerobic infections?

A. Penicillin **B.** Clindamycin
C. Chloramphenicol **D.** Gentamicin

Ans. D. Gentamicin

Ref: Basic and Clinical Pharmacology, 2012, 12th Ed, Tata McGraw Hill, Katzung BG, Masters SB, Trevor AJ P 813- 816

Explanation:

- **Aminoglycosides** are **transported actively across** the **cell** by an **oxygen dependent process**. Hence they are effective only in **aerobic gram** negative bacterial infection and **ineffective in anaerobic infection.**
- **Chloramphenicol** is against **both aerobic** and **anaerobic** organisms.
- **Clindamycin** is effective against **anaerobes, gram positive, negative organisms.**
- **Penicillins** can be used in the treatment of **anaerobic infections** of **oral cavity.**

19. Which of the following drugs is used to treat Chlamydia infection in pregnancy?

A. Doxycyclin **B.** Erythromycin
C. Mirepenam **D.** Tetracyclin

Ans. B. Erythromycin

Ref: Goodman & Gillman's The Pharmacological Basis of Therapeutics, 2011, 12th Edition, McGraw Hill, Burton LL,P 1533

Explanation:

- **Erythromycin base 500mg 6th hrly for 7 days** is the **first choice** for the treatment of **Chlamydial infection in pregnancy.**
- **Azithromycin** 1g single dose being the alternate drug.

- **Tetracyclines** are **contraindicated** because of their **Teratogenic potential.**

20. Troglitazone is the drug used in the treatment of:

A. Petit mal epilepsy
B. Type 2 diabetes mellitus
C. Hyperlipidaemia
D. Osteoporosis

Ans. B. Type 2 diabetes mellitus

Ref: *Goodman & Gillman's The Pharmacological Basis of Therapeutics, 2011, 12th Edition, McGraw Hill, Burton LL,P 1261-62*

Explanation:

Troglitazone

- As a **Monotherapy** it is **not useful in Type 1 diabetes** because it needs **presence of insulin** for its action.
- Troglitazone is **withdrawn** from the **market** because it is known to cause **severe fatal hepatic failure.**
- The newer thiazolidenidiones like **Pioglitazone** and **rosiglitazone** are known to cause **CHF** as a result of **fluid retention.**
- **Rosiglitazone** is found to be associated with **increased risk of cardiovascular events.**
- **Pioglitazone** can reduce the **TG levels** by **10-15%** because of its action **on PPAR³.**

21. Which of the following is not an alpha-2 stimulant?

A. Guanabenz
B. Guanadrel
C. Clonidine
D. Alpha methyl dopa

Ans. B. Guanadrel

Ref: *Goodman & Gillman's The Pharmacological Basis of Therapeutics, 2011, 12th Edition, McGraw Hill, Burton LL, P 297,775*

Explanation:

- Guanadrel **inhibits** the **peripheral post-ganglionic receptor** after reaching the adrenergic neuron by the reuptake of NE transport mechanism.
- It **acts** as a **false neurotransmitter** after **displacing** the **stored NE** from the vesicle.
- **Guanabenz, Guanfacine, Clonidine** and **alpha methyl dopa** are **centrally active.**
- **Alpha2 agonist** which inhibits the release of **NE** from the vasomotor centre.

22. 99% of degradation of ^{131}I occurs in:

A. 26 days
B. 36 days
C. 46 days
D. 56 days

Ans: D. 56 days

Ref: *Goodman & Gillman's The Pharmacological Basis of Therapeutics, 2011, 12th Edition, McGraw Hill, Burton LL, P 1154*

Explanation:

- **^{131} I** has a t1/2 **of 8 days, emits ? and Y particles.**
- More than **99% radiation** is degraded in **56 days.**
- This has been used in **therapeutic destruction of overactive or enlarged thyroid gland.**

Note: **^{123} I** is used mainly in **diagnostic studies** to measure the **24 hr uptake** and thyroid imaging studies. Its half life being **13 hrs.** It emits **Y particles.**

23. Niacin toxicity causes all *except:*

A. Hepatitis
B. Diabetes
C. Hypertriglyceridemia
D. Macular edema

Ans: C. Hypertriglyceridemia

Ref: *Harrison's Principles of Internal Medicine, 18th edition*

Explanation:

Niacin Toxicity

- **Prostaglandin-mediated flushing.**
- Flushing always starts in the face and may be accompanied by skin dryness, itching, paresthesia and headache.
- **Nausea, vomiting, and abdominal pain** also occur at similar doses of niacin.
- **Hepatic toxicity** is the most serious toxic reaction caused by niacin and may present as jaundice with elevated aspartate aminotransferase (AST) and alanine aminotransferase (ALT) levels.
- A few cases of **fulminant hepatitis requiring liver transplantation** have been reported at doses of 3–9 g/d. Other toxic reactions include **glucose intolerance, hyperuricemia, macular edema** and **macular cysts.**
- The combination of nicotinic acid preparations for dyslipidemia with 3-hydroxy-3-methylglutaryl coenzyme A (HMG-CoA) reductase inhibitors may increase the risk of **rhabdomyolysis.**
- The upper limit for daily niacin intake has been set at **35 mg.**

PATHOLOGY

1. **Which of the following is not a feature of anemia of chronic disease?**
   A. Increased TIBC
   B. Increased serum iron
   C. Increased serum ferritin
   D. Increased bone marrow iron

   Ans: B. Increased serum iron

   Ref: *Robbins Pathologic Basis of Disease, 8th edition*

   Explanation: (See Table-1)

2. **Which among the following does not secrete Interleukin 1 alpha?**
   A. Lymphocyte B. Fibroblast
   C. Macrophage D. Endothelium

   Ans: A. Lymphocyte

   Ref: *Robbins Pathologic Basis of Disease, 8th edition,*

   Explanation:
   - **Interleukin-1 alpha** (IL-1α) is a protein of the interleukin-1 family that in humans is encoded by the *IL1A* gene.
   - Interleukin 1 is responsible for the production of inflammation, as well as the promotion of fever and sepsis.
   - IL-1α is produced mainly by:
     - Activated macrophages
     - Neutrophils
     - Epithelial cells
     - Endothelial cells
     - Fibroblast **(See Table-2)**

3. **'Pseudopalisading' arrangement of malignant cells is characteristic of:**

Table-1

	Normal values	Iron deficiency anemia	Thalassemia	Sideroblastic anemia	Anemia of chronic disease
Peripheral smear		Microcytic Hypochromic	Microcytic Hypochromic	Microcytic Hypochromic	Normocytic Normochromic > >Microcytic Hypochromic
Serum iron	50 – 150 microg/dl	Low	Normal or ↑	Normal or ↑	↓
Total iron binding capacity (TIBC)	300 – 600 microg/dl	High ↑↑	Normal	Normal or ↑	↓
% Saturation	30 – 50%	<10 (↓)	Normal or ↑	Normal or ↑	↓
Serum ferritin (microgram/L)	50 – 200	<15	↑	↑	Normal or ↑
Hemoglobin pattern	HbA2 – 1.5 – 3.5% total Hb	Normal	Abnormal	Normal	Normal

Table-2 List of the common interleukines, their source and function

Interleukin	Source	Function
IL1	Macrophages, Neutrophils, Epithelial cell and Endothelial cells	Proliferation and differentiation of T, B and other cells; pyrogenic
IL2	T cells	Promote growth and differentiation of T and B cells, cytotoxicity of T and NK cells
IL4	TH cells	Proliferation of B; increase IgG1 and IgE production
IL5	TH cells	Proliferation of ***eosinophils***, stimulate IgA and IgM production
IL7	Spleen, bone marrow stromal cells	B and T cell growth factor
IL8	Macrophages	***Neutrophil chemotactic factor***
IL10	T cells, B cells, macrophages	Inhibit IFN production and mononuclear cell functions
IL11	Bone marrow stromal cells	Induce acute phase proteins
IL13	T cells	Inhibit mononuclear cell functions

A. Glioblastoma **B.** Ependymoma
C. Oligodendroglioma **D.** Medulloblastoma

Ans: A. Glioblastoma

Ref: *Robbins and Cotran, 'Pathologic Basis of Disease', 8th Edition, Elsevier, 2011, Page 1331*

Explanation:

"The highest grade tumor of astrocytoma, known as glioblastoma, has a histologic appearance similar to anaplastic astrocytoma with the additional features of ***necrosis and vascular or endothelial cell proliferation and pseudo-palisading nuclei."***

- Glioblastoma is type of infiltrating astrocytoma (Classified as Grade 4).
- Necrosis in glioblastoma often results in a SERPENTINE pattern in areas of hypercellularity.
- Tumor cells collect along the edges of the necrotic regions, producing histologic pattern referred to as pseudopalisading pattern.

GLIOMAS

Gliomas are tumors of the brain parenchyma that histologically resemble different types of glial cells. The major types of tumor in this category are:

a. ***Astrocytomas***
b. ***Oligodendrogliomas***
c. ***Ependymomas.***

ASTROCYTOMAS

- Two major categories of astrocytoma, infiltrating and non-infiltrating types.
- Infiltrating astrocytomas account for about 80% of adult primary brain tumors.
- They are most frequent in the fourth through sixth decades.
- They are usually found in the cerebral hemispheres.
- The most common presenting signs and symptoms are seizures, headaches and focal neurologic deficits related to the anatomic site of involvement.
- Infiltrating astrocytomas show a spectrum of histologic differentiation that correlates well with clinical course and outcome.

Based on the degree of differentiation, they are classified into four groups:

- Pilocytic astrocytoma - Grade 1 - Most common
- Astrocytoma - Grade 2
- Anaplastic astrocytoma - Grade 3
- Glioblastoma multiforme - Grade 4 - Least differentiated

PILOCYTIC ASTROCYTOMA

- Pilocytic astrocytomas are relatively benign tumors, often cystic, that typically occur in children and young adults.
- They are usually located in the cerebellum; also in the floor and walls of the third ventricle, the optic nerves, and occasionally the cerebral hemispheres.
- A pilocytic astrocytoma is often cystic, with a mural nodule in the wall of the cyst; if solid, it is usually well circumscribed.
- The tumor is composed of areas with bipolar cells with long, thin "**hairlike**" processes that are **GFAP positive; Rosenthal fibers, eosinophilic granular bodies**, and **microcysts** are often present.
- Necrosis and mitoses are absent.

OLIGODENDROGLIOMAS

- These tumors constitute about 5% to 15% of gliomas and are most common in the fourth and fifth decades.
- Patients may have had several years of neurologic complaints, often including seizures. The lesions are found mostly in the cerebral hemispheres, with a predilection for white matter.
- Oligodendrogliomas are infiltrative tumors that form gelatinous, gray masses, and may show cysts, focal hemorrhage and calcification.
- On microscopic examination, the tumor is composed of sheets of regular cells with spherical nuclei containing finely granular chromatin (similar to normal oligodendrocytes) surrounded by a **clear halo of cytoplasm**.
- The tumor typically contains a delicate network of anastomosing capillaries. **Calcification**, present in as many as **90%** of these tumors, ranges from microscopic foci to massive depositions.
- With increasing cell density, nuclear anaplasia, increased mitotic activity and necrosis, the tumor becomes higher grade (anaplastic oligodendroglioma.
- Patients with oligodendrogliomas have a better prognosis than do patients with astrocytomas.
- Current treatment with surgery, chemotherapy, and radiotherapy yields an average survival of 5 to 10 years.
- Patients with anaplastic oligodendroglioma have a worse prognosis.

EPENDYMOMAS

- Ependymomas most often arise next to the ependyma-lined ventricular system, including the central canal of the spinal cord.

- In the first two decades of life, they typically occur near the fourth ventricle and constitute 5% to 10% of the primary brain tumors in this age group.
- In adults, the spinal cord is their most common location; tumors in this site are particularly frequent in the setting of neurofibromatosis type 2.
- Because ependymomas usually grow within the ventricles, CSF dissemination is a common occurrence.
- In the fourth ventricle, ependymomas are typically solid or papillary masses extending from the floor of the ventricle.
- These tumors are composed of cells with regular, round to oval nuclei with abundant granular chromatin.
- Between the nuclei there is a variably dense fibrillary background.
- Tumor cells may form round or elongated structures (**rosettes,** canals) that resemble the embryologic ependymal canal, with long, delicate processes extending into a lumen. More frequently present are **perivascular pseudo-rosettes** in which tumor cells are arranged around vessels with an intervening zone consisting of thin ependymal processes directed toward the wall of the vessel.
- Anaplastic ependymomas show increased cell density, high mitotic rates, necrosis and less evident ependymal differentiation.
- The clinical outcome for completely resected supratentorial and spinal ependymomas is better than for those in the posterior fossa.

4. Metastatic calcification of the gastrointestinal tract commonly affects the mucosa of:

A. Stomach **B.** Esophagus
C. Ileum **D.** Rectum

Ans: A. Stomach

Ref: *Robbins and Cotran, 'Pathologic Basis of Disease', 8th Edition, Elsevier, 2011, Page 38-9*

Explanation:

Pathologic calcification is the abnormal tissue deposition of calcium salts, together with smaller amounts of iron, magnesium, and other mineral salts.

There are two forms of pathologic calcification:

Dystrophic Calcification

- Deposition occurs locally in dying tissues.
- It occurs despite normal serum levels of calcium and in the absence of derangements in calcium metabolism.
- Dystrophic calcification is encountered in areas of necrosis, whether they are of coagulative, caseous, or liquefactive type, and in foci of enzymatic necrosis of fat.
- Calcification is almost always present in the atheromas of advanced atherosclerosis. It also commonly develops in aging or damaged heart valves, further hampering their function.
- Calcium salts appear macroscopically as fine, white granules or clumps, often felt as gritty deposits.
- On H & E stain, calcium salts have a basophilic, amorphous granular, sometimes clumped appearance. They can be intracellular, extra-cellular, or in both locations.
- In the course of time, heterotopic bone may be formed in the focus of calcification. On occasion single necrotic cells may constitute seed crystals that become encrusted by the mineral deposits. The progressive acquisition of outer layers may create lamellated configurations, called **psammoma bodies** because of their resemblance to grains of sand.
- Some types of papillary cancers (e.g., thyroid are apt to develop psammoma bodies.
- In asbestosis, calcium and iron salts gather about long slender spicules of asbestos in the lung, creating exotic, beaded dumbbell forms.
- In dystrophic calcification, the final common pathway is the formation of crystalline calcium phosphate mineral in the form of an apatite similar to the hydroxyapatite of bone.

Metastatic Calcification

- The **deposition of calcium** salts in otherwise **normal tissues.**
- It almost always results from **hypercalcemia** secondary to some disturbance in calcium metabolism.
- Metastatic calcification may occur in normal tissues whenever there is hypercalcemia.
- Hypercalcemia **also accentuates dystrophic calcification.**
- There are four principal causes of hypercalcemia:
- Increased **secretion of parathyroid hormone (PTH)** with subsequent bone resorption, as in hyperparathyroidism due to parathyroid tumors, and ectopic secretion of PTH-related protein by malignant tumors.
- **Destruction of bone tissue**, secondary to primary tumors of bone marrow (e.g., multiple myeloma, leukemia or diffuse skeletal metastasis (e.g., breast cancer), accelerated bone turnover (e.g., Paget disease), or immobilization.

- **Vitamin D-related disorders**, including **vitamin D intoxication, sarcoidosis** (in which macrophages activate a vitamin D precursor), and **idiopathic hypercalcemia** of infancy (Williams syndrome), characterized by abnormal sensitivity to vitamin D; **and** Renal **failure**, which causes retention of phosphate, leading to **secondary hyperparathyroidism**.
- Less common causes include **aluminum intoxication**, which occurs in patients on **chronic renal dialysis**, and **milk-alkali syndrome**, which is due to excessive ingestion of calcium and absorbable antacids such as milk or calcium carbonate.
- **Metastatic calcification** may occur widely throughout the body but principally affects the interstitial tissues of the **gastric mucosa, kidneys, lungs, systemic arteries, and pulmonary veins.**
- Though quite different in location, all of these tissues excrete acid and therefore have an internal alkaline compartment that predisposes them to metastatic calcification.
- In all these sites the calcium salts morphologically resemble those described in dystrophic calcification.
- Thus, they may occur as **noncrystalline amorphous deposits** or, at other times, as **hydroxyapatite crystals.**
- Usually the mineral salts cause no clinical dysfunction, but on occasion massive involvement of the lungs produces remarkable X-ray films and respiratory deficits.
- Massive deposits in the kidney (**nephrocalcinosis**) may in time cause renal damage.

5. SS-A (Ro) and SS-B (LA) antibodies found in Sjögren syndrome are targeted against:

A. DNA topoisomerase 1
B. Histones
C. Ribonucleoproteins
D. Native DNA

Ans: C. Ribonucleoproteins

Ref: *Robbins and Cotran, 'Pathologic Basis of Disease', 8th Edition, Elsevier, 2011, Page 221-3.*

Explanation:

SJÖGREN SYNDROME

- It is a immune-mediated destruction of the lacrimal and salivary glands characterized by dry eyes (keratoconjunctivitis sicca) and dry mouth (xerostomia), resulting from immune-mediated destruction of the lacrimal and salivary glands.
- It occurs as an isolated disorder (primary form), also known as the **sicca syndrome**, or more often in association with another autoimmune disease (secondary form).
- Associated with **Rheumatoid Arthritis (**Most common SLE, **polymyositis, systemic sclerosis, vasculitis**, or **thyroiditis**.
- The **ductal epithelial cells** of the **exocrine glands** are the **primary target** for auto-antibodies.
- There is also **systemic B-cell hyperactivity**, as evidenced by the presence of ANAs and RF (even in the absence of associated RA).
- Most patients with primary Sjögren syndrome have **autoantibodies to the RNP antigens SS-A (Ro) and SS-B (La)** (These are **also present in SLE**).
- Other secretory glands, including those in the nasopharynx, upper airway, and vagina, may also be involved.
- Involved tissues show an intense **lymphocyte** (primarily activated CD4+ T cells) and **plasma-cell infiltrate**.
- There is associated destruction of the native architecture.
- **Lacrimal gland destruction** results in a **lack of tears**, leading to drying of the corneal epithelium, with subsequent inflammation, erosion, and ulceration (**keratoconjunctivitis sicca**).
- Similar changes may occur in the oral mucosa as a result of loss of salivary gland output, giving rise to mucosal atrophy, with inflammatory fissuring and ulceration (**xerostomia**).
- Dryness and crusting of the nose may lead to ulcerations and even perforation of the nasal septum.
- When the respiratory passages are involved, secondary laryngitis, bronchitis, and pneumonitis may appear.
- Approximately 25% of the patients (especially those with anti-SS-A antibodies) develop **extraglandular disease affecting** the **CNS, skin, kidneys** and **muscles**.
- Renal lesions take the form of mild interstitial nephritis associated with tubular transport defects; unlike in SLE, glomerulonephritis is rare.
- Approximately 90% of Sjögren syndrome cases occur in women between the ages of 35 and 45 years.
- Extraglandular manifestations include **synovitis, pulmonary fibrosis** and **peripheral neuropathy.**

- Notably, there is a 40-fold increased **risk** of developing a **non-Hodgkin B-cell lymphoma**, arising in the setting of the initial robust polyclonal B-cell proliferation.

6. **Which of the following subtype of Hodgkin lymphoma is not associated with Ebstein Barr virus infection?**
   A. Lymphocyte rich
   B. Mixed cellularity
   C. Lymphocyte depletion
   D. Nodular sclerosis

   Ans: D. Nodular sclerosis

Ref: *Robbins and Cotran 'Pathologic Basis of Disease', 8th Edition,Elsevier, 2011, Page 618*

Explanation:

The WHO classification recognizes five subtypes of HL:

1. Nodular sclerosis
2. Mixed cellularity
3. Lymphocyte rich
4. Lymphocyte depletion
5. Lymphocyte predominance

- In the first four subtypes—nodular sclerosis, mixed cellularity, lymphocyte rich and lymphocyte depletion—the Reed-Sternberg cells have a similar immuno-phenotype. These subtypes are often lumped together as *classical* forms of HL.
- In the remaining subtype, lymphocyte predominance, the Reed-Sternberg cells have a distinctive B-cell immunophenotype that differs from that of the "classical" types.

(See Table-3)

7. **Which statement best describes the tears seen in Mallory-Weiss syndrome?**
   A. Longtitudinal tears in lower 1/3 esophagus
   B. Circumferential tears in lower 1/3 esophagus
   C. Longtitudinal tears in middle 1/3 esophagus
   D. Circumferential tears in middle 1/3 esophagus

   Ans: A. Longtitudinal tears in lower 1/3 esophagus

Ref: *Robbins and Cotran, 'Pathologic Basis of Disease', 8th Edition, Elsevier, 2011, Page 768*

Explanation:

Mallory-Weiss Syndrome

- **Longitudinal tears** in the **esophagus near the gastroesophageal junction** are termed *Mallory-Weiss tears*, and are
- Most often associated with **severe retching or vomiting** secondary to **acute alcohol intoxication.**

Table-3

Subtype	Morphology and immunophenotype	Typical clinical features
Nodular sclerosis	Frequent lacunar cells and occasional diagnostic RS cells; background infiltrate composed of T lymphocytes, eosinophils, macrophages, and plasma cells; fibrous bands dividing cellular areas into nodules. RS cells CD15+, CD30+; usually **EBV-**	Most common subtype; usually stage I or II disease; frequent mediastinal involvement; equal occurrence in males and females (F = M), most patients young adults
Mixed cellularity	Frequent mononuclear and diagnostic RS cells; background infiltrate rich in T lymphocytes, eosinophils, macrophages, plasma cells; RS cells CD15+, CD30+; 70% **EBV+**	More than 50% present as stage III or IV disease; M greater than F; biphasic incidence, peaking in young adults and again in adults older than 55
Lymphocyte rich	Frequent mononuclear and diagnostic RS cells; background infiltrate rich in T lymphocytes; RS cells CD15+, CD30+; 40% **EBV+**	Uncommon; M greater than F; tends to be seen in older adults
Lymphocyte depletion	Reticular variant: Frequent diagnostic RS cells and variants and a paucity of background reactive cells; RS cells CD15+, CD30+; **most EBV+**	Uncommon; more common in older males, HIV-infected individuals, and in developing countries; often presents with advanced disease
Lymphocyte predominance	Frequent L&H (popcorn cell) variants in a background of follicular dendritic cells and reactive B cells; RS cells CD20+, CD15-, C30-; **EBV-**	Uncommon; young males with cervical or axillary lymphadenopathy; mediastinal

- Normally, a reflex relaxation of the gastro-esophageal musculature precedes the anti-peristaltic contractile wave associated with vomiting.
- It is speculated that this relaxation fails during prolonged vomiting, with the result that refluxing gastric contents overwhelm the gastric inlet and cause the esophageal wall to stretch and tear.
- The roughly **linear lacerations** of Mallory-Weiss syndrome are **longitudinally oriented** and range in length from **millimeters** to **several centimeters**.
- These tears usually cross the **gastroesophageal junction** but may also be located in the proximal gastric mucosa.
- Upto **10%** of upper GI bleeding, which often presents as **hematemesis**, is due to superficial esophageal lacerations such as those associated with Mallory-Weiss syndrome.
- These do not generally require surgical intervention, and healing tends to be rapid and complete.
- In contrast, **Boerhaave syndrome**, characterized by **distal esophageal rupture** and **mediastinitis**, occurs rarely and is a catastrophic event.

8. Subendothelial deposits in glomerulus are characteristically seen in:

A. Lupus nephritis
B. IgA nephropathy
C. Post infectious nephritis
D. Goodpasture disease

Ans: A. Lupus nephritis

Ref: *Robbins and Cotran, 'Pathologic Basis of Disease', 8th Edition, Elsevier, 2011, Pg 918*

Explanation:

Subepithelial Deposits

- Post infectious Glomerulonephritis (Lumpy bumpy deposits)
- Membranous Glomerulopathy

Subendothelial Deposits

- Membranoproliferative glomerulonephritis (MPGN) type I
- Lupus nephritis
- Post infectious glomerulonephritis (Rarely)

9. Pauci-immune glomerulonephritis is seen in:

A. Post-transplantation in Alport's syndrome
B. Microscopic polyangitis
C. Henoch-Schölein purpura
D. Lupus Nephritis

Ans: B. Microscopic polyangitis

Ref: *Robbins and Cotran, 'Pathologic Basis of Disease', 8th Edition, Elsevier, 2011, Pg 920*

Explanation:

Rapidly Progressive Glomerulonephritides (RPGN)

TYPE I (Anti-GBM Antibody)

- Goodpasture syndrome

TYPE II (Immune Complex)

- Idiopathic
- Post-infectious glomerulonephritis
- Lupus nephritis
- Henoch-Schönlein purpura (IgA nephropathy)

TYPE III (Pauci-Immune)

- ANCA-associated
- Idiopathic
- Wegener granulomatosis
- Microscopic polyangiitis

10. All the following are signs of aging heart *except:*

A. Increased atrial size
B. Increased ventricular size
C. Increased subepicardial fat
D. Increased myocardial mass

Ans: B. Increased ventricular size

Ref: *Robbin's Pathologic Basis of Disease, 8th ed, Pg. 532*

Explanation:

- Aging cases decrease in ventricular size.

Changes in the Aging Heart

CHAMBERS
• Increased left atrial cavity size • Decreased left ventricular cavity size • Sigmoid-shaped ventricular septum
VALVES
• Aortic valve calcific deposits • Mitral valve annular calcific deposits • Fibrous thickening of leaflets • Buckling of mitral leaflets toward the left atrium • Lambl excrescences
EPICARDIAL CORONARY ARTERIES
• Tortuosity • Increased cross-sectional luminal area • Calcific deposits • Atherosclerotic plaque
MYOCARDIUM
• Increased mass • Increased subepicardial fat • Brown atrophy

Contd.

• Lipofuscin deposition • Basophilic degeneration • Amyloid deposits
AORTA
• Dilated ascending aorta with rightward shift • Elongated (tortuous) thoracic aorta • Sinotubular junction calcific deposits • Elastic fragmentation and collagen accumulation • Atherosclerotic plaque

11. Translocation of t(8:14) is characteristic of:

A. Burkitt's lymphoma
B. Hairy cell leukemia
C. Mantle cell lymphoma
D. Follicular lymphoma

Ans: A. Burkitt's lymphoma

Ref: *Robbin's Pathologic Basis of Disease, 8th ed, Pg. 601*

Explanation: (See Table-4)

Table-4

Summary of Major Types of Lymphoid Leukemias and Non-Hodgkin Lymphomas

Diagnosis	Cell of Origin	Genotype	Salient Clinical Features
NEOPLASMS OF IMMATURE B AND T CELLS			
B-cell acute lymphoblastic leukemia/lymphoma	Bone marrow precursor B cell	Diverse chromosomal translocations; t(12;21) involving *CBFα* and *ETV6* present in 25%	Predominantly children; symptoms relating to marrow replacement and pancytopenia; aggressive
T-cell acute lymphoblastic leukemia/lymphoma	Precursor T cell (often of thymic origin)	Diverse chromosomal translocations, *NOTCH1* mutations (50% to 70%)	Predominantly adolescent males; thymic masses and variable bone marrow involvement; aggressive
NEOPLASMS OF MATURE B CELLS			
Burkitt lymphoma	Germinal-center B cell	Translocations involving c-*MYC* and Ig loci, usually t(8;14); subset EBV-associated	Adolescents or young adults with extranodal masses; uncommonly presents as "leukemia"; aggressive
Diffuse large B-cell lymphoma	Germinal-center or post–germinal-center B cell	Diverse chromosomal rearrangements, most often of *BCL6* (30%), *BCL2* (10%), or c-*MYC* (5%)	All ages, but most common in adults; often appears as a rapidly growing mass; 30% extranodal; aggressive
Extranodal marginal zone lymphoma	Memory B cell	t(11;18), t(1;14), and t(14;18) creating *MALT1-IAP2*, *BCL10-IgH*, and *MALT1-IgH* fusion genes, respectively	Arises at extranodal sites in adults with chronic inflammatory diseases; may remain localized; indolent
Follicular lymphoma	Germinal-center B cell	t(14;18) creating *BCL2-IgH* fusion gene	Older adults with generalized lymphadenopathy and marrow involvement; indolent
Hairy cell leukemia	Memory B cell	No specific chromosomal abnormality	Older males with pancytopenia and splenomegaly; indolent
Mantle cell lymphoma	Naive B cell	t(11;14) creating *CyclinD1-IgH* fusion gene	Older males with disseminated disease; moderately aggressive
Multiple myeloma/solitary plasmacytoma	Post–germinal-center bone marrow homing plasma cell	Diverse rearrangements involving *IgH*; 13q deletions	Myeloma: older adults with lytic bone lesions, pathologic fractures, hypercalcemia, and renal failure; moderately aggressive Plasmacytoma: isolated plasma cell masses in bone or soft tissue; indolent
Small lymphocytic lymphoma/chronic lymphocytic leukemia	Naive B cell or memory B cell	Trisomy 12, deletions of 11q, 13q, and 17p	Older adults with bone marrow, lymph node, spleen, and liver disease; autoimmune hemolysis and thrombocytopenia in a minority; indolent

Contd.

Contd.

NEOPLASMS OF MATURE T CELLS OR NK CELLS			
Adult T-cell leukemia/lymphoma	Helper T cell	HTLV-1 provirus present in tumor cells	Adults with cutaneous lesions, marrow involvement, and hypercalcemia; occurs mainly in Japan, West Africa, and the Caribbean; aggressive
Peripheral T-cell lymphoma, unspecified	Helper or cytotoxic T cell	No specific chromosomal abnormality	Mainly older adults; usually presents with lymphadenopathy; aggressive
Anaplastic large-cell lymphoma	Cytotoxic T cell	Rearrangements of *ALK*	Children and young adults, usually with lymph node and soft-tissue disease; aggressive
Extranodal NK/T-cell lymphoma	NK-cell (common) or cytotoxic T cell (rare)	EBV-associated; no specific chromosomal abnormality	Adults with destructive extranodal masses, most commonly sinonasal; aggressive
Mycosis fungoides/Sézary syndrome	Helper T cell	No specific chromosomal abnormality	Adult patients with cutaneous patches, plaques, nodules, or generalized erythema; indolent
Large granular lymphocytic leukemia	Two types: cytotoxic T cell and NK cell	No specific chromosomal abnormality	Adult patients with splenomegaly, neutropenia, and anemia, sometimes, accompanied by autoimmune disease

12. Predominant osteoblastic secondaries are seen in: (Repeat)

A. Prostate Ca **B.** Breast Ca
C. Bone Ca **D.** Stomach Ca

Ans: A. Prostate Ca

Ref: *Robbins Pathologic Basis of Disease, 8th edition, Bone misc tumors chapter Pg. 1205*

Explanation:

- The radiographic manifestations of metastases may be **purely lytic, purely blastic, or mixed lytic and blastic.**
- **In lytic lesions**, the metastatic cells secrete substances such as **prostaglandins, cytokines,** and **PTH-related protein** that stimulate **osteoclastic bone resorption**; the tumor cells themselves do not directly resorb bone.
- Lysis of bone tissue rich in growth factors such as **TGF-β, IGF-1, FGF, PDGF**, and **bone morphogenetic proteins**, in turn helps create an environment conducive to tumor cell growth.
- **Prostate adenocarcinoma** secretes **WNT proteins** that stimulate **osteoblastic bone formation.**
- Most metastases induce a mixed lytic and blastic reaction.

Primaries which produce predominantly lytic bone lesions

- Carcinoma of the kidney
- Carcinoma of the lung
- Carcinoma of the gastrointestinal tract
- Malignant melanoma

Primaries which produce predominantly Sclerotic/Osteoblastic lesions

- Prostate adenocarcinoma
- Ca Colon
- Ca Breast

13. All are true regarding oral hairy leukoplakia *except:* (Repeat)

A. It is premalignant
B. Associated with EBV infection
C. Seen in HIV infected patients
D. Hyperkeratosis on HPE

Ans: A. It is premalignant

Ref: *Robbin's Pathologic Basis of Disease, 8th ed*

Explanation:

- Leukoplakia is premalignant, not OHL.

ORAL HAIRY LEUKOPLAKIA (OHL)

- Hairy leukoplakia is a distinctive oral lesion that is usually seen in immunocompromised patients.
- Approximately 80% of patients with hairy leukoplakia are infected with the human immunodeficiency virus (HIV).
- 20% of lesions are seen in patients who are immunocompromised for other reasons, such as cancer therapy or transplant immunosuppression.
- Hairy leukoplakia takes the form of white, confluent patches of fluffy ("hairy"), hyperkeratotic thickenings, almost always situated on the lateral border of the tongue.
- Unlike thrush, the lesion cannot be scraped off. The distinctive microscopic appearance consists of hyperparakeratosis and acanthosis with "balloon cells" in the upper spinous layer.
- There is no dysplasia (It is not premalignant).

- Sometimes there is **koilocytosis** of the superficial, nucleated epidermal cells, suggesting **human papillomavirus (HPV)** infection, and HPV transcripts have occasionally been found within the cells.
- However, **EBV** is present in most cells and is now accepted as the cause of the condition.
- Sometimes there is superimposed **candidal infection** on the surface of the lesions, adding to the "hairiness."
- In HIV-positive individuals, with hairy leukoplakia, symptoms of AIDS follow in 2 to 3 years.

MICROBIOLOGY

1. **Which of the following cell has both T lymphocyte and B lymphocyte function:**

A. Plasma cell
B. T-lymphoblast cell
C. B-lymphoblast cell
D. NK cell

Ans. B. T-lymphoblast cell

Ref: *Ananthanarayan R, Paniker CKJ. Textbook of Microbiology. 8th Edition. Hyderabad: Universities Press; 2009. Pg. 130*

Explanation:

Plasma Cell

- Plasma cell is the antibody secreting cell.
- It is structurally designed to be an immunoglobulin producing factory.
- Plasma cells are end cells and have a short life span of two or three days.
- A plasma cell makes an antibody of a single specificity.

Lymphoblasts

- While plasma cell is the best antibody producing cell lymphoblasts may also synthesise Ig to some extent.
- B lymphoblasts will have only B cell function. However, T lymphoblasts primarily have T cell function, but they can also synthesise Ig to some extent.

NK Cell

- Natural killer cells possess spontaneous cytotoxicity towards various target cells mainly malignant and virus infected cells.
- Their cytotoxicity is not antibody dependent or MHC restricted.
- NK activity is 'natural' or 'nonimmune' as it does not require sensitisation by prior antigenic contact.
- NK cells form part of the innate immune.

2. **Gram negative antigen is injected in a rabbit intradermally followed by a second intravenous injection 24 hours later. It developed a hemorrhagic and necrotic lesion at the site of the first injection. What is this reaction?**

A. Schwartzman reaction
B. Schultz-dale phenomenon
C. P-K-reaction
D. Arthus reaction

Ans. A. Schwartzman reaction

Ref: *Ananthanarayan R, Paniker CKJ. Textbook of Microbiology. 8th Edition. Hyderabad: Universities Press; 2009. Pg.121, 166*

Explanation:

Schwartzman Reaction

- A localized cutaneous reaction following intradermal injection of endotoxin (lipopolysaccharide, a component of gram negative cell wall) followed 24 hours later by intravenous injection of endotoxin.
- It is marked by hemorrhage, necrosis, and white blood cell infiltration at the site of first injection.

Schultz-Dale Phenomenon

Isolated tissues, such as intestinal or uterine muscle strips from sensitised guinea pigs held in a bath of Ringer's solution will contract vigorously on addition of the specific antigen to the bath. This is known as the Schultz-Dale phenomenon.

Prausnitz-Kustner (PK) Reaction

- Serum containing IgE antibodies is drawn from the allergic (atopic) patient. This serum is injected intradermally into a non-allergic person. The suspected antigens are then intradermally injected into the non-allergic person 24–48 hours later. This will cause a local reaction in the non-allergic person.

Arthus Reaction

- Arthus observed that when rabbits were repeatedly injected subcutaneously with normal horse serum, the initial injections had no local effect but with later injections, there occurred intense local reaction consisting of edema, induration and hemorrhagic necrosis. This is known as the Arthus reaction.

3. **Which of the following is an oncogenic retrovirus?**
A. HTLV-1
B. HPV
C. EBV
D. HBV

Ans. A. HTLV-1

Ref: *Jawetz, Melnick & Adelberg's Textbook of Medical Microbiology, 25th Edition. 2010*

Explanation:

- Viruses which produce tumors in either their natural host or experimental animals or induce malignant transformation in cell cultures are called oncogenic viruses.

RNA viruses	**CANCER**
HCV	Hepatocellular cancer
HTLV 1	Adult T cell leukemia
HIV	AIDS related malignancies
DNA viruses	**CANCER**
HPV	Genital tumours Oropharyngeal cancer
EBV	Burkitt's lymphoma Nasopharyngeal carcinoma B cell lymphoma
HHV 8	Kaposi's sarcoma
HBV	Hepatocellular cancer

4. **Which of the following activates the alternate complement pathway?**
A. IgA
B. IgG
C. IgM
D. IgD

Ans. A. IgA

Ref: *Ananthanarayan R, Paniker CKJ. Textbook of Microbiology. 8th Edition. Hyderabad: Universities Press; 2009. Pg. 98*

Explanation:

Comparison of the ability of different classes of antibodies to cause complement activation

Complement activation	IgG	IgA	IgM	IgD	IgE
Classical pathway	++	-	+++	-	-
Alternate pathway	-	+	-	-	-

5. **The disease called "lumpy jaw" is produced by:**
A. Actinomyces israelii
B. Streptomyces
C. Nocardia asteroids
D. Rhizopus nigricans

Ans: A. Actinomyces israelii

Ref: *Ananthanarayan, Paniker CJ. Textbook of Microbiology. 8th Edition. London: John Wiley & Sons; 2009. Pg. 391-392*

Explanation:

- Lumpy jaw refers to actinomycosis caused by *Actinomyces israelii.* It is a chronic granulomatous infection occurring in humans and animals.
- It is characterized by indurated swelling with multiple sinuses discharging sulphur granules.
- It is an endogenous infection caused by anaerobic actinomycetes.
- The 4 clinical types of actinomycosis are:
  – Cervicofacial actinomycosis
  – Thoracic actinomycosis
  – Abdominal actinomycosis
  – Pelvic actinomycosis

6. **Which of the following statement is true about bacteroides?**
A. It is gram positive bacilli
B. It is strictly aerobic
C. It may cause peritonitis
D. Presence in stool culture indicates need for treatment

Ans. C. It may cause peritonitis

Ref: *Ananthanarayan, Paniker CJ. Textbook of Microbiology. 8th Edition. London: John Wiley & Sons; 2009. Pg. 265*

Explanation:

Classification of Non-sporing Anerobes

I. COCCI

A. Gram positive
- Peptostreptococcus
- Peptococcus

B. Gram negative
- Veillonella

II. BACILLI

A. Gram positive
- Eubacterium
- Propionibacterium
- Lactobacillus
- Mobiluncus
- Bifidobacterium
- Actinomyces

B. Gram negative
- Bacteroides
- Prevotellla

- Porphyromonas
- Fusobacterium

Bacteroides

- The Bacteroides (B. fragilis) is the **most common non-sporing anaerobe** isolated from clinical specimens.
- They are **non-sporing, non-motile, strict anaerobes**, usually very **pleomorphic**, appearing as **slender rods**.
- They possess **capsular polysaccharides** which appear to be a virulence factor.
- They are **normal inhabitants** of the **intestinal, respiratory and female genital tracts**.
- It is often recovered from blood, pleural and peritoneal fluids, CSF, brain abscesses, wounds and urogenital infections.

7. **MHC II is present in:**

A. Langhans cell **B.** Dendritic cell
C. T cell **D.** NK cell

Ans. B. Dendritic cell

Ref: *Ananthanarayan, Paniker CJ. Textbook of Microbiology. 8th Edition. London: John Wiley & Sons; 2009. Pg. 134*

Explanation:

- **HLA class I antigens (A, B and C)** are found on the surface of virtually **all nucleated cells.** They are the principal antigens involved in **graft rejection** and **cell mediated cytolysis**. Class I molecules may function as **components of hormone receptors**.
- **HLA class II antigens** are more restricted in distribution, being found only on **antigen presenting cells** of the immune system such as **macrophages, dendritic** cells, **B cells** and **activated T cells.**
- T cells normally do not possess MHC II, **only activated T cells** may express **MHC II** molecules.
- Langhans giant cells are large cells found in granulomatous conditions. They are formed by the fusion of epithelioid cells (macrophages), and contain nuclei arranged in a horseshoe-shaped pattern in the cell periphery.
- **Langerhans cells are dendritic cells** (antigen-presenting immune cells) of the skin and mucosa, and contain large granules.

8. **False regarding NK cells:**

A. NK cell activity is augmented by interferons
B. Initial response in viral infection
C. Active against tumour cells
D. MHC restricted

Ans. D. MHC restricted

Ref: *Ananthanarayan, Paniker CJ. Textbook of Microbiology. 8th Edition. London: John Wiley & Sons; 2009. Pg. 131*

Explanation:

Natural Killer Cells

- Natural killer cells possess **spontaneous cytotoxicity** towards various target cells such as **malignant** and **virus infected cells.**
- Their **cytotoxicity** is **NOT antibody dependent** or **MHC restricted.**
- NK cell activity is **'natural' or 'nonimmune'** as it **does not require sensitisation** by prior antigenic contact.
- NK cells form part of the **innate** immune set-up.
- They belong to a different lineage from T and B cells.
- They have **CD16** and **CD56** on their surface.
- NK cell activity is augmented by **interferons**.

9. **Which agent is effective in killing spores?**

A. Alcohol **B.** Phenol
C. Chlorine **D.** Formaldehyde

Ans. D. Formaldehyde

Ref: *Ananthanarayan R, Paniker CKJ Textbook of Microbiology. 8th Edition. Hyderabad: Universities Press; 2009. Pg. 35-8*

Explanation:

- Formaldehyde is active against the amino group in the protein molecule.
- In aqueous solutions, it is markedly bactericidal and sporicidal and also has a lethal effect on viruses.
- It is used to preserve anatomical specimens, and for destroying anthrax spores in hair and wool

Disinfectant	Effective against	Characteristic
Alcohols Compounds	Active against bacteria and fungal spores	Good general use disinfectant
Aldehydes	Active against bacteria and virus and spores	Good activity against bacteria, virus and spores
Chlorine	Good disinfectant for blood and body fluid spills	Active against bacteria, virus and moderate action against spores

10. The cyclic trend seen with influenza is due to:

A. Antigenic drift B. Antigenic shift
C. Endemicity D. Virulence

Ans. A. Antigenic drift

Ref: *Ananthanarayan R, Paniker CKJ. Textbook of Microbiology. 8th Edition. Hyderabad: Universities Press; 2009. Pg. 496*

Jawetz, Melnick & Adelberg's, Textbook of Medical Microbiology, 25th Edition. 2010

Explanation:

- A unique feature of the **influenza virus** is its ability to undergo **antigenic variation**.
- Antigenic variability is highest in **influenza virus type A** and **less in type B**, while it has **not been demonstrated in type C.**
- Antigenic variation is of two types: **antigenic drift** or **antigenic shift**.
- **Antigenic Drift**
  - The gradual sequential change in antigenic structure occurring **regularly at frequent intervals** is known as antigenic drift. Here, the new antigens, though different from the previous antigens, are yet **related to them**, so that they react with antisera to the predecessor virus strains, to varying degrees.
  - Antigenic drift is due to mutation and selection, the process being influenced by the presence of antibodies to the predecessor strains in the host population.
  - Antigenic drift accounts for the periodical epidemics of influenza. Influenza outbreaks occur in waves, which depends on the interplay between extent of antigenic drift of the predominant virus and waning immunity in the population.
- **Antigenic Shift**
  - Antigenic shift is an **abrupt, drastic, discontinuous variation** in the antigenic structure, resulting in a **novel virus strain unrelated antigenically** to predecessor strains.
  - Such changes may involve hemagglutinin, neuraminidase or both.
  - Antibodies to predecessor viruses do not neutralise the new variants and can, therefore, spread widely in the population causing major epidemics or pandemics.
  - The changes involved in antigenic shift are due to **genetic re-assortment.**

11. Most common cause of traveller's diarrhea is:

A. EHEC B. ETEC
C. EPEC D. EIEC

Ans. B. ETEC

Ref: *Ananthanarayan, Paniker CJ. Textbook of Microbiology. 8th Edition. London: John Wiley & Sons; 2009. Pg 276-7*

Explanation:

There are 5 classes of *E. coli* that cause diarrheal diseases:

- Enterotoxigenic *E. coli* (ETEC)
- Enteroinvasive *E. coli* (EIEC)
- Enterohemorrhagic *E. coli* (EHEC)
- Enteropathogenic *E. coli* (EPEC)
- Enteroaggregative *E. coli* (EAggEC).

ETEC

- Fimbrial adhesins e.g. CFA I, CFAII, K88, K99
- Non invasive
- Produce labile toxine (LT) and/or Stable toxin (ST) toxin
- Watery diarrhea in travelers **(Traveller's Diarrhea).**
- No inflammation, No fever

EIEC

- Nonfimbrial adhesins, possibly outer membrane protein
- Invasive, penetrate and multiply within epithelial cells
- Does not produce shiga toxin
- Dysentery-like diarrhea (mucous, blood)
- Severe inflammation, Fever

EPEC

- Non fimbrial adhesin (intimin)
- Moderately invasive (not as invasive as Shigella or EIEC.
- Does not produce LT or ST; some reports of shiga-like toxin
- Usually **infantile diarrhea**; watery diarrhea similar to ETEC
- Some inflammation, no fever

EAggEC

- Produce ST-like toxin (EAST) and a hemolysin
- **Persistent diarrhea** in young children without inflammation, no fever

EHEC

- Moderately invasive
- Produce shiga toxin

- Pediatric diarrhea,
- Copious bloody discharge (hemorrhagic colitis)
- Intense inflammatory response, may be complicated by **hemolytic uremic synrome**

Shiga Toxin-Producing *Escherichia coli* (STEC)

- A type of **enterohemorrhagic *E. coli* (EHEC)** bacteria
- Hemolytic Uremic Syndrome

12. **All mycobacteria produces pigment *except:***
 A. M. kansasii
 B. M. simiae
 C. M. avium
 D. M. scrofulaceum

Ans. C. M. avium

Ref: *Ananthanarayan, Paniker CJ. Textbook of Microbiology. 8th Edition. London: John Wiley & Sons; 2009. Pg 360-1*

Explanation:

Classification of Atypical Mycobacteria (Runyons Classification)

Atypical mycobacteria/Non-tuberculous mycobacteria/Mycobacteria other than tubercle bacilli

- **Group I – photochromogens**
  - Produce pigment when exposed to light but not in dark
  - E.g. *M marinum, M simiae, M kansasii*
- **Group II – scotochromogens**
  - Form pigment even in dark
  - E.g. *M scrofulaceum, M gordonae*
- **Group III – non photochromogens**
  - Do not form pigment even on exposure to light
  - E.g. *M avium, M intracellulare, M xenopi, M ulcerans*
- **Group IV – rapid growers**
  - Capable of rapid growth, colonies developing within 7 days
  - E.g. *M fortuitum, M chelonae*

FORENSIC MEDICINE

1. **Subpoena is a:**
 A. Legal document
 B. Medicolegal document
 C. Medical document
 D. First information report (FIR)

Ans: A. Legal document

Ref: *The Essentials of Forensic Medicine and Toxicology by KS Narayan Reddy.29th edition. 2010.Pg. 7*

Explanation:

SUBPOENA OR SUMMONS

- Section **61 to 69 Cr PC** deals with summons.
- Sub-poena means **Sub - Under**; **Poena - Penalty**
- It is a **legal document** compelling the attendance of a witness in a Court of Law under penalty, or a particular day, time and place, for the purpose of giving evidence
- It may also require him to bring with him any books, documents or other things under his control, that he is bound by law to produce as evidence.
- It is **issued by the Court in writing**, in duplicate, **signed** by the presiding officer of the Court and bears the seal of the Court.
- Crime number and name of the accused person is mentioned.
- It is served on the witness by a police officer, by a officer of the Court or other public servant by delivering one of the copies of summons.
- The person should sign a receipt on the back of the other copy.
- It can also be served by **registered post, or fixed on some conspicuous part of the house** in which the person resides.
- For **Government servants**, summons send in duplicate to the **head of the office** in which such person is employed.
- The witness will be excused from attending the Court, if he has a valid and urgent reason.
- **If witness fails to attend the court**
  - In **Civil Case,** he or she is liable to pay damages.
  - In **Criminal Case**, he or she can be fined or court may issue bailable or non-bailable warrant.
- If witness is summoned by 2 courts one criminal and civil on the same day, he or she should attend criminal court and intimate the civil court of his inability to attend.
- If witness is summoned by 2 courts, higher court has priority over lower courts.
- If witness is summoned by 2 courts of same status, then priority is given for the summon he received first.

2. **Which of the following is most useful for sex determination?**
 A. Skull **B.** Femur
 C. Pelvis **D.** Tibia

Ans: C. Pelvis

Ref: *The Essentials of Forensic Medicine and Toxicology by KS Narayan Reddy. 29th edition. 2010. Pg. 57-61*

Explanation:

According to **Krogman theory**, the degree of accuracy in sexing adult skeletal remains is:

Entire Skeleton	100 %
Pelvis alone	95 %
Skull alone	90 %
Pelvis + Skull	98 %
Long bones alone	80 %

Some Important Difference Between Male and Female Pelvis (See Table-5)

3. **Which of the following is diagnostic of drowning?**
   A. Froth in the nostrils
   B. Cutis anserina
   C. Water in the stomach
   D. Mud in the respiratory passages

Ans. A. Froth in the nostrils **D.** Mud in the respiratory passages

Ref: *The Essentials of Forensic Medicine and Toxicology by KS Narayan Reddy. 29th edition. 2010. Pg:328*

Explanation:

Postmortem Changes in Drowning

External Changes

- The postmortem signs are variable and **none of them** are **Pathognomonic**
- **A fine, white, lathery froth or foam** is seen at the **mouth** and **nostrils**, which is one of the most characteristic signs of **external drowning**
- **Cutis Anserina** or **goose skin or goose flesh**: Skin has granular and puckered appearance, which is most prominent in thighs.
- It is produced by **spasm of the erector pilae muscles**, attached to each hair follicle.
- **Weeds, sticks, leaves etc firmly grasped by hands** due to **cadaveric spasm**. (Suggests **antemortem drowning**)
- Wrinkling of skin - **Washerwoman hands**

Internal Changes

- Drowning fluid penetrates tissues from alveoli — **Emphysema aquosum**
- The alveolar walls may ruputre due to increased pressure during forced expirations, produce **subpleural hemorrhages (Paltauf's hemorrhage)**

Others

- **Stomach** contains water in 70% cases
- **Diatoms** in **blood** and **bone marrow**
  - Diatoms are unicellular algae suspended in water.
  - Diatoms in BM and brain have maximum medicolegal significance.
  - BM of long bones (femur, tibia, humerus) and sternum is highly suitable and reliable.
  - Diatoms resist putrefaction.
  - Test is negative in cases of postmortem drowning.

Reliable Signs of Drowning at Autopsy

1. Fine, white froth at the mouth and nose
2. The presence of weed, leaves , twigs etc firmly grasped in hand
3. The presence of fine froth in lung passages
4. The voluminous water logged lungs
5. The presence of water in stomach and intestines
6. Finding of diatoms in the tissues

Table-5

Trait	Male pelvis	Female pelvis
Bony framework	Massive, rougher, marked muscle sites Stands higher and more erect	Less massive, slender, smoother
Preauricular sulcus (attachment of anterior sacroiliac ligament	Not frequent; narrow, shallow	More frequent, broad and deep
Greater sciatic notch	Smaller, narrower, deeper	Larger, wider, shallower
Subpubic angle	V-shaped, sharp angle 70-75 degree	U-shaped, rounded, broader angle, 90-100 degree
Pelvic brim or inlet	Heart shaped	Circular or elliptical More spacious Diameters longer
Ischiopubic index	73 - 94	91 -115
Sciatic notch index	4 - 5	5 - 6

4. **Mummification refers to:**
   A. Hardening of muscle following death
   B. Colliquative putrifaction
   C. Saponification of subcuatenous fat
   D. Desiccation of dead body

Ans: D. Desiccation of dead body

Ref: *The Essentials of Forensic Medicine and Toxicology by KS Narayan Reddy. 29th edition. 2010*

Explanation:

Mummification

- It is **dessication/dehydration** or drying and **shriveling of body tissue** and viscera after death
- Common in **infants (neonates and still births)**
- Ideal conditions for its formation are:
  - **High temperature**
  - **Devoid of moisture**
  - **Free circulation of air around the body**
- **Chronic arsenic or antimony poisoning** favour mummification
- First involves exposed body parts like **lips, nose, fingers, toes** etc
- The natural appearances and body features are preserved, but **face is grossly distorted** due to shrinkage of skin.
- The skin is **contracted**, **shruken** and **dry** (rusty brown in colour)
- The body is **odourless** and helps in **estimation of time since death**

5. **Rigor mortis starts in:**
   A. Heart **B.** Brain
   C. Right iliac fossa **D.** Left iliac fossa

Ans: A. Heart

Ref: *The Essentials of Forensic Medicine and Toxicology by KS Narayan Reddy. 29th edition. 2010*

Explanation:

Rigor Mortis

- This is the state of **stiffening** and sometimes **shortening of muscles** following death
- It occurs due to **lack of ATP** after birth.
- When the ATP is reduced to a critical levels of **85%** of normal, the overlapping portions of **myosin and actin filaments combine as rigid link of actomyosin**, which is viscous and inextensible causing hardness and rigidity of muscles
  - Order of appearance: **Heart** (left) → **eyelids → facial muscles → neck and trunk → upper extremities → legs → muscles of fingers and toes.**
  - It passes off in the same order. In India, it commences by **2-3 hrs**, develops for **12 hrs,** and usually lasts for **18-36 hrs in summer**, and **24-48 hrs in winter.**

Time of Onset: In India, it begins 1 - 2 hours after birth.

Duratin of RM: In India, it usually lasts for 24 - 36 hours during winter and 16 - 24 hours during summer.

Medico-legal Importance

a. It is a **definite sign of death**
b. Its extent helps in estimating the time since death
c. It indicates the position of body at the time of death

Conditions Simulating RM

a. Heat stiffening
b. Cold stiffening
c. Cadaveric spasm or instantaneous rigidity

Secondary Relaxation

- Flaccidity following RM is caused by action of the alkaline liquids produced by putrefaction.

6. **MTP Act was introduced in:**
   A. 1961 **B.** 1971
   C. 1981 **D.** 1991

Ans: B. 1971

Ref: *The Essentials of Forensic Medicine and Toxicology by KS Narayan Reddy. 29th edition. 2010.*

Explanation:

The Medical Termination of Pregnancy (MTP) Act of India

It clearly states the conditions under which a pregnancy can be **ended or aborted**, the persons who are qualified to conduct the abortion and the place of implementation.

- Women whose **physical and/or mental health** were endangered by the **pregnancy**
- Women facing the **birth of a potentially handicapped** or **malformed child**
- **Rape**
- Pregnancies in **unmarried girls** under the **age of eighteen** with the **consent** of a **guardian**
- Pregnancies in "**lunatics**" with the consent of a guardian
- Pregnancies that result are a result of **failure in sterilisation**
- The length of the pregnancy must not exceed **twenty weeks** in order to qualify for an abortion.

MTP Act of 1971 legalizes abortion on the following grounds:

- Therapeutic
- Eugenic
- Humanitarian
- Social

7. **The first permanent tooth to appear is:**
   A. 1st molar **B.** Lateral incisor
   C. Upper canine **D.** 1st premolar

   Ans: A. 1st molar

Ref: *The Essentials of Forensic Medicine and Toxicology by KS Narayan Reddy. 29th edition. 2010.*

Explanation:

Appearance of temporary teeth:

- Lower central incisor (6 mths)
- Upper central incisor (7 M)
- Upper lateral incisor (8 M)
- Lower lateral incisor (9 M)
- 1st molar (1 yr)
- Canine (1 ½ yr)
- 2nd molar (2 yr)

Appearance of permanent teeth:

- 1st molar (6 yr)
- Central incisors (7 yr)
- Lateral incisors (8 yr)
- 1st premolar (9 yr)
- 2nd premolar (10 yr)
- Canine (11 yr)
- 2nd molar (12-14 yr)
- 3rd molar (17-25 yr)

8. **Which of the following is not present in dhatura? (Repeat)**
   A. Hyoscine
   B. Hyoscyamine
   C. Muscarine
   D. Atropine

   Ans: C. Muscarine

Ref: *The Essentials of Forensic Medicine and Toxicology by KS Narayan Reddy. 29th edition. 2010*

Explanation:

Dhatura Poisoning

- Dhatura contain alkaloids such as ***Hyoscine (scopolamine)***, ***hyoscyamine*** and ***atropine***
- Dhatura poisoning symptoms are essentially due to atropine poisoning

The classical description of clinical features in datura poisoning is:

- **Dry as a bone** – Dryness of mouth and throat
- **Red as a beat** – Flushing of face
- **Blind as a bat** – Dilated pupils, sluggish light and accommodation reflex
- **Hot as a hare** – Raised body temperature
- **Mad as a wet hen** – Delirium with gait disturbances.

Symptoms of Dhatura Poisoning

- Dryness of mouth and throat
- Flushing of face
- Dilated pupils
- Sluggish light and accommodation reflex
- Raised body temperature
- Delirium
- Gait disturbances
- Slurred speech
- Dysphagia
- Drowsiness
  - Most of these features are also seen in alcohol intoxication (like drowsiness, irrelevant speech, dilated pupils, staggering gait and slurred speech).
  - Differentiating features are hot skin and dry mouth and lack of alcohol smell in breath.

Treatment

- **Gastric lavage** and the administration of **activated charcoal** can be used to reduce the stomach's absorption of the ingested material.
- The drug **physostigmine** is used to reverse the effect.
- **Benzodiazepines** to decrease patient's agitation, and supportive care with oxygen, hydration, and symptomatic treatment.

Muscarine is a natural product found in certain **mushrooms**, particularly in **Inocybe** and **Clitocybe** species.

9. **The lowest court that can give life imprisonment verdict is: (Repeat)**
   A. Chief metropolitan magistrate
   B. Metropolitan magistrate
   C. High court
   D. First class judicial magistrate

   Ans: C. High court

Ref: *The Essentials of Forensic Medicine, KS. Narayan Reddy. 24th edition*

Explanation:

Courts of Law: There are 4 types of criminal courts in India.

A. Supreme Court:
  a. Highest judicial tribunal
  b. Located at New Delhi
  c. Has **power to supervise all courts** in India

B. High Court:
  a. Located in **capital of every state**
  b. Highest tribunal for state
  c. It may try any offence and **pass any sentence authorised by law**

C. Sessions Court:
  a. Located at district headquarters
  b. Can only try cases which have been committed to it by a Magistrate
  c. It can pass any sentence authorised by law, but a death sentence passed must be confirmed by High court
  d. **Assistant Sessions Court:** Can pass all sentences except:
    1. **Death sentence** and
    2. Imprisonment for more than 10 years

D. Magistrates: There are three types:
  a. Chief judicial magistrate – Up to 7 years imprisonment
  b. First class judicial magistrate – Up to 3 years imprisonment
  c. Second class judicial magistrate – Up to 1 year imprisonment

PSM

1. **Following are louse borne disease:**
   A. Endemic typhus
   B. KFD
   C. Lyme's disease
   D. Trench fever

Ans: D. Trench fever

Louse borne diseases

Disease	Vector	Causative organism	Reservoir
Epidemic typhus	Pediculus humanus	R. prowazeki	Man
Epidemic relapsing fever	Pediculus humanus	Borrelia recurrentis	Man
Trench fever	Pediculus humanus	Bartonella quintana	Man/animals
Dermatitis	Pediculus humanus/ capitis	Secondary organisms	Man

Control measures:
Insecticide: DDT resistant, hence 0.5-1% Malathion dusting to be done on inner side of clothing.

Disease	Vector	Causative organism	Reservoir
Endemic typhus	Rat flea	R typhi	Rat
KFD	Hard tick	Arbovirus group B	Monkeys/Birds
Lymes disease	Hard Tick	Spirochete	

Ref: *Textbook of Preventive and Social Medicine, K. Park, 22nd edition page no 722*

Lice transmits disease by both direct and indirect contact

(See the following tables)

2. **Point prevalence of a chronic disease is studied best by:**
   A. Case control study
   B. Cross sectional study
   C. Historical cohort
   D. Cohort

Ans: B. Cross sectional study

Ref: *Textbook of Preventive and Social Medicine, K. Park, 22nd edition page no 59*

Explanation:

- **Prevalence** is an important measure of burden of disease in the community at a point of time or during a period of time. Accordingly they are called **point prevalence** and **period prevalence.**

Study design and important measurements done

Study design	Measurement
Cross sectional study	Prevalence (any one of point prevalence and period prevalence) Generation of hypothesis
Case control study	Odds ratio
Cohort	Incidence Relative risk Attributable risk Population attributable risk

3. **In Revised National TB Control Program mainstay of diagnosis of pulmonary tuberculosis is:**
   A. Sputum AFB **B.** CXR
   C. Clinical examination **D.** PCR

Ans: A. Sputum AFB

Ref: Textbook of Preventive and Social Medicine, 22nd edition page no 396

& Flowchart is by Textbook of Community Medicine, 1st edition, Armed Force Medical College, Pune

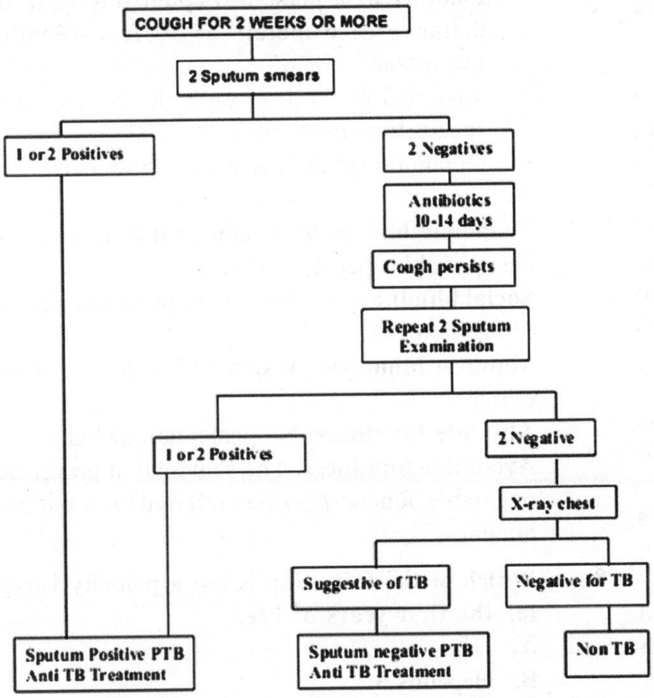

4. **Yellow fever is not present in India because of absence of:**
   - **A.** The virus
   - **B.** The vector mosquito aedes
   - **C.** Suitable atmospheric condition
   - **D.** Susceptible individuals

Ans: A. The virus

Ref: Textbook of Preventive and Social Medicine, K. Park, 22nd edition page no 257

Explanation:

- **Virus**: flavi virus fibricus.
- **Vector**: aedes egypti.
- **Reservoir**: man and monkey.
- Has both **domestic** and **sylvatic** cycle.
- **Incubation period.**
- **Vaccination certificate** is essential for those who travel to India or even have transit through India international travel. It is also compulsory for those who travel to South American countries.
- Certificate is valid for 10 years. Validity starts from one week after taking vaccination.
- **17-D** is **vaccine** given 0.5ml, subcutaneous
- Only **virus** is **not there** in **India**, otherwise all other favorable conditions are present (host and environment).

5. **The approximate magnitude of completed family size from demographic point view is given by:**
   - **A.** TFR
   - **B.** GFR
   - **C.** NRR
   - **D.** GRR

Ans: A. TFR

Ref: Textbook of Preventive and Social Medicine, K. Park, 22nd edition page no 450

Explanation:

Total Fertility Rate (TFR)

- The number of children who would be born per woman (or per 1,000 women) if she/they were to pass through the childbearing years bearing children according to a current schedule of age-specific fertility rates.
- **TFR** = Σ ASFR $_a$(for single year age groups)
- **TFR** = 5 Σ ASFR $_a$(for 5-year age groups)
- **TFR** is given importance because
  - It is not affected by differences/changes in age-gender composition,
  - It provides an easily understandable measure of completed family size.
- **Current TFR** of **India** is **2.5.**

General Fertility rate (GFR)

- Number of live births per 1000 women aged 15-49 in a given year.
- As per 2005 value All India 95.8/1000 women of 15-49 years.

GRR-Gross Reproduction Rate (GRR)

- Average number of daughters that would be born to a woman during her lifetime if she passed through her child-bearing years **experiencing the age specific fertility rates of a given year.**
- As per 2005 it is 1.4 per woman.

NRR: Net Reproduction Rate

- Average number of daughters that would be born to a woman if she passes through her life-time during her reproductive years **experiencing the age-specific fertility and mortality rates** of a given year.
- NRR is always lower than GRR, as it takes into account of the fact that some women will die before entering and/or completing their child-bearing years. Correspondingly NRR will be less than half the magnitude of the TFR.
- Currently it is 1.2 (UN Source: World Population Prospects: The 2010 Revision United Nations Population Division).
- Goal of national population policy is to reach TFR of 2.1 and NRR of 1.

6. **According to WHO the minimum number of antenatal visits to prevent maternal mortality is:**
A. 3 **B.** 6 **C.** 9 **D.** 12

Ans: A. 3

Ref: *Textbook of Preventive and Social Medicine, K. Park, 22nd edition, page 483*

Explanation:

- (Earlier editions mentioned **3 visits; latest edition mentions 4 visits as per 2010, guidelines** of GoK, since the nearest answer is given is option 3).
- Ideally the mother should attend the antenatal clinic **once** a month during the **first 7 months; twice** a **month**, during the **next month**: and thereafter, **once a week**, if everything is **normal.**
- Since many mothers are of lower socio-economic status and work for daily wages. Attendance at the antenatal clinic may mean loss of wages. Hence, it is difficult for them to attend antenatal clinic so often.
- In these cases, a **minimum of 4 visits** covering the entire period of pregnancy should be done.
- **First** visit **within 12 weeks, second** at around **14-26 weeks, third 28-34 weeks** and **fourth** visit **around 36 weeks** to term has to be done.
- **Third visit** should be preferably with **medical officer.**

7. **What is the definition of blindness according to WHO ?**
A. Vision less than 3/60
B. <6/60
C. <6/18
D. Only no light perception

Ans: A. Vision less than 3/60

Ref: *Textbook of Preventive and Social Medicine, K. Park, 22nd edition, page 371 & NPCB website*

Explanation:

WHO definition

Presenting distance visual acuity		
Category	**Worse than**	**Equal to or better than**
Mild or no visual impairment 0		6/18
Moderate visual impairment 1	6/18	6/60
Severe visual impairment 2	6/60	3/60
Blindness 3	3/60	1/60
Blindness 4	1/60	Light perception
Blindness 5	No light perception	
9	Undetermined or unspecified	

Category 0,1&2, are **Low vision**
Category 3,4&5 are **Blindness**
Note: WHO definition is different from NPCB definition.

NPCB definition of blindness is either of three:

- Inability of a person to count fingers from a distance of 6 meters or 20 feet Technical Definition.
- Vision 6/60 or less with the best possible spectacle correction.
- Diminution of field vision to 20° or less in better eye.

Economic blindness: Vision 6/60 or less with the best possible spectacle correction.
Social blindness: Vision 3/60 or diminution of field of vision to 10°.
Manifest blindness: Vision 1/60 to just perception of light.
Absolute blindness: No perception of light.
Avoidable blindness: The sum total of preventable or curable blindness is often referred to as avoidable blindness.

8. **Which of the following is not a priority vaccine for the first years of life?**
A. Hib
B. Hepatitis B
C. DPT
D. BCG

Ans: B. Hepatitis B

Ref: *Textbook of Preventive and Social Medicine, K. Park, 22nd edition*

Explanation:

- Hib causes meningitis, pneumonia which is common in first year of life.
- Diphtheria, pertussis and tetanus are though not common under one year, it is essential to start within first year to develop adequate immune response by 2nd year.
- BCG protects from severe form of neonatal, infantile tuberculosis (also TB Meningitis and Miliary TB.
- Hepatitis is largely given for prevention of hepatitis in future life exposure as it is less common in less than one year age, except for maternal transmission.

9. **Which of the following rates is not only an indicator of mortality but also of the living standard of a community ?**
A. IMR **B.** PNMR
C. MMR **D.** CDR

Ans: A. IMR

Ref: Textbook of Preventive and Social Medicine, K. Park, 22nd edition, page 525

Explanation:

- **IMR** is most important indicator of health status.
- Latest IMR is **48/1000** live birth in **2011**.
- Infant mortality is largest single age category mortality.
- Deaths at this age are due to peculiar set of diseases and conditions to which adult population is exposed or less vulnerable.
- It is affected quickly and directly by specific health programs and hence change rapidly compared to crude death rate.

10. Which of the following is a parametric test of significance?

A. U test
B. t-test
C. Chi-square test
D. Kruskal-Wallis test

Ans: B. t-test

Ref: Textbook of Preventive and Social Medicine, K. Park, 21st ed.

Explanation:

Parametric tests are used for normal distribution observations.

Parametric	Non-parametric
Independent t test	Mann Whitney U test
Paired t test	Wilcoxon signed rank test
Repeated measure ANOVA	Chi-square test
ANOVA one way	Kruskal-Wallis test
Pearson's correlation	Friedman test
	Spearman's correlation

11. Most common cause of blindness in India is:

A. Cataract
B. Refractive error
C. Glaucoma
D. Diabetes

Ans: A. Cataract

Ref: Textbook of Preventive and Social Medicine, K. Park, 22nd edition, page 372

Explanation:

- The national survey on blindness **2006-07**
- Cause for blindness in India
  - **Cataract** 62.6%
  - **Refractive error** 19.7%
  - **Glaucoma** 5.8%

12. Mininimum educational requirement for ASHA:

A. Class eight or higher
B. Class ten or higher
C. Completed 10+2
D. No educational qualification required

Ans: A. Class eight or higher

Ref: Textbook of Preventive and Social Medicine, K. Park, 22nd edition

Explanation:

ASHA (Accredited social health activist) are involved in health care of community under the National Rural health Mission.

- Accredited social health activists (ASHAs) are community health workers instituted by the Government of India's Ministry of Health and Family Welfare (MoHFW) as part of the National Rural Health Mission (NRHM).
- The mission began in 2005; full implementation was targeted for 2012. Once fully implemented, there is to be "an ASHA in every village" in India, a target that translates into 250,000 ASHAs in 10 states.

Roles and Responsibilities

ASHAs are local women trained to act as health educators and promoters in their communities. Their tasks include:

- Motivating women to give birth in hospitals
- Bringing children to immunization clinics
- Encouraging family planning (e.g., surgical sterilization)
- Treating basic illness
- Injury with first aid
- Keeping demographic records
- Improving village sanitation.
- ASHAs are also meant to serve as a key communication mechanism between the healthcare system and rural populations.

Selection

- ASHAs must primarily be **female residents of the village** that they have been selected to serve, who are likely to remain in that village for the foreseeable future.
- **Married, widowed or divorced women are preferred** over women who have yet to marry since Indian cultural norms dictate that upon marriage a woman leaves her village and migrates to that of her husband.
- ASHAs must have **class eight education or higher**, preferably be between the ages of **25 and 45**, and are selected by and accountable to the gram panchayat (local government).

- If there is no suitable literate candidate, a semi-literate woman with a formal education lower than eighth standard, may be selected.

Remuneration

- Although ASHAs are considered volunteers, they receive outcome-based remuneration and financial compensation for training days.
- For example, if an ASHA facilitates an **institutional delivery** she receives Rs. **600** and the mother receives **Rs. 1400**.
- ASHAs also receive Rs. **150** for each child **completing an immunization session** and **Rs. 150** for each individual who undergoes family planning.

13. **A patient with cervical cancer is missed by a screening test and later diagnosed to have advanced disease. This time interval is called: (Repeat)**

A. Lead time **B.** Screening time
C. Serial interval **D.** Generation time

Ans: A. Lead time

Ref: *Textbook of Preventive and Social Medicine, K. Park, 22th edition. P 127; Textbook of Public Health and Community Medicine. Armed Force Medical College, Pune. First edition 2009 p 136, 224*

Explanation:

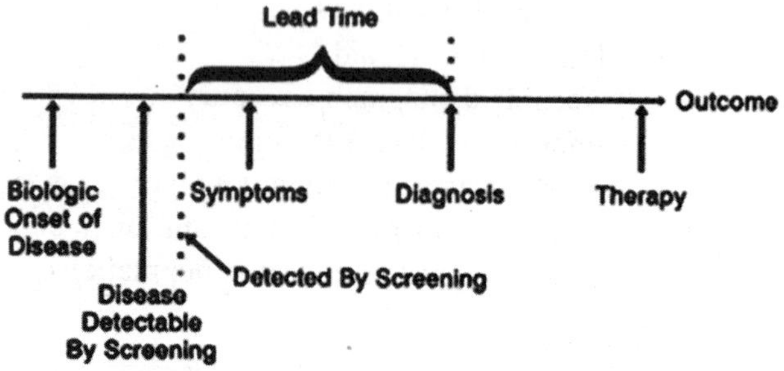

Lead time:

- Lead time is defined as the interval between the point a condition is detected through screening and the time it would normally have been detected due to appearance and reporting of signs and symptoms.
- It is the advantage gained by screening.

Screening time:

- The time interval between the point a condition is detected through screening and final critical diagnosis by other means before usual time of diagnosis.

Serial interval:

- The gap in time between the onset of the primary case and the secondary case is called the "serial interval".

Generation time:

- It is defined as "the interval of time between receipt of infection by a host and maximal infectivity of that host."

14. **Sickness absenteeism is a useful index to assess:**

A. Workers-management relationship
B. Working environment
C. State of health of workers
D. Sincerity of the workers

Ans: C. State of health of workers

Ref: *Textbook of Preventive and Social Medicine, K. Park, 20th edition, page 715*

Explanation:

- Sickness absenteeism is a useful index in industry to assess the state of health of workers, and their physical, mental and social well-being.
- Sickness absence is an important health problem in industry. The other options such as workers management relationship will impact the mental health of the workers; working environment will impact the physical and mental well-being of the individual. So option C indirectly includes A, B.

ENT

1. **Which among the following is not true about otosclerosis?**

A. Hearing better in louder conditions
B. Eustachian tube is always abnormal
C. Tympanic membrane is normal
D. Bilateral progressive conductive deafness

Ans. B. Eustachian tube is always abnormal

Ref: *Diseases of the Ear, Nose and Throat by PL Dhingra 5th edn.2010. P. 98*

Explanation:

Eustachian tube function is normal in otosclerosis.

Otosclerosis

- **Irregular spongy bone** replaces the **dense endochondral layer** of the **bony labyrinth.**
- Hereditary.
- Associated with **Van der hoove's syndrome-osteogenesis imperfecta, otosclerosis** and **blue sclera.**

- More common in **females.**
- Hearing loss **worsens** during **pregnancy.**
- **Cochlear type** presents with **SNHL.**
- **Stapedial type** has COHL and may have anterior (most common) posterior, circumferential, biscuit or obliterative focus.
- C/F **Hearing loss, Paracusis willisi** and **tinnitus** (indicates an active focus).
- O/E **Schwartze** sign— reddish hue over the promontory because of increased vasculature in active lesions.
- PTA will show the type of hearing loss and **Carhart's** notch which is a dip in the bone conduction at 2kHz.
- Impedance audiometry will show a **As type curve.**
- Medical treatment with **sodium fluoride** can be tried.
- **Surgery** is the **treatment of choice** and includes **stapedotomy or stapedectomy** followed by replacement with a piston made of Teflon or stainless steel or titanium.

2. **For Grommet tube insertion in serous otitis media, the incision on tympanic membrane is made on:**
   A. Anteroinferior quadrant
   B. Anterosuperior quadrant
   C. Posterosuperior quadrant
   D. Posteroinferior quadrant

Ans: A. Anteroinferior quadrant

Ref: *Diseases of the Ear, Nose and Throat by PL Dhingra. 5th edn.2010.Page 407*

Explanation:

- **Myringotomy** is a surgical procedure in which incision is made on the tympanic membrane to drain suppurative or non suppurative effusion of the middle ear or to provide aeration of middle ear in case of malfunctioning Eustachian tube.

Indications are:

- Asom with severe earache, incomplete resolution or with complications like mastoiditis.
- Secretory otitis media.
- Aero-otitis media.
- Atelectatic ear.

Incision used are:

- **Radial incision:** Made in the anteroinferior quadrant in secretory otitis media.
- **Circumferential incision**: Made in the posteroinferior quadrant in acute suppurative otitis media.

3. **Bezold's abscess is seen at: (Repeat)**
   A. Petrous tip
   B. Mastoid tip
   C. Digastric triangle
   D. Subdurally

Ans. B. Mastoid tip

Ref: *Diseases of the Ear, Nose and Throat by PL Dhingra 5th edn .2010Page 87*

Explanation:

Bezold's Abscess

- **Follows acute coalescent mastoiditis.**
- Pus breaks through the medial side of the mastoid tip and present with a swelling in the neck
- It may lie
  - Deep to sternocleidomastoid muscle
  - May reach parapharyngeal space
  - Track along the carotid into mediastinum
- There will be history of purulent otorrhea followed by pain, fever
- On examination there will be torticollis and tender swelling in the neck
- Treatment is with IV antibiotics, drainage of abscess and cortical mastoidectomy.

Other Abscess are:

- **Post aural abscess**: Most common.
  Displaces the pinna forwards, outwards and downwards.
- **Meatal abscess:** Luc's abscess.
  Pus breaks into the bony osseous external auditory meatus.
- **Citelle's abscess**:
  Pus tracks along the digastric muscle and presents in the digastric triangle.
- **Zygomatic abscess:** Presents at the root of zygoma.
  Swelling seen in front and above the pinna.

4. **Which of the following is not a feature of Rhinosporidiosis?**
   A. Bleeding polyp
   B. Russell bodies are seen
   C. Oral dapsone is useful in treatment
   D. Bleeding is present

Ans: B. Russell bodies are seen

Ref: *Diseases of the Ear, Nose and Throat by PL Dhingra 5th edn.2010 Page 172*

Explanation:

- **Russell bodies** are seen in **Rhinoscleroma** and not **Rhinosporidiosis**

- **Rhinoscleroma** is caused by **gram negative bacilli - Klebsiella rhinoscleromatis** also called **Frisch bacillus.**
- Histopathological features are:
  - **Russell bodies**– Homogenous eosinophilic inclusion bodies found in plasma cells.
  - **Mikulicz cells** – Large foam cells with a central nucleus and vacuolated cytoplasm containing the bacilli.

5. True statement about antrochoanal polyp is:

A. Often bilateral
B. Usually multiple
C. Arises from lateral wall
D. Recurrence is less common

Ans: D. Recurrence is less common

Ref: *Diseases of the Ear, Nose and Throat by PL Dhingra 5th edn.2010. pg 186-188*

Explanation:

Antrochoanal Polyp

It is a polyp which arises from the **maxillary sinus** and extends into **the nasal cavity** and **choana**.

- Etiology is **infection+/- allergy.**
- Seen in **children and young adults.**
- **Unilateral** may be bilateral.
- Presents with **nasal block and hypo nasal voice.**
- O/E **single pale polyp seen** in the **middle meatus.**
- **X-ray lateral view** of the skull shows a **mass in nasopharynx** with air column behind it.
- Can be done is surgical; **Endoscopic polypectomy.**
  For **recurrent case - Caldwell luc surgery.**
- Recurrence is uncommon.

6. A patient hears better in noise. Most likely diagnosis is:

A. Hyperacusis
B. Presbyacusis
C. Hypoacusis
D. Paracusis

Ans: D. Paracusis

Ref: *Diseases of the Ear, Nose and Throat by PL Dhingra 5th edn.2010. pg 98*

Explanation:

Paracusis willisii - Patient hears better in noisy environment.

- This is because people raise their voice in noise which will be near the patients hearing threshold.
- Seen in otosclerosis.

Presbycousis - Decreased hearing associated with aging.

7. Which of the following is not true about secretory otitis media?

A. Tympanic membrane is intact, retracted and lusterless
B. Hairline fluid level seen inside the tympanic cavity on otoscopy
C. Fistula test is positive
D. Politzerization affords relief

Ans: C. Fistula test is positive

Ref: *Diseases of the Ear, Nose and Throat by PL Dhingra 5th edn .2010.pg 47, 71-73*

Explanation:

Secretory otitis media

- Also called **glue ear, serous otitis media.**
- Most commonly seen in **school going age.**
- There accumulation of **'sterile' fluid** in the middle ear.
- Due to decreased function of the Eustachian tube or increased secretion of the middle ear.
- Presents with decreased hearing and delayed speech.
- O/E dull **opaque tympanic membrane**, maybe **blue in color, air fluid level** and bu**bbles may also be seen** in the middle ear.
- **PTA** shows **conductive hearing loss.**
- **Impedance audiometry** shows a **flat 'B' type curve.**
- Medical treatment consists of antihistaminics, decongestants and valsalva maneuver.
- Surgical drainage of the **fluid- myringotomy +/- grommet insertion** may be done in patients not responding to conservative measures.

Fistula test

- Performed by applying **Intermittent pressure** on the **tragus** or **using Siegles speculum.**
- **Positive test** is when patient complains of **vertigo or nystagmus** is induced.
- **Positive test** is seen in:
  - Erosion of horizontal semicircular canal by cholesteatoma.
  - Surgical window in the HSCC like post fenestration surgery.
  - Abnormal opening in oval window (post stapedectomy).
  - Rupture of round window.
- **False negative test** is seen in a **dead labyrinth** or when **cholesteatoma covers the site of fistula.**
- False positive test is seen in **hypermobile foot plate, Meniere's disease** and in **congenital syphilis (Hennebert's sign).**

OPHTHALMOLOGY

1. **Earliest manifestation of vitamin A deficiency is:**
   A. Conjunctival xerosis
   B. Corneal xerosis
   C. Bitot's spot
   D. Night blindness

Ans: D. Night blindness

Ref: *Basak Diseases of the Eye 5th edition, pg 474-476*

Explanation:

- The characteristic ocular manifestations of vitamin A deficiency is called **Xerophthalmia**.
- **WHO Classification of Xeropthth-Almia** [in chronological order]

XN	Night blindness
X1A	Conjunctival xerosis
X1B	Bitot's spots
X2	Corneal xerosis
X3A	Keratomalacia < 1/3rd corneal surface
X3B	Keratomalacia > 1/3rd corneal surface
XS	Corneal scar
XF	Xerophthalmic fundus

- **Night Blindness**: Earliest manifestation; responds rapidly to vitamin A therapy.
- **Conjunctival xerosis**: First appears at the temporal side in the interpalpebral area.
- **Bitot's Spot:** In the xerotic areas, keratin and corynebacterium xerosis accumulate giving it a foamy or cheesy appearance.
- **Corneal xerosis**: Dry and lustreless cornea
- **Keratomalacia**: Colliquative necrosis [sterile corneal melting.
- **Scarring** of the cornea.
- **Xerophthalmic fundus [Uyemura's fundus]**

Treatment:

Day	Oral	I.M.
Immediately, Day 1	2 lakh I.U.	1 lakh I.U.
Day 2	2 lakh I.U.	1 lakh I.U.
Within 1-4 weeks	2 lakh I.U.	1 lakh I.U.

- Children between 6-11 months - half the above dose.
- Children < 6 months – one-quarter of the above dose.

2. **Sunflower cataract is seen in:**
   A. Blunt trauma **B.** Diabetes
   C. Chalcosis **D.** Argyriosis

Ans: C. Chalcosis

Ref: *Parson's Diseases of the Eye 22nd edition pg.258 259*

Explanation:

Cause	Type of cataract
Diabetes	**Snow flake** cataract
Myotonic dystrophy	**Christmas tree** cataract
Galactosemia	**Oil droplet** cataract
Alport syndrome	**Anterior polar** cataract
Atopic dermatitis	**Shield** cataract
Traumatic cataract	**Rosette** cataract
Complicated cataract	**Posterior subcapsular** cataract [PSCC] with bread crumb appearance and polychromatic luster
Steroid induced	**PSCC** – discoid
Chalcosis / copper	**Sunflower** cataract
Siderosis/iron	**Brown** discoloration

3. **Steroid may be used in the treatment of which of the following type of herpes keratitis?**
   A. Superficial punctate keratitis
   B. Dendritic ulcer
   C. Geographic ulcer
   D. Disciform keratitis

Ans: D. Disciform keratitis

Ref: *Parson's Diseases of the Eye 22nd edition pg.202*

Explanation:

Treatment of Viral Keratitis:

- Epithelial keratitis: Topical antivirals, cycloplegic, mechanical debridement.
  Steroids are Contraindicated in the presence of active viral infections as it may in geographical ulcer.
- Stromal keratitis [disciform keratitis], endothelitis and iridocyclitis are treated with topical antivirals, topical steroids and cycloplegic.

Herpetic Eye Disease Study [HEDS]:

- In the absence of accompanying HSV epithelial keratitis, stromal keratitis improves more rapidly when steroid eyedrops are used along with topical antiviral drugs.
- **Oral acyclovir** 400 mg 5 times/day does not seem to prevent the occurrence of iridocyclitis or stromal keratitis following epithelial keratitis.
- In HS iridocyclitis, oral acyclovir may be added along with topical antiviral agent and corticosteroid.
- Low dose oral acyclovir 400mg BD reduce the rate of recurrent herpetic eye disease.

4. **Which of the following is the cause of blindness in partial retinal branch vein occlusion?**
A. Cystoid macular edema
B. Macular hemorrhage
C. Vitreous hemorrhage
D. All the above

Ans: D. All the above

Ref: *Kanski Clinical Ophthalmology, 7th edition p. 553-554; Basak: Essentials of Ophthalmology, 5th edition,pg. 313*

Explanation:

Branch Retinal Vein Occlusion (BRVO):

- **Classification :**
  – Occlusion at the disc – due to increased IOP.
  – Occlusion away from the disc – due to hypertension at the arteriovenous crossings.

Macular Branch Occlusion

- The **most common branch** involved in branch retinal vein occlusion is **superotemporal branch** because the no of AV crossings are more in that branch.
- If > 5 disc diameter capillary non-perfusion areas are seen in BRVO, then it is of ischemic type.
- Neovascularisation of the disc is more common in BRVO than neovascularisation of iris.
- So vitreous hemorrhage is more common than neovascular glaucoma.

Causes of Defective Vision in BRVO:

- **Macular edema – the most common**
- Macular ischemia
- Macular hemorrhage
- Vitreous hemorrhage

5. **In a patient, highest visual morbidity is seen in:**
A. Nuclear cataract
B. Intumescent cataract
C. Posterior subcapsular
D. Cuneiform cataract

Ans: C. Posterior subcapsular cataract

Ref: *Basak Essentials of Ophthalmology, 5th edition, pg. 248; Parson's Diseases of the Eye 21st edition pg no 262.*

Explanation:

Posterior subcapsular cataract or posterior cortical cataract:

- The **opacity** in the **posterior cortex** is close to the **nodal point of the lens**.
- Nodal point **7.08 mm** from the anterior surface of the cornea.
- Posterior cortical cataract is at the visual axis so during day time pupil constricts → **Day Blindness.**

6. **For the treatment of a patient with after cataract which laser is used?**
A. LASIK
B. Nd-YAG
C. Excimer
D. Argon

Ans: B. Nd – YAG

Ref: *Parson's Diseases of the Eye 21st edition pg. 584.*

Explanation:

Lasers	Frequency	Uses
Nd:YAG [Neodymium – Yttrium- Aluminium – Garnet]	1064	Posterior capsulotomy, iridotomy, vitreolysis
Frequency doubled Nd:YAG	532	Retinal photocoagulation, cyclophotocoagulation
Argon green	514	Trabeculoplasty, iridoplasty, pupillomydriasis, retinal photocoagulation
Diode laser	800	Retinal photocoagulation
Krypton Red	714	Retinal photocoagulation
Excimer (Argon fluoride)	193	Photorefractive keratectomy, phototherapeutic keratectomy, LASIK, LASEK
Femto second laser [neodymium glass]	1053	In refractive surgeries and lamellar and full thickness corneal transplants to create flaps

7. **Reversible cataract is seen in which of following:**
A. Galactosemia
B. Hypoparathyroidism
C. Diabetes mellitus
D. Trauma

Ans: C. Diabetes mellitus

Ref: *Parson's Diseases of the Eye 21st edition pg. 263.*

Explanation:

DIABETES:

Two types of cataract are seen in diabetic patients:

1. **Senile Cataract** – tends to develop at an early age and progress more rapidly.
2. **True Diabetic Cataract** – usually seen in young patients with acute onset of diabetes which disturbs the water balance in the lens.

- Large number **fluid vacuoles** are seen under the **anterior** and **posterior lens** capsule leading to **diffuse opacity (cataract)**.
- At an **early stage**, with the control of blood sugars, the **cataract is reversible**.
- **Snow flake cataract.**
- In **hyperglycemia**, the refractive status of the eyes become **myopic**.
- In **hypoglycaemia**, it becomes **hypermetropic**.

8. **Extorsion is a primary action of which of the following extra ocular muscle?**

A. Medial rectus **B.** Lateral rectus
C. Superior oblique **D.** Inferior oblique

Ans: D. Inferior oblique

Ref: *Kanski; Clinical Ophthalmology 7th edition; pg. 736 -737*

Explanation:

Remember a simple Mnemonic: **SIN RAD**
ALL **SUPERIORS** ARE **INTORTERS**
ALL **RECTI** ARE **ADDUCTORS**

Muscle	Primary action	Subsidiary action
Medial rectus	Adduction	None
Lateral rectus	Abduction	None
Superior rectus	Elevation	Intorsion and adduction
Inferior rectus	Depression	Extorsion and adduction
Superior oblique	Depression	Intorsion and abduction
Inferior oblique	Elevation	Extorsion and abduction

9. **Gonioscopy is used to study:**

A. Anterior chamber
B. Posterior chamber
C. Angel of anterior chamber
D. Retina

Ans: C. Angel of anterior chamber

Ref: *Kanski, Clinical Ophthalmology 6th edition; pg. 11*

Explanation:

GONIOSCOPY – To study the angle of the anterior chamber:
Structures: From anterior to posterior
S – Schwalbe line
T – trabecular meshwork
S – sclera spur
C – ciliary body

Uses:

Diagnostic – Abnormal angle structure [tumors, neovascularisation], estimation of the width of the chamber angle.
Surgical gonioscopy – While doing goniotomy, laser trabeculoplasty.

Types of Lenses:

Direct – Gonioprism – Direct view of the angle – **KOEPPE LENS.**
Indirect – Goniomirror – Image of the opposite angle – **GOLDMANN, ZEISS, POSNER and SUSSMAN.**

10. **Anterior Staphyloma is seen in:**

A. Sloughing corneal ulcer
B. Scleritis
C. Glaucoma
D. Pathological myopia

Ans: A. Sloughing corneal ulcer

Ref: *Parson's Disease of the Eye 21st edition, pg. 222–223*

Explanation:

Staphyloma

- Staphyloma is characterized by an **ectasia of the outer coats** [cornea, sclera or both] of the eye with an incarceration of the uveal tissue

Types	Site	Causes
Anterior	Involving part or the whole of the cornea; lined by iris	Sloughing corneal ulcer
Intercalary	Limbus and 2 mm from the limbuslined by ciliary body	Perforating injuries Marginal corneal ulcer Anterior scleritis Scleromalacia perforans Post surgical wound site Secondary glaucoma
Equatorial	2-8 mm from the limbus [vortex vein entry] lined by the choroid	Scleritis, Pathological myopia Chronic uncontrolled glaucoma
Posterior	Posterior pole; lined by the choroid	Same as equatorial

Management:

- Treat the cause
- IOP control
- Observation
- Local excision with sclera or corneal patch graft

MEDICINE

1. **All are causes of acute tubulointerstitial nephritis *except:***
   A. Methicillin
   B. Sjögren syndrome
   C. SLE
   D. Down's syndrome

Ans: D. Down's syndrome

***Ref**: Harrison's Principles of Internal Medicine. 18th edition. 2012. Chapter 285. (Table 285-1)*

Explanation:

Acute Tubulointerstitial Disorders

Therapeutic agents
Antibiotics (Beta-lactams, sulfonamides, quinolones, vancomycin, erythromycin, minocycline, rifampin, ethambutol, acyclovir)
Nonsteroidal anti-inflammatory drugs, COX-2 inhibitors
Diuretics (rarely thiazides, loop diuretics, triamterene)
Anticonvulsants (phenytoin, valproate, carbamazepine, phenobarbital)
Miscellaneous (proton pump inhibitors, H_2 blockers, captopril, mesalazine, indinavir, allopurinol)
Infection
Bacteria (*Streptococcus, Staphylococcus, Legionella, Salmonella, Brucella, Yersinia, Corynebacterium-diphtheriae*)
Viruses (EBV, CMV, hantavirus, polyomavirus, HIV)
Miscellaneous (*Leptospira, Rickettsia, Mycoplasma*
Autoimmune
Tubulointerstitial nephritis with uveitis (TINU)
Sjögren's syndrome
Systemic lupus erythematosus
Granulomatous interstitial nephritis
IgG4-related systemic disease
Idiopathic autoimmune interstitial nephritis
Acute obstructive disorders
Light chain cast nephropathy ("myeloma kidney")
Acute phosphate nephropathy
Acute urate nephropathy

2. **The minimum possible score in "Glasgow coma scale" is:**
   A. 0 **B.** 1
   C. 3 **D.** 5

Ans: C. 3

***Ref:** Harrison's Principles of Internal Medicine. 18th edition. 2012. Chapter 267 (Table 267-1)*

Explanation:

Glasgow Coma Scale for Head Injury

Eye opening (E)		Verbal response (V)	
Spontaneous	4	Oriented	5
To loud voice	3	Confused, disoriented	4
To pain	2	Inappropriate words	3
Nil	1	Incomprehensible sounds	2
		Nil	1
Best motor response (M)			
Obeys	6		
Localizes	5		
Withdraws (flexion)	4		
Abnormal flexion posturing	3		
Extension posturing	2		
Nil	1		

Note: Coma score = E + M + V.
The lowest possible score = 1+1+1 = 3

3. **MENKES disease due to defective absorption of:**
   A. Zinc **B.** Manganese
   C. Copper **D.** Selenium

Ans: C. Copper

***Ref**: Harrison's Principles of Internal Medicine. 17th edition. 2008. Chapter 71. Pg.449*

Explanation:

- Dietary copper deficiency is relatively rare, although it has been described in premature infants who are fed milk diets and in infants with malabsorption.
- **Copper-deficiency anemia** has been reported in patients with **malabsorptive diseases** and **nephrotic syndrome** and in patients treated for **Wilson's disease** with chronic high doses of **oral zinc,** which can interfere with copper absorption.
- **Menkes' kinky hair syndrome** is an X-linked metabolic disturbance of copper metabolism characterized by mental retardation, **hypocupremia** and **decreased circulating ceruloplasmin.**
  - It is caused by mutations in the copper-transporting *ATP7A* gene.
  - Children with this disease often die within 5 years because of dissecting aneurysms or cardiac rupture.
- **Aceruloplasminemia** is a rare autosomal recessive disease characterized by tissue iron overload, mental deterioration, microcytic anemia, and low serum iron and copper concentrations.

- The diagnosis of copper deficiency is usually made on the basis of low serum levels of copper (<65 microg/dL) and low ceruloplasmin levels (<20 mg/dL).
- Serum levels of copper may be elevated in pregnancy or stress conditions since ceruloplasmin is an acute-phase reactant and 90% of circulating copper is bound to ceruloplasmin.

4. **Recurrent meningococcal meningitis occurs in:**
   A. C1 esterase deficiency
   B. C2 deficiency
   C. C3 deficiency
   D. C5-9 deficiency

Ans: D. C5-9 deficiency

Ref: *Harrison's Principles of Internal Medicine. 17th edition. 2008. Chapter 136. Pg.911*

Explanation:

Host defect	Disease or therapy associated with Defect	Common etiologic agent of infection
Complement system		
C3	Congenital liver disease, SLE, nephrotic syndrome	S. aureus, S. pneumoniae, Pseudomonas spp., Proteusspp.
C5	Congenital	Neisseria spp., gram-negative rods
C6, C7, C8	Congenital, SLE	Neisseria meningitidis, N. gonorrhoeae
Alternative pathway	Sickle cell disease	S. pneumoniae, Salmonella spp.

5. **68 years old chronic alcoholic presents with ecchymotic patches in the lower extremities. He also has perifollicular hemorrhages, fragmented hairs, splinter hemorrhages in nail beds and multiple red tender swellings in the muscle. What is the likely diagnosis?**
   A. Vitamin K deficiency
   B. Vitamin C deficiency
   C. Pyridoxine deficiency
   D. Chronic myelogenous leukemia

Ans: B. Vitamin C deficiency

Ref: *Harrison's Principles of Internal Medicine. 18th edition. 2012. Chapter 74*

Explanation:

Vitamin C deficiency

- Causes **scurvy**.
- This is seen primarily among the **poor and elderly**, in **alcoholics** and in individuals **consuming macrobiotic diets**.
- Vitamin C deficiency also can occur in **young adults** who eat **severely unbalanced diets**.
- In addition to **generalized fatigue**, symptoms of scurvy primarily reflect impaired formation of mature connective tissue and
- Clinical features include generalized fatigue, **bleeding into skin** (petechiae, ecchymoses, perifollicular hemorrhages); **inflamed** and **bleeding gums**; and manifestations of **bleeding into joints**, the **peritoneal cavity**, the **pericardium**, and the **adrenal glands**.
- In children, vitamin C deficiency may cause **impaired bone growth**.

Vitamin K Deficiency

- Clinically manifests as **hemorrhage**, and **newborns** are particularly susceptible because of low fat stores, low breast milk levels of vitamin K, sterility of the infantile intestinal tract, liver immaturity, and poor placental transport.
- **Intracranial bleeding**, as well as **gastrointestinal and skin bleeding**, can occur in vitamin K–deficient infants 1–7 days after birth.
- Thus, vitamin K (1 mg IM) is given prophylactically at the time of delivery.
- Vitamin K deficiency in adults may be seen in patients with chronic small-intestinal disease (e.g., celiac disease, Crohn's disease), in those with obstructed biliary tracts, or after small-bowel resection.
- Broad-spectrum antibiotic treatment can precipitate vitamin K deficiency by reducing gut bacteria, which synthesize menaquinones, and by inhibiting the metabolism of vitamin K.
- In patients with warfarin therapy, the antiobesity drug orlistat can lead to international normalized ratio (INR) changes due to vitamin K malabsorption.

Vitamin B6 (Pyridoxine) Deficiency

- Symptoms of include **epithelial changes**, as seen frequently with other B vitamin deficiencies.
- In addition, severe vitamin B6 deficiency can lead to **peripheral neuropathy, abnormal electroencephalograms**, and **personality changes** that include **depression** and **confusion.**
- In infants, **diarrhea, seizures, and anemia** have been reported.
- **Microcytic hypochromic anemia** is due to diminished hemoglobin synthesis, since the first

enzyme involved in heme biosynthesis (aminolevulinate synthase) requires PLP as a cofactor.

- In some case reports, **platelet dysfunction** has been reported.
- Since vitamin B6 is necessary for the conversion of **homocysteine to cystathionine**, it is possible that chronic low-grade vitamin B6 deficiency may result in hyperhomocysteinemia and increased risk of cardiovascular disease.
- Independent of homocysteine, low levels of circulating vitamin B6 have been associated with inflammation and elevated levels of C-reactive protein.
- Certain medications, such as **isoniazid, l-dopa, penicillamine, and cycloserine**, interact with **PLP** due to a reaction with carbonyl groups.

6. **All the following are supplemented in cystic fibrosis with gastrointestinal disease *except:***
   A. Vitamin E **B.** Vitamin K
   C. Vitamin B_{12} **D.** Pancreatic lipase

Ans: C. Vitamin B_{12}

Ref: *Harrison's Principles of Internal Medicine. 18th edition. 2012. Chapter 259*

Explanation:

GIT Involvement in Cystic Fibrosis

Clinical Features

- **Meconium ileus** in infants presents with **abdominal distention, failure to pass stool and emesis.**
- The **abdominal flat plate** can be diagnostic, with small intestinal air-fluid levels, a granular appearance representing meconium, and a small colon.
- In children and young adults, a syndrome termed **distal intestinal obstruction syndrome (DIOS)** occurs, which presents with right lower quadrant pain, loss of appetite, occasionally emesis, and often a palpable mass.
- DIOS can be confused with appendicitis, whose frequency is not increased in CF patients.
- **Exocrine pancreatic insufficiency** occurs in >90% of patients with CF.
- Insufficient pancreatic enzyme secretion yields protein and fat malabsorption, with frequent, bulky, foul-smelling stools.
- Signs and symptoms of malabsorption of fat-soluble vitamins, including **vitamins E and K,** are also noted.
- Pancreatic beta cells are spared early, but function decreases with age.
- This effect, plus inflammation-induced insulin resistance, causes **hyperglycemia** and a **requirement for insulin in >29%** of older patients with CF (>35 years).

Treatment

- Maintenance of **adequate nutrition** is critical for the health of the CF patient.
- Most (>90%) CF patients require **pancreatic enzyme replacement**.
- Capsules generally contain between **4000 and 20,000 units of lipase.**
- The dose of enzymes (typically no more than 2500 units/kg per meal, to avoid risk of fibrosingcolonopathy) is adjusted on the basis of weight, abdominal symptomatology, and stool character.
- Replacement of **fat-soluble vitamins**, particularly **vitamins E and K**, is usually required.
- **Hyperglycemia** most often becomes manifest in the adult and typically requires insulin treatment.
- For treatment of **acute distal intestinal obstruction, megalodiatrizoate** or other **hypertonic radiocontrast materials** delivered by enema to the terminal ileum are used.
- For control of symptoms, adjustment of pancreatic enzymes and solutions containing osmotically active agents, (e.g., propyleneglycol) is recommended. Persistent symptoms may indicate a gastrointestinal malignancy, which is increased in incidence in patients with CF.
- **Cholestatic liver disease** occurs in about 8% of CF patients.
- Treatment with **urodeoxycholic acid** is often initiated, but has not been shown to influence the course of hepatic disease.
- **End-stage liver disease** occurs in about **5%** of CF patients and is treated by **transplantation.**

7. **Clinical manifestation of thalamus lesion hemorrhage (Repeat):**
   A. Head bobbing **B.** Gaze palsy
   C. Miosis **D.** Ataxia

Ans: B. and D. Gaze palsy and miosis

Ref: *Harrison's Principles of Internal Medicine, 18th edition, pg 3295*

Explanation:

– **Common sites of ICH** are: **Putamen (most common)**, thalamus, cerebellum and pons.

- **Thalamic hemorrhage:**
  - Contralateral hemiparesis, hemisensory loss
  - Aphasia, constructional apraxia, mutism
  - Ocular: Deviation of eyes as if looking at the nose, unequal pupils, skew deviation, ipsilateral Horner's syndrome, absence of convergence, paralysis of vertical gaze, retraction nystagmus
  - **Dejerine-Roussy syndrome**-chronic, contralateral pain syndrome
- **Putamen bleed**:
  - Contralateral hemiparesis, facial palsy, slurring.
  - Deviation of eyes away from the side of hemiparesis.
  - Coma due to brainstem involvement.
  - Dilated and fixed ipsilateral pupil, decerebrate rigidity.
- **Pontine hemorrhage**:
  - Deep coma with quadriplegia, decerbrate rigidity.
  - Pin point pupils, absent dolls eye movement.
  - Hyperpnea, hypertension and hyperhidrosis.
- **Cerebellar hemorrhage:**
  - Occipital headache, repeated vomiting, gait ataxia, vertigo.
  - Eyes-ipsilateral horizontal gaze palsy, deviation to opposite side, ipsilateral 6th N palsy, blepharospasm, ocular bobbing, skew deviation.
  - Dysarthria, dysphagia, hydrocephalus due to 4th ventricular obstruction, coma.
  - Hematoma >3 cm needs surgery, <1 cm no treatment needed if patient is alert and oriented; 1-3 cm needs observation.
- **'Dot-sign' in contrast CT** indicates hematoma is actively bleeding, bad prognosis.
- **Dural AV fistula**: Produces pulse –synchronous cephalic bruit (pulsatile tinnitus).

Causes of ICH

- Cerebral amyloid angiopathy
- Cocaine
- Methamphetamine
- Reversible posterior leukoencephalopathy
- Brain tumor (metastatic chorioca, malignant melanoma, renal cell ca, bronchogenic ca; glioblastoma multiforme in adults and medulloblastoma in children).
- Moyamoya disease
- Vasculitis
- Sepsis
- Hematological disorders.

8. **All are true regarding Tumor lysis syndrome except (Repeat):**

A. Hypercalcemia
B. Hypocalcemia
C. Hyperphosphatemia
D. Hyperkalemia

Ans: A. Hypercalcemia

Ref: Harrison's Principles of Internal Medicine, 18th edition, pg 2274

Explanation:

Tumor Lysis Syndrome (TLS)

- Characteristic biochemical changes in tumor lysis syndrome
  - Hyperuricemia
  - Hyperkalemia
  - Hypocalcemia
  - Hyperphosphatemia
  - Acidosis
  - Acute renal failure
- Caused by destruction of large number of rapidly multiplying neoplastic cells: During Burkitt's lymohoma, ALL, CLL on chemotherapy.
- Chemotherapy commonly associated are:
  - Fludarabine
  - Letrozole
  - Tamoxifen
  - Glucocorticoids
  - Rituximab
  - Gemtuzumab
- Acute hyperurecemic nephropathy- **urinary uric acid / urine creatinine > 1**
- High calcium:phosphate ratio→ renal failure
- Tumor burden, hyperuricemia and high LDH→ high risk for TLS

Treatment

- Allopurinol
- **Rasburicase** (recombinant urate oxidase): contraind in G6PD deficiency, can cause bronchospasm, hypotension and hypoxia
- Aggressive hydration with ½ NS
- Urinary alkalinization with pH > 7 with IV sodium bicarbonate
- **Hemodialysis/hemofiltration:**
  - If S. potassium > 6
  - S. Uric acid > 10
  - S. Phosphate >10
  - S. Creat > 10 with severe hypocalcemia

Causes of hypercalcemia: VITAMINS TRAP

- Vitamin D, A intoxication, VIPoma

- Immobilisation
- Thiazide, TPN
- Addison's
- Milk-alkali syndrome
- Infection: Tuberculosis
- Neoplasm: Myeloma, secondary deposits
- Sarcoidosis
- Tuberculosis, Thyrotoxicosis
- Radiation
- AIDS
- Parathyroid excess primary/tertiary; Pagets

9. A single retrocardiac air-fluid level on a chest radiograph typically implies the presence of:

A. Sliding hiatal hernia
B. Gastric volvulus
C. Pericardial effusion
D. Lung abscess

Ans: A. Sliding hiatal hernia

Ref: *Canadian Asso Radiology Journal, 1986*

Explanation:

Sliding hiatus hernia is the most common type of hiatus hernia:

- The GE junction is displaced upwards
- The gastric fundus is also displaced above the diaphragm → retrocardiac mass with air fluid level
- A differential (2 airfluid levels at different interfaces) retrocardiac air-fluid level → gastric volvulus
- Pericardial effusion produces **'water bottle'** appearance of cardiac silhouette on CXR
- Lung abscess produces a cavity with airfluid level

10. Anti-Saccharomyces cerevisiae antibodies (ASCA) are seen in which of the following condition?

A. Ulcerative colitis
B. Behcet's syndrome
C. Primary biliary cirrhosis
D. Cryoglobulinemia

Ans: B. Behcet's syndrome

Ref: *Harrison's Principles of Internal Medicine. 18th edition. 2012. Chapter 327*

Explanation:

Behcet Disease

Behçet's syndrome is a multisystem disorder presenting with recurrent oral and genital ulcerations as well as ocular involvement.

Diagnostic Criteria of Behcet's Disease

Recurrent oral ulceration plus two of the following:
• **Recurrent genital ulceration**
• **Eye lesions**
• **Skin lesions**
• **Pathergy test**

Pathogenesis

- The etiology and pathogenesis of this syndrome remain obscure.
- The main pathologic lesion is systemic **perivasculitis** with **early neutrophil infiltration** and endothelial swelling.
- In some patients, diffuse inflammatory disease, involving all layers of large vessels and resulting to formation of **pseudoaneurysms**, suggests **vasculitis of vasa vasorum**. Apart from neutrophils, increased numbers of infiltrating CD4+ T cells are observed.
- Circulating **autoantibodies against–enolase of endothelial cells, selenium binding protein** and **anti-Saccharomyces cerevisiae antibodies (ASCA)**—characteristic of **Crohn's.**
- A recent genome-wide association study, confirmed the known association of Behçet's disease with **HLA-B*51** and identified a second, independent association within the MHC Class I region.
- An association with **IL10** and the **IL23R-IL12RB2** locus were also observed.

Clinical Features

- The **recurrent aphthous ulcerations** are a sine qua non for the diagnosis.
- The ulcers are usually painful, are shallow or deep with a central yellowish necrotic base, appear singly or in crops, and are located anywhere in the oral cavity.
- Small ulcers, less than 10 mm in diameter are seen in 85% of patients, while large or herpetiform lesions are less frequent.
- The ulcers persist for 1–2 weeks and subside without leaving scars.
- The genital ulcers are less common but more specific, are painful, do not affect the glans penis or urethra, and produce scrotal scars.
- **Skin involvement** is observed in 80% of patients and includes **folliculitis, erythema nodosum, an acne-like exanthem, and, infrequently, vasculitis, Sweet's syndrome and pyodermagangrenosum.**
- Nonspecific skin inflammatory reactivity to any scratches or intradermal saline injection

(**pathergy test**) is a common and specific manifestation.

- Eye involvement with **scarring** and **bilateral panuveitis** is the most dreaded complication, since it occasionally progresses rapidly to **blindness**.
- The eye disease, occurring in 50% of patients, is usually present at the onset but may also develop within the first few years.
- In addition to **iritis**, **posterior uveitis**, **retinal vessel occlusions**, and **optic neuritis** can be seen in some patients with the syndrome.
- **Non-deforming arthritis or arthralgias** are seen in a 50% of patients and affects the knees and ankles.
- **Superficial or deep peripheral vein thrombosis** is seen in 30% of patients.
- **Pulmonary emboli** are a rare complication.
- The **superior vena cava is obstructed** occasionally, producing a dramatic clinical picture.
- Arterial involvement occurs in less than 5% of patients and presents with aortitis or peripheral arterial aneurysm and arterial thrombosis.
- **Pulmonary artery vasculitis** presenting with dyspnea, cough, chest pain, hemoptysis, and infiltrates on chest roentgenograms has been reported in 5% of patients and should be differentiated from thromboembolic disease since it warrants anti-inflammatory and not thrombolytic therapy.
- **Neurologic involvement** (5–10%) appears mainly in the **parenchymal** form (80%); it is associated with brainstem involvement and has a serious prognosis (CNS-Behçet's syndrome).
- **IL-6** is persistently raised in cerebrospinal fluid of these patients.
- **Dural sinus thrombi (20%)** are associated with headache and increased intracranial pressure.
- MRI and/or proton magnetic resonance spectroscopy (MRS) are very sensitive and should be employed if CNS-Behçet's syndrome is suspected.
- Gastrointestinal involvement is seen more frequently in patients from Japan and consists of mucosal ulcerations of the gut, resembling Crohn's disease.
- Epididymitis is seen in 5% of patients, while amyloidosis of AA type and glomerulonephritis are uncommon.
- Laboratory findings are mainly nonspecific indices of inflammation, such as leukocytosis and elevated erythrocyte sedimentation rate, as well as C-reactive protein levels.

Treatment:

- Mucous membrane involvement may respond to topical glucocorticoids in the form of mouthwash or paste.
- In more serious cases, **thalidomide (100 mg/d** is effective. Thrombophlebitis is treated with aspirin, 325 mg/d.
- **Colchicine** can be beneficial for the mucocutaneous manifestations and arthritis. Uveitis and CNS-Behçet's syndrome require **systemic glucocorticoid therapy** (prednisone, 1 mg/kg per day) and azathioprine (2–3 mg/kg per day).
- **Cyclosporin** (5 mg/kg) has been used for sight-threatening uveitis, alone or in combination with azathioprine.
- **Pulse doses of cyclophosphamide** are useful early in the course of the disease, for pulmonary or peripheral arterial aneurysms.
- Recent recommendations for **anti–tumor necrosis factor** therapy suggest that they may serve as an add-on immunosuppressive therapy in patients with panuveitis refractory or intolerant to other immunosuppressives.

11. Which of the following is not seen in Parkinsonism?

A. Preserved postural reflexes
B. Hypokinesia
C. Rigidity
D. Static tremors

Ans: A. Preserved postural reflexes

Ref: *Harrison's Principles of Internal Medicine. 18th edition. 2012. Chapter 372. (Table 372-3)*

Explanation:

Clinical Features of Parkinson's Disease

Cardinal Features	Other Motor Features	Nonmotor Features
Bradykinesia Rest tremor Rigidity Gait disturbance/ postural instability	Micrographia Masked facies (hypomimia equalize Reduced eye blink Soft voice (hypophonia) Dysphagia Freezing	Anosmia Sensory disturbances (e.g., pain) Mood disorders (e.g., depression) Sleep disturbances Autonomic disturbances Orthostatic hypotension Gastrointestinal disturbances

Contd.

Contd.

	Genitourinal disturbances Sexual dysfunction Cognitive impairment/ Dementia

12. **All of the following are features of Guillian-Barré syndrome *except:***
    - **A.** Predominant motor involvement
    - **B.** Facial nerve involvement
    - **C.** Absence of pleocytosis in CSF
    - **D.** Bladder and bowel involvement

Ans: **D.** Bladder and bowel involvement

Ref: *Harrison's Principles of Internal Medicine. 18th edition. 2012. Chapter 385. (Table 385-3)*

Explanation:

Guillian-Barré Syndrome

- GBS manifests as a **rapidly evolving areflexic motor paralysis** with or without sensory disturbance.
- The usual pattern is an **ascending paralysis** that may be first noticed as **rubbery legs.** Weakness typically evolves over hours to a few days and is frequently accompanied by **tingling dysesthesias** in the extremities.
- The legs are usually more affected than the arms, and facial diparesis is present in 50% of affected individuals.
- The lower cranial nerves are also frequently involved, causing **bulbar weakness** with **difficulty handling secretions and maintaining an airway**; the diagnosis in these patients may initially be mistaken for brainstem ischemia.
- **Pain in the neck, shoulder, back, or diffusely over the spine** is also common in the early stages of GBS, occurring in 50% of patients.
- Most patients require hospitalization, and in different series upto 30% require ventilatory assistance at some time during the illness.
- **Fever and constitutional symptoms are absent** at the onset.
- **Deep tendon reflexes attenuate or disappear** within the first few days of onset.
- Cutaneous sensory deficits (e.g., loss of pain and temperature sensation) are usually relatively mild, but functions subserved by large sensory fibers, such as deep tendon reflexes and proprioception, are more severely affected.
- **Bladder dysfunction** may occur in severe cases but is usually **transient.**
- If **bladder dysfunction** is a **prominent feature** and comes early in the course, diagnostic possibilities other than GBS should be considered, particularly **spinal cord disease.**
- Once clinical worsening stops and the patient reaches a plateau (almost always within 4 weeks of onset), further progression is unlikely.
- Autonomic involvement is common and may occur even in patients whose GBS is otherwise mild.
- The usual manifestations are loss of vasomotor control with wide fluctuation in blood pressure, postural hypotension and cardiac dysrhythmias.
- **Pain** is another common feature of GBS; in addition to the acute pain described above, a deep aching pain may be present in weakened muscles that patients like to having overexercised the previous day.
- Other pains in GBS include **dysesthetic pain** in the extremities as a manifestation of sensory nerve fiber involvement. These pains are self-limited and often respond to standard analgesics.

13. **Following cranial nerve is most commonly involved in patients with sarcoidosis:**
    - **A.** II Cranial nerve
    - **B.** III Cranial nerve
    - **C.** VII Cranial nerve
    - **D.** IX Cranial nerve

Ans: C. VII Cranial nerve

Ref: *Harrison's Principles of Internal Medicine 18th edition. 2012. Chapter 329*

Explanation:

Nervous System Involvement in Sarcoidosis

- Neurologic disease is reported in **5–10%.**
- Any part of the central or peripheral nervous system can be affected.
- The presence of **granulomatous inflammation** is often visible on **MRI studies.**
- The MRI with gadolinium enhancement may demonstrate space-occupying lesions, but the MRI can be negative due to small lesions or the effect of systemic therapy in reducing the inflammation.
- The cerebral spinal fluid (CSF) findings include lymphocytic meningitis with a mild increase in protein.
- The CSF glucose is usually normal but can be low.
- Certain areas of the nervous system are more commonly affected in **neurosarcoidosis.**
  - **Cranial nerve involvement**
  - **Basilar meningitis**

- Myelopathy
- **Anterior hypothalamic disease** with associated diabetes insipidus

- **Seizures** and **cognitive** changes also occur.
- Of the cranial nerves, **seventh nerve paralysis** can be transient and mistaken for Bell's palsy (idiopathic seventh nerve paralysis).
- **Optic neuritis** is another cranial nerve manifestation of sarcoidosis. This manifestation is more chronic and usually requires long-term systemic therapy. It can be associated with both anterior and posterior uveitis.

14. Features of large orange tonsils and very low HDL levels are characteristic of:

A. Familial hypobetalipoproteinemia
B. Abetalipoproteinemia
C. Hypoalphalipoproteinemia
D. Tangier disease

Ans: D. Tangier disease

Ref: *Harrison's Principles of Internal Medicine. 18th edition. 2012. Chapter 356*

Explanation:

Tangier Disease (ABCA1 Deficiency)

- Tangier disease is a very rare **autosomal codominant** form of **extremely low plasma HDL-C** caused by mutations in the gene encoding **ABCA1**, a cellular transporter that facilitates efflux of **unesterified cholesterol and phospholipids** from **cells to apoA-I.**
- **ABCA1** in the **liver** and **intestine** rapidly **lipidates** the **apoA-I** secreted from these tissues.
- In the absence of ABCA1, the nascent, poorly **lipidated apoA**-I is immediately **cleared from the circulation.**
- Thus, patients with Tangier disease have **extremely low circulating plasma levels of HDL-C (<5 mg/dL) and apoA-I (<5 mg/dL).**
- **Cholesterol accumulates** in the **reticulo-endothelial** system of these patients, resulting in hepatosplenomegaly and pathognomonic enlarged, grayish **yellow or orange tonsils.**
- An intermittent **peripheral neuropathy (mononeuritis multiplex)** or a sphingomyelia-like neurologic disorder can also be seen in this disorder.
- Tangier disease is probably associated with some increased risk of **premature atherosclerotic disease,** although the association is not as robust as might be anticipated, given the very low levels of HDL-C and apoA-I in these patients.

15. Endocrine causes for hypertension are all the following *except:*

A. Cushing's syndrome
B. Hypopituitarism
C. Hyperaldosteronism
D. Gigantism

Ans: B. Hypopitutarism

Ref: *Harrison's Principles of Internal Medicine. 17th edition. 2008. Chapter 241. Pg.1554. Table 241-3*

Explanation:

Secondary Causes of Hypertension

Renal	• Parenchymal diseases • Renal cysts (including polycystic kidney disease) • Renal tumors (including renin-secreting tumors) • Obstructive uropathy
Renovascular	Arteriosclerotic, Fibromuscular dysplasia
Adrenal	• Primary aldosteronism • Cushing's syndrome • 17-alpha-hydroxylase deficiency • 11-alpha-hydroxylase deficiency • 11-hydroxysteroid dehydrogenase deficiency (licorice), pheochromocytoma
Aortic coarctation	
Obstructive sleep apnea	
Preeclampsia/ eclampsia	
Neurogenic	• Psychogenic • Diencephalic syndrome • Familial dysautonomia • Polyneuritis (acute porphyria, lead poisoning) • Acute increased intracranial pressure • Acute spinal cord section
Miscellaneous endocrine	• Hypothyroidism • Hyperthyroidism • Hypercalcemia • Acromegaly
Medications	• High-dose estrogens • Adrenal steroids • Decongestants • Appetite suppressants • Cyclosporine • Tricyclic antidepressants • Monamine oxidase inhibitors • Erythropoietin • Nonsteroidal anti-inflammatory agents • Cocaine

16. Patient presents with rhabdomyolysis and acute renal failure. What should be done next?

A. Mannitol
B. Forced alkaline diuresis
C. Dopamine
D. Hemodialysis

Ans: B. Forced alkaline diuresis

Ref: *Harrison's Principles of Internal Medicine, 18th edition 2012*

Explanation:

Though, all options are used in the management of rhabdomyolysis with ARF. The first line of management would be **Foreced alkaline diuresis** since it can **reverse** or **prevent ARF.**

Rhabdomyolysis

Causes

- Traumatic crush injuries
- Muscle ischemia during vascular or orthopedic surgery
- Compression during coma or immobilization
- Prolonged seizure activity
- Excessive exercise
- Heat stroke
- Malignant hyperthermia
- Infections
- Metabolic disorders (e.g., **hypophosphatemia**, severe **hypothyroidism**)
- Myopathies (drug-induced, metabolic, or inflammatory)

Clinical Manifestations

- In adults, rhabdomyolysis is characterized by the triad of:
  - Muscle weakness
  - Myalgias
  - Dark urine
- **Myalgias** and **generalized muscle weakness** are the most common presenting symptoms.
- Life-threatening **renal failure.**
- Disseminated intravascular coagulation (**DIC**).
- Sensitive laboratory **markers of myocyte injury** include elevated **plasma creatine kinase** (CK) levels (often in excess of 4- to 5-fold the upper limit of normal).

Management

- ***Fluid Resuscitation***
  - Expansion of extracellular volume is the cornerstone of treatment and must be initiated as soon as possible.
- ***Prevention of Acute Kidney Injury and Renal Failure***
  - Acidic urine is necessary to cause ATN. Therefore, **Alkalization of urine** in preventing ATN and renal failure and also reduces cast formation.
  - If urine output is adequate, consider the use of **diuretics** such as **mannitol** (in adults) and furosemide.
- ***Correction of Electrolyte, Acid-Base and Metabolic Abnormalities***
  - Hyperkalemia
  - Hypocalcemia
- ***Other Medical Treatment Measures***
  - **Dialysis** may be required in patients with **oliguric renal failure**, **persistent hyperkalemia**, other **electrolyte** abnormalities, **pulmonary edema**, **congestive heart failure**, and **persistent metabolic acidosis.**
  - The free-radical scavengers and antioxidants (e.g, pentoxifylline, vitamin E and vitamin C) may have some effect.
- **Fasciotomy,** if there is raised intracompartmental pressure and muscle ishcemia.

17. Causes of Type 2 renal tubular acidosis are all *except:*

A. Cystinosis
B. Lowe syndrome
C. Essential fructosuria
D. Galatosemia

Ans: C. Essential fructosuria

Ref: *Nelson's Textbook of Pediatrics 18th edition: pg.2197*

Explanation:

Renal Tubular Acidosis (RTA)

- It is a disease state characterized by a **normal anion gap metabolic acidosis** resulting from either **impaired bicarbonate reabsorption or impaired urinary acid (hydrogen ion) excretion.**
- There are 3 main forms of RTA:
  - Proximal (type II) RTA
  - Distal (type I) RTA and
  - Hyperkalemic (type IV) RTA
- Mixed lesions (those with elements of type I and II RTA), which occur primarily in patients with inherited carbonic anhydrase deficiency, are designated as type III RTA by some authors.
- Proximal RTA usually occurs as a component of global proximal tubular dysfunction or **Fanconi syndrome,** which is characterized by low molecular weight proteinuria, glycosuria, phosphaturia, aminoaciduria and proximal RTA.

Classification of Renal Tubular Acidosis

Proximal (Type II)	Distal (Type I)	Hyperkalemic (Type IV)
Primary	Interstitial nephritis	Hypoaldosteronism
Cystinosis	Obstructive uropathy	Addison disease
Lowe syndrome	Vesicoureteral reflux	Congenital adrenal hyperplasia
Galactosemia	Pyelonephritis	Pseudo hypoaldosteronism
Tyrosinemia	Sickle cell nephropathy	Obstructive uropathy
Hereditary fructose intolerance	Lupus nephritis	Pyelonephritis
Fanconi-Bickel syndrome	Nephrocalcinosis	Interstitial nephritis
Wilson disease	Medullary sponge kidney	Diabetes mellitus
Mitochondrial diseases	Amphotericin B	Sickle cell nephropathy
	Lithium	Trimethoprim/sulfamethoxazoie
Secondary	Toluene	ACE inhibitors
Heavy metals	Cisplatin	Cyclosporine
Outdated tetracycline		
Gentamicin		
Ifosfamide		
Cyclosporine/tacrolimus		

18. Antibiotic prophylaxis is indicated in:

A. Cardiac catheterisation
B. Prostectomy
C. Cystoscopy
D. Dental procedures

Ans: D. Dental procedures

Ref: *Harrison's Principles of Internal Medicine, 18th ed. and http://emedicine.medscape.com/article/Antibiotic Prophylactic Regimens for Endocarditis*

Explanation:

- The antibiotic prophylactic regimens below are recommended by the American Heart Association (AHA) only for patients with underlying cardiac conditions associated with the highest risk of adverse outcome from infective endocarditis.

High-Risk Cardiac Conditions

Antibiotic prophylaxis is indicated for the following high-risk cardiac conditions:

- **Prosthetic cardiac valve**
- History of **infective endocarditis**
- **Congenital heart disease (CHD)** (*except for the conditions listed, antibiotic prophylaxis is no longer recommended for any other form of CHD).*
  (1) Unrepaired cyanotic CHD, including palliative shunts and conduits;
  (2) Completely repaired congenital heart defect with prosthetic material or device, whether placed by surgery or by catheter intervention, during the first 6 months after the procedure; and
  (3) Repaired CHD with residual defects at the site or adjacent to the site of a prosthetic patch or prosthetic device (which inhibits endothelialization)
- **Cardiac transplantation recipients** with cardiac **valvular disease.**

Dental Procedures

- For patients with high cardiac risk, antibiotic prophylaxis is recommended for **all** dental procedures that involve **manipulation of gingival tissue** or the **periapical region** of teeth or **perforation of the oral mucosa**.

The following dental procedures do not require endocarditis prophylaxis:

- Routine anesthetic injections through noninfected tissue
- Taking dental radiographs
- Placement of removable prosthodontic or orthodontic appliances
- Adjustment of orthodontic appliances
- Placement of orthodontic brackets
- Shedding of deciduous teeth
- Bleeding from trauma to the lips or oral mucosa

Respiratory Tract, Infected Skin, Skin Structures, or Musculoskeletal Tissue Procedures:

- Antibiotic prophylaxis is **recommended.**
- Invasive respiratory tract procedures that involve incision or biopsy of the respiratory mucosa (e.g., tonsillectomy, adenoidectomy).
- Antibiotic prophylaxis is **not recommended.**
- Bronchoscopy unless the procedure involves incision of the respiratory tract mucosa.
- For invasive respiratory tract procedures to **treat** an **established infection** (e.g., **drainage** of **abscess, empyema**), administer an **antibiotic** that is **active against Streptococcus viridans**.
- Patients with high cardiac risk who undergo a **surgical procedure that involves infected**

skin, skin structure, or musculoskeletal tissue should receive an agent active against staphylococci and beta-hemolytic streptococci (e.g., antistaphylococcal penicillin, cephalosporin).

- If the causative organism of respiratory, skin, skin structure, or musculoskeletal infection is known or suspected to be ***Staphylococcus aureus***, administer an **antistaphylococcal penicillin** or **cephalosporin**, or **vancomycin** (if patient is unable to tolerate beta-lactam antibiotics).
- Vancomycin is recommended for known or **suspected methicillin-resistant strains of *S aureus*.**

Genitourinary or GI Tract Procedures

- Antibiotics are **no longer recommended** for endocarditis prophylaxis for patients undergoing **genitourinary or gastrointestinal tract procedures**.

  All doses shown below are administered once as a single dose 30-60 min before the procedure.

Standard General Prophylaxis

- **Amoxicillin**
- Adult dose: 2 g PO
- Pediatric dose: 50 mg/kg PO; not to exceed 2 g/dose.

Unable to take oral medication

- **Ampicillin**
- Adult dose: 2 g IV/IM
- Pediatric dose: 50 mg/kg IV/IM; not to exceed 2 g/dose

Allergic to Penicillin

- **Clindamycin**
- Adult dose: 600 mg PO
- Pediatric dose: 20 mg/kg PO; not to exceed 600 mg/dose
- **Cephalexin** or other first- or second-generation oral cephalosporin in equivalent dose (do not use cephalosporins in patients with a history of immediate-type hypersensitivity penicillin allergy, such as urticaria, angioedema, anaphy-laxis).
- Adult dose: 2 g PO
- Pediatric dose: 50 mg/kg PO; not to exceed 2 g/dose
- **Azithromycin or clarithromycin**
- Adult dose: 500 mg PO
- Pediatric dose: 15 mg/kg PO; not to exceed 500 mg/dose.

Allergic to penicillin and unable to take oral medication

- **Clindamycin**
- Adult dose: 600 mg IV
- Pediatric dose: 20 mg/kg IV; not to exceed 600 mg/dose
- **Cefazolin or ceftriaxone** (do not use cephalosporins in patients with a history of immediate-type hypersensitivity penicillin allergy, such as urticaria, angioedema, anaphy-laxis)
- Adult dose: 1 g IV/IM
- Pediatric dose: 50 mg/kg IV/IM; not to exceed 1 g/dose

19. Dorsal column lesions are associated with loss of:

A. Ankle jerk
B. Knee jerk
C. Proprioception
D. Superficial abdominal reflexes

Ans: C. Proprioception

Ref: *Harrison's Principles of Internal Medicine, 18 ed.*

Explanation:

The Posterior Column (Dorsal Column)

- It refers to the area of white matter in the dorsomedial side of the spinal cord.
- It is made up of the **fasciculus gracilis** and **fasciculus cuneatus**
- It is part of an **ascending pathway** that is important for **well-localized fine touch** and conscious **proprioception** called the **posterior column-medial lemniscus** pathway.
- **Joint capsules, tactile** and **pressure receptors** send a signal through the **dorsal root ganglia** up through the **fasciculus gracilis** for **lower body** sensory impulses and the **fasciculus cuneatus** for **upper body impulses**.
- Once the fasciculus gracilis reaches the nucleus gracilis and the fasciculus cuneatus reaches the nucleus cuneatus in the **lower** medulla, they begin to **cross over** the medulla as the **internal arcuate** fibers.
- When they reach the **contralateral side**, they become the **medial lemniscus**, which is the **second part** of the **posterior column-medial lemniscus** pathway.
- Lesions in this pathway can diminish or completely abolish **tactile sensations** and **movement** or **position sense** below the lesion.

Tests of sensation

Modality	Pathway
Light touch	Large fast-conducting axons
Proprioception	Dorsal columns
Vibration	Medial lemniscus
Two-point discrimination	
Pinprick (superficial pain)	Smaller slower-conducting axons
Deep pain	Spinothalamic tracts
Temperature	
Stereognosis	Parietal cortex (only valid if peripheral sensory function intact)
Graphaesthesia	
Two-point discrimination	

20. Reiter's disease is associated with (Repeat):

A. Pseudomonas aeruginosa
B. Shigella flexneri
C. Streptococcus pyogenes
D. Pneumococcus

Ans: B. Shigella flexneri

Ref: *Harrison's Principles of Internal Medicine, 18th ed.*

Explanation:

Causes of Reiter's Syndrome (Reactive Arthritis)

- Reactive arthritis is associated with the HLA-B27 gene on chromosome 6 and by the presence of enthesitis as the basic pathologic lesion and is triggered by a preceding infection.
- **Shigella flexneri** (Most common, both epidemic and sporadic.
- **Shigella sonnei**
- **Shigella dysenteriae**
- **Salmonella** spp
- **Yersinia enterocolitica**
- Y. pseudotuberculosis
- **Campylobacter** jejuni
- **Chlamydia** trachomatis
- **Ureaplasma** urealyticum

21. Microcytic anemia is seen in deficiency of:

A. Vitamin B2 **B.** Vitamin B5
C. Pyridoxine **D.** Folic acid

Ans: C. Pyridoxine

Ref: *Davidson 21st edn, pg 127*

Explanation

Pyridoxine (Vitamin B6) Deficiency

- It is seen with **INH, Penicillamine**
- Pyridoxine is used in INH induced **peripheral neuropathy, sideroblastic anemia**
- Therapeutic uses:
  - **Antiemetic** in **radiation induced nausea.**
  - **Nausea in pregnancy**
  - **Carpal tunnel syndrome**
  - **Premenstrual syndrome**
- Chronic high doses can cause **sensory polyneuropathy**

Nutrient	Clinical finding	Contributing factors
Thiamine- B1	• Dry and wet beriberi • Wernicke's encephalopathy Korsakoff's psychosis	• Alcoholism • Chronic diuretic use • Hyperemesis
Riboflavin- B2	• Seborrhea • Magenta tongue • Angular stomatitis • Cheilosis	
Niacin- B3	• **Pellagra:** • Diarrhea • Dementia • Dermatitis • Death • Glossitis	• Alcoholism • B2 deficiency • B6 deficiency
Pyridoxine- B6	• Seborrhea • Glossitis • Neuropathy • Depression • Convulsions • Microcytic anemia	• Alcoholism • INH
Folate	• Megaloblastic anemia • Atrophic glossitis • Depression • ↑ homocysteine	• Alcoholism • Sulfasalazine • Pyrimethamine • Triamterene
Vitamin B12	• Megaloblastic (pernicious) anemia Subacute combined degeneration of the cord ↑ homocysteine • ↑ methylmalonic acid	• Gastric atrophy • Terminal ileal disease • Vegans • H2 blockers • Chronic metformin use

Sideroblastic Anemia

- It results from defective incorporation of iron into heme molecule in the cytoplasm of cells
- **Causes:** Congenital or Acquired
  - Myelodysplastic syndromes
  - Copper
  - B6 deficiencies
  - Zinc overdose
  - Alcohol
  - ATT
- Microcytic hypochromic picture, siderocytes with basophilic iron deposits (**Pappenheimer bodies**).
- Serum **iron** is **high** and **TIBC** is **low**, **S. Ferritin** is **high.**
- **Ringed sideroblasts** are seen in bone marrow with **Prussian blue** staining.

22. All except are features of Plummer-Vinson syndrome: (Repeat)

A. Hypertrophy of oral mucosa
B. Dysphagia
C. Glossitis
D. Iron deficiency anemia

Ans: A. Hypertrophy of oral mucosa

Ref: *Harrison's Principles of Internal Medicine, 18th ed.*

Explanation:

Plummer-Vinson syndrome (PVS)

- Also called **Paterson – Brown – Kelly syndrome** or **sideropenic dysphagia**
- **It is premalignant**
- Presents as a triad of
  - Dysphagia
  - Esophageal webs
  - Iron deficiency anemia
- It most usually occurs in postmenopausal women.

Clinical Features

- Burning sensation with the tongue and oral mucosa
- **Atrophy of lingual papillae** produces a smooth, shiny, red dorsum of the tongue
- Dysphagia
- Pain
- Weakness
- Odynophagia
- **Atrophic glossitis**
- Angular stomatitis
- The condition is associated with **koilonychia, glossitis, cheilitis** and **splenomegaly**.
- Hemogram – **Microcytic hypochromic** anemia suggestive of iron deficiency.
- Increased risk of **squamous cell carcinoma of esophagus.**

23. Most common Ig seen in multiple myeloma (Repeat):

A. IgG **B.** IgM
C. IgA **D.** IgE

Ans: A. IgG

Ref: *Harrison's Principles of Internal Medicine, 18th edition*

Explanation:

Also refer Medicine 2013 question explanation.

Multiple Myeloma

- Multiple myeloma is a malignant proliferation of plasma cells derived from a single clone.
- **Characteristics:**
  - *Lytic bone lesions*
  - Anemia with high ESR
  - Roulex formation of red cells
  - Renal failure
  - Infections
  - Hypercalcemia
- **Triad of Multiple Myeloma:**
  - *Marrow plasmacytosis* >10%
  - Lytic bone lesions
  - Serum and/or urine M component
- Monoclonal plasma cells (κ,λ light chain restricted) in BM or as a tumor (solitary plasmacytoma)
- **End organ damage**:
  - Lytic bony lesions
  - Anemia
  - Hypercalcemia
  - Renal failure with paraprotenemia (mostly IgG or IgA)
- S. electrophoresis for M band (β, γ); Urine Bence Jones protein for light chains.
- Non secretory myeloma– no paraproteins, poor prognosis.
- X-rays axial skeleton–skull, spine, long bones, ribs for lytic lesions.
- PET or MRI useful for early lesions.
- Radionuclide scan not useful.
- Must be differentiated from smoldering myeloma and MGUS.
- **Treatment:** Thalidomide/lenolidamide + high dose dexamethasone.
- Bortezomib, autologous hematopoietic SCT
- Localized RT for vertebral collapse.

- Bisphosphonates for malignant hypercalcemia (beware of their osteonecrosis jaw!).
- **Prognosis**

Stage	β2 microglobulin	Albumin	Survival
Stage 1	<3.5 mg/L	≥3.5 g/dL	> 5yrs
Stage 2	3.5-5.5 mg/L		
Stage 3	>5.5 mg/L		< 2yrs

24. Niacin deficiency occurs in:

A. Prolonged antibiotic use
B. Hartnups disease
C. Carcinoid syndrome
D. Isoniazid use

Ans: B. Hartnups disease

Ref: *Harrison's Principles of Internal Medicine, 18th edition*

Explanation:

Niacin Deficiency

- Causes clinical syndrome called Pellagra
- **Risk factors**
  - Alcoholics
  - Congenital defects of intestinal and kidney absorption of tryptophan (Hartnup disease)
  - Carcinoid syndrome (↑conversion of tryptophan to serotonin)

Early Symptoms

- Loss of appetite
- Generalized weakness
- Irritability
- Abdominal pain
- Vomiting

Other Features

- Bright red glossitis
- Characteristic skin rash that is **pigmented** and **scaling**, particularly in skin areas exposed to sunlight.
- This rash is known as **Casal's necklace** because it forms a ring around the neck.
- Vaginitis
- Esophagitis
- Diarrhea (due to **proctitis** and **malabsorption**)
- Depression
- Seizures
- Dementia
- Pellagra syndrome—the **four Ds: dermatitis, diarrhea** and **dementia** leading to **death**.

Note:

- Several **therapeutic drugs** can provoke pellagra.
- These include the antibiotics **isoniazid** and **chloramphenicol**, the anti-cancer agent **fluorouracil**, and the immunosuppressant **mercaptopurine.**

SURGERY

1. Trendelenburg's procedure in treatment of varicose veins is:

A. Ligation of short saphenous vein
B. Stripping of superficial varicose veins
C. Sapheno-femoral ligation
D. Ligation of perforators

Ans: C. Sapheno-femoral ligation

Ref: *Bailey & Love's Short Practice of Surgery, 25th Edition, pg. 929-932 and Sabiston Textbook of Surgery,19th Edition pg. 1805-11*

Explanation:

Indications for Intervention in Varicose Veins

- Cosmesis
- Symptoms refractory to conservative therapy
- Bleeding from a varix
- Superficial thrombophlebitis
- Lipodermatosclerosis
- Venous stasis ulcer

The Principles are to:

- Ligate the point of communication, the sapheno-femoral and/or saphenopopliteal junctions.
- Remove the major part of the incompetent trunk to prevent connections to the tributaries.
- Individually remove tributaries by making minor cut-downs and teasing them out from under the skin (avulsions).

Management of Great Saphenous Varicosity

Surgery

- Saphenofemoral junction ligation and greater saphenous stripping

Non Operative Methods

- Ultrasound Guided Foam Sclerotherapy
- Radiofrequency ablation
- Endovenous laser ablation

Management of Short Saphenous Vein Varicosity

- Saphenopopliteal junction ligation and lesser saphenous stripping

Management of Minor Varicosities

- Injection sclerotherapy using sodium tetradecyl sulphate

Management of Perforator Incompetence

- Subfascial endoscopic perforator surgery

Also Know

CEAP Classification

C	Clinical signs (Grade 0-6), supplemented by "A" for asymptomatic and "S" for symptomatic presentation
E	Classification by cause (Etiology)—congenital, primary, secondary
A	Anatomic distribution—superficial, deep, or perforator, alone or in combination
P	Pathophysiologic dysfunction—reflux or obstruction, alone or in combination
CLASS	**FEATURES**
0	No visible or palpable signs of venous disease
1	Telangiectasia, reticular veins, malleolar flare
2	Varicose veins
3	Edema without skin changes
4	Skin changes ascribed to venous disease (e.g., pigmentation, venous eczema, lipodermatosclerosis)
5	Skin changes as defined above with healed ulceration
6	Skin changes as defined above with active ulceration

2. In an intussusception, the term intussuscipiens refers to:

A. The inner tube
B. The middle tube
C. The outer tube
D. The entire complex of intussusception

Ans: C. The outer tube

Ref: *Bailey & Love's Short Practice of Surgery, 25th Edition pg. 1191*

Explanation:

- **Intussuscipiens** refers to the sheath or outer tube of **intussusception**

Intussusception

- Portion of the gut becomes invaginated within an immediately adjacent segment.
- Usually the proximal segment gets invaginated into the distal.
- Most commonly in children.
- Peak incidence - 5 to 10 months of age.

Aetiology and Risk Factors

- 90% of cases are idiopathic.
- Upper respiratory tract infection or gastroenteritis may precede the condition.
- Hyperplasia of peyer's patches in the terminal ileum may be the initiating event.

Risk Factors in Infants

- Weaning
- Loss of passively acquire maternal immunity
- Common viral pathogens

Risk Factors in Older Children

- Pathological lead points are common in children more than 2 years of age.
- After the age of 2 years, a pathological lead point is found in at least one-third of affected children.
- Meckel's diverticulum
- Polyp
- Duplication
- Henoch-Schönlein purpura
- Appendix

Risk Factors in Adults

- Invariably associated with a lead point
- Polyp (e.g. Peutz-Jeghers syndrome)
- Submucosal lipoma
- Other tumours

Pathology

An intussusception is composed of three parts:

- The entering or inner tube
- The returning or middle tube
- The sheath or outer tube (intussuscipiens).

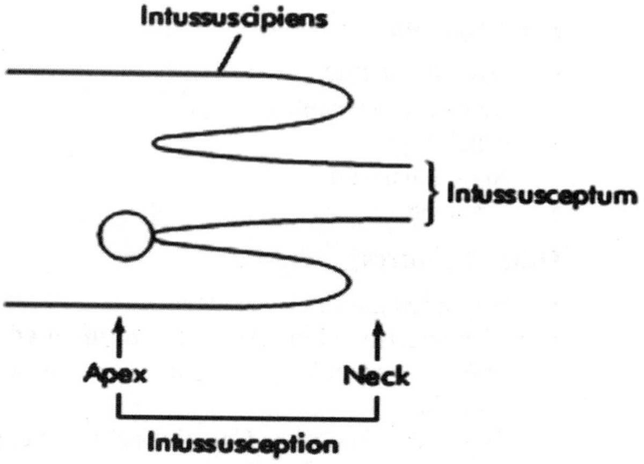

- The part that advances is the apex, the mass is the intussusceptions and the neck is the junction of the entering layer with the mass.
- An **intussusception** is a strangulating obstruction as the blood supply of the inner layer is usually impaired.
- The degree of ischaemia is dependent on the tightness of the invagination, which is usually greatest as it passes through the ileocaecal valve.
- **Most common** intussusception in **children** is **ileocolic.**
- **Most common** intussusception in **adults** is **colocolic.**

Clinical Features

- The classical presentation is with episodes of screaming and drawing up of the legs in a previously well male infant.
- The attacks last for a few minutes and recur repeatedly.
- During attacks the child appears pale, whereas between episodes he may be listless.
- Initially vomiting may or may not occur but becomes conspicuous and bile-stained with time.
- In early stage the passage of stool may be normal, later, blood and mucus are evacuated – the **'red currant jelly'** stool.

Physical Examination

- Child should be examined between episodes of colic.
- Classically, the abdomen is *not* initially distended.
- Lump that hardens on palpation is present in **60%** of cases.
- Emptiness in the right iliac fossa– **the sign of Dance.**
- Rectal examination– blood stained mucus may be found on the finger.
- Occasionally, in extensive intussusception, the apex may be palpable or even protrude from the anus.
- Progressive dehydration and abdominal distension from small bowel obstruction ensues without treatment, followed by peritonitis secondary to gangrene.
- Rarely, natural cure may occur as a result of sloughing of the intussusceptions.

Imaging

Plain Abdominal X-ray

- Evidence of small or large bowel obstruction with an absent caecal gas shadow in ileocolic cases.
- A soft tissue opacity is often present.

Barium Enema

- **Claw sign** in ileocolic intussusception.
- Does not demonstrate small bowel intussusception.

Ultrasound

- **Doughnut appearance** of concentric rings in transverse section.

Computerised Tomography (CT)

- Used in equivocal cases.

Treatment

In infants with ileocolic intussusception non-operative reduction is tried first. More than 70% of intussusceptions can be reduced non-operatively.

- Resuscitation with intravenous fluids
- Broad-spectrum antibiotics
- Naso-gastric drainage

Non-Operative Reduction

- Non-operative reduction is attempted using an air or barium enema.
- Successful reduction can only be accepted if there is free reflux of air or barium into the small bowel, together with resolution of symptoms and signs.

Contraindications for Non-Operative Reduction

- Signs of peritonitis or perforation
- Known pathological lead point
- Shock.

Problems with Non-Operative Reduction:

- Strangulated bowel and pathological lead points are unlikely to reduce.
- Perforation of the colon - rare.
- Recurrent intussusception occurs in upto 10%.

Surgical Management

- Indicated when radiological reduction has failed or is contraindicated.

3. **True statement regarding Follicular carcinoma of thyroid is:**

A. Spreads hematogenously
B. Multifocal
C. FNAC is diagnostic
D. Frequent bony metastasis

Ans: A. Spreads hematogenously **& D.** Frequent bony metastasis

Ref: *Sabiston Textbook of Surgery, 19th Edition, Pg. 890*

Explanation:

- **Multifocal lesions** are seen in **papillary thyroid carcinoma.**
- **Follicular cancer** can be diagnosed **ONLY** by **histopathological examination.**
- **FNAC cannot differentiate** between **follicular adenoma and carcinoma.**

Follicular Cancer

- Second most common thyroid malignancy (Most common Papillary)

Clinical Features

- 40-60 years
- Female: Male =3:1
- Most commonly presents as **asymptomatic thyroid nodule**
- Can be associated with **Multinodular Goitre in 10%**
  - Hoarseness and firm fixation of the mass on clinical evaluation suggest advanced disease and a poor prognosis, these circumstances are again found in a minority of cases.
  - **Associated with iodine deficiency**
  - **Not** strongly associated with radiation exposure.
- A subtype of follicular cancer, known as ***Hürthle cell carcinoma***, consists of ***oxyphilic cells*** and tends to occur in ***older patients***, usually ***60 to 75*** years of age.

Pathology

- Histologic diagnosis of follicular cancer depends on the demonstration of follicular cells occupying abnormal positions, including **capsular, lymphatic and vascular invasion**.
- If these findings are absent, the diagnosis is benign follicular adenoma.
- Using these criteria, two types of follicular carcinoma are usually described, minimally invasive and widely invasive.
- **Lymph node involvement** is **unusual**, occurs in < **10%** of cases.
- Typically spreads via **hematogenous routes**, which occurs in **10% to 15%** of cases.
- The most common sites for **metastatic deposits** are **lytic bone lesions** and **lung**.

Prognostic Factors

- Prognosis is **less favorable** for **follicular** than for **papillary** cancer.
- Best prognosis in **young patients** with **limited capsular or vascular invasion**.
- Age is the most important predictor of survival, with a 95% 10-year survival in those younger than 40 years and an 80% 10-year survival between 40 and 60 years.
- Follicular cancers in **older patients** also are less likely to respond to radioiodine therapy.
- **Size of the primary tumor** is also an important prognostic factor.

Diagnosis

- **Only on Histopathological examination**
- The distinction between a follicular carcinoma and an adenoma can only be made by histological examination
  - **Invasion of the capsule** or of **pericapsular blood vessels** is necessary to diagnose carcinoma which can be demonstrated only by histopathology.
  - Intraoperative frozen section is not useful

Management

Based on size of the lesion

If Size <2cm – **Hemithyroidectomy** followed by **Histopathological examination.**

If HPE Shows:

- **Adenoma** – No further treatment
- **Carcinoma** – Proceed with total thyroidectomy
- **Size >2 cm**–Total thyroidectomy

Adjuvant Therapy

- Radioiodine ablation with iodine 131
- Long-term monitoring of thyroglobulin.

4. All the following are true about branchial cyst *except:*

A. It occurs at lower 2/3rd of sternocleidomastoid
B. It is lined by squamous epithelium
C. It develops from remnants of 2nd branchial cyst
D. Usually presents in early or middle adulthood

Ans: A. It occurs at lower 2/3rd of sternocleidomastoid

Ref: *Bailey & Love's Short Practice of Surgery, 25th Edition, pg. 728*

Explanation:

Branchial cyst is located at the junction of the upper third and middle third of the sternomastoid muscle at its anterior border.

BRANCHIAL CYST

Aetiopathology

- Develops from the vestigial remnants of the second branchial cleft
- Lined by squamous epithelium.
- Contents - thick, turbid fluid full of cholesterol crystals.

Clinical Features

- Presents in the upper neck in early or middle adulthood.
- At the junction of the **upper third and middle third of the sternomastoid muscle** at its **anterior border**.

- **Soft**, **fluctuant** swelling
- **Transillumination** may be present
- May be difficult to palpate in early stages because of soft consistency.

Complications

- May get infected–becomes erythematous and tender may be difficult to differentiate from a tuberculous abscess.

Investigations

- Ultrasound neck
- Fine-needle aspiration

Treatment

- Complete surgical excision.
- Surgery is best done when the lesion is quiescent.

Technical Details

- Anterior aspect of the cyst is easy to dissect.
- Passes backwards and upwards through the bifurcation of the common carotid artery as far as the pharyngeal constrictors.
- It passes superficial to the hypoglossal and glossopharyngeal nerves, but deep to the posterior belly of the digastric.
- These structures and the spinal accessory nerve are at risk of injury during surgery.

5. **Commonly done surgery in sarcoma is:**

A. Wide excision
B. Compartmental excision / exentration
C. Excision
D. Enucleation

Ans: A. Wide excision

Ref: *Devita Cancer: Principles & Practice of Oncology, 7th edn.*

Explanation:

- **Wide *en bloc* resection** is used most often.
- Historical attempts to resect all muscle bundles from origin to insertion have now been supplanted by an encompassing resection, aiming to obtain a 2-cm margin of uninvolved tissue in all directions.
- The limiting factor is usually neurovascular or, occasionally, bony juxtaposition.
- Because most soft tissue **sarcomas** tend not to invade **bone directly**, only rarely does bone need to be resected.
- Soft tissue sarcomas **uncommonly** involve the **skin, so major skin resection** should be limited.
- In situations of primary or recurrent tumors in which skin is involved, or in which the tumor is so extensive that skin is involved, and then consideration of free flap or rotational flap closure becomes important.
- Extent of surgical resection
- The most extensive resection is clearly **amputation**. This should be only rarely indicated in soft tissue sarcoma because **limb-sparing operations** are possible in at least **90%** of patients.
- Amputation should be reserved for tumors not able to be resected by any other means, without evidence of metastatic disease and the potential for good long-term functional rehabilitation.

6. **Management of cystosarcoma phylloides in a young female:**

A. Wide excision with a margin
B. Wide excision and chemotherapy
C. Wide excision and radiotherapy
D. Modified mastectomy

Ans: A. Wide excision with a margin

Ref: *Robbins Pathologic Basis of Disease, 8th edition & Bailey and Love's Short Practice of Surgery 25th Edition*

Explanation:

PHYLLODES TUMOR

- They are a **fibroepithelial** tumor composed of an **epithelial** and a **cellular stromal** component.
- Phyllodes tumors arise from intralobular stroma
- Most patients present in the sixth decade.
- The majority is detected as palpable masses, but a few are found by mammography.
- Aka **cystosarcoma phyllodes** and **serocystic disease of brodie.**
- However, the term **phyllodes tumor** is preferred, since most are benign and are not cystic.
- Around **70%** are benign.

Morphology

- The tumors vary in size from a few centimeters to massive lesions.
- The larger lesions have bulbous protrusions (phyllodes "leaflike") due to the presence of nodules of proliferating stroma covered by epithelium.
- In some tumors these protrusions extend into a cystic space.
- **Low-grade lesions** resemble **fibroadenomas** but contain more cellular and contain mitotic figures. High-grade lesions have foci of mesenchymal differentiation (DD: soft-tissue sarcomas).

- The frequent chromosomal mutation is **amplification of EGFR**.

Treatment

- **Excision with wide margins** or by **mastectomy** (to **avoid local recurrences**).
- Axillary lymph node dissection is not indicated, because of nodal metastases is rare.
- The majority are low-grade tumors that may recur locally but only rarely metastasize.
- Rare high-grade lesions behave aggressively, with frequent local recurrences and distant hematogenous metastases in about one third of cases.
- **Malignant Phyllodes – Total Mastectomy.**

7. **All are complications of gall stones *except:* (Repeat)**

A. Hepatocellular Ca
B. Acute cholangitis
C. Mucocele
D. Empyema of gallbladder

Ans: A. Hepatocellular Ca

Ref: *Bailey and Love's Short Practice of Surgery 25th Edition & Schwartz's Principles of Surgery, 9th Edition*

Explanation:

Complications of Gall Stones

- Acute and chronic cholecystitis
- Jaundice
- Mucocele of GB
- Empyema of GB
- Gangrene of GB
- Sepsis
- Ca gallbladder
- Cholangitis
- Pancreatitis
- **Mirrizi syndrome**: Biliary duct obstruction secondary to stone impaction in hartman's pouch of GB
- Gallstone ileus

8. **True statement about pseudocyst of pancreas is:**

A. Contains a wall of fibrous connective tissue
B. Develops immediately after acute pancreatitis
C. Requires laparotomy
D. Preceded by trauma in 90% cases

Ans: A. Contains a wall of fibrous connective tissue

Ref: *Sabiston Textbook of Surgery, 19th Edition, pg. 1524-25*

Explanation:

Pancreatic Pseudocysts

- Pancreatic pseudocysts occur **in 5% to 15%** of patients who have peripancreatic fluid collections after **acute pancreatitis**.
- By definition, the **capsule** of a pseudocyst is composed of **collagen** and **granulation tissue** and it is **not lined by epithelium**.
- The fibrotic reaction typically **requires at least 4 to 8 weeks** to develop.

Clinical Features

- Upto 50% develop symptoms
- Abdominal pain
- Early satiety
- Nausea
- Weight loss

Diagnosis

- Elevated pancreatic enzyme levels in plasma is suggestive
- CT or MRI can confirm the diagnosis
- EUS with FNA is indicated for patients in whom the diagnosis is not clear
- Cyst fluid analysis
- **High amylase**
- **Absence of mucin**
- Low carcinoembryonic antigen (CEA) levels

Management

Asympomatic Patients

- Only **observation** is indicated because spontaneous regression has been documented in upto 70% of asymptomatic patients.
- Factors favoring spontaneous regression
  - Pseudocysts smaller than 4 cm in diameter
  - Located in the tail
  - No evidence of pancreatic duct obstruction or communication with the main pancreatic duct.

Symptomatic Patients

- Management options are

Endoscopic Management

- **Transgastric/transduodenal endoscopic drainage** – for pseudocysts in close contact (defined **as <1 cm)** with the stomach and duodenum.
- **Transpapillary drainage** can be attempted in pancreatic pseudocysts communicating with the main pancreatic duct.
- For pancreatic duct stricture is associated with a pancreatic pseudocyst, endoscopic dilation and stent placement are indicated.

Surgery

- Indicated for patients with pancreatic pseudocysts that cannot be treated with endoscopic techniques and patients who fail endoscopic treatment.
- Depends on the location of the cyst.
- Pancreatic pseudocysts closely attached to the stomach should be treated with a cyst-gastrostomy.
- Pancreatic pseudocysts located in the head of the pancreas that are in close contact with the duodenum are treated with a cystoduodenostomy.
- For pseudocysts are not in contact with the stomach or duodenum the surgical treatment is a roux-en-y cystojejunostomy.

Percutaneous Drainage

- Percutaneous drainage is only indicated for septic patients secondary to pseudocyst infection
- High incidence of external fistula

Complications of Pseudocyst

- Bleeding
- Pancreaticopleural fistula
- Bile duct obstruction
- Duodenal obstruction
- Rupture into the abdominal cavity
- Infection

9. Tissue reaction is minimal with:

A. Dexon **B.** Catgut
C. Silk **D.** Chromic catgut

Ans: A. Dexon

Ref: *Bailey & Love's Short Practice of Surgery, 25th Edition, pg. 237-8*

Explanation:

Sutures with Maximal Tissue Reaction

- Plain catgut
- Silk

Sutures with Moderate Tissue Reaction

- Linen
- Chromic catgut

Sutures with Mild Tissue Reaction

- Nylon
- Surgical steel
- Polyester
- Polybutester
- Polypropelene
- Polyglactin
- Polyglyconate
- Polyglycolic acid
- Polyglycaprone
- Polydioxanone (PDS)

10. All the following form the boundaries of Calot's triangle during cholecystectomy *except:*

A. Inferior surface of liver
B. Cystic duct
C. Lateral border of rectus sheath
D. Common hepatic duct

Ans: C. Lateral border of rectus sheath

Ref: *Shackelford's Surgery* of the *Alimentary Tract, 7th edition, pg. 1289; Blumgart's Surgery* of the *Liver, Biliary Tract,* and *Pancreas 5th edition, pg. 513. Sabiston Textbook of Surgery, 19th Edition, pg. 1477*

Explanation:

Boundaries of Calot's Triangle

- **Superiorly** - Inferior border of liver
- **Medially** - Common hepatic duct
- **Laterally** - Cystic duct

Contents

- Cystic artery
- Cystic lymph node

Indications for Laparoscopic Cholecystectomy

- Symptomatic cholelithiasis
- Biliary colic
- Acute cholecystitis
- Asymptomatic cholelithiasis
- Sickle cell disease
- Total parenteral nutrition
- Chronic immunosuppression
- No immediate access to health care facilities
- Incidental cholecystectomy for patients undergoing laparoscopic procedure for other indications

Others

- Acalculous cholecystitis (biliary dyskinesia).
- Gallstone pancreatitis
- Gallbladder polyps greater than 1 cm in diameter
- Porcelain gallbladder

Contraindications to Laparoscopic Cholecystectomy

- Absolute
- Unable to tolerate general anesthesia
- Refractory coagulopathy
- Suspicion of carcinoma
- Relative

- Previous upper abdominal surgery
- Cholangitis
- Diffuse peritonitis
- Cirrhosis or portal hypertension
- Chronic obstructive pulmonary disease
- Cholecystenteric fistula
- Pregnancy

11. The triad of diverticulosis, gall stones and hiatus hernia is termed as:

A. Saint's triad **B.** Beck's triad
C. Whipple's triad **D.** Murphy's triad

Ans: A. Saint's triad

Ref: *Sabiston Textbook of Surgery, 19th Edition, pg. 951*

Explanation:

Saint's Triad

- Diverticulosis
- Gall stones
- Hiatus hernia

Whipple's Triad

- Seen in insulinoma (most common functioning tumor of the endocrine pancreas).
- Fasting-induced neuroglyopenic symptoms of hypoglycemia (diaphoresis, shaking, mental confusion, obtundation and seizures).
- Low blood glucose levels (40 to 50 mg/dl).
- Relief of symptoms after the administration of glucose.

Beck's Triad

- Seen in cardiac tamponade
- Hypotension
- Soft or absent heart sounds
- Jugular venous distention (increased JVP)

Murphy's Triad

- Seen in acute appendicitis
- Pain
- Fever
- Vomiting

Murphy's Sign

- Right upper quadrant tenderness exacerbated during inspiration

Charcot' Triad

- Seen in cholangitis
- Pain
- Jaundice
- Fever

Reynold's Pentad

- Seen in severe cholangitis. Charcot's triad with
- Shock
- Mental obtundation

12. The most common site for ectopic testis is:

A. Above superficial inguinal ring
B. Perineum
C. Root of penis
D. Femoral triangle

Ans: A. Above superficial inguinal ring

Ref: *A Textbook on Surgical Short Cases-S Das. 2nd edition 303, Sabiston Textbook of Surgery, 19th Edition, pg. 1857*

Explanation:

- An ectopic testis is one in which the testis fails to descend into the scrotum and is deviated from its normal path of descent.
- The Gubernaculum testis is essential for the descent of testis. The Gubernaculum testis has five tails:
  - The Scrotal tail - the main one
  - The Pubic tail - attached to pubic tubercle
  - Perineal tail – attached to perineum
  - Inguinal tail- attached to front of inguinal canal
  - Femoral tail – attached to saphenous opening
- The scrotal tail is the strongest and the other tails disappear. So, normally testis descends into scrotum.
- In case one of the accessory tail becomes stronger, the testis reaches an ectopic position.

Sites of Ectopic Testis

- Superficial Inguinal Pouch- **most common**
- Perineal
- Pubupenile
- Crural or Femoral

Characteristics of Ectopic Testis

- Testis is normally developed
- Scrotum is usually fully developed
- Spermatogenesis is normal
- Not associated with indirect inguinal hernia
- Treatment is surgery
- Main complication is risk of trauma.

Undescended Testis

Cryptorchidism (undescened testis) is a condition in which one or both testes fail to descend into the scrotum before birth.

- Occurs in upto 30% of preterm infants.
- 3% of full-term infants.
- Some undescended testes eventually descend by

1 year of age, but are unlikely to descend after this time.

- The undescended testis is associated with histologic and morphologic changes as early as 6 months of age.
- Atrophy of Leydig cells, decrease in tubular diameter, and spermatogenesis can also occur by 2 years of age.
- A true undescended testis has had its descent halted somewhere along the path of normal descent and can be found in the inguinal canal at exploration.

Diagnoses and Management

- Ultrasound is used evaluate for undescended testis, however an examination by an experienced surgeon has a higher sensitivity for locating an undescended testis.
- For unilateral palpable testis in the inguinal canal, standard dartos pouch orchidopexy is performed.
- The recommended timing for this procedure is at or **near 1 year of age.**
- Nonpalpable unilateral testis, diagnostic laparoscopy is useful.
- If the testicular vessels are seen exiting the internal ring, an open inguinal orchidopexy is performed.
- For an intra-abdominal testis, two-stage **Fowler-Stephen orchidopexy** can be considered, in which testicular vessels are ligated as a first stage to allow collateral circulation to develop for 6 months before performing orchidopexy as a second stage of the procedure.
- If both testes are nonpalpable, a **human chorionic gonadotropin (hCG) stimulation test** is carried out to confirm the presence of functioning testicular tissues. If present, diagnostic laparoscopy is performed to determine surgical therapy.

Retractile Testis

- A retractile testis is a **normally descended testis** that **retracts into the inguinal canal**, but can be brought down into the scrotal sac during the **examination**.
- Does not require any management except for reassurance.

(See the following figure)

13. **One of the following is termed as Troissier's sign:**
    A. Migratory superficial thrombophlebitis seen in pancreatic Ca
    B. Carpopedal spasm seen in hypoparathyroidism
    C. Mediastinal crunch seen in esophageal rupture
    D. Enlargement of left supraclavicular node in occult gastric Ca

Ans: D. Enlargement of left supraclavicular node in occult gastric Ca

Ref: *Sabiston Textbook of Surgery, 19th Edition, pg. 1147 Bailey and Love's Short Practice of Surgery, 25th Edition, pg. 806, 1067*

Explanation:

Troissier's sign

Enlargement of left supraclavicular node (Virchow's node) in occult gastric Ca.

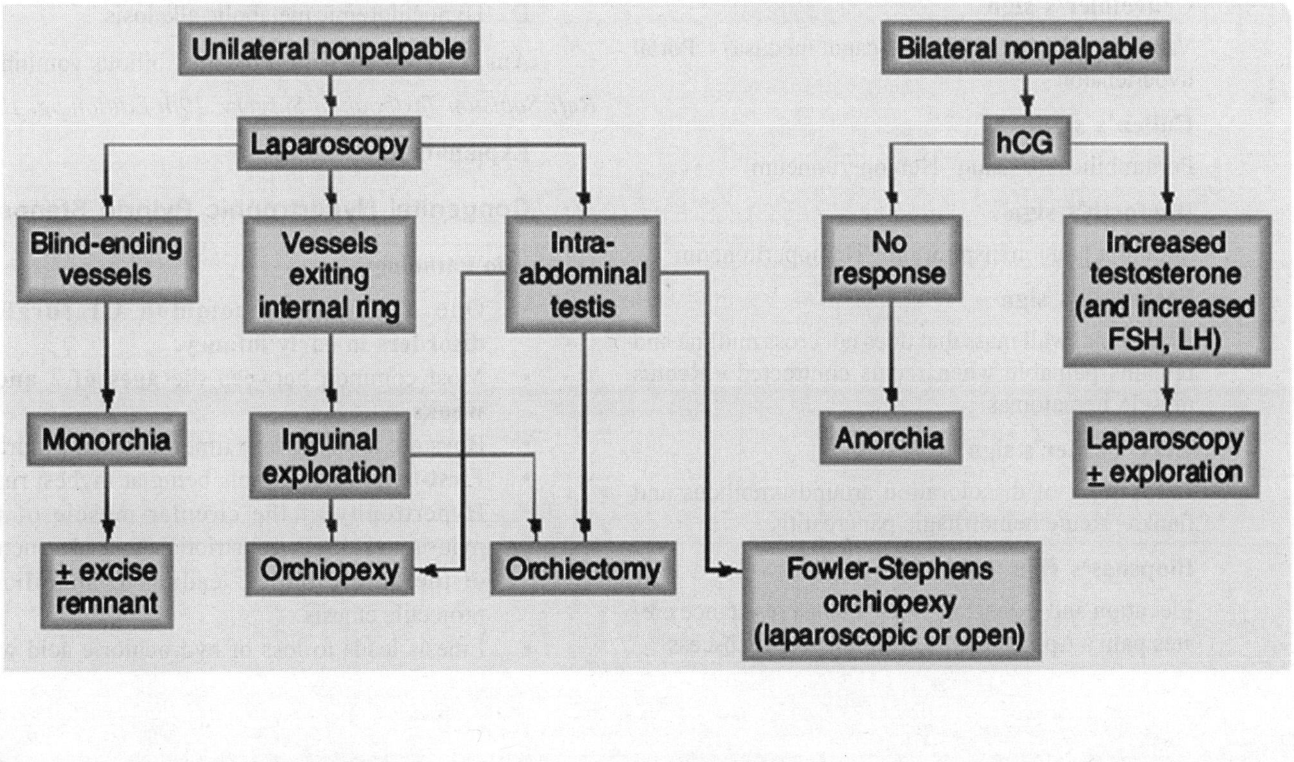

Trousseau's sign

Carpopedal spasm seen in hypoparathyroidism

Aaron's sign

Pain or pressure in epigastrium or anterior chest with persistent firm pressure applied to McBurney's point –Acute appendicitis

Bassler's sign

Sharp pain created by compressing appendix between abdominal wall and Iliacus-Chronic appendicitis

Blumberg's sign

Transient abdominal wall rebound tenderness-Peritoneal inflammation

Carnett's sign

Loss of abdominal tenderness when abdominal wall muscles are contracted– Intra-abdominal source of abdominal pain

Chandelier's sign

Extreme lower abdominal and pelvic pain with movement of cervix - Pelvic inflammatory disease

Charcot's sign

Intermittent right upper abdominal pain, jaundice and fever – Choledocholithiasis

Claybrook's sign

Accentuation of breath and cardiac sounds through abdominal wall - Ruptured abdominal viscus

Courvoisier's sign

Palpable gallbladder in presence of jaundice - Periampullary tumor

Cruveihier's sign

Varicose veins at umbilicus (caput medusa) - Portal hypertension

Cullen's sign

Periumbilical bruising –Hemoperitoneum

Danforth's sign

Shoulder pain on inspiration – Hemoperitoneum

Fothergill's sign

Abdominal wall mass that does not cross midline and remains palpable when rectus contracted - Rectus muscle hematomas

Grey Turner's sign

Local areas of discoloration around umbilicus and flanks– Acute hemorrhagic pancreatitis

Iliopsoas's sign

Elevation and extension of leg against resistance creates pain - Apppendicitis with retrocecal abscess

Kehr's sign

Left shoulder pain when supine and pressure placed on left upper Abdomen - Hemoperitoneum (especially from splenic origin)

Mannkopf's sign

Increased pulse when painful abdomen palpated - Absent if malingering

Murphy's sign

Pain caused by inspiration while applying pressure to right upper abdomen - Acute cholecystitis

Obturator's sign

Flexion and external rotation of right thigh while supine creates hypogastric
Pain - Pelvic abscess or inflammatory mass in pelvis

Ransohoff's sign

Yellow discoloration of umbilical region - Ruptured common bile duct

Rovsing's sign

Pain at McBurney's point when compressing the left lower abdomen- Acute appendicitis

Ten Horn's sign

Pain caused by gentle traction of right testicle- Acute appendicitis

14. One of the following is not true about congenital hypertrophic pyloric stenosis:

A. Common in first born males
B. Manifests between 3-6 weeks of life
C. Presents with projectile, bilious vomiting
D. Hypochloremic metabolic alkalosis

Ans: C. Presents with projectile, bilious vomiting

Ref: *Sabiston Textbook of Surgery, 19th Edition,pg. 1841*

Explanation:

Congenital Hypertrophic Pyloric Stenosis

Etio Pathology

- One of the **most common GI surgical disorders in early infancy.**
- Most common between the **ages of 2 and 8 weeks.**
- Boys are affected four times as often as girls.
- **First-born male** infants being at highest risk.
- Hypertrophy of the circular muscle of the pylorus results in constriction and obstruction of the gastric outlet, leading to nonbilious, projectile emesis.
- Emesis leads to loss of hydrochloric acid with

the onset of **hypokalemic hypochloremic metabolic alkalosis and dehydration**.

- Exact cause for HPS remains unknown; a **lack of nitric oxide synthase** in pyloric tissue has been implicated.

Clinical Presentation

- Progressively worsening nonbilious emesis.
- With time, the emesis becomes more frequent, forceful, and projectile in nature.
- Occasionally, visible gastric peristalsis may be observed as a wave of contractions from the left upper quadrant to the epigastrium.
- Shortly after emesis, infants usually crave additional feedings.
- Palpation of the pyloric tumor (**olive-shaped**) in the epigastrium or right upper quadrant by an experienced examiner is pathognomonic for the diagnosis. If the olive is palpated, no additional diagnostic testing is necessary.

Investigations

Abdominal Radiograph

- Upper abdominal gas bubble in the stomach.

Ultrasound

- A persistent pyloric muscle thickness more than 3 to 4 mm or a pyloric length more than 15 to 18 mm in the presence of functional gastric outlet obstruction is diagnostic. When the olive is non-palpable, the diagnosis of HPS can be made by ultrasound.

Upper GI Contrast

- With equivocal clinical history, an upper GI contrast study is useful to evaluate for other causes of vomiting.

Treatment

Surgical Management

- The treatment of HPS is pyloromyotomy.
- Incising through thickened pyloric musculature while preserving the underlying mucosa.
- Right upper quadrant or periumbilical incision is used.
- Laparoscopic pyloromyotomy has better cosmesis, with similar outcomes to those of the open technique.

Perioperative Management

- Before surgery, it is important that the infant be fully rehydrated with IV fluids to establish an adequate urine output and correct electrolyte disturbances such as metabolic alkalosis.
- Because the infant with underlying metabolic alkalosis will compensate with respiratory acidosis, postoperative apnea may occur. Thus, the serum HCO_3 level needs to be normalized before surgery.
- Postoperatively, infants are usually allowed to resume enteral feedings.
- Complications include incomplete myotomy, mucosal perforation and wound infection.

15. What type of metabolic change is seen in a burns patient?

A. Hyperkalemic metabolic acidosis
B. Hyperkalemic metabolic alkalosis
C. Hypokalemic metabolic acidosis
D. Hypokalemic metabolic alkalosis

Ans: A. Hyperkalemic metabolic acidosis

Ref: *Sabiston Textbook of Surgery, 19th Edition, pg 536, 522 & Bailey & Love's Short Practice of Surgery, 25th Edition, pg 381-384*

Explanation:

- Renal failure is a common complication in burns patients; it leads to hyperkalemic metabolic acidosis.

Also Know:

Depths of Burn Injury

- **First degree**—injury localized to the epidermis
- **Superficial second degree**—injury to the epidermis and superficial dermis
- **Deep second degree**—injury through the epidermis and deep into the dermis
- **Third degree**—full-thickness injury through the epidermis and dermis into subcutaneous fat
- **Fourth degree**—injury through the skin and subcutaneous fat into underlying muscle or bone

Rule of Nines

- Each upper limb 9% TBSA
- Each lower limb 18%
- The torso 18% each side (anterior and posterior)
- The head and neck 9%
- Genitalia 1%

Parkland's Formula

- **Total percentage body surface area × weight (kg) × 4 = volume (ml)**
- Half this volume is given in the first 8 hours, and the second half is given in the next 16 hours.

16. Trendlenburg's test done for varicose veins is for detection of:

A. Perforator incompetency
B. Deep veins patency
C. Saphenofemoral incompetency
D. Site of perforators

Ans: C. Saphenofemoral incompetency

Ref: *74 A Manual on Clinical Surgery S. Das*

Explanation:

Clinical Examination of Varicose Veins

Brodie–Trendelenberg Test

- Done to determine the incompetency of Saphenofemoral valve.
- Patient is placed in recumbent position.
- Limbs are raised to empty the veins. Veins are milked proximally for further emptying.
- Saphenofemoral junction is compressed either with the thumb of the examiner/tourniquet and the patient is asked to stand up quickly.
- There are two variants of this test.
- The first method is to assess saphenofemoral incompetency. The pressure is released and if the column of blood fills up quickly from above downwards it indicates saphenofemoral incompetency.
- The second method is to assess the perforators. Here, the pressure is maintained for one minute. Gradual filling of the veins during this period indicates incompetent perforators allowing reflux of blood from deep veins to superficial veins.
- *Positive Brodie–Trendelenberg test is an indication for surgery.*

1. **Tests to Assess Saphenofemoral Incompetency**
   - Brodie –Trendelenberg test
   - Morrisey's cough impulse test
2. **Tests to Assess Deep Veins**
   - Perthe's test
   - Modified Perthe's test
3. **Tests to Assess Perforators**
   - Multiple tourniquet test
   - Pratt's test
   - Fegan's test
   - Brodie –Trendelenberg test
4. **Test to Assess Valves in Superficial Vein**
   - Schwartz test

Note:

- Even though Brodie–Trendelenberg test is used to assess both saphenofemoral incompetency and incompetent perforators its primary purpose is to assess saphenofemoral incompetency.

ORTHOPAEDICS

1. **In supra condylar fracture, after a close reduction and plaster application, assessment of which parameter helps to evaluate the reduction and decide the next line of management?**

A. Q - angle
B. Cobb's angle
C. Bohler's angle
D. Baumann's angle

Ans: D. Baumann's angle

Ref: *Watson-Jones Fractures and Joint Injuries, 7th edition, pg 526-527*
http://www.wheelessonline.com/ortho/bohlers_angle
http://www.wheelessonline.com/ortho/9738
Apley's System of Orthopaedics and Fractures, 9th edition, pg 460

Explanation:

Baumann's Angle

- After closed reduction of a supracondylar fracture of the humerus, the **elbow is kept flexed** to stabilise the reduction.
- So an AP view is not possible and one has to take a **shoot through view**, which superimposes the radius and ulna over the humerus.
- The lower end of humerus is seen in sharp focus as it is near the X-ray plate.
- Provided rotation is not present as shown on a lateral view residual mediolateral displacements correct by moulding.
- Tilt of the distal fragment will not correct by moulding.
- To assess this one uses the **Baumann's Angle** which is the angle **subtended between a transverse line drawn along the lower border of the lateral humeral metaphysis and a line drawn at right angles to long axis of humerus.**
- It is also called **humero-capitellar angle**.
- A deviation of **more than 5 degrees** compared to the opposite side is considered **unacceptable**.

The Cobb's Angle

- It was originally used to **measure coronal plane deformity on antero-posterior plane radiographs** in the classification of **scoliosis**.
- It has subsequently been adapted to **classify sagittal plane deformity**, especially in the setting of **traumatic thoracolumbar spine fractures**.

- In the **assessment of scoliosis** in the AP X-rays a line is drawn along the superior end plate of the superior end vertebra and a second line drawn along the inferior end plate of the inferior end vertebra of a scoliosis curve.
- If the end plates are indistinct the line may be drawn through the pedicles.
- The angle between these two lines (or lines drawn perpendicular to them) is measured as the **Cobb angle**.
- In the setting of spine trauma and assessing sagittal plane deformity, the **Cobb angle** is defined as the angle formed between a line drawn parallel to the superior endplate of one vertebra above the fracture and a line drawn parallel to the inferior endplate of the vertebra one level below the fracture.

Q Angle

- It is the **angle formed by a line drawn from the ASIS to central patella and a second line drawn from central patella to tibial tubercle**; an increased Q angle is a risk **factor for patellar subluxation** – used in assessing **recurrent patellar subluxations or dislocations.**

Bohler's Angle or "Tuber Angle"

- It is a normal anatomic landmark seen in **lateral radiographs of the ankle**. It is formed by the intersection of:
  - **a.** A line from the highest point of the **posterior calcaneal articular facet** to the highest point of the **posterior tuberosity** of the calcaneum, and
  - **b.** A line from the highest point of the **posterior calcaneal articular facet** to the highest point on the **anterior articular facet. An angle < 20° suggests a depression of posterior facet and possible calcaneal fracture.**

2. A young woman, 30 years old complains of pain in the left knee joint which increases after exercise since 4 months. An X-ray shows eccentric bone cyst. The likely diagnosis is:

A. Aneurysmal bone cyst
B. Unicameral bone cyst
C. Hydatid cyst
D. Fibrous dysplasia.

Ans: A. Aneurysmal bone cyst

Ref: *Apley's System of Orthopaedics and Fractures, 9th edition - Tumours*

Explanation:

Aneurysmal Bone Cyst

- It may be encountered at **any age** and in almost **any bone**, though more often in **young adults** and in the **long-bone metaphyses.**
- Usually it arises spontaneously but it may appear after degeneration or haemorrhage in some other lesion.
- With expanding lesions, patients may complain of **pain.**
- Occasionally, a large cyst may cause a visible or palpable swelling of the bone.
- X-rays show a well-defined **radiolucent cyst,** often **trabeculated** and **eccentrically placed.**
- In a growing tubular bone it is always situated in the **metaphysis** and therefore may resemble a **simple cyst** or one of the other cyst-like lesions.
- Occasional sites include **vertebrae** and the **flat bones.**
- In an **adult** an aneurysmal bone cyst **may be mistaken for a giant-cell tumour.**

Unicameral Bone Cyst

- Also called as **simple bone cyst,** appears during **childhood,** typically in the **metaphysis** of one of the long bones and most commonly in the **proximal humerus or femur.**
- It is **not a tumour,** it tends to **heal spontaneously** and it is **seldom seen in adults.**
- The condition is usually **discovered after a pathological fracture** or as an **incidental finding** on X-ray.
- X-rays show a **well-demarcated radiolucent area in the metaphysis,** often extending up to the physeal plate; the cortex may be thinned and the bone expanded.

Hydatid Cyst

- It is disease, is caused by the **tapeworm Echinococcus.**
- Parasitic infestation is common among **sheep farmers,** but **bone lesions are rare.**
- The bones most commonly affected are the **vertebrae, pelvis, femur, scapula** and **ribs.**
- The patient may complain of **pain and swelling,** or may present for the first time with a **pathological fracture** or **compression of the spinal cord.**
- Infestation sometimes starts in **childhood** but the cysts take so long to enlarge that clinical symptom and signs may not become apparent for many years.

- X-rays show **solitary or multiloculated bone cysts**, but only moderate expansion of the cortices. However, **cortical thinning** may lead to a pathological fracture.
- In the spine, hydatid disease may involve adjacent vertebrae, with large cysts extending into the paravertebral soft tissues.
- These features are best seen on **CT and MRI**, which should always be performed if operative excision of the lesion is contemplated.

Fibrous Dysplasia

- It is developmental disorders in which areas of trabecular bone are replaced by cellular fibrous tissue containing flecks of osteoid and woven bone.
- It may affect one bone (**monostotic**) one limb (**monomelic**) or many bones (**polyostotic**).
- If the lesions are large, the bone is considerably weakened and pathological fractures or progressive deformity may occur.
- The **most common sites of** occurrence are the **proximal femur, tibia, humerus, ribs and craniofacial bones.**
- **Small, single lesions** are **asymptomatic**.
- Large, monostotic lesions may cause pain or may be discovered only when the patient develops a **pathological fracture**.
- Patients with polyostotic disease present in childhood or adolescence with **pain, limp, bony enlargement, deformity or pathological fracture**.
- Untreated, the characteristic **deformities** persist through **adult life**.
- **Occasionally the bone disorder is associated with café-au-lait patches on the skin and (in girls) precocious sexual development (Albright's syndrome).**
- X-rays show **radiolucent 'cystic' areas** in the metaphysis or shaft; because they contain fibrous tissue with diffuse spots of immature bone, the **lucent patches** typically have a **slightly hazy or 'ground-glass' appearance.**
- The weight bearing bones may be bent, and one of the classic features is the '**shepherd's crook**' deformity of the proximal femur.
- **Radioscintigraphy** shows marked activity in the lesion.

3. **In the following conditions, bone mass is reduced *except:* (Repeat)**

A. Osteoporosis
B. Osteomalacia
C. Hyperparathyroidism
D. Osteopetrosis

Ans: D. Osteopetrosis

Ref: *Apley's System of Orthopaedics and Fractures, 9th edition, pg. 131-136, 167*

Explanation:

- Almost half the bone volume is mineral matter – mainly calcium and phosphate in the form of crystalline hydroxyapatite which is laid down in osteoid at the calcification front.
- In mature bone the proportions of calcium and phosphate are constant and the molecule is firmly bound to collagen.
- It is important to appreciate that in life 'demineralization' of bone occurs only by resorption of the entire matrix.

Osteoblasts

- These cells are concerned with **bone formation** and **osteoclast activation.**
- They are derived from mesenchymal precursors in the bone marrow and the deep layer of the periosteum.
- Differentiation is controlled by a number of interacting growth factors, including bone morphogenetic proteins.
- They are responsible for the production of type I collagen as well as the non-collagenous bone proteins and for the mineralization of bone matrix.

Osteoclasts

- These are large multinucleated cells and are the principal mediators of bone resorption.
- They develop from mononuclear precursors in the haemopoietic marrow (the same lineage as macrophages) under the influence of local osteoblastic stromal cells that generate an essential osteoclast differentiating factor – receptor activator of nuclear factor-κβ ligand (**RANKL**) – which binds with a specific receptor site (**RANK**) on the osteoclast precursors.

Osteoporosis

- It is characterized by an **abnormally low bone mass,** normal mineral to matrix ratio and defects in bone structure, a combination which renders the bone unusually fragile and at greater than normal risk of fracture in a person of that age, sex and race.
- In X-rays characteristic signs of osteoporosis are loss of trabecular definition, thinning of the cortices and insufficiency fractures.

- Compression fractures of the vertebral bodies, wedging at multiple levels or biconcave distortion of the vertebral end-plates due to bulging of intact intervertebral discs are typical of severe postmenopausal osteoporosis.

Osteomalacia

- It is a manifestation of **Vitamin D deficiency** in adults.
- There is **inadequate mineralisation of bone**.
- It is characterized by a **decreased ratio of bone mineral to matrix**. Thus there is a decrease in bone mineral mass.

Hyperparathyroidism

- It is characterized by a general loss of bone substance.
- In severe cases, osteoclastic hyperactivity produces subperiosteal erosions, endosteal cavitation and replacement of the marrow spaces by vascular granulations and fibrous tissue (**osteitis fibrosa cystica**).
- Haemorrhage and giant-cell reaction within the fibrous stroma may give rise to brownish, tumour-like masses, whose liquefaction leads to fluid-filled cysts.

Osteopetrosis

- It is characterized by **sclerosis** and **thickening** of the **bones** which appear with **increased radiographic density.**
- This is the result of an **imbalance between bone formation and bone resorption**; in the most common form, osteopetrosis, there is failed bone resorption due to a defect in osteoclast production and/or function.
- As a result of this bone mass is increased in this condition.
- This does not translate into increased strength but causes increased brittleness and susceptibility to pathological fractures.
- This condition is also called **marble bones disease** or **Albers–Schönberg Disease**.

4. **In osteomalacia, all the following seen *except:***
   A. Looser zones
   B. High alkaline phosphate levels
   C. Increased resistance to pathological fractures
   D. Diminished urinary excretion of calcium.

Ans: C. Increased resistance to pathological fractures

***Ref:** Apley's System of Orthopaedics and Fractures, 4th edition, pg. 137-8*

Explanation:

Osteomalacia

- The **classical lesion** is the **Looser zone**, a thin transverse band of rarefaction in an otherwise normal-looking bone.
- These zones, seen especially in the shafts of long bones and the axillary edge of the scapula, are due to incomplete stress fractures which heal with callus lacking in calcium.
- More often, however, there is simply a slow fading of skeletal structure, resulting in biconcave vertebrae (from disc pressure), lateral indentation of the acetabula (**'trefoil' pelvis**) and spontaneous fractures of the ribs, pubic rami, femoral neck or the metaphyses above and below the knee.
- Features of **secondary hyperparathyroidism** characteristically appear in the middle phalanges of the fingers, and in severe cases so-called **'brown tumours'** are seen in the long bones.
- Biochemical changes common to almost all types of **vitamin D related rickets** and **osteomalacia** are **diminished levels of serum calcium and phosphate, increased alkaline phosphatase and diminished urinary excretion of calcium.**
- In vitamin D deficiency 25-OH D levels also are low.
- The **'calcium phosphate product'** (derived by multiplying calcium and phosphorus levels expressed in mmol/L), normally about 3, is diminished in rickets and osteomalacia, and values of less than 2.4 are diagnostic.

6. **Housemaid knee is inflammation of: (Repeat)**
   A. Prepatellar bursa
   B. Suprapatellar bursa
   C. Infrapatellar bursa
   D. Anserine bursa

Ans: A. Prepatellar bursa

***Ref:** Apley's System of Orthopaedics and Fractures, 9th edition, pg. 578-9*
http://en.wikipedia.org/wiki/Knee_bursae

Explanation:

Housemaid's Knee

- This is a friction bursitis of the **pre-patellar bursa.**
- The fluctuant **swelling** is confined to the **front of the patella** and the joint itself is normal.
- This is an **uninfected bursitis** due not to pressure but to constant friction between skin and bone.

- It is seen mainly in **carpet layers, paving workers, floor cleaners and miners** who do not use protective knee pads.
- Treatment consists of firm bandaging, and kneeling is avoided; occasionally aspiration is needed.
- In **chronic** cases the **lump is best excised.**

INFRAPATELLAR BURSITIS ('CLERGYMAN'S KNEE')

- The swelling is **below the patella** and **superficial to the patellar ligament**, being more distally placed than prepatellar bursitis
- Treatment is similar to that for prepatellar bursitis.
- Occasionally the bursa is affected in **gout**.

Other Bursa

- The **anserine bursa** lies between the medial (tibial) collateral ligament and the tendons of the sartorius, gracilis, and semitendinosus (i.e. the pes anserinus).
- Theoretically, bursitis results from stress to this area (e.g. stress may result when an obese individual with anatomic deformity from arthritis ascends or descends stairs).
- An occurrence of **pes anserine bursitis** commonly is characterized by pain, especially when climbing stairs, tenderness, and local swelling.
- The **suprapatellar bursa** or recess between the anterior surface of the lower part of the femur and the deep surface of the quadriceps femoris.
- It allows for movement of the quadriceps tendon over the distal end of the femur.
- The suprapatellar bursa extends superiorly from beneath the patella under the quadriceps femoris muscle and its tendon.
- The bursa is held in place by a small portion of the vastus intermedius muscle called the **articularis genus muscle**.
- The suprapatellar bursa may exist as a single bursal sac or, in some patients, as a multisegmented series of loculated sacs.
- The suprapatellar bursa is vulnerable to injury from both acute trauma and repeated micro-trauma.
- Acute injuries may be caused by direct trauma to the bursa during falls onto the knee or patellar fractures.

6. **Calcification in calcific supraspinatus tendinitis is due to deposition of:**

A. Calcium pyrophosphate
B. Calcium hydroxyapatite
C. Calcium oxalate
D. Calcium sulphate

Ans: B. Calcium hydroxyapatite

Ref: *Apley's System of Orthopaedics and Fractures, 9th edition, pg. 348-349*

Explanation:

Calcific Supraspinatus Tendinitis

- Acute shoulder pain may follow deposition of **calcium hydroxyapatite crystals**, usually in the **'critical zone'** of the supraspinatus tendon slightly medial to its insertion, occasionally elsewhere in the **rotator cuff**.
- The condition is **not unique to the shoulder**, and similar lesions are seen in **tendons** and **ligaments around the ankle, knee, hip and elbow**.
- The cause is unknown but it is thought that **local ischaemia** leads to **fibrocartilaginous metaplasia** and **deposition of crystals by the chondrocytes**.
- **Calcification** alone is probably not painful; symptoms, when they occur, are due to the florid vascular reaction which produces swelling and tension in the tendon.
- **Resorption of the calcific material is rapid** and it may soften or disappear entirely within a few weeks.

7. **Median nerve involvement is most common with:**

A. Elbow dislocation
B. Supracondylar fracture
C. Lateral condyle fractrue
D. Olecranon fracture

Ans: B. Supracondylar fracture

Ref: *Practical Fracture Treatment by Ronald McRae 4th edition, p 147-148, 159*

Explanation:

- **Median nerve injury** is common with **supracondylar fractures in children** with an incidence of **6 to 16%.**
- The **Anterior Interosseos distribution** of the nerve is **more commonly affected**.
- This nerve is injured in **elbow dislocations** less often, though it can occur.

8. **Earliest bone to ossify is:**

A. Clavicle **B.** Tibia
C. Sternum **D.** Ribs

Ans: A. Clavicle

Ref: 1. Moore, Keith L.; Dalley, Arthur F. (1999). Clinically Oriented Anatomy (4th ed.). Lippincott Williams & Wilkins. and

2. http://medind.nic.in/jae/t02/i2/jaet02i2p199.pdf

Explanation:

- The **clavicle** is the **first bone** to begin the process of **ossification** (laying down of minerals onto a preformed matrix) during development of the embryo, during the **fifth and sixth** weeks of gestation. However, it is one of **the last bones to finish ossification** at about **21–25 years** of age.
- Its lateral end is formed by intramembranous ossification while medially it is formed by endochondral ossification.
- It consists of a mass of cancellous bone surrounded by a compact bone shell.
- The cancellous bone forms via two ossification centres, one medial and one lateral, which fuse later on.
- The compact forms as the layer of fascia covering the bone stimulates the ossification of adjacent tissue. The resulting compact bone is known as a **periosteal collar**.
- Even though it is classified as a long bone, the clavicle has no medullary (bone marrow) cavity like other long bones.
- It is made up of **spongy (trabecular) bone** with a shell of compact bone.

9. **Baker's cyst is a swelling which occurs in:**
   A. Popliteal fossa **B.** Cubital fossa
   C. Lateral malleolus **D.** Medial malleolus

Ans: A. Popliteal fossa

Ref: Apley's System of Orthopaedics and Fractures. 9th Edition

Explanation:

- A **Baker's cyst** is produced by bulging of the **posterior capsule** of the **knee** and synovial herniation which produce a swelling in the popliteal fossa.
- The lump, which is usually seen in **older people**, is in the **midline** of the limb and at or below the level of the joint.
- It **fluctuates** but is **not tender**. It becomes **less prominent on knee flexion** as opposed to semimembranosus bursa.
- It is more likely to be caused by **rheumatoid or osteoarthritis**.

OBS AND GYNE

1. **Which of the following is the most common cause of urethritis with leucorrhea?**
   A. Chlamydia trachomatis
   B. H. vaginalis
   C. Trichomonas
   D. Candida

Ans: A. Chlamydia trachomatis

Ref: DC Dutta's Textbook of Gynaecology, 6th edition, Pg 144

Explanation:

- **Chlamydial** and **gonococcal infections** are the most common infections that cause **vulvovaginitis** and **urethritis.**
- **Chlamydia** affects the **columnar** and **transitional epithelium** of the genitourinary tract.
- **Chlamydia** causes
  - Urethritis
  - Bartholinitis
  - Cervicitis
  - Endometritis
  - Salpingitis
  - Perihepatitis
- **Tubal scarring** caused by **Chlamydia** results in infertility and ectopic pregnancy.
- **Fitz Hugh Curtis syndrome** – **Perihepatitis** caused by **Chlamydia trachomatis** (Violin string adhesions).

2. **A pregnant woman presents with a placenta previa of a major degree. The fetus is malformed. Which of the following will be the best line on management?**
   A. Cesarean section
   B. Oxytocin drip
   C. Rupture of membranes
   D. Instillation of PG E2

Ans: A. Cesarean section

Ref: DC Dutta's Textbook of Obstetrics, 7th edn, Pg 248

Explanation:

Placenta Previa - Management

- **Type II B, III and IV** are the **major degree placenta previa.**
- Criteria for expectant management:
  - Gestational age < 37 weeks
  - Hemodynamicallly stable patient
  - Bleeding has stopped

 – No evidence of fetal distress/congenital mal formations/intrauterine death.
- **Expectant management** includes **tocolysis, steroids for lung maturity.**
- In this scenario, baby is congenitally malformed. Hence, there is no question of expectant management. Now, the question is to whether to induce labor or directly go for caesarean section.
- Whatever is the condition of the baby, **caesarean section** is the mode of delivery for **major degree placenta previa.**

Also Note:

- **Dangerous type** of placenta previa – **Type II B.**
- **Stallworthy sign** is seen in – Type II B placenta previa.

3. **Transverse lie is most likely to occur in:**

A. Subseptate uterus **B.** Uterus didelphys
C. Hypoplastic uterus **D.** Unicornuate uterus

Ans: A. Subseptate uterus

Ref: *DC Dutta's Textbook of Obstetrics, 7th edn, Pg 395*

Explanation:

- **Transverse lie** is common in **subseptate** and **arcuate uterus.**
- **Breech** is common in **septate** and **bicornuate** uterus.

4. **What is Osiander's sign?**

A. Pulsation in the lateral vaginal fornix
B. Bluish colour change in the vagina
C. Softening of the cervix
D. On bimanual palpation the fingers can be approximated as if nothing is in between

Ans: A. Pulsation in the lateral vaginal fornix

Ref: *DC Dutta's Textbook of Obstetrics, 7th edn*

Explanation:

- **Osiander's sign:** Increased pulsation felt through the lateral fornices. Felt at 8th week.
- **Jacquemier's or Chadwick's sign:** Dusky hue at the vestibule and the anterior vaginal wall. Visible at 8th week.
- **Goodell's sign**: Cervix becomes soft. Felt at 6th week.
- **Piskacek's sign**: Asymmetrical enlargement of the uterus if there is lateral implantation of the placenta. Felt at 12 weeks.
- **Hegar's sign**: Variation in consistency of the uterus at 12 weeks.
- **Palmer's sign**: Regular and rhythmic contractions of uterus demonstrated during bimanual examination at 4 – 8 weeks.

5. **In 'after coming head', best forceps used for delivery is:**

A. Piper's forceps **B.** Kielland's forceps
C. Wrigley' forceps **D.** Kocher's forceps

Ans: A. Piper's forceps

Ref: *DC Dutta's Textbook of Obstetrics, 7th edn*

Explanation:

- Delivery of ACH in breech is **by flexion.**
- **Piper's forceps** – specially designed forceps for delivery of after coming head in assisted breech delivery.

Other Techniques for Delivery of After Coming Head are:

- **Burn Marshall Method** – legs held at ankle joint and trunk is taken in a wide arc across the maternal abdomen.
- **Mauriceau Smellie Veit Technique** – malar flexion and shoulder traction.
- **Prague's maneuver** – technique to deliver the ACH if bank is posterior in vaginal breech delivery.
- **Durhssen's incision** – incision made on the cervix to deliver the ACH if cervix is not fully dilated.
- **Star gazing sign** – hyperextended head in breech noted in USG.
- **Pinard's maneuver** – converting frank breech into a flexed breech by pressure on popliteal fossa with slight abduction after which legs can be delivered.
- **Lovset's maneuver** – procedure to deliver the extended arms or nuchal arm in vaginal breech delivery.

Breech

- Most common malpresentation
- Most common cause – prematurity
- **Types of Breech**
  - **Complete breech**
    - More common in multi with lax abdominal wall
  - **Incomplete breech**
    - Frank breech (extended breech) – Most common in primi
    - Footling breech / knee presentation
  - **Cord prolapse** — **Incidence**
    - Frank breech - 0.5%
    - Flexed breech - 5%
    - Footling breech - 15%

6. **Longest diameter of the skull is:**
   A. Suboccipital bregmatic
   B. Occipital frontal
   C. Bitemporal
   D. Biparietal

Ans: B. Occipital frontal

Ref: *DC Dutta's Textbook of Obstetrics, 7th edn p 85*

Explanation:

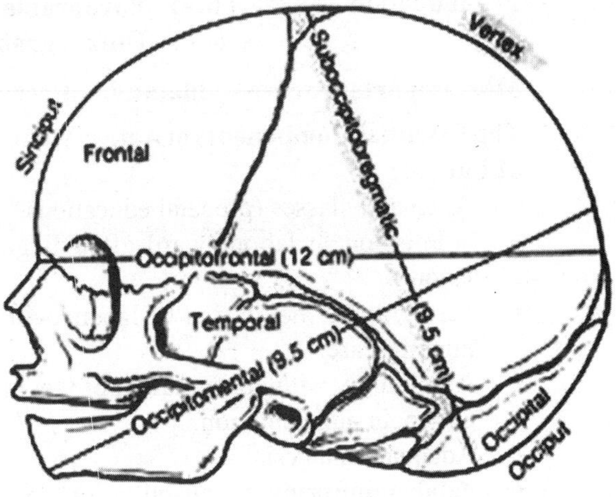

DIAMETERS OF FETAL SKULL

Fetal Skull Diameter	Borders	Length
Suboccipito-bregmatic	From **nape of neck** to **center of bregma**	9.5 cm
Suboccipito-frontal	From **nape of neck** to **anterior fontanelle** or center of sinciput	10 cm
Occipito-frontal	From **occipital eminence** to **root of nose**	11.5cm
Mentovertical	From **midpoint of chin** to **highest point of sagittal suture**	14 cm
Submentovertical	From **junction of floor of the mouth and neck** to **highest point of sagittal suture**	11.5 cm
Submentobregmatic	From **junction of mouth** and **neck to center of bregma**	9.5 cm
Biparietal	Extends **between two parietal eminences**	9.5 cm
Super sub-parietal	From a point placed **below one parietal eminence** to a point placed above the **other parietal eminence on opposite side**	8.5 cm
Bitemporal	Distance **between two anterior ends of coronal suture**	8 cm
Bimastoid	Distance between **tips of mastoid processes**	7.5 cm

Presentation	Engaging diameter
Submento bregmatic	Suboccipito bregmatic
Mento vertical	Suboccipito frontal / occipito frontal
Submento bregmatic	Submento bregmatic
Mento vertical	Mento vertical

7. **Bishop score is used to evaluate:**
   A. Cervix status
   B. Uterine contraction
   C. Fetal well being
   D. Pelvic assessment

Ans: A. Cervix status

Ref: *DC Dutta's Textbook of Obstetrics, 7th edn, pg 522*

Bishop's pre-induction cervical scoring system

Score	0	1	2	3	Max Score
Cx position	Posterior	Central	Anterior		2
Cx consistency	Firm	Medium	Soft		2
Cx effacement	0-30 %	40-50%	60-70%	80%+	3
Cx dilatation	0	1-2	3-4	5+	3
Station of head	-3	-2	-1,0	+1.+2	3
Max Total Score					13

Pre-induction score >= 6 → Favourable
< 6 → Unfavourable

Most important score – dilatation of cervix

The Essential Components of Active Management of Labour:

- Antenatal classes (prenatal education).
- Admission in labour ward after diagnosis of labour.
- Partographic monitoring of labour with 1 to 1 nursing care.
- Amniotomy with confirmation of labour.
- Oxytocin augmentation.
- Adequate analgesia.
- Fetal monitoring by auscultation/continuous EFM.
- **AIM** –To accomplish delivery within 12 hours of admission without increasing maternal and perinatal morbidity.

8. **The management of eclampsia includes all *except:***
   A. Control of convulsion
   B. Prolongation of pregnancy
   C. Control of BP
   D. Delivery of fetus

Ans: B. Prolongation of pregnancy

Ref: *DC Dutta's Textbook of Obstetrics, 7th edn, p232*

Explanation:

Eclampsia

- Convulsions/coma occurring in a women with preeclampsia
- Ante partum eclampsia – **Most common type** of eclampsia (50%)
- Postpartum eclampsia – occurs within 48 hours after delivery
- Intercurrent eclampsia – pregnancy continues beyond 48 hours after recovery

PRINCIPLES OF MANAGEMENT IN ECLAMPSIA

- Maintain airway, breathing and circulation
- Oxygen administration
- Prevention of injury
- **Arrest of convulsions**
- **Control BP**
- **Deliver by 6-8 hours**
- Prevention of complications
- Ventilatory support (if required)
- Postpartum care

Drug of Choice

- Magnesium sulphate
- **Pritchard regimen**
  - Loading dose - 4 gm slow IV (20%) + 10 gm IM
  - Maintenance dose - 5 gm IM q 4 hours
- Monitor
  - Urine output
  - Respiratory rate
  - Knee jerks
- Therapeutic level of serum $MgSO_4$ - 4-7 meq/L.
- **$MgSO_4$** continued for **24 hours** after the last seizure or delivery whichever is later.

Status Eclampticus

- Fits occurring in quick succession
- Management
  - **Thiopentone sodium**
  - Muscle relaxation and assisted ventilation

9. **The most common cause of vesicovaginal fistula in developing countries is: (Repeat)**
   A. Pressure necrosis of urethra during obstructed labor
   B. Forceps delivery
   C. Abdominal hysterectomy
   D. Tuberculosis

Ans: A. Pressure necrosis of urethra during obstructed labor

Ref: *DC Dutta's Textbook of Gynaecology 6th edition P401*

Explanation:

Refer: *2010 Obs & Gyne question explanation.*

10. **Treatment of primary ovarian failure is:**
    A. FSH
    B. GnRH
    C. LH
    D. Estrogen/progesterone

Ans: D. Estrogen/progestrone

Ref: *DC Dutta's Textbook of Gynaecology, 6th edition, P401*

Explanation:

Hypergonadotropic Hypogonadism

Causes

- **Primary ovarian failure/premature ovarian failure**
  - Ovarian failure before 40 years
  - Failure of germ cell migration or accelerated germ cell depletion
  - Causes
    - Genetic

Turner's
Gonadal dysgenesis
- Autoimmune disorders
- Infections: mumps, TB
- Iatrogenic: RT, chemotherapy
- Metabolic: galactosemia (follicles destroyed by toxic effects of galactose)

- **Resistant ovarian syndrome**
  - FSH receptor defect or absence (Savage syndrome)
  - Follicles are present

Diagnosis

- History of amenorrhoea in < 35 years
- **Increased FSH levels**
- **Decreased E2 levels**
- Karyotyping abnormality (Turner's)
- Organ specific Ab (anti thyroid Ab most common)
- Ovarian biopsy
  - Autoimmune disorders – perifollicular infiltration
  - Premature ovarian failure – Follicles are **absent**
  - Resistant ovarian syndrome – follicles are **present** (FSH rec. Defect)
  - Menopausal symptoms

Management

- **HRT**
  - To prevent/minimize post menopausal symptoms
  - Prevention of osteoporosis
  - Specific group of women for prescription of HRT
    - Premature ovarian failure
    - Gonadal dysgenesis
    - Surgical or radiation menopause
  - Preparations for HRT
    - **Estrogen + progesterone combination**
    - Estrogen: conjugated estrogen/micronized estradiol
    - Progestins: mpa/micronized p/dydrogesterone

Flowchart for evaluation of primary amenorrhoea

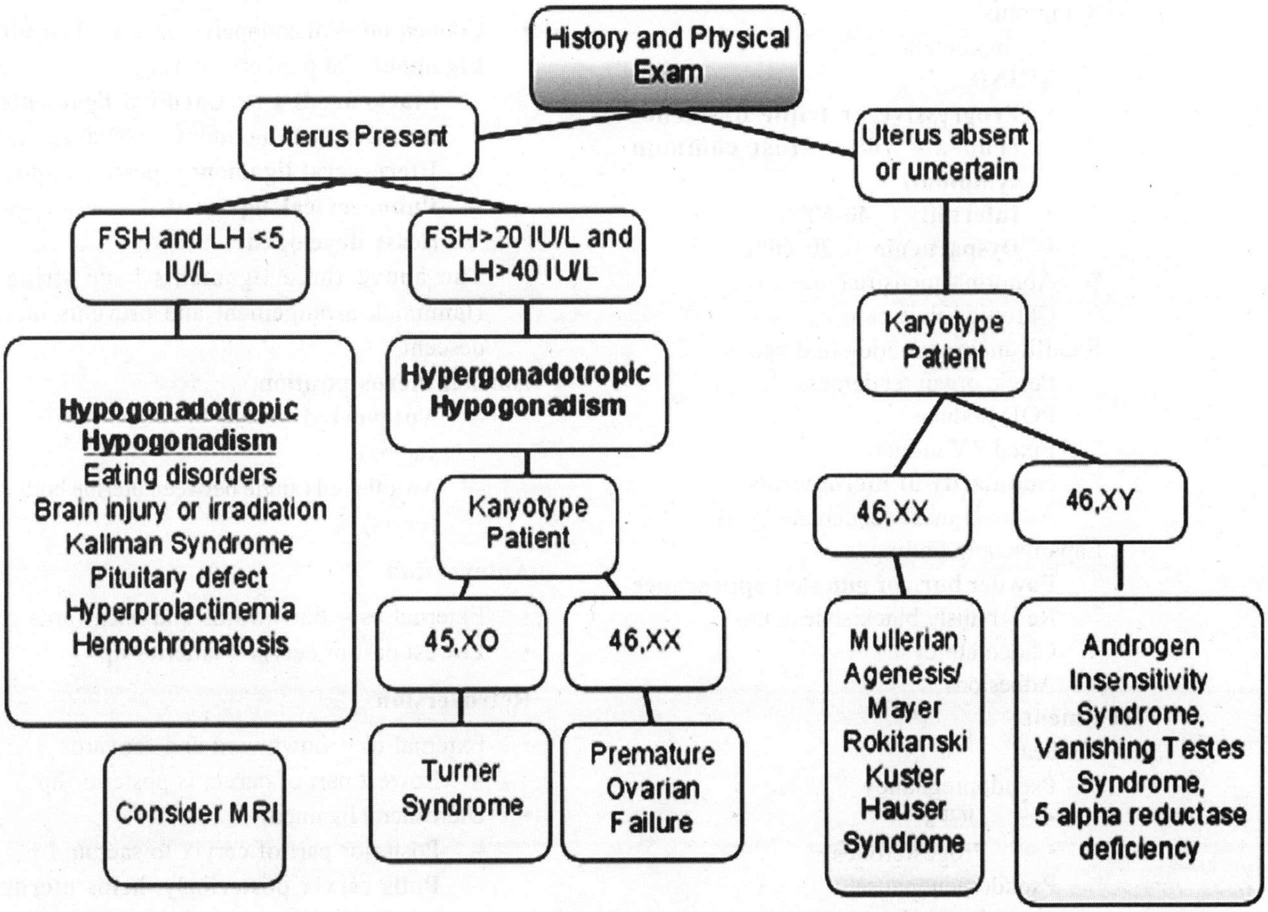

11. The characteristic symptom of dysmenorrhea, menorrhagia, recurrent abdominal pain and infertility is suggestive of:

A. Endometriosis
B. Ectopic pregnancy
C. Endometritis
D. Endometrial carcinoma

Ans: A. Endometriosis

Ref: DC Dutta's Textbook of Gynaecology 6th edition p 293

Explanation:

Endometriosis

- **Most common site** – ovary
- **Theories**
  - **Sampsons** – Retrograde menstruation
  - **Halbans** – Metastasis via blood and lymphatics
  - **Meyer and Ivanoff** – Coelomic metalasia
  - **Merill's** – Histogenesis by induction
- **Clinical features**
  - 30-45 years
  - Mostly nulliparous
  - Symptoms
    - Asymptomatic -25%
    - **TRIAD**
      - **Progressive or triple dysmenorrhoea – 70% (Most common symptom)**
      - **Infertility – 40-60%**
      - **Dysparuenia – 20-40%**
    - Abnormal menstruation–20%
    - Chronic pelvic pain
  - Significant examination findings
    - Pelvic organ tenderness
    - POD nodules
    - Fixed RV uterus
    - **Nodularity of uterosacrals**
    - Adnexal mass (chocolate cyst)
  - Laparoscopic findings
    - **Powder burn or gun shot appearance**
    - Red/ bluish/ blackish lesions
    - Chocolate cyst
    - Adhesions
- **Treatment**
  - **Medical**
    - Pseudopregnancy
      - OCPs
      - Progesterones
    - Pseudomenopause
      - Danazole
      - Gestrinone
    - Oopherectomy
      - *GnRH analogues : leuprolide, naferelin, Goserelin*
  - **Surgical**
    - Conservative
      - Laparoscopic endometrial ablation and adhesiolysis
      - Chocolate cyst removal
    - Definitive
      - TAH + BSO

12. Anteversion of uterus is due to following ligament:

A. Uterosacral ligament
B. Mackenrodt's ligament
C. Round ligament
D. Pubocervical ligament

Ans: A. Uterosacral ligament

Ref: DC Dutta's Textbook of Gynaecology 6th edition, Pg 192

Explanation:

Supports of Uterus

- Condensation of endopelvic fascia – **Triradiate Ligament** – at pericervical ring
  - **Mackenrodt's or Cardinal ligaments** or **transcervical ligament** – lateral spoke
  - **Uterosacral ligament** – posterior spoke
  - **Pubocervical ligament** – anterior spoke **(least developed)**
- The above three ligaments have string of Hammock arrangement and prevents uterine descent

Normal uterus position
  - **Anteverted** (angle between cervix and vagina)
  - **Anteflexed** (angle between uterine body and cervix)

Anteversion

- External os – downwards and backwards
- Lowest part of cervix – anterior lip

Retroversion

- External os – downward and forwards
  - Lowest part of cervix is posterior lip
- Uterosacral ligament
  - Posterior part of cervix to sacrum
  - **Pulls cervix posteriorly, helps uterus to fall forward – maintains anteversion and anteflexion**

DE LANCEY'S SUPPORTS OF VAGINA

- Level I - Triradiate ligament
- Level II- Pelvic fascia, recto vaginal septum
- Level III- levator ani, perineal body, urogenital diaphragm.

13. A nulliparous female aged 30 years develops IInd degree UV prolapse. The operative procedure done is:

A. Cervicopexy
B. LeForte repair
C. Manchester repair
D. Ward Mayo surgery

Ans: A. Cervicopexy

Ref: *Dutta's Textbook of Gynaecology, 5th ed. Pg 211*
Shaw's Textbook of Gynaecology, 15th ed. Pg 338

Explanation:

Surgeries for Prolapse

- **Ward Mayo's operation**
  - Women > 40 years
  - Completed family
  - Not desirous of retaining menstruation
- **Components of Ward Mayo Surgery**
  - Anterior colporraphy
  - Colpoperineorraphy
  - Vaginal hysterectomy
  - Anterior colporraphy and colpoperineorraphy is known as pelvic floor repair
- **Manchester / Fothergill's operation**
  - Women < 40 years
  - Completed family
  - Desirous of retaining menstrual function
- **Fothergill's Repair/ Manchester Repair**
  - Anterior colporraphy
  - Amputation of cervix
  - Suturing cut ends of Meckendrodt's ligaments in front of cervix
  - Covering the raw area on amputated cervix with vaginal mucosa
  - Colpoperineorraphy
- **Shirodkar's Repair (Modified Fothergill's Repair)**
  - No cervical amputation
  - POD is opened
  - Uterosacral ligaments identified and divided close to cervix and the stumps are crossed and situated together in front of cervix
  - High closure of POD
- **Abdominal Sling Surgery (Cervicopexy)**
  - Young women
  - Nulliparous prolapse
  - Desirous of retaining child bearing function
    - ° Shirodkar's sling – to anterior longitudinal ligament of sacrum
    - ° Khanna's sling – to ASIS
    - ° Purandrare's sling – to rectus sheath
- **Lefort's Repair**
  - Very elderly post menopausal bedridden patients
  - Approximation of anterior and posterior vaginal flaps with two channels in vagina for drainage
- **Pregnancy with Prolapse**
  - Pessary inserted
  - Surgery 3-4 months after delivery

14. In minilap procedure, the most common method successfully used is:

A. Uchida's
B. Pomeroy's
C. Irving's
D. Parkland's

Ans: B. Pomeroy's

Ref: *DC Dutta's Textbook of Gynaecology 6th edition, pg 476*

Explanation:

Tubectomy Methods

A. Abdominal Methods

1. **Conventional laparotomy** – abdominal incision 3-5 cms
2. **Minilaparotomy** – abdominal incision 2 - 2.5 cms
   - Techniques
     - **Modified Pomeroy's**
       - o Recommended by Govt. of India
       - o Most common method
       - o 1 -1.5 cms tube excised
       - o Isthumus portion of tube
       - o No. 1-0 chr. catgut used for ligation of tube
       - o Adv. –
         - Failure rate : 0.1- 0.5%
         - Simple procedure
     - Parkland method – another commonly employed method with similar success rates
     - Other uncommon methods
       - o Uchida method
       - o Irving's method
       - o Madlener method
       - o Kroener's method
3. **Laparoscopy**
   - Single / double puncture

- **C/I during PUERPEREUM**
- Fallope ring (silicon rubber with 5% barium sulphate)
- Filshie clip (titanium lined with silicon rubber)
  - Only 4 mm of tube is destroyed
  - Failure rate –0.1%
  - Chances of tubal recanalisation – BEST with filshie clips laparoscopic sterilization
- Hulka – Clemens spring clip
- Electrosurgical method – bipolar cautery preferred over unipolar

B. Vaginal Methods

- Through posterior colpotomy incision.
- Hysteroscopic electrocoagulation of tubes.
- **ESSURE** – 4 cms long, 2 mm dm microcoil made of nickel titanium steel alloy containing polyethylene fibres within it.
  - Introduced into the corneal end of tubed under hysteroscopy guidance.
  - Tubes blocked permanently by scar tissue growing into the device.
  - Additional contraceptive method used for first 3 months.

15. Mesonephric duct remnant presenting as swelling in anterior vaginal wall is:

A. Nebothian cyst **B.** Gartner's cyst
C. Bartholin's cyst **D.** Inclusion cyst

Ans: B. Gartner's cyst

Ref: *Shaw's Textbook of Gynecology 15th ed pg 136*

Explanation:

VAGINAL CYSTS

- Vaginal cysts are rare and are located more commonly in **anterior vaginal wall**
- **Gartner's cyst**
  - Arises from remnants of mesonephric duct
  - Lies in anterolateral aspect of vaginal wall
  - Small cyst is asymptomatic
  - Large cyst causes dyspareunia
  - Large symptomatic cysts requires excision
- **Inclusion cyst**
  - Seen in lower end of vagina on its posterior surface.
  - It is caused by tags of mucosa embedding inside the scar that later forms a cyst.
- **Bartholin cyst**—extends into vagina
- **Endometriotic cyst**
  - Bluish bulge in posterior fornix.
  - It is treated with either danazol or surgical excision.

A Nabothian Cyst (or Nabothian Follicle)

- It is a mucus-filled cyst on the surface of the **cervix.**
- They are most often caused when stratified squamous epithelium of the ectocervix grows over the simple columnar epithelium of the endocervix (Metaplasia).
- This tissue growth can block the cervical crypts, trapping cervical mucus inside the crypts.

PEDIATRICS

1. Juvenile idiopathic arthritis includes all the following categories *except:*

A. Psoriatic arthritis
B. Enthesitis related arthritis
C. Systemic arthritis
D. Reactive arthritis

Ans: D. Reactive arthritis

Ref: *Nelson Textbook of Pediatrics, 19th edition. Pg 830*

Explanation:

- Juvenile rheumatoid arthritis (JRA) was recently re-termed as Juvenile idiopathic arthritis (JIA) by International League of Associations for Rheumatology (ILAR).

ILAR Classification of Juvenile Idiopathic Arthritis (JIA) *(See Table on the next Page)*

2. An infant presents with cardiac failure. Examination reveals a weaker femoral pulse when compared to the radial pulse. What is the probable diagnosis?

A. PDA **B.** COA
C. Aorto-iliac vasculitis **D.** VSD

Ans: B. COA

Ref: *Nelson's Textbook of Pediatrics. 19th Edition, Page 1567*

Explanation:

Weak femoral pulse is indicative of coarctation of aorta. Normally, the femoral pulse occurs slightly before the radial pulse. Weak femoral pulse or femoral pulse felt after radial pulse is a characteristic feature of COA.

Coarctation of Aorta (COA)

- Constrictions of the aorta of varying degrees may occur at any point from the transverse arch to the iliac bifurcation, but **98%** occur just **below the origin of the left subclavian** artery at the origin of the **ductus arteriosus (juxtaductal coarctation)**.

ILAR Classification of Juvenile Idiopathic Arthritis (JIA)

Category	Definition	Exclusions
Systemic-onset JIA	Arthritis in ≥1 joints with, or preceded by, fever of at least 2 wk in duration that is documented to be daily ("quotidian"*) for at least 3 days and accompanied by ≥1 of the following: 1. Evanescent (nonfixed) erythematous rash. 2. Generalized lymph node enlargement. 3. Hepatomegaly or splenomegaly or both. 4. Serositis.	**a.** Psoriasis or a history of psoriasis in the patient or a 1st-degree relative. **b.** Arthritis in an HLA-B27–positive boy beginning after the 6th birthday. **c.** Ankylosing spondylitis, enthesitis-related arthritis, sacroiliitis with inflammatory bowel disease, Reiter syndrome, or acute anterior uveitis, or a history of one of these disorders in a 1st-degree relative. **d.** Presence of immunoglobulin M RF on at least 2 occasions at least 3 months apart.
Oligoarticular JIA	Arthritis affecting 1-4 joints during the 1st 6 mo of disease. Two subcategories are recognized: 1. Persistent oligoarthritis—affecting ≤4 joints throughout the disease course. 2. Extended oligoarthritis—affecting >4 joints after the 1st 6 mo of disease.	a, b, c, d (above) **plus** e. Presence of systemic JIA
Polyarthritis (RF-negative)	Arthritis affecting ≥5 joints during the 1st 6 mo of disease; a test for RF is negative.	a, b, c, d, e
Polyarthritis (RF-positive)	Arthritis affecting ≥5 joints during the 1st 6 mo of disease; >2 tests for RF at least 3 mo apart during the 1st 6 mo of disease are positive.	a, b, c ,e
Psoriatic arthritis	Arthritis and psoriasis, or arthritis and at least 2 of the following: 1. Dactylitis. 2. Nail pitting and onycholysis. 3. Psoriasis in a 1st-degree relative.	b, c, d, e
Enthesitis-related arthritis	Arthritis and enthesitis, or arthritis or enthesitis with at least 2 of the following: 1. Presence of or a history of sacroiliac joint tenderness or inflammatory lumbosacral pain or both. 2. Presence of HLA-B27 antigen. 3. Onset of arthritis in a male > 6 yr old. 4. Acute (symptomatic) anterior uveitis. 5. History of ankylosing spondylitis, enthesitis-related arthritis, sacroiliitis with inflammatory bowel disease, Reiter syndrome, or acute anterior uveitis in a 1st-degree relative.	a, d, e
Undifferentiated arthritis	Arthritis that fulfills criteria in no category or in ≥2 of the above categories.	

- The anomaly occurs twice as often in males as in females.
- Coarctation of the aorta may be a feature of **Turner syndrome** and is associated with a **bicuspid aortic valve in** more than 70% of patients.
- Mitral valve abnormalities (a supravalvular mitral ring or parachute mitral valve) and subaortic stenosis are potential associated lesions.
- When this group of left-sided obstructive lesions occurs together, they are referred to as the ***Shone complex.***

Clinical Manifestations

- Mostly asymptomatic
- Some children or adolescents complain about weakness or pain in the legs after exercise.
- Silent hypertension diagnosed on routine physical examination.
- Disparity in pulsation and blood pressure in the arms and legs.
- The **femoral, popliteal, posterior tibial and dorsalis pedis pulses** are **weak** (or absent in up to 40% of patients), in contrast to the bounding pulses of the arms and carotid vessels.
- The radial and femoral pulses should always be palpated simultaneously for the presence of a radial-femoral delay.

- Normally, the femoral pulse occurs slightly before the radial pulse. A radial-femoral delay occurs when blood flow to the descending aorta is dependent on collaterals, in which case the femoral pulse is felt after the radial pulse.
- In normal persons, systolic blood pressure in the legs obtained by the cuff method is 10-20 mm Hg higher than that in the arms.
- In coarctation of the aorta, **blood pressure** in the **legs** is **lower than** that in the **arms**.
- The precordial impulse and heart sounds are usually normal.
- The presence of a systolic ejection click or thrill in the suprasternal notch suggests a bicuspid aortic valve (present in 70% of cases).
- A short systolic murmur is often heard along the left sternal border at the 3rd and 4th intercostal spaces.
- In older patients with well-developed collateral blood flow, systolic or continuous murmurs may be heard over the left and right sides of the chest laterally and posteriorly (**Suzman sign**).
- In these patients, a palpable thrill can occasionally be appreciated in the intercostal spaces on the back.

Diagnosis

- Cardiac enlargement and pulmonary congestion are noted in infants with severe coarctation.
- The enlarged left subclavian artery commonly produces a prominent shadow in the left superior mediastinum.
- **Notching** of the **inferior border of the ribs** from pressure erosion by enlarged collateral vessels is common by late childhood.
- In most instances, the descending aorta has an area of **poststenotic dilatation**.

3. **What percentage of weight loss in infants constitutes severe dehydration?**
 A. > 10% loss of body weight
 B. > 6% loss of body weight
 C. 5% loss of body weight
 D. 7% loss of body weight

Ans: A. > 10% loss of body weight

Ref: *Nelson's Textbook of Pediatrics. 19th Edition, Chapter on 'Deficit Therapy'. Page 245*

Explanation:

- In an **older child** with diarrhea, **6% loss of body weight** amounts to **Severe dehydration** whereas **10% loss of body weight** is required to cause the same in **infants** (Ref: Nelson).

CLINICAL EVALUATION OF DEHYDRATION

- **Mild dehydration** (<5% in an infant; <3% in an older child or adult):
  - Normal or increased pulse
  - Decreased urine output
  - Thirsty
  - Normal physical findings
- **Moderate dehydration** (5-10% in an infant; 3-6% in an older child or adult):
  - Tachycardia
  - Little or no urine output
  - Irritable/lethargic
  - Sunken eyes and fontanel
  - Decreased tears
  - Dry mucous membranes
  - Mild delay in elasticity (skin turgor)
  - Delayed capillary refill (>1.5 sec)
  - Cool and pale
- **Severe dehydration** (>10% in an infant; >6% in an older child or adult):
  - Peripheral pulses either rapid and weak or absent
  - Decreased blood pressure
  - No urine output
  - Very sunken eyes and fontanel
  - No tears
  - Parched mucous membranes
  - Delayed elasticity (poor skin turgor)
  - Very delayed capillary refill (>3 sec)
  - Cold and mottled
  - Limp, depressed consciousness

4. **All the following are indicated in the long term therapy of children with coronary abnormalities in kawasaki disease *except:***
 A. Intravenous immunoglobulins
 B. Aspirin
 C. Clopidogrel
 D. Warfarin

Ans: A. Intravenous immunoglobulins

Ref: *Nelson Textbook of Pediatrics, 19th edition. Pg 867*

Explanation:

Treatment of Kawasaki Disease

Acute Stage
Intravenous immunoglobulin 2 g/kg over 10–12 hr with aspirin 80–100 mg/kg/day divided every 6 hr orally until 14th illness day.
Convalescent Stage
Aspirin 3–5 mg/kg once daily orally until 6–8 wk after illness onset.

Contd.

Long-Term Therapy for Those with Coronary Abnormalities
Aspirin 3–5 mg/kg once daily orally ± clopidogrel 1 mg/kg/day (max 75 mg/day) (most experts add warfarin for those patients at particularly high risk of thrombosis).
Acute Coronary Thrombosis
Prompt fibrinolytic therapy with tissue plasminogen activator, streptokinase, or urokinase under supervision of a pediatric cardiologist.

5. **All the following drugs are indicated in the treatment of complicated typhoid fever in children *except:***

A. Ceftriaxone B. Oral azithromycin

C. Ciprofloxacin D. Chloramphenicol

Ans: D. Chloramphenicol

Ref: *Nelson Textbook of Pediatrics, 19th edition. Pg 958*

Explanation:

Treatment of Typhoid Fever in Children **(See the following Table)**

6. **A 6-year-old boy presents with complaints of hyperactivity, excessive shoulder shrugging, throat clearing and eye blinking. During examination, he is not cooperative, uses obscene words and runs around in the consultation room. What is the most probable diagnosis?**

A. Attention deficit hyperactivity disorder

B. Tic disorder

C. Psychomotor seizures

D. Childhood psychosis

Ans: B. Tic Disorder

Ref: *Nelson Textbook of Pediatrics, 19th edition. Pg 77*

Explanation:

The clinical vignette describes a classical case of **Tourette syndrome (Tic Disorder)**

- **Tics** involve sudden, rapid, repetitive, involuntary movements of muscle groups or vocalizations and represent discharges of tension related to central nervous system electrochemical signals.
- Parts of the body that are most frequently involved are the muscles of the face, neck, shoulders, trunk and hands.
- Simple tics involve only 1 muscle group, as in eye blinking, shoulder shrugging or neck jerking, whereas complex tics may include multiple muscle groups and cause more complex motions.
- Simple vocalizations include grunting and throat clearing; complex vocalizations include the use of repetitive obscenities (**coprolalia**).
- Motor or vocal tics lasting <1 yr are transient; those lasting >1 yr are chronic.

Tourette Syndrome

- It is characterized by a history of motor **and** vocal tics (may not present concurrently).

Treatment of Typhoid Fever in Children

	OPTIMAL THERAPY			ALTERNATIVE EFFECTIVE DRUGS
Susceptibility	**Antibiotic**	**Daily dose (mg/kg/day)**	**Days**	**Antibiotic**
Uncomplicated Typhoid Fever				
Fully sensitive	Chloramphenicol	50–75	14–21	Fluoroquinolone
	Amoxicillin	75–100	14	
Multidrug resistant	Fluoroquinolone or cefixime	15	5–7	Azithromycin
		15–20	7–14	Cefixime
Quinolone resistant[†]	Azithromycin or ceftriaxone	8–10	7	Cefixime
		75	10–14	
Severe / Complicated Typhoid Fever				
Fully sensitive	Ampicillin or ceftriaxone	100	14	Fluoroquinolone
		60–75	10–14	
Multidrug resistant	Fluoroquinolone	15	10–14	Ceftriaxone or cefotaxime
Quinolone resistant	Ceftriaxone	60–75	10–14	Azithromycin

- Tourette syndrome has a lifetime prevalence rate of 0.5/1,000 individuals and commonly presents in childhood, beginning with simple motor tics, often before age 7 years.
- In many cases, multiple tics and complex vocal sounds, such as barking and grunting, develop over time and peak in severity by age 10–12 years.
- Shouting obscene words **(coprolalia)** is characteristic, but is seen in only 10% of affected patients. It affects boys 3–4 times more often than girls.
- In some families, it is an autosomal dominant disorder with greater penetrance in males.

Criteria for the diagnosis of Tourette syndrome include:

1.	Multiple motor and vocal tics lasting >1 year, with no tic-free interval lasting >3 months
2.	Onset before age 18 years.
3.	No medical causes (drugs, central nervous system disease).

- Children with Tourette syndrome often have behavioral, emotional, and academic problems.
- In particular, these children have higher rates of obsessive-compulsive disorder, attention-deficit/hyperactivity disorder, and oppositional-defiant disorder.
- Neuroimaging studies suggest that there is a lack of normal asymmetry within the striatum and a decrease in the size of the cavum septum pellucidum.
- Single-photon emission computed tomography scan data implicate **dysfunction in dopamine receptor** binding in severely affected children.
- Studies have also implicated systemic and local cytokine responses in Tourette syndrome and in the exacerbation of symptoms.
- Lyme disease may rarely present with clinical manifestations of Tourette syndrome.
- Laboratory studies are nonspecific; upto 80% of patients with Tourette syndrome have nonspecific abnormal electroencephalographic findings.

Treatment

- Many children with Tourette syndrome require medication for obsessive-compulsive symptoms or attention and impulsivity problems.
- Pharmacotherapy, targeting the tics themselves, is indicated when tics interfere with social development or classroom function.
- For 1st-line treatment, **neuroleptics** have the strongest track record in controlled trials.
- **Haloperidol** and **pimozide, dopaminergic antagonists**, have been shown to reduce the severity of tics by 65%.
- Because potentially severe side effects are associated with traditional neuroleptics, most clinicians recommend risperidone.
- **Risperidone** is equivalent to clonidine in reducing tics.
- **Clonidine**, an α2 agonist, is effective; sedation and low blood pressure are common side effects of clonidine and require careful monitoring.

7. **Areola and papilla forming secondary mound in adolescent girls is classified under which stage of sexual maturity rating (SMR)?**

A. SMR Stage 2 B. SMR Stage 3
C. SMR Stage 4 D. SMR Stage 5

Ans: C. SMR Stage 4

Ref: *Nelson Textbook of Pediatrics, 19th edition. Pg 651*

Explanation:

Classification of Sex Maturity States in Girls

SMR Stage	Pubic Hair	Breasts
1	Preadolescent	Preadolescent
2	Sparse, lightly pigmented, straight, medial border of labia	Breast and papilla elevated as small mound; diameter of areola increased
3	Darker, beginning to curl, increased amount	Breast and areola enlarged, no contour separation
4	Coarse, curly, abundant, but less than in adult	Areola and papilla form secondary mound
5	Adult feminine triangle, spread to medial surface of thighs	Mature, nipple projects, areola part of general breast contour

Classification of Sex Maturity States in Boys

SMR Stage	Pubic Hair	Penis	Testes
1	None	Preadolescent	Preadolescent
2	Scanty, long, slightly pigmented	Minimal change/ enlargement	Enlarged scrotum, pink, texture altered
3	Darker, starting to curl, small amount	Lengthens	Larger
4	Resembles adult type, but less quantity; coarse, curly	Larger; glans and breadth increase in size	Larger, scrotum dark
5	Adult distribution, spread to medial surface of thighs	Adult size	Adult size

8. **Daily maintanence fluid for a child weighing 10 kg is:**

A. 1000 ml/day **B.** 800 ml/day
C. 500 ml/day **D.** 1200 ml/day

Ans: A. 1000 ml/day

Ref: *Nelson's Textbook of Pediatrics. 19th Edition*

Explanation:

The Holliday-Segar Method

- In the Holliday-Segar Method, fluid and electrolyte requirements are empirically based on the caloric needs of the average hospital patient.
- The same formula is used for calculating **calorie requirement** as well as **fluid requirement.**

Relation of Body Weight to Maintenance Fluids	
For each kilogram in this range	Daily fluid requirement per kilogram
First 1-10 kg	100 ml/kg/day
Next 11-20 kg	50 ml/kg/day
For >20 kg	20 ml/kg/day

- For **10 kg** child, Maintanence fluid for 24 hours = **10** × 100 = **1000 ml/day**
- For **15 kg** child, Maintanence fluid for 24 hours = **10** × 100 + **5**× 50 = **1250 ml/day**
- For **25 kg** child, Maintanence fluid for 24 hours = **10** × 100 + **10**× 50 + **5**× 20 = **1600 ml/day**

9. **Definition of extremely low birth weight: (Repeat)**

A. Wt <2.5 kg **B.** Wt <2 kg
C. Wt <1.5 kg **D.** Wt <1 kg

Ans: D. Wt < 1kg

Ref: *Nelson's Textbook of Pediatrics. 19th Edition*

Explanation:

Some Important Definitions in Neonatology

Low birth weight: Birth weight of less than 2.5 kg irrespective of gestational age.
Very low birth weight: Birth weight of less than 1.5 kg irrespective of gestational age.
Extremely low birth weight: Birth weight of less than 1.0 kg irrespective of gestational age.
Neonatal: First 28 days of postnatal life.
Preterm: Less than 37 completed weeks of gestations.
Term: After 37 completed weeks of gestations.
Post term: After 42 completed weeks of gestations.
Past dates: After 40 completed weeks of gestations.
Still birth: Delivering dead fetus after 28 weeks of gestation (Defn changes with country).
Abortion: Expulsion of products of conception before 28 weeks of gestation.
Small for Gestational Age (SGA): Weight below the 10th percentile for the gestational age.
Large for Gestational Age (LGA): Weight above the 90th percentile for the gestational age.
Appropriate for Gestational Age (AGA): Weight between 10th and 90th percentile for the gestational age.

10. **Nocturnal enuresis should be investigated and treated after:**

A. 2 years **B.** 3 years
C. 4 years **D.** 5 years

Ans: D. 5 years

Ref: *Nelson's Textbook of Pediatrics. 19th Edition, Page. 71*

Explanation:

Enuresis (Bed-Wetting)

Enuresis is defined as the repeated voiding of urine into clothes or bed at least twice a week for at least 3 consecutive months in a child who is at least 5 years of age.
Diurnal enuresis - Wetting while awake.
Nocturnal enuresis - Voiding during sleep.
Primary enuresis - In children who have never been consistently dry through the night.
Secondary enuresis - Resumption of wetting after at least 6 months of dryness.

Normal Voiding and Toilet Training

- Urine storage consists of sympathetic and pudendal nerve–mediated inhibition of detrusor contractile activity accompanied by closure of the bladder neck and proximal urethra with increased activity of the external sphincter.
- The infant has coordinated reflex voiding as often as 15-20 times per day. Over time, bladder capacity increases.
- At **2-4 years**, the child is developmentally ready to begin toilet training.
- To achieve conscious bladder control, several conditions must be present: awareness of bladder filling, cortical inhibition (suprapontine modulation) of reflex (unstable) bladder contractions, ability to consciously tighten the external sphincter to prevent incontinence, normal bladder growth, and motivation by the child to stay dry.

- The transitional phase of voiding is the period when children are acquiring bladder control.
- Girls typically acquire bladder control before boys, and bowel control typically is achieved before bladder control.

Organic Causes of Secondary Enuresis

- Urinary tract infections
- Chronic kidney disease
- Spinal cord disorders
- Constipation
- Diabetes (thirst, polyuria and polydipsia)

Laboratory Evaluation Should Include

- Urinalysis to check for glycosuria or a low specific gravity.
- Bladder ultrasonography - to check residual urine in bladder after voiding.

Treatment

- The treatment of monosymptomatic nocturnal enuresis should be marked by a conservative, gentle and patient approach.
- Treatment can begin with **parent-child education**, charting with rewards for dry nights, voiding before bedtime, and night awakening 2-4 hr after bedtime, while at the same time making sure that parents do not punish the child for enuretic episodes.
- In addition, the child should be encouraged to avoid holding urine and to void frequently during the day (to avoid day wetting).
- If this approach fails, **urine alarm treatment** is recommended.
- Application of an alarm for a period of 8-12 wk can be expected to result in a 75-95% success in the arrest of bedwetting.
- The underlying conditioning principle likely lies in the alarm's being an annoying awakening stimulus that causes the child to awaken in time to go to the bathroom and/or retain urine in order to avoid the aversive stimulus.
- Urine alarm treatment has been shown to be of equal or superior effectiveness when compared to all other forms of treatment.
- Relapse rates are approximately 40%, with the simplest response being a second alarm course as well as considering the addition of intermittent schedules of reinforcement or the use of overlearning (drinking just before bedtime).

Pharmacotherapy for Nocturnal Enuresis is second-line Treatment:

- **Desmopressin acetate (DDAVP)** is a synthetic analog of the antidiuretic hormone (ADH) vasopressin, which decreases nighttime urine production.
- The relapse rate is high when DDAVP is discontinued.
- DDAVP is also associated with rare side effects of hyponatremia and water intoxication, with resulting seizures.
- Although **imipramine** has some usefulness, less than 50% of children respond, and most relapse when the medication is discontinued.
- Much less commonly used, **oxybutynin** and **tolterodine** are **antimuscarinic** drugs, which may be effective by reducing bladder spasm and increasing bladder capacity.

11. Child with recurrent fractures and wormian bones is most likely to have:

A. Osteogenesis imperfecta
B. Rickets
C. Battered baby syndrome
D. Shaken baby syndrome

Ans: A. Osteogenesis imperfecta

Ref: *Nelson's Textbook of Pediatrics. 19th Edition*

Explanation:

- **Soft areas (craniotabes)** are occasionally found in the **parietal bones** at the vertex near the sagittal suture; they are more common in **premature infants** and in infants who have been exposed to **uterine compression**. Though such soft areas are usually insignificant.
- Soft areas in the **occipital region** suggest the irregular calcification and **wormian bone formation.**

Conditions Associated with Wormian Bones

- Osteogenesis imperfecta
- Cleidocranial dysostosis
- Lacunar skull
- Hypophosphatasia
- Cretinism
- Down syndrome
- Healing rickets
- Chronic hydrocephalus
- Pyknodysostosis
- Pachydermoperiostosis

Osteogenesis Imperfecta (OI) (Brittle bone Disease)

- It is the most common genetic cause of osteoporosis in children

- It is a generalized disorder of connective tissue matrix of bone

Etiology

- Structural or quantitative defects in **type I collagen**.
- Type I collagen is the primary component of the extracellular matrix of bone and skin.
- Other cases are caused by recessive null mutations in a collagen-modifying enzyme, **prolyl 3-hydroxylase 1** (coded by the *LEPRE1* gene on chromosome 1p34.1) or its associated protein, **CRTAP.**

Pathology

- The bone matrix contains **abnormal type I collagen fibrils.**
- Relatively **increased** levels of **types III and V collagen**.
- Several non-collagenous proteins of bone matrix are also reduced.
- The **hydroxyapatite crystals** deposited on matrix are poorly aligned with the long axis of fibrils.

Clinical Manifestations

OI has the triad of:

- Fragile bones
- Blue sclerae
- Early deafness.

The **Sillence classification** divides OI into four types based on clinical and radiographic criteria.

Osteogenesis Imperfecta Type I (Mild)

- Mild disease
- Families have blue sclerae
- Recurrent fractures in childhood
- Presenile hearing loss (30-60%)
- **Dentinogenesis imperfecta**
- Easy bruising
- Joint laxity
- Mild short stature

Osteogenesis Imperfecta Type II (Perinatal Lethal)

- Infants may be **stillborn or die** in the 1st yr of life.
- Birthweight and length are small for gestational age.
- There is extreme fragility of the skeleton and other connective tissues.
- There are **multiple intrauterine fractures** of long bones.
- **Crumpled appearance** on radiographs.
- **Micromelia** and bowing of extremities.
- The legs are held abducted at right angles to body **(frog-leg position).**
- **Multiple rib fractures** create a beaded appearance.
- **Small thorax** leading to respiratory insufficiency.
- The skull is large for body size, with enlarged anterior and posterior fontanels.
- **Sclerae are dark blue-gray**.

Osteogenesis Imperfecta Type III (Progressive Deforming)

- Most severe nonlethal form of OI.
- Results in significant physical disability.
- Birthweight and length are often low normal.
- Fractures usually occur in utero.
- Relative **macrocephaly** and **triangular facies**
- Fractures occur from inconsequential trauma and heal with deformity.
- Disorganization of the bone matrix results in a **"popcorn" appearance** at the **metaphyses.**
- Basal flaring of rib cage has and pectal deformity.
- **Scoliosis** and **vertebral compression**.
- **Extreme short stature**.
- Scleral hue ranges from white to blue.

Osteogenesis Imperfecta Type IV (Moderately Severe)

- In utero fractures and congenital bowing of lower long bones.
- Recurrent fractures after ambulation.
- Fracture rates decrease after puberty.
- X-ray: Osteoporosis metaphyseal flaring and vertebral compressions.
- Moderate short stature.
- Scleral hue may be blue or white.

Osteogenesis Imperfecta Type V (Hyperplastic Callus) and Type VI (Mineralization Defect)

- Have distinct findings on bone histology.
- Hyperplastic callus.
- Calcification of the interosseous membrane of the forearm.
- Radiodense metaphyseal band.
- The genetic etiology is unknown (No collagen defect).
- They constitute <5% of OI populations.

Osteogenesis Imperfecta Types VII and VIII (Recessive Form)

- Types VII and VIII patients have null mutations in **P3H1** and **CRTAP,** respectively.
- Clinically they **overlap types II and III OI.**
- Distinct features including.

– **White sclerae**
– **Rhizomelia**

- Small to normal head circumference
- Surviving children have **severe osteochondro-dysplasia**
- Extreme short stature
- Dual energy X-ray absorptiometry (DEXA) L1-L2 z-score in the–6 to–7 range

12. Cleft palate is repaired at: (Repeat)

A. 2 - 4 months **B.** 1 - 4 weeks
C. 6 - 12 months **D.** 12 - 38 months

Ans: C. 6 - 12 months

Ref: *Nelson's Textbook of Pediatrics, 19th Edition*

Explanation:

*"In an otherwise healthy child, **closure of the palate** is usually done **before 1 yr of age** to enhance normal speech development." Ref: Nelson*

*"Surgical closure of a **cleft lip** is usually performed by **3 mo of age**, when the infant has shown satisfactory weight gain and is free of any oral, respiratory, or systemic infection." Ref: Nelson*

DERMATOLOGY

1. Epidermolysis bullosa is due to:

A. Autoimmune disease
B. Atopic disease
C. Infective agent
D. Genetic fragility of skin

Ans: D. Genetic fragility of skin

Ref: *Rook's Dermatology, 8th ed.*

Explanation: (See the following Table)

HEREDITARY TYPES

- Congenital absence of components

ACQUIRED TYPES

- Autoantibodies (IgG; sometimes IgA) to type VII collagen.

CLINICAL FEATURES

1. **Epidermolysis Bullosa Simplex**
   - Autosomal dominant
   - Mutation in keratin 5,14
   - Sites of trauma/friction
   - Involve hands, feet and neck; occ. knees and elbows
   - Teeth not affected; intraoral blisters seen
   - Appears during infancy
   - No scarring
2. **Junctional Epidermolysis Bullosa**
   - Autosomal recessive
   - Mutation in **uncein, laminin 5, BPAg 2** (anchoring filaments)
   - Haemorrhagic blisters; loss of nails, large blisters of face, trunk and extremities
   - Generalized scarring and atrophy
   - Intraorally-haemorrhagic blisters of palate, perioral and perinasal areas
   - Erupted teeth exhibit hypoplastic and severely pitted enamel prone to caries
3. **Dystrophic Epidermolysis Bullosa**
   - Both autosomal dominant and recessive; recessive is severe
   - Lesions are birth; arise at pressure sites
   - Blisters rupture leaving painful ulcers which heal with large scars that undergo contractures, leading to loss of motility and claw-like hands (**Mitten Deformity**)
   - Teeth exhibit delayed eruption and enamel hypoplasia with rapid caries development
   - Scarring around mouth leads to diminished opening, **ankyloglossia**
   - Mutation in type 7 collagen (anchoring fibrils)

Skin Structure

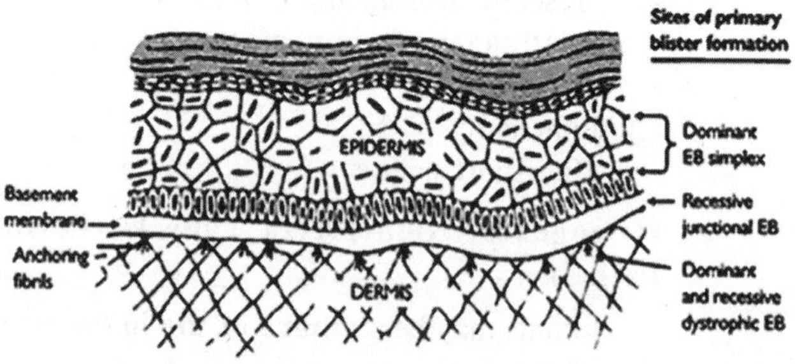

Type	Genetic Pattern	Separation Level	Defective Structure
Hereditary			
Simplex	AD	Intraepithelial	Linking proteins
Junctional	AR	Lamina lucida	Anchoring filaments
Dystrophic	AD	Sublamina densa	Type VII collagen
Acquired			
Acquisita	None/autoimmune	Sublamina densa	Type VII collagen

2. **Ridley-Jopling classification includes all *except:***
   A. Lepromatous leprosy
   B. Borderline borderline
   C. Tuberculoid
   D. Neuritic

   Ans: D. Neuritic

Ref: Thappa, Essentials in Dermatology, 1st ed. Pg 236

Explanation:

- Ridley and Jopling classified leprosy taking into account the immunological and histopathological basis in addition to clinical and bacteriological findings.

Classification

- Tuberculoid Tuberculoid (TT)
- Borderline Tuberculoid (BT)
- Borderline Borderline/ Mid Borderline/ Dimorphous leprosy (BB)
- Borderline Lepromatous (BL)
- Lepromatous Lepromatous (LL)

Note: Two other types of leprosy which are not classified under Ridley-Jopling classification (but included in Indian Leprologist Association classification) are:

- **Indeterminate leprosy**
- **Polyneuritic leprosy**

3. **Most common nerve affected in leprosy is:**
   A. Radial nerve **B.** Ulnar nerve
   C. Median nerve **D.** Axillary nerve

   Ans: B. Ulnar nerve

Ref: The Disease. In Jopling WH, McDougall AC, editors. Handbook of Leprosy, 5th edn., New Delhi: CBS Publishers and Distributors 2005;10-53.
Clinical Leprosy. In: Thappa DM, editor. Essentials in Dermatology, 2ndedn., New Delhi: Jaypee Brothers Medical Publishers (P) Ltd 2009;333-50.

Explanation:

- Nerves invaded by leprosy bacilli are either dermal (cutaneous nerves) or nerve trunks
- Nerves that are most vulnerable are those:
  - That are in **cooler regions** of the body – nerves that are more superficial are more cooler
  - That are subject to repeated trauma
- These include:
  - **Ulnar nerves** just above the elbow – palsy causes ulnar claw hand – **most common to be involved in leprosy**
  - **Median nerves** at wrist – ape thumb deformity
  - **Lateral popliteal** or **common peroneal nerves** as they wind around neck of fibula – palsy causes foot drop
  - **Posterior tibial nerve** behind medial malleoli – palsy causes clawing of toes or hammer toes
  - **Facial nerve** - facial palsy
  - Others – radial cutaneous nerve at wrist, greater auricular nerves in neck, supraclavicular nerves as they cross the clavicles, sural nerves at back of legs, superficial peroneal nerves in front of ankles
- **Radial nerve** is **very rarely affected** as it is located at a higher and deeper level and does not lie superficial. Only the peripheral branch–the radial cutaneous nerve is affected commonly due to its superficial location.
- **Axillary nerve** is **never** affected in **leprosy**.

4. **Apple jelly nodules are seen in:**
   A. Ichthyosis vulgaris **B.** Lichen planus
   C. Lupus vulgaris **D.** Lupus erythematous

   Ans: C. Lupus vulgaris

Ref: Principles of Diagnosis in Dermatology. In: Thappa DM, editor. Essentials in Dermatology, 2ndedn., New Delhi: Jaypee Brothers Medical Publishers (P) Ltd 2009;16-30
Mycobacterial Diseases. In: James WD, Berger TG, Elston DM, editors. Andrew's Diseases of the Skin: Clinical Dermatology, 11th edn., Saunders Elsevier 2011; 322-33)

Explanation:

- **Lupus vulgaris** is a type of **progressive cutaneous tuberculosis.**
- Occurs in people with moderate to **high immunity.**
- Single plaque composed of grouped redbrown papules with peripheral extension on one side and scarring on the other side.
- On diascopy of active edge-translucent pale brownish yellow or **apple jelly colour** in the periphery – **apple jelly nodules** – **granulomatous nodules.**
- **Diascopy/vitropression:**
  - Compression with a glass slide useful in.
  - Differentiating purpura (no blanching) from erythema (blanches).
  - Differentiating nevus anemicus (margins blurred) from nevus depigmentosus (no change).

ANESTHESIOLOGY

1. **Which of the following mechanism prevents fitting of wrong gas cylinder to the anaesthesia machine in operation theatre? (Repeat)**

   A. Pin index system **B.** Yolk assembly
   C. Bodock seal **D.** Gas analyser

   Ans: A. Pin index system

   Ref: *Miller Textbook of Anaesthesia. 6th edition*

   Explanation:

   - The **Pin Index Safety System,** or PISS, is a safety system that uses geometric features on the yoke to ensure that pneumatic connections between a gas cylinder and a machine that uses pressurized gases are not connected to the wrong gas yoke.
   - This system can be seen on an anesthesia machine.
   - Each gas cylinder has a pin configuration to fit its respective gas yoke.

   PIN Index of Commonly Used Gases in Anesthesia

   - **O_2: 2-5**
   - **N_2O: 3-5**
   - **Air: 1-5**
   - **CO_2: 1-6**
   - **Heliox: 2-4**
   - **Entonox: 7**

2. **Centrineuraxial anaesthesia is not contra-indicated in:**

   A. Platelets <80,000
   B. Patient on aspirin
   C. Patient on anticoagulants
   D. Raised intracranial pressure

   Ans: B. Patient on aspirin

   Ref: *Miller Textbook of Anaesthesia. 6th edition*

   Explanation

   - Patients on **Single antiplatelet drug** is **not a contraindication to central neuraxial blockade,** whereas patients on **multiple antiplatelet drugs** are contraindicated for neuraxial anesthesia.
   - Patients on **Anticoagulants, Fibrinolytic agents and Thrombocytopenia** (platelet count <80,000) are at risk of bleeding and neuraxial hematoma with a possibility of spinal cord compression. Such patients are contraindicated for neuraxial anesthesia.
   - Patients with **raised Intracranial pressure** carry a risk of coning of the brainstem and death. Such patients are contraindicated for neuraxial anesthesia.

   Contraindications for Centrineuraxial Anesthesia

   - Anticoagulants
   - Fibrinolytic agents
   - Thrombocytopenia
   - Raised intracranial pressure
   - Multiple antiplatelet drugs

3. **All are true about ether *except:***

   A. It has additional sympathomimetic effect
   B. Can undergo spontaneous decomposition when exposed to light
   C. It has additional bronchodilator and analgesic effects
   D. It inhibits salivation

   Ans: D. It inhibits salivation

   Ref: *Miller Textbook of Anaesthesia. 6th edition*

   Explanation:

Ether

Physical Properties:

- It is a pungent smelling liquid, decomposes in the presence of light, air and heat. So stored in amber coloured bottles.
- Highly inflammable and explosive.
- Highly irritant vapour.

Anesthetic Properties:

- Induction is very slow (Blood gas coefficient 12.0).
- Very unpleasant smelling -> Increased chances of laryngospasm.
- Potency is moderate (MAC – 1.92).
- Very good analgesic.
- Usually required concentration is 5 – 15%.
- Very good muscle relaxation.
- Delivery method: By open drop, EMO inhaler, copper kettle vaporizer.

Systemic Effects

CVS

- It does not depress myocardium rather it stimulates sympathetic system causing tachycardia and hypertension.
- Baroreceptor reflex is preserved with ether so it can be used safely in shock.

Resp System

- It does not depress respiration; infact it stimulates it.
- Ventilatory response to hypoxia and hypercarbia are preserved.
- Potent bronchodilator.
- It preserves ciliary activity (*Only inhalational agent to do so).
- Increases tracheobronchial secretions markedly – so atropine premedication is required.

GIT

- Highest incidence of nausea and vomiting among inhalational agents

CNS

- Increased intracranial pressure

Metabolic

- It releases catecholamines and can cause hyperglycemia. Avoided in diabetics.

Uteroplacental Barrier

- It readily crosses placenta and can cause respiratory depression in newborn

4. **Dead space is increased by all *except:***
   A. Anticholinergic drugs
   B. Standing
   C. Hyperextention of neck
   D. Endotracheal intubation

Ans: D. Endotracheal intubation

Ref: *Miller Textbook of Anaesthesia. 6th edition*

Explanation:

Dead Space

- **Endotracheal intubation** bypasses the gases from upper respiratory tract thereby **decreasing the anatomical dead space.**
- **Dead space increases** with **standing** and **hyperextension** of the **neck** as the volume of the upper respiratory tract increases.
- **Anticholinergics** increase the diameter of the upper airway by **bronchodilatation** and **antisialagogue action** thereby increasing the dead space.
- **Normal dead space-150 ml (1/3rd of the normal tidal volume).**

5. **Anesthetic which increases intracranial tension: (Repeat)**
   A. Ketamine **B.** Propofol
   C. Etomidate **D.** Ether

Ans: A. Ketamine

Ref: *Ajay Yadav, Short Textbook of Pediatrics 1st edition pg. 76 & Miller Textbook of Anaesthesia. 6th edition*

Explanation:

Ketamine

- Causes **Dissociative anesthesia**
- Phencyclidine derivative
- **NMDA receptor agonist**
- **Anesthetic Properties**
  - Onset of Action: 30 – 60 seconds.
  - Early regain of consciousness after 15 – 20 min due to **Redistribution.**
  - Elimination half life: 2-3 hours.
  - **Strong analgesic property.**
  - Metabolised in **Liver** and products excreted in **urine.**
  - Not a muscle relaxant.
- Primary site of action – **Thalamo-neo-cortical projections.**

Cardiovascular System

- Increases arterial BP.
- Increases heart rate.
- Increases cardiac output.
- IV agent of choice in **SHOCK.**

Respiratory System

- **Potent bronchodilator.**
- Good induction agent for asthmatics.
- **Upper airway reflexes remain largely intact.**
- Increases salivatory and tracheobronchial secretions.
- Using glycopyrollate or atropine becomes necessary.

Central Nervous System

- **Increases intracranial pressure** and can precipitate **seizures.**
- **Emergence reactions:**
  - These are seen at emergence.
  - Vivid dreaming.
  - Illusions.
  - Extracorporeal experiences like floating.
  - Excitement.
  - Confusión.
  - Euphoria.
  - Fear.
- **Hallucinations:**
  - Auditory and visual hallucinations (Most Common side effect of Ketamine).
  - Treated with Benzodiazepine.

Other Systems

- **Eye**
  - Increase intraocular tensión.
  - Pupils dilate moderately.
  - Nystagmus.
- **GIT**
  - Increases intragastric pressure.
  - Salivary secretions increased.
- **Muscular**
  - Increases muscle tone.
  - Increased non-purposeful movements.

Dose

Can be given IV, IM, oral, rectal and intrathecal route.
IV – 2 mg/kg.
IM – 5-10 mg/kg.

Advantages

- **Induction Agent of Choice in:**
  - Asthmatics.
  - Shock.
  - Children (Now Sevoflurance is DOC).
  - Constrictive pericarditis.
  - Cardiac tamponade.
- Can be used as **SOLE** agent.
- Can be used safely at remote places and in inexperienced hands since does not depress heart or respiration.
- Preferred agent when patient is in FULL STOMACH (Preserves laryngo-pharyngeal reflexes).

Contraindicated in:

- Head injury.
- ICSOL.
- Eye injury.
- Opthal pathology.
- Ischemic heart disease.
- Vascular aneurysm.
- Psychiatric diseases.
- Drug addicts.
- Hypertensives.

RADIOLOGY

1. **Thymus is rarely discovered in chest X-ray after the age of:**

   A. 6 months **B.** 2 years
   C. 4 years **D.** 8 years

   Ans: D. 8 years

   Ref: *Arthur R. Interpretation of the Paediatric Chest X-ray; Current Paediatrics (2003) 13, 438—447*

   Explanation:

Thymus Gland

- The thymus gland gives rise to a **prominent anterior mediastinal shadow** in **infancy** which is quite variable in size and can be recognized by its characteristic **'sail' shape** or **wavy margins** resulting from the interdigitation of the soft thymic tissue in the intercostal spaces.
- The thymus gradually becomes less evident between the **ages of 2-8 years**, after which it cannot be visualized on the frontal chest X-ray.
- At times, the normal thymus can appear very large, and may need to be differentiated from a mediastinal mass or an area of pulmonary consolidation.
- A **lateral decubitus view** of the chest may accentuate the **scalloped appearance** of the thymic outline and help to clarify the nature of an anterior mediastinal shadow.

2. **Causes of thickened gallbladder wall on ultra-sound examination are all *except:***

   A. Postprandial state
   B. Cholecystitis
   C. Congestive cardiac failure
   D. Kawasaki disease

   Ans: D. Kawasaki disease

   Ref: *Manual of Emergency Critical Care Ultrasound. Vicke E Noble. 2nd ed. Pg 156*

   Explanation:

- Kawasaki disease is associated with hydrops of gallbladder.

Gallbladder Wall Thickening

- A gallbladder wall that is thickened is a sign of inflammation. This is a non-specific finding, and many other pathologic processes, as well as a postprandial gallbladder, can give you falsely elevated measurements.
- It is important to measure the wall of the anterior gallbladder surface because of the acoustic enhancement artifact mentioned.
- Because sound waves travel through a fluid-filled structure, no attenuation occurs. Thus, when those sound waves hit the back of the gallbladder, they will be so strong that they will obscure an accurate picture of the wall thickness.
- For gallbladder wall thickness, greater than **3 mm** is abnormal.

Differential for Thickened Gallbladder Wall

- Postprandial

- Renal failure
- Ascites
- Hepatitis
- Hypoalbuminemia
- HIV/AIDS
- Adenomyomatosis
- Multiple myeloma
- Cholecystitis
- Congestive heart failure

3. **Popcorn calcification in lung is characteristic of:**
   A. Congenital adenoid malformation
   B. Hamartoma
   C. Small cell Ca lung
   D. Bronchial carcinoids

Ans: B. Hamartoma

Ref: *Multiple Sources*

Explanation:

Chest X-Ray Findings

Heart and Blood Vessels

- Flask-shaped / Pear-shaped / Leathe- bottle / Money-bag shaped heart - Pericardial effusion
- Boot-shaped heart / Coer-en-sabot - Fallot's tetralogy
- Box shaped appearance - Tricuspid atresia
- Jug Handle appearance - Primary pulmonary artery hypertension
- "3" like appearance - Coarctation of Aorta
- Egg on side appearance - Transposition of great vessels
- Egg in cup appearance - Constrictive pericarditis
- Snow-man heart - TAPVC (total anomalous pulmonary venous connection)
- Figure of '8' - TAPVC (total anomalous pulmonary venous connection)
- Cottage leaf appearance - TAPVC
- Pericardial calcification - Constrictive pericarditis
- Calcification in heart wall - is seen in - Carcinoid syndrome
- Calfication of ascending aorta - Atherosclerosis, Syphilis
- Hilar dance on fluoroscopy - Atrial Septal Defect
- X-ray finding in Ebstein's anomaly - Pulmonary oligemia
- Posterior displacement of trachea - seen in - aneurysm of aorta
- Obliteration of left border of heart (PA view of chest) is - suggestive of - Lingular pathology (left lung)
- Bat's wings appearance - Pulmonary oedema
- Pruned tree appearance (of pulmonary circulation) - Pulmonary artery hypertension

Lungs

- Ground glass appearance - Hyaline membrane disease.
- Solitary pulmonary mass lesion > 4 cms - is most commonly due to - Bronchial adenoma.
- Honey Comb appearance.
- SarcoidosisQ.
- Histiocytosis X.
- Interstitial lung diseaseQ.
- TuberculosisQ.
- Collagen disordersQ.
- PneumoconiosisQ.
- Drugs - bleomycin, busulphan, melphalan, cyclophosphamide.
- Meniscus sign / Crescent sign (mobile mass in pulmonary cavity) is most commonly seen in - Aspergilloma (fungal ball lesion).
- Egg-Shell calcification - SilicosisQ, SarcoidosisQ, Coal miner's pneumoconiosisQ, Lymphoma following radiotherapyQ.
- Pop-corn calcification / Craggy pop-corn calcification - Pulmonary Hamartoma.
- Pleural calcification - most common cause is - Tuberculosis (Asbestosis).
- Diaphragmatic pleura calcification - is due to - Asbestosis.
- Calcification in a pulmonary metastasis - is most commomly due to - Osteosarcoma.
- Coin shadow in the lung (single), with calcification in the centre - Epidermoid carcinoma.
- For radiologically evident pleural effusion - the minimal amount of pleural fluid that should be present is - 250 ml.
- Plethoric lung fields - seen in - L-R shunts (VSD, PDA, ASD).
- Oligemic lung fields - Pulmonary atreisa, Stenosis; Ebstein's anomaly.
- Perihilar fluffy opacities - seen in - Pulmonary venous hypertension.

Ribs

- Superior surface notch of ribs - seen in - Hyper-parathyroidsm, Neurofibromatosis, Connective tissue disorders.
- Inferior surface notch of ribs - seen in - Coarctation of Aorta, SVC obstruction, Chest wall AV fistula, Aortic Thrombosis.
- Unilateral notching of ribs - Coarctation of Left subclavian artery, Subclavian artery block, Blalock-Taussig Operation.

Others

- Displacement of tracheal shadow - most common cause is - Thyroid swelling.
- Water Lily sign - Ruptured hydatid cyst.

4. **All are characteristic radiological features of cardiogenic pulmonary edema *except:***
A. Bilateral infiltrates **B.** Cardiomegaly
C. Kerley B lines **D.** Oligemia

Ans: D. Oligemia

Ref: *Harrison's Principles of Internal Medicine 18th ed.*

Explanation:

- There are two basic types of pulmonary edema. One is cardiogenic edema caused by increased hydrostatic pulmonary capillary pressure.
- The other is termed non-cardiogenic pulmonary edema, and is caused by either altered capillary membrane permeability or decreased plasma oncotic pressure.

A helpful mnemonic for noncardiogenic pulmonary edema is NOT CARDIAC (near-drowning, oxygen therapy, transfusion or trauma, CNS disorder, ARDS, aspiration, or altitude sickness, renal disorder or resuscitation, drugs, inhaled toxins, allergic alveolitis, contrast or contusion.

Chest X-ray Findings in Cardiogenic Pulmonary Edema

- Cephalization of the pulmonary vessels
- Kerley B lines or septal lines
- Peribronchial cuffing
- "Bat wing" pattern
- Patchy shadowing with air bronchograms
- Increased cardiac size
- Unilateral, miliary and lobar or lower zone edema are considered atypical patterns of cardiac pulmonary edema.
- A unilateral pattern may be caused by lying preferentially on one side.
- Unusual patterns of edema may be found in patients with COPD who have predominant upper lobe emphysema.

PSYCHIATRY

1. **In a patient with strikingly abnormal behaviour, the most likely diagnosis is:**
A. Paranoid schizophrenia
B. Catatonic schizophrenia
C. Hebephrenic schizophrenia
D. Simple schizophrenia

Ans: B. Catatonic schizophrenia

Ref: *Synopsis of Psychiatry, Kaplan & Sadock, 10th edition*

Explanation:

- Schizophrenia is one of most severe mental disorders. It is basically a disorder of thought.
- The term was coined by "Bleuler".
- His idea about schizophrenia centered around 4As – Loosening of Associations (between thoughts and feelings, between thoughts themselves), Ambivalence, Affective flattening and Avolition.
- Kraeplein used the term "dementia precox" (meaning dementia in younger age) for patients with symptoms suggestive of schizophrenia.
- Schneider gave an account of "first rank symptoms" which are characteristic (but not pathognomonic) of schizophrenia.

Currently DSM-IV reserve this term to denote a syndrome characterized by:

1. Hallucinations
2. Delusions
3. Disorganized speech
4. Disorganized behaviour
5. Negative symptoms.

- ICD-10 lays heavy emphasis on Schneider's first rank symptoms.
- Both classificatory systems use sub-typing of schizophrenia
  - **Paranoid** – Delusions and hallucinations are marked
  - **Hebephrenic** – Disorganized speech (word salad) and behaviour (mannerisms and stereotypy) are marked
  - **Catatonic** – Stupor / **excitement**, mutism, starring, posturing, waxy flexibility, negativism, echolalia/echopraxia are presenting features. Carries best prognosis (means symptoms resolve rapidly with ECT)
  - **Simple** – Chronic negative symptoms (alogia, avolition, amotivation, affective blunting) without conspicuous positive symptoms. Carries worst prognosis.

2. **Wernicke Korsakoff's syndrome is due to the deficiency of which of the following (Repeat):**
A. Pyridoxine
B. Thiamine
C. Vitamin B^{12}
D. Riboflavin

Ans. B. Thiamine

Ref: *Synopsis of Psychiatry, Kaplan & Sadock, 10th edition*

Explanation:

See 2010 Psychiatry question explanation.

3. **Infantile autism is seen as a:**
A. Dysthymic personality disorder
B. Personality disorder
C. Paranoid personality
D. Behavioral disorder

Ans: D. Behavioural disorder

Ref: *Synopsis of Psychiatry, Kaplan & Sadock, 10th edition*

Explanation:

- **Personality disorders** are entirely different group of disorders.
- They are diagnosed ONLY after the age of 18 (the age at which one's personality might have developed well).
- Personality is a unique way of perceiving, experiencing, thinking, feeling and behaving.
- Based on the similarities, the entire population of the world are typed into two – A & B.
- **Type A personality** people are high energy packed whereas **B type people** are cool. Such typing is physiological, hence normal.

Personality disorder is used when one's personality is inflexible, resulting in distress for self and others and/or dysfunction. Both ICD-10 and DSM-IV code personality disorders.

In the latter, they have been grouped as "clusters"– there are 3 clusters viz.

Cluster A (ODD)

1. **Paranoid** – suspiciousness is the hallmark
2. **Schizoid** – self-imposed social isolation
3. **Schizotypal** – both paranoid and schizoid traits present in the same person

Cluster B (DRAMATIC)

1. **Antisocial** – psychopaths with no empathy for fellow humans, seen in most of the criminals
2. **Borderline** – empty feelings resulting in "micro-psychotic" episodes, impulsivity, rapid formation as well as rapid dissolution of relationships, self-injurious behaviour (wrist-slashing), mostly seen in females
3. **Narcissistic** – self-loving, boasting and projecting oneself as the best in the world, seen in men.
4. **Histrionic** – same as narcissistic along with attention seeking and seductive behaviour, seen in females

Cluster C (ANXIOUS)

1. **Dependent** – needs someone always for support
2. **Avoidant** – exactly opposite to dependent, shy and not mingling with others
3. **Anankastic** (obsessive-compulsive) – perfectionist, time-bound, rule-bound. (Don't get confused with OCD, since there is neither obsession nor compulsion here, efforts to erase such misnomer are underway!)

Others / Unspecified

1. **Depressive** – chronic low mood state and unrelishing anything / everything in life.
2. **Passive-aggressive** – showing the anger by indirect means (coming late to class, sickness absenteeism).
3. **Sadistic** – getting pleasure by hurting others, Masochistic – getting pleasure by being hurt.

4. **Systematic desensitization as form of therapy is done in (Repeat):**
A. Phobia
B. Obsessive compulsive disorder
C. Generalized anxiety disorder
D. Hypochondriasis

Ans: A. Phobia

Ref: *Synopsis of Psychiatry, Kaplan & Sadock, 10th edition*

Explanation:

Systematic Desensitization

It is a type of '**Behavior therapy**' (which in turn is a type of **Psychotherapy**).

It is based on the principle of "**Respondent Conditioning**".

It was first elaborated by **Wolpe**.

It is used to treat 'Phobias' (Specific and Social).

It consists of three steps- [**HCG**-pneumonic]

1. **Hierarchy chart** (where anxiety/fear provoking stimuli are identified and charted from lowest to highest level of potency in inducing the anxiety/fear)
2. **Coping skills** (learning to relax, by various methods like – paced breathing exercises, Jacobson's progressive muscle relaxation, applied relaxation by meditation)
3. **Graded exposure** (applying the relaxation techniques after exposing oneself to the anxiety/fear provoking stimuli in graded manner, i.e., from weakest stimulus to strongest stimulus)

Other Forms of Exposure Therapy

1. **Flooding**- Sudden exposure and making one to cope up at one go.
2. **Virtual Reality Exposure** – Useful for PTSD

3. **ERP: Exposure and Response Prevention-** Unlike other exposure therapies, here, the escape is not allowed completely and even in between the sessions. Used in OCD.

Psychotherapy

- It is one of three forms of therapy (the other two are – chemical, i.e., drugs and physical, i.e., ECT, Psychosurgery, VNS, rTMS).
- It involves patient –therapist co-operation and usually conducted in sessions.
- The following is an outline of psychotherapies practiced worldwide.
  1. **Supportive psychotherapy** (often termed as counseling), is the most widely used method
  2. **Cognitive therapy** (for depression, anxiety disorders, eating disorders, sexual disorders)
  3. **Behavior therapy** (anxiety disorders like OCD, childhood behavioral problems)
  4. **Cognitive-Behavior therapy (CBT)-** Highly useful and often an alternative to substance abuse (a special form called Motivation Enhancement Therapy used here), depres-sion, anxiety disorders, eating disorders, sexual disorders.
  5. **Dialectical** – Behavior therapy– useful for BPD (Borderline personality disorder).
  6. **Psychoanalytical / Psychodynamic therapy-** Not used as before, however useful in conversion / dissociative disorders.

5. **Morbid jealousy is seen in:**
   A. Alcoholism
   B. Persons who are isolated from society
   C. Social phobia
   D. Depression

Ans: A. Alcoholism

Ref: *Synopsis of Psychiatry, Kaplan & Sadock, 10th edition*

Explanation:

- **Morbid jealousy** is pathological suspiciousness of **fidelity of close ones**, usually **spouse**.
- It is one of "overvalued ideas".
- An overvalued idea is also a false belief, but contrary to delusion, the person is less convinced and not sure/firm (i.e., shakeable).
- **Morbid jealousy** is seen in **chronic alcoholics**.

6. **Electroconvulsive therapy not useful on *except:***
   A. Delirium **B.** Seizures
   C. Depression **D.** Panic attacks

Ans: C. Depression

Ref: *Synopsis of Psychiatry, Kaplan & Sadock, 10th edition*

Explanation:

Electro-Convulsive Therapy [ECT]

- It is one of the physical methods of treatment in psychiatry.
- Psychosurgery, Vagal Nerve Stimulation [VNS], Repetitive Transcranial Magnetic Stimulation [rTMS], Deep Brain Stimulation [DBS] are other physical methods.
- ECT is very effective in treating:
  - **Severe depression with suicidality**
  - **Catatonia**
  - **Mania/Excitement**
  - **OCD** (intractable cases)
- The exact mechanism of action of ECT is not known but it has been hypothesized that direct stimulation of neurons by current and / or activation of HPA axis / HPT axis or enhancement of certain neurotransmitters like serotonin are proposed.
- Whatever the mechanism, ECT is not only effective but also rapid in its effect (drugs might take days and psychotherapy might take months to show efficacy) and safe also.

Contraindications:

1. ***Absolute contraindication***
   Raised intracranial pressure (the ONLY absolute contraindication) as evidenced by papilledema clinically.
2. ***Relative contraindications*** (which means, the following conditions should be treated adequately and patient should be fit) – *Hypertension, Diabetes, Sepsis,* etc.

Types of ECT:

1. Unmodified (No anaesthesia).
2. Modified (under general anaesthesia) [Note - In many countries, including India, unmodified ECT is illegal and banned].

Drugs Used in ECT:

1. IV anaesthetic agents like **methohexiatone, thiopentone sodium** and **propofal**
2. Muscle relaxants like **succinylcholine**
3. Anti-secretary agents like **atrophine, glycopyrrolate**

Side Effects of ECT:

- Transient delirium

- Headache
- Nausea
- Body aches
- *Reversible memory loss (both retrograde and anterograde)*

7. **True statement regarding Ganser's syndrome is:**
   A. Involuntary
   B. Psychotic symptoms absent
   C. Memory symptoms absent
   D. Approximate answers

   Ans: D. Approximate answers

   Ref: *Bhatia's Textbook of Psychiatry, P.185*

   Explanation:

Ganser's Syndrome

- It is a **voluntary** production of **psychotic**, **memory symptoms** and **approximate answers**.
- It is common in **males**, especially seen in **prison inmates/ hospitalized persons**.
- It is a form of **malingering** (voluntary and wilful production of symptoms with the aim of *materialistic gain*) [Note–Voluntary production of symptoms for *immaterial gains-Factitious disorder*].
- E.g., if a female complains of headache to get money from her husband and spending it on movies – malingering. If the female complains of headache get attention and affection from her ever-running husband– factitious disorder.
- **Approximate answers**- Vorbeireden
- **Verbegeration**- Meaningless repetition of words (syn. *Cataphasia)*
- **Neologism**- New word with only self-referential meaning.
- **Word salad**- Mixing up of syllables resulting in un-understandable words.
- All three are seen in **Schizophrenia**.

JIPMER–2008

ANATOMY

1. **Hassall's corpuscles are present in:**
   A. Bone marrow **B.** Thymic Cortex
   C. Medulla of Thymus **D.** Splenic sinusoids

   Ans: C. Medulla of Thymus

   Ref: *Wheater's functional histology: A text and colour atlas.5th edition,2007,Page.217*

   Explanation:

   Hassall's corpuscles:
   - Are present in the **medulla** of **thymus.**
   - **Round or oval bodies** made up of **concentric cells** derived from epithelial reticular cells which surround the central pink stained hyaline mass, represent a degenerative phenomenon.
   - **3 types :**
     (a) ***Concentric*** type giving onion peel appearance
     (b) ***Cystic*** type where the cysts are filled with degenerated material or dead cells
     (c) ***Compound*** type
   - **3 stages** in the formation & maturation of Hassall's corpuscle:
     (a) Stage of **secretion**
     (b) Stage of **absorption**
     (c) Stage of **hyalinization**
   - *Time of appearance:* **8th week** of intrauterine life, number increased during **17th to 24th week** of IUL.
   - *Functions:* Act as a **grave yard** for **T-lymphocytes** which are **not immunocompetent.**

2. **True statement regarding bare area of liver:**
   A. Covered by visceral peritoneum
   B. Supplied by phrenic nerve
   C. Present in the left lobe of liver
   D. Attached to the diaphragm

   Ans: D. Attached to the diaphragm

   Ref: *Gray's Anatomy, 39th edition, 2008.Page.1222*

   Explanation:

   Bare area of liver:
   - The "bare area" of the liver is the part of its surface not covered by peritoneum.
   - It is situated **posteriorly on the right lobe** and is in contact with the diaphragm.
   - Between the 2 layers (superior & inferior) of coronary ligament there is a large triangular area of liver
   - Which is devoid of peritoneal covering i.e. bare area
   - Here the liver is attached to the diaphragm by **areolar tissue**
   - The parietal peritoneum, particularly in the area of the bare area and superior surface is supplied by **lower intercostal nerves** (lower six)

   Note: Superior & inferior coronary ligament is formed by the reflection peritoneum from the diaphragm onto the posterior surfaces of the **right lobe of liver**.

   Other areas not covered with peritoneum are:
   (a) Fossa for gallbladder
   (b) Fissure for the ligamentum venosum
   (c) Groove for inferior vena cava

3. **Which of the following artery gives rise to posterior gastric artery? (Repeat)**
   A. Left gastric artery
   B. Right gastric artery
   C. Splenic artery
   D. Left gastroepiploic artery

   Ans: C. Splenic artery

   Ref: *Gray's Anatomy, 39th edition, 2008.Page 1147*

   Explanation:
   - Posterior gastric artery arises from the **splenic artery** in its middle section posterior to the body of the stomach.
   - It ascends behind the peritoneum of the lesser sac towards the fundus.
   - It reaches the posterior surface of the stomach in the gastrophrenic fold.

STOMACH

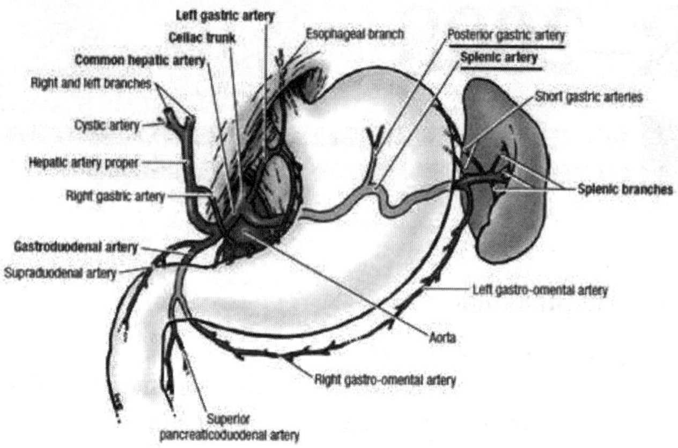

4. **Hypoglossal nerve supplies all the following muscles *except:*:**

A. Styloglossus B. Hyoglossus
C. Palatoglossus D. Genioglossus

Ans: C. Palatoglossus

Ref: *Gray's Anatomy, 39th edition, 2008.Page 628*

Explanation:

Palatoglossus:

- It is supplied by cranial part of **accessory nerve** via pharyngeal plexus (Some books mention as **Vagus** nerve via pharyngeal plexus and accessory nerve)
- ***Origin:*** from the palatine aponeurosis,passes downwards in front of tonsil (palatoglossal arch)
- ***Insertion:*** into the sides of tongue
- ***Action:*** elevates the root of tongue
- ***Blood supply:*** ascending palatine branch of facial artery and ascending pharyngeal artery.
- **Remember**:
  (a) All the muscles of **tongue** is supplied by **hypoglossal nerve** except **palatoglossus** which is supplied by accesory nerve
  (b) All the muscles of **pharynx** is supplied by cranial part of **accessory nerve** except **stylopharyngeus** which is supplied by **glossopharyngeal** nerve
  (c) All the muscles of **larynx** is supplied by **recurrent laryngeal nerve** except **cricothyroid** which is supplied by **external laryngeal nerve**

5. **All the following extra ocular muscles are supplied by 3rd nerve *except:***

A. Lateral rectus B. Medial rectus
C. Superior rectus D. Inferior oblique

Ans: A. Lateral rectus

Ref: *Gray's Anatomy, 39th edition, 2008.Page 693*

Explanation:

- **Oculomotor nerve (3rd nerve)** has 2 divisions (superior & inferior) supplies the following muscles:
  (a) Levator palpebrae superioris (superior division)
  (b) Superior rectus (superior division)
  (c) Medial rectus (inferior division)
  (d) Inferior rectus (inferior division)
  (e) Inferior oblique (inferior division)
- **Superior oblique** is supplied by **trochlear nerve** (4th nerve)
- **Lateral rectus** is supplied by **abducens nerve** (6th nerve)
- **Mnemonics for nerve supply to extraocular muscles: $SO_4LR_6R_3$** (SO-sup oblique, LR-lateral rectus, R-remaining muscles)

6. **Which of the following muscle produces abduction of vocal cord? (Repeat)**

A. Transverse arytenoid
B. Posterior cricoaryteniod
C. Lateral cricoarytenoid
D. Oblique arytenoid

Ans: B. Posterior cricoarytenoid

Ref: *Gray's Anatomy, 39th edition, 2008.Page 642*

Explanation:

Posterior cricoarytenoid :

- The only muscle produce **abduction of vocal cord** (open the rima glottides and it becomes triangular in shape)
- So called the **Safety muscle of larynx**
- ***Origin:*** Posterior surface of lamina of cricoid cartilage
- ***Insertion:*** Muscular process of arytenoid cartilage
- ***Nerve supply:*** **Recurrent laryngeal nerve** (branch of vagus)
- ***Blood supply:*** Laryngeal branches of superior & inferior thyroid arteries

To remember :

- Safety muscle of tongue is **genioglossus**

7. **Nutrient artery to tibia arises from which of the following arteries?**

A. Popliteal artery
B. Anterior tibial artery
C. Peroneal artery
D. Posterior tibial artery

Ans: D. Posterior tibial artery

Ref: *Gray's Anatomy, 39th edition, 2008.Page 1493*

Explanation:

- Tibia has proximal end, shaft and distal end
- **Proximal end (2 condyles)** is supplied by **metaphyseal** arteries arising from **genicular** arterial anastomosis around knee
- **Shaft** has nutrient foramen near soleal line which transmits a branch from **posterior tibial artery**
- **Periosteum** of **shaft** receives blood supply from **anterior tibial artery** and from muscular branches
- Distal end (2 malleolus) is supplied by branches from the anastomosis around the ankle

Note: Nutrient artery to tibia may arise from popliteal artery at the level of bifurcation or from anterior tibial artery. Option a or b may be considered if posterior tibial artery is not in the option.

8. Right superior intercostal vein drains into:

A. Right brachiocephalic vein
B. Azygos vein
C. Hemiazygos vein
D. Accessory hemiazygos vein

Ans: B. Azygos vein

Ref: *Gray's Anatomy, 39th edition, 2008, Page 966*

Explanation:

- Right second, third and sometimes fourth posterior intercostal veins unite to form **superior intercostal vein**
- Right superior intercostal vein joins with **azygos vein**

To remember:

- **Left superior intercostal** vein formed by the union of **second, third** and sometimes **fourth** left **posterior intercostal veins**
- **Left superior intercostal vein** open into **left brachiocephalic vein.**
- **Azygos vein:**
  – Formed by union of **right ascending lumbar vein** and **right subcostal vein** opposite to L1 or L2 vertebra
  – Enters the thorax by passing through **aortic opening** of diaphragm
  – At the level of T4 arches over the root of right lung and opens into extra pericardial part of superior vena cava
- **Tributaries of azygos vein:**
  (a) Right superior intercostal vein
  (b) 5th to 11th right posterior intercostal veins
  (c) Hemiazygos vein
  (d) Accessory hemiazygos vein
  (e) Oesophageal veins
  (f) Pericardial veins
  (g) Right bronchial veins

9. All are true regarding tensor tympani muscle *except:*

A. Origin from cartilaginous part of auditory tube
B. Innervated by facial nerve
C. Related to processus trochleariformis
D. Inserted on handle of malleus

Ans: B. Innervated by facial nerve

Ref: *Gray's Anatomy, 39th edition, 2008.Page 658*

Explanation:

Tensor tympani: It is a long slender muscle occupies the bony canal (canal for tensor tympani)
Origin: Cartilaginous part of auditory tube, adjoining region of greater wing of sphenoid and from the canal for
tensor tympani.
Insertion: Slim tendon round the pulley –Processus trochleariformis and inserted in to the handle of malleus.
Blood supply: Superior tympanic branch of middle meningeal artery.
Nerve supply: **Mandibular nerve** (branch of the nerve to medial pterygoid which traverses the otic ganglion without interruption to reach tensor tympani)
Actions: Tenses the tympanic membrane and helps to damp sound vibrations, also pushes the base of stapes more tightly into fenestra vestibuli.

10. Vocalis is a part of which of the following muscle?

A. Thyroarytenoid
B. Cricoarytenoid
C. Transverse arytenoid
D. Posterior cricoarytenoid

Ans: A. Thyroarytenoid

Ref: *Gray's Anatomy, 39th edition, 2008.Page.642*

Explanation:

Thyroarytenoid :

- ***Anterior attachment:*** To the inner aspect of angle of thyroid cartilage & cricothyroid membrane
- ***Posterior attachment:*** Arytenoid cartilage (anterolateral surface)
- ***Vocalis muscle:*** Lower & deeper fibres of thyroarytenoid form a bundle which attached to the lateral surface of vocal process and anterolateral surface of arytenoid cartilage.
- This bundle is **vocalis muscle**, which lies lateral to vocal ligament.
- Vocalis muscle is thicker posteriorly than anteriorly

- ***Blood supply:*** Laryngeal branches of superior and inferior thyroid arteries.
- ***Nerve supply:*** **Recurrent laryngeal nerve**
- ***Action:*** **Shortening** and **relaxing** the **vocal ligaments**
- Approximate the vocal cord/closure of **rima glottides**
- **Vocalis** can change the **pitch of voice**

11. False statement regarding adductor pollicis muscle:

A. Has 2 heads
B. Supplied by Median nerve
C. Causes Adduction of thumb
D. Arterial supply is from Arteria priceps pollicis

Ans: B. Supplied by Median nerve

Ref: *Gray's Anatomy, 39th edition, 2008.Page.918*

Explanation:

Adductor pollicis:

- **Has 2 heads**, i) Oblique head ii) Transverse head
- **Oblique head**: Origin from capitate, bases of 2nd & 3rd metacarpal bones
- **Transverse head**: Origin from palmar surface of 3rd metacarpal bone
- ***Insertion:*** Two heads united by a tendon which attached to the ulnar side of base of proximal phalanx of thumb
- ***Blood supply:*** **Arteria princeps pollicis** & **Arteria radialis indicis** and **branches from deep palmar arch**
- ***Nerve supply:*** Deep branch of **ulnar nerve** (C8 & T1 fibres)
- ***Action:*** **Adduction of thumb** i.e. approximates the thumb to the palm of hand
- ***Testing:*** With the thumb lying along the palmar aspect of the index finger, the subject is asked to retain a strip of paper between the thumb and palm against resistance.

To remember:

- There are **20 muscles** in the hand. Out of this **only 5 muscles** supplied by **median nerve** and remaining **15 muscles** are supplied **by ulnar nerve**.
- Muscles supplied by **MEDIAN NERVE** are:
  i. Flexor pollicis brevis
  ii. Abductor pollicis brevis
  iii. Opponens pollicis
  iv. First lumbrical
  v. Second lumbrical
- Muscles supplied by **ULNAR NERVE** are:
  *By its **superficial** branch*
  i. Palmaris brevis
  By its deep branch
  i Adductor pollicis
  ii. Flexor digiti minimi
  iii. Abductor digiti minimi
  iv. Opponens digiti minimi
  v. Third & fourth lumbrical
  vi. 4 Dorsal interosseous
  vii. 4 Palmar interosseous

12. False regarding Klumpke's paralysis is:

A. Claw hand deformity
B. Intrinsic muscles of hand involved
C. Horner's syndrome
D. Upper trunk of brachial plexus involved

Ans: D. Upper trunk of brachial plexus involved

Ref: *Gray's Anatomy, 39th edition, 2008.Page.848*

Explanation:

Klumpke's paralysis:
Site of injury: Lower trunk of brachial plexus (mainly T1& partly C8)
Cause of injury: Forcible breech delivery, Pancoast tumour, thoracic surgery involving sternal split & cervical rib (thoracic outlet syndrome)
Muscles paralysed: **Intrinsic muscles** of hand (T1) & **Ulnar side flexors** of **wrist** and **fingers** (C8)
Deformity:

1. *Motor fibres involved :*
   – **Claw hand** (hyper extension at MCP joint & flexion at IP joint)
2. *Sensory fibres involved:*
   – Anaesthesia & analgesia along the ulnar border of forearm and hand
   – Trophic changes (long standing cases)– dry & scaly skin, nail cracks and atrophy of pulp of fingers
3. *Sympathetic fibres involved:*
   – **Horner's syndrome** (sympathetic fibres from T1)
   Consists of Ptosis, Miosis, Enophthalmos, Anhydrosis & Loss of Ciliospinal reflex.
   – Vasomotor changes – skin warm & dry (arteriolar dilatation)

Note: Erb's paralysis: Upper trunk of brachial plexus involved. i.e. **Erb's point (C5 & C6)**

13. The opening transmitting Azygos vein in the diaphragm is at the level of: (Repeat)

A. T10 **B.** T12
C. T6 **D.** T8

Ans: B. T12

Ref: *Grays Anatomy 40 th Ed Pg 1007*

Explanation:

Level	Openings	Structures
T8	Vena caval opening	IVC Right phrenic nerve
T10	Oesophageal opening	Oesophagus, ant & post vagal nerves Small oesophageal arteries
T12	Aortic opening	Aorta Azygos vein Thoracic duct
T12	2 lesser aperture of right crus	Greater and lesser right splanchnic nerves
T12	3 lesser aperture of left crus	Greater and lesser left splanchnic nerves and the hemiazygos vein

Note:

Foramen of Morgagni- areolar tissue between the sternal and costal parts

Mneumonic:

Indian- **I**nferior vena cava (T8)
Overseas - **O**esophagus (T10)
BAnk - **A**orta (T12)

14. **Which of the following is not a content of the pudendal canal?**
   A. Pudendal nerve
   B. Internal pudendal artery
   C. Internal pudendal vein
   D. Nerve to obturator internus

Ans: D. Nerve to obturator internus

Ref: *Gray's Anatomy 40th Ed pg.1140*

Explanation:

Pudendal canal

- It is a **fascial canal** in the **lateral wall of ischiorectal fossa** 2.5 cm above ischial tuberosity
- It extends from **lesser sciatic foramen** to **deep perineal pouch**
- The pudendal canal (**Alcock's canal**) is formed by the **obturator internus fascia**.

It encloses the following:
- Internal pudendal artery
- Internal pudendal veins
- Pudendal nerve

Pudendal nerve block
- The pudendal nerve block given in the canal in perineal surgery *(See the following figure)*

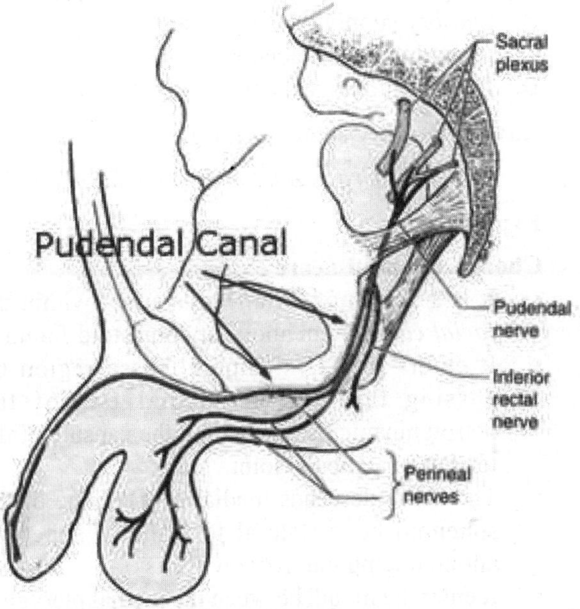

15. **All the following are general visceral efferent *except:***
   A. Nucleus ambiguous
   B. Dorsal nucleus of vagus
   C. Salivatory nucleus
   D. Edinger Westphal nucleus

Ans: A. Nucleus ambiguous

Ref: *Grays Anatomy 40th Ed pg.225*

Explanation:

1. **General Somatic Afferent (GSA)** fibers are related to receptors for pain temperture and mechanical receptors in the skin, muscles and joints.
2. **General Visceral Afferent (GVA)** fibers are related to receptors in visceral structures.
3. **General Visceral Efferent (GVE)** fibers are preganglionic autonomic fibers.
4. **General Somatic Efferent (GSE)** fibers innervate skeletal muscle (these are axons of alpha and gamma motor neurons).

Formation:
- The cell bodies on which spinal afferents synapse and the cell bodies of the spinal efferent fibers are located in portions of the spinal gray matter that are predictable from embryological development.
- Embryologically ,the sulcus limitans separates the alar plate (which becomes the posterior horn) from the basal plate (which becomes the anterior horn).

- Within both plates the cells concerned with visceral function are located near the sulcus limitans.
- For each of the four spinal functions there is a corresponding column of cells in the spinal gray matter.
- GSA and GSE extend the length of the cord.
- GVA and GVE columns are found at T1 to L2-3 and T1 to S2-4.

16. All are true about Chorda tympani nerve *except:* (Repeat)

A. Supplies anterior 2/3rd tongue
B. Sensory supply of face
C. It is a branch of facial nerve
D. It joins with lingual nerve

Ans: B. Sensory supply of face

Ref: *Gray's Anatomy 40th edition pg, 543*

Explanation:

Chorda tympani nerve

- It is a branch of ***facial nerve*** arises within the ***facial canal*** 6mm above stylomastoid foramen
- It enters the infratemporal fossa region by passing through the medial end of the petrotympanic fissure behind the capsule of the temporomandibular joint.
- The nerve descends medial to the spine of the sphenoid bone (lateral to spine of sphenoid auriculo temporal nerve will pass).
- It enter the mouth between the medial pterygoid muscle and ramus of the mandible
- It is crossed medially by the middle meningeal artery, the roots of the auriculotemporal nerve and by the inferior alveolar nerve .
- The chorda tympani joins the posterior aspect of the lingual nerve at an acute angle
- It carries **taste fibres** for the **anterior two-thirds of the tongue** and **efferent pre-ganglionic parasympathetic (secretomotor) fibres** destined for the **submandibular ganglion** in the floor of the mouth.It carries secretomotor fibers for both submandibular gland and sublingual gland.
  (See the following figure)

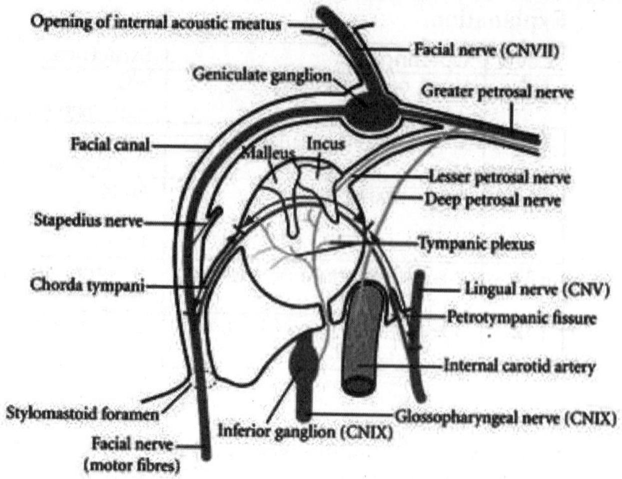

17. All the following veins drain into internal jugular vein *except:* (Repeat)

A. Facial vein
B. Lingual vein
C. Superior thyroid vein
D. Retromandibular vein

Ans: D. Retromandibular vein

Ref: *Grays Anatomy 40 th edition pg: 400*

Explanation:

Retromandibular Vein

- The **superficial temporal vein** joins with the ***maxillary vein*** to form retromandibular vein.
- It divides into anterior and posterior division.
- ***Anterior division*** joins with the ***facial vein*** to form ***common facial vein*** which drains into ***internal jugular vein.***
- The ***posterior division*** joins with the ***posterior auricular vein*** to form ***external jugular vein.***

Internal Jugular Vein

- The internal jugular vein collects blood from the **skull, brain, superficial parts of face** and **neck**.
- It begins at the cranial base in the posterior compartment of the jugular foramen, where it is **continuous with the sigmoid sinus.**
- At its origin it is dilated as the **superior bulb,** which lies below the posterior part of the tympanic floor.
- The internal jugular vein descends in the **carotid sheath**, and **unites with the subclavian vein,** posterior to the sternal end of the clavicle, to form the **brachiocephalic vein** .
- Near its termination the vein dilates into the **inferior bulb.**

Tributaries

- The inferior petrosal sinus
- Facial vein
- Lingual vein
- Pharyngeal vein
- Superior and middle thyroid veins
- Occipital vein (Occasionally)
- The internal jugular vein may communicate with the external jugular vein.
- The thoracic duct opens near the union of the left subclavian and internal jugular veins, and the right lymphatic duct opens at the same site on the right.

PHYSIOLOGY

1. **Equilibrium potential of potassium is:**

A. +90 mv B. - 90 mv
C. +70 mv D. -70 mv

Ans: B. - 90 mv

Ref: Pal GK. Transport across cell membrane. In: Textbook of medical physiology. Ahuja publishing house. 2007; 4: 44.

Explanation:

Equilibrium potential of

- K^+ (-90) mV
- Na^+ (+60) mV
- Cl^- (-70) mV
- HCO_3^- (-25) mV

2. **Major cation in intracellular space:**

A. Proteins B. Potassium
C. Sodium D. Chloride

Ans: B. Potassium

Ref: Guyton & Hall. The Body Fluid Compartments: Extracellular and Intracellular Fluids. In: Textbook of Medical Physiology. 12th ed. Philadelphia: Saunders Elsevier; 2012. P288.

Explanation: *(See the following table)*

3. **Which of the following parts of brain contains dopaminergic neurons?**

A. Locus ceruleus system
B. Cerebellum
C. Nigro striatal system
D. Midline raphe nucleus

Ans: C. Nigro striatal system

Ref: Pal GK. Limbic system. In: Textbook of medical physiology. Ahuja publishing house. 2007; 120: 910-13.

Explanation:

Dopaminergic system
- Meso-cortical system
- Tubero-infundibular system
- Nigro-striatal system
- Incerto-hypothalamic system

Noradrenergic system
- Locus ceruleus system
- Tegmental system

Adrenergic system
- From Medulla to spinalcord, hypothalamus, thalamus, periaqueductal gray

Serotonergic system
- Midline raphe nucleus of hypothalamus

Histaminergic system
- Tubero-mamillary nucleus of posterior hypothalamus

Cholinergic system
- Nucleus basalis of Meynert to amygdala and neocortex

	Plasma ($mOsm/L\ H_2O$)	Interstitial ($mOsm/L\ H_2O$)	Intracellular ($mOsm/L\ H_2O$)
Na^+	142	139	14
K^+	4.2	4.0	140
Ca^{++}	1.3	1.2	0
Mg^{++}	0.8	0.7	20
Cl^-	108	108	4
HCO_3^-	24	28.3	10
HPO_4^{2-}, $H_2PO_4^-$	2	2	11
SO_4^-	0.5	0.5	1
Phosphocreatine			45
Carnosine			14
Amino acids	2	2	8
Creatine	0.2	0.2	9
Lactate	1.2	1.2	1.5
Adenosine triphosphate			5
Hexose monophosphate			3.7
Glucose	5.6	5.6	
Protein	1.2	0.2	4
Urea	4	4	4
Others	4.8	3.9	10
Total mOsm/L	**301.8**	**300.8**	**301.2**
Corrected osmolar activity (mOsm/L)	**282.0**	**281.0**	**281.0**
Total osmotic pressure at 37 °C (mm Hg)	**5443**	**5423**	**5423**

4. **Most important sensory organ in the ampulla is:**
A. Organ of corti **B.** Macula
C. Otolith **D.** Crista

Ans: D. Crista

Ref: *Pal GK. Vestibular apparatus. In: Textbook of medical physiology. Ahuja publishing house. 2007; 116: 886-88.*

Explanation:

Receptor structure	Receptor organ	Detected stimuli
Otolith organs		
Saccule	Macula	Gravitation & linear acceleration
Utricle	Macula	Gravitation & linear acceleration
Semicircular canals		
Horizontal canal	Ampulla	Rotational acceleration
Anterior canal	Ampulla	Rotational acceleration
Posterior canal	Ampulla	Rotational acceleration

Note:
- **Macula** – Sensory epithelium in **saccule** and **utricle** which contain **hair cells**
- **Otolith (or) otoconia** – calcium carbonate **crystals** in **otolith membrane**
- Each **ampulla** contains **Crista ampularis** in which hair cells are located. These hair cells are embedded in a gelatinous mass '***cupula***' (which does ***not*** contain otoliths)
- **Organ of corti** – locaed in **middle** ear; involved in **audition**

5. **The incisura of arterial pulse corresponds with:**
A. S1 **B.** S2
C. Opening snap **D.** S3

Ans: B. S2

Ref: *1. Pal GK. Cardiac cycle. In: Textbook of medical physiology. Ahuja publishing house. 2007; 73: 601.*

Explanation:

*"The **dicrotic notch** recorded directly from the central aorta is termed the **incisura** (from the Latin, a cutting into). The **incisura** is sharply defined and undoubtedly is related to **aortic valve closure**."*
(See the following figure)

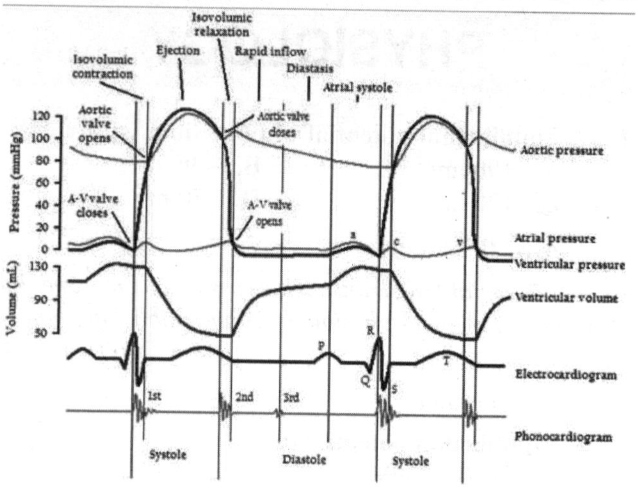

6. **Instrumental conditioning in learning was introduced and demonstrated by:**
A. Pavlov **B.** Skinner
C. Freud **D.** Watson

Ans: B. Skinner

Ref: *Pal GK. Physiology of Learning and memory. In: Textbook of medical physiology. Ahuja publishing house. 2007; 121: 919.*

Explanation:
- **Operant conditioning** (or **instrumental conditioning**) is a type of learning in which an individual's behavior is modified by its consequences; the behaviour may change in form, frequency, or strength
- Operant conditioning is a term that was coined by B. F. **Skinner in 1937**
- Operant conditioning is distinguished from **classical conditioning** (or respondent conditioning) in that operant conditioning deals with the modification of **"voluntary behaviour"** or **operant behaviour**.
- Operant behavior operates on the environment and is maintained by its consequences, while classical conditioning deals with the conditioning of **reflexive (reflex) behaviours** which are elicited by antecedent conditions

7. **Endothelium derived relaxation factor is supposed to be: (Repeat)**
A. Nitric oxide B. Angiotensin
C. Serotonin D. Norepinephrine

Ans: A. Nitric oxide

Ref: *Pal GK. Synaptic transmission in CNS; and Neurotransmitters. In: Textbook of medical physiology. 2nd ed. Ahuja publishing house. 2011; 100: 794.*

Explanation:
- Nitric oxide is also called as **EDRF** (Endothelial derived relaxation factor)
- Formed from **arginine** by **NO synthase** which needs **NADPH**
- It mediates the action of many other **vasodilators – Histamine, Ach, bradykinin, VIP, substance P**

8. **All the following are involved in the control of posture *except:***

A. Anterior corticospinal tract
B. Lateral corticospinal tract
C. Tectospinal
D. Vestibulospinal

Ans: B. Lateral corticospinal tract

Ref: *Pal GK. Descending pathways. In: Textbook of medical physiology. Ahuja publishing house. 2007; 113: 844-45.*

Explanation:

Lateral system pathways – regulation of ***skilled voluntary movements***
- Lateral cortico-spinal tract
- *Rubro-spinal tract*

Medial system pathways – Regulation of posture
- Reticulo-spinal tract
- Vestibulo-spinal tract
- Tecto-spinal tract
- Anterior cortico-spinal tract
- Interstitio-spinal tract

9. **All are true regarding withdrawal reflex *except:* (Repeat)**
A. Has long latency
B. Poly synaptic
C. Carried by 1a fibers
D. Has after-discharge

Ans: C. Carried by 1a fibers

Ref:

1. Guyton & Hall. Flexor Reflex and the Withdrawal Reflexes. In: Textbook of Medical Physiology.12th ed. Philadelphia: Saunders Elsevier; 2012. p 661-663.

2. W F Ganong. Excitable Tissue: Nerve. In: Review of Medical Physiology. 21st ed. California: McGraw-Hill Companies; 2003.

Explanation:

Refer 2013 Physiology question explanation

Withdrawal Reflex

It is a typical **polysynaptic reflex** that occurs in response to a noxious and usually painful stimulation of the skin or subcutaneous tissues and muscle.
- The response is flexor muscle contraction and inhibition of extensor muscles, so that the part stimulated is flexed and withdrawn from the stimulus.
- When a strong stimulus is applied to a limb, the response includes not only flexion and withdrawal of that limb but also extension of the opposite limb. This **crossed extensor response** is properly part of the withdrawal reflex.
- Withdrawal reflexes are **prepotent;** i.e., they preempt the spinal pathways from any other reflex activity taking place at the moment.

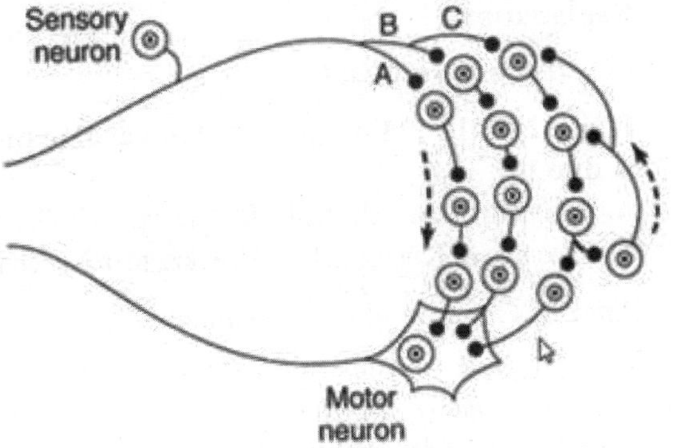

Fig. Polysynatic reflex

10. **Function of ubiquitin in the cell is: (Repeat)**
A. Degradation of intracellular protein
B. Endocytosis
C. Exocytosis
D. Plays an important role in acute inflammation

Ans: A. Degradation of intracellular protein

Ref: *Koeppen BM, Stanton BA. Skeletal Muscle Physiology. In: Berne & Levy Physiology 6th ed. Mosby; 2008 p 250. & Hershko A, Ciechanover A. The ubiquitin system. Annu Rev Biochem. 1998;67:425-79.*

Explanation:

*"One factor thought to contribute to the decreased protein synthesis and increased protein degradation during periods of mechanical inactivity is the release of a **ubiquitin ligase** (MuRF2) from titin. **MuRF2** also promotes protein degradation through **ubiquitination**"*

The ubiquitin system
- The ***selective degradation*** of many ***short-lived proteins*** in eukaryotic cells is carried out by the ubiquitin system.
- In this pathway, proteins are targeted for degradation by ***covalent ligation*** to ubiquitin, a highly conserved small protein.
- UBIQUITIN-mediated degradation of regulatory proteins plays important roles in
  - Cell-cycle progression
  - Signal transduction
  - Transcriptional regulation
  - Receptor down-regulation
  - Endocytosis
  - Immune response
  - Development
  - Programmed cell death (Apoptosis)

11. **Most common cell type in anterior pituitary is:**
A. Corticotroph
B. Gonadotroph
C. Lactotroph
D. Somatotrope

Ref: *W F Ganong.Review of Medical Physiology.23rd Edn.Chapter 24.The Pituitary Gland.Page 379.*

Ans: D. Somatotrope

Explanation:

(See the following table)

12. Phase 2 of the action potential in cardiac muscle is due to:

A. Opening of Ca^{2+} channels B. Opening of Na^+ channels
C. Opening of K^+ channels D. Closure of Na^+ channels

Ans: A. Opening of Ca^{2+} channels

Ref: *W F Ganong. Origin of heart beat & The electrical activity of the heart . In: Review of Medical Physiology. 21st ed. California: McGraw-Hill Companies; 2003. p 550.*

Explanation:

The trans-membrane action potential of single cardiac muscle cells is characterized by

- **Rapid depolarization (phase 0)** - due to Na^+ influx through rapidly opening Na+ channels (the Na+ current, I_{Na})
- **Initial rapid repolarization (phase 1)** - inactivation of Na+ channels and K+ efflux
- **Plateau (phase 2)** - Ca^{2+} influx through more slowly opening Ca^{2+} channels (the Ca^{2+} current, I_{Ca})
- **Slow repolarization process (phase 3)** - net K^+ efflux through multiple types of K^+ channels
- Return to the resting membrane potential **(phase 4)**

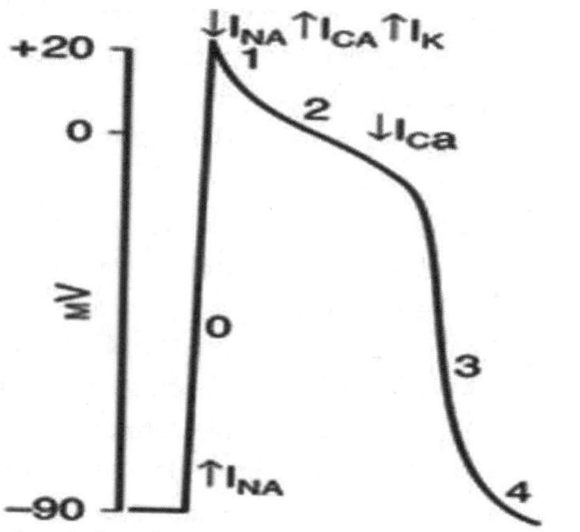

13. Which of the following has least effect on the metabolic rate?

A. TSH B. TRH
C. TBG D. Free T_4

Ans: C. TBG

Ref: *Guyton & Hall. Thyroid Metabolic Hormones. In: Textbook of Medical Physiology.12th ed. Philadelphia: Saunders Elsevier; 2012. p 907-910.*

Explanation:

- TSH, TRH stimulate thyroid gland for synthesis and release of thyroid hormones
- T_4 is secreted more into the circulation; T_3 is the active form in ta rget tissues
- **Thyroid hormones increase basal rate of metabolism**
- On entering the blood, more than 99 % of the thyroxine and triiodothyronine combines immediately with several of the plasma proteins, (mainly with **thyroxine-binding globulin (TBG)** and much less so with thyroxine-binding prealbumin and albumin)
- Thyroid hormones are **functionally active** only in **free form; not in bound form (binding with TBG, etc)**

14. Each kidney contains about___ nephrons: (Repeat)

A. One million B. Two million
C. Four million D. Half million

Ans: A. One million

Ref: *Guyton & Hall. Physiologic Anatomy of the Kidneys. In: Textbook of Medical Physiology.12th ed. Philadelphia: Saunders Elsevier; 2012. p 305.*

Explanation:

- Each kidney in the human contains about **800,000 to 1,000,000 *nephrons*,** each capable of forming urine
- The kidney ***cannot regenerate*** **new nephrons.**
- ***After age 40,*** the number of functioning nephrons usually ***decreases about 10 % every 10 years***
- At **age 80**, many people have **40 % fewer functioning nephrons** than they did at age 40.
- This loss is *not life threatening* because ***adaptive changes*** in the remaining nephrons allow them to excrete the proper amounts of water, electrolytes, and waste products

15. Election fraction of the ventricle refers to the ratio of:

A. Amount of blood received/amount of blood ejected

Hormone Secreting Cells of the Human Anterior Pituitary Gland

Cell Type	Hormones Secreted	% of Total Secretory Cells	Stain Affinity	Diameter of Secretory Granules (nm)
Somatotrope	Growth hormone	50	Acidophilic	300–400
Lactotrope	Prolactin	10–30	Acidophilic	200
Corticotrope	ACTH	10	Basophilic	400–550
Thyrotrope	TSH	5	Basophilic	120–200
Gonadotrope	FSH, LH	20	Basophilic	250–400

B. Stroke volume/end-diastolic volume
C. End-systolic volume/end diastolic volume
D. Stroke volume/end-systolic volume

Ans: B. Stroke volume/end-diastolic volume

Ref: Pal GK. Cardiac Output . In: Textbook of medical physiology. New Delhi: Ahuja publishing house; 2007. 607.

Explanation:

- Ejection fraction is the **percentage of end diastolic volume, ejected with each beat**
- **EF = SV/ EDV**
- EF is an **index** of myo-cardial **performance**
- Normal EF is **~65%**

BIOCHEMISTRY

1. **Folic acid deficiency can be estimated by:**
A. Histidine load test
B. Dexa suppression test
C. Isovaleric acid levels
D. Aminoleuvelinic acid levels

Ans: A. Histidine load test

Ref: Harper's Illustrated biochemistry,28th edition

Explanation:

Histidine load test (Figlu Excretion)

- **Folates** are involved in the **histidine metabolism** during the conversion of **formiminoglutamate** to **glutamate**.
- During the breakdown of **histidine (to a-ketoglutarate)** in the liver, a first nitrogen atom is split off as ammonia with a second one being released from the produced formiminoglutamate as part of a formimino group and passed on to THF
- This is deaminated to 5-Formyl-THF and subsequently converted into 5,10-methylene-THF.
- During **folic acid deficiency**, this **conversion** of the **formimino group** is **disturbed**.
- After a **histidine load test** (oral intake of 15 or 20 g of histidine), patients secrete **more N-formimino glutamate** in the urine; hence, this test is **suitable to diagnose folic acid deficiency**.
- Normally, less than 30 µg/mL or 0.1 to 18 mg/day are excreted.
- In cases of active folate deficiency, this excretion is greatly increased **(up to 2 g/day)**.
- However, this test is **obsolete** and **rarely carried out**.

2. **Solubility of cholesterol depends on:**
A. Water
B. Phosphatidul choline
C. Bile salts
D. Cholesterol

Ans: C. Bile salts?

Ref: Harper's Illustrated biochemistry,28th edition & Ganong's Physiology & Bandyopadhyay A et al. Cholesterol solubility by bile salts in pure and mixed states. J Phys Chem: 1991; 95: 4529-34

Explanation:

*"**Bile salts** are metabolic products which together with **phospholipids solubilize cholesterol** forming **bile***

- **Cholesterol** is only **slightly soluble** in water; it can dissolve and travel in the water-based bloodstream at exceedingly small concentrations.
- Since cholesterol is insoluble in blood, it is transported in the circulatory system within **lipoproteins**, complex discoidal particles that have an exterior composed of amphiphilic proteins and lipids whose outward-facing surfaces are water-soluble and inward-facing surfaces are lipid-soluble; triglycerides and cholesterol esters are carried internally.
- Phospholipids and cholesterol, being amphipathic, are transported in the surface monolayer of the lipoprotein particle.

3. **Enzyme catalysing urea formation: (Repeat)**
A. Arginase
B. Ornithine trans carbamoylase
C. Carbamoyl phosphate synthase
D. Arginosuccinate synthase

Ans: A. Arginase

Ref: Harper's illustrated biochemistry,28th edition, chapter-28,pp-244

Explanation: *(See the figure on the next page)*

4. **Marker of lysosome is: (Repeat)**
A. Acid Phosphatase
B. Lactate dehydrogenase
C. Oxidase
D. Na K ATPase

Ans: A. Acid Phosphatase

Ref: Harper's illustrated biochemistry, 28th edition.

Explanation:

Markers of Intracellular organelles

- **Plasma Membrane**: Na^{+} K^{+} ATPase & 5' Nucleotidase

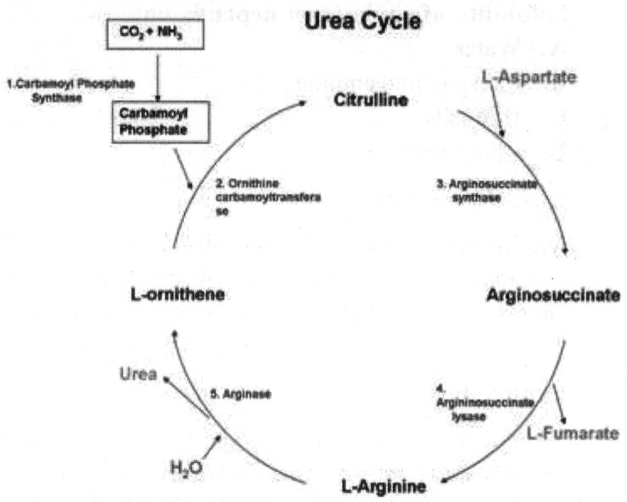

- **Cytoplasm**: Lactate dehydrogenase
- **Mitochondria**: Glutamate dehydrogenase
- **Ribosome**: RNA
- **Endoplasmic reticulum**: Glucose-6 phosphatase
- **Lysosome**: Acid phosphatase
- **Golgi Apparatus**: Galactosyl transferase
- **Peroxisomes**: Catalase & Uric acid oxidase
- **Nucleus**: DNA
- **Peroxisome**: Oxidase & catalase

5. **Vitamin K required for which of the following reaction?**
   A. Hydroxylation **B.** Chelation
   C. Transamination **D.** Carboxylation

Ans: D. Carboxylation

Ref: *Harper's Illustrated Biochemistry, 28th edition, Chapter 44, pp 473*

Explanation:

- Co-enzyme like activity for **protein carboxylases**
  - Formation of active clotting factors **II, VII, IX & X** in the **liver**
  - Formation of **Protein C and Protein S** – Anticoagulants
  - Formation of some of the bone matrix proteins
- The reaction is **inhibited by dicumarol**, an anticoagulant occurring naturally and by **warfarin** a synthetic analog of vitamin K.
- The **Gamma carboxy glutamate** residues of **prothrombin** are **good chelators** of positively charged **calcium ions,** because of the two adjacent, negatively charged carboxylate groups.
- The **prothrombin–calcium complex** is then able to bind to phospholipids essential for blood clotting on the surface of platelets.
- Attachment to the platelet increases the rate at which the proteolytic conversion of prothrombin to thrombin can occur.

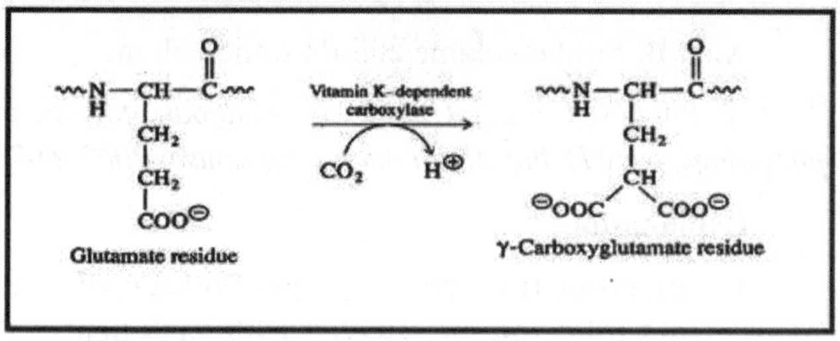

6. **Fructose is absorbed by:**
   A. Simple diffusion **B.** Facilitated diffusion
   C. Cotransport **D.** Symport

Ans: B. Facilitated diffusion

Ref: *Textbook of Biochemistry for Medical Students by DM Vasudevan, 6th edition, Chapter 9, pp-91.*

Explanation:

- The **GLUT 5** Na+-independent facilitative transporter allows **fructose**, as well as **glucose** and **galactose**, to be transported down their concentration gradients
- Exit from the cell for all sugars is via the **GLUT 2** facilitative transporter.

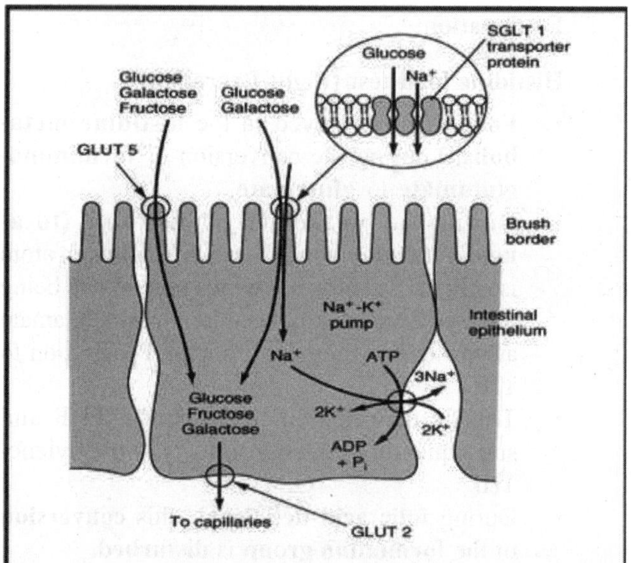

7. **Enzyme deficiency responsible for gout are all** ***except:*** **(Repeat)**
   A. PRPP synthase
   B. Pseudogout enzyme
   C. 5 – phosphoribosyl amido transferase
   D. Glucose 6 phosphatase

Ans: B. Pseudogout enzyme

Ref: *Harper's Illustrated Biochemistry, 28th edition*

Explanation:

- **Hyperuricemia**–Uric acid level: **Males >7 mgdL Females > 6 mg/dL**
- Accumulation of insoluble monosodium urate crystals in the synovial fluid causes inflammation – **Acute arthritis.**
- Deposition in cooler areas – **Tophi**
- **Renal lithiasis.**

PRIMARY GOUT- Causes

- Abnormality **in 5 – phosphoribosyl amido transferase.**
- Abnormality in **PRPP synthetase.**
- Deficiency of enzymes of salvage pathway.
- **Glucose-6-phosphatase deficiency.**
- Increased activity of **Glutathione reductase**

SECONDARY GOUT- Causes

- ***Increased turnover rate of nucleic acids.***
  - Leukemias, polycythemia.
  - Treatment of Malignant tumors.
  - Psoriasis.
- ***Reduced excretion rate.***
  - Renal failure.
  - Thiazide diuretics.
  - Lactic acidosis and Ketoacidosis.

8. In starvation, least common change seen is: (Repeat)

A. Depletion of buccal fat
B. Increased lipogenesis
C. Increased gluconeogenesis
D. Increased glycogenolysis

Ans: B. Increased lipogenesis

Ref: *Harper's illustrated biochemistry, 28th edition.*

Explanation:

Metabolic Fuel Reserves Are Mobilized in the Fasting State

- There is a small **fall in plasma glucose** in the **fasting state**, then little change as fasting is prolonged into starvation.
- **Plasma free fatty acids increase** in **fasting,** but then rise little more in starvation; as fasting is prolonged, so the plasma concentration of **ketone bodies** (acetoacetate and-hydroxybutyrate) **increases** markedly

Plasma Concentrations of Metabolic Fuels (mmol/L) in the Fed and Fasting States

	Fed	40 Hours Fasting	7 Days Starvation
Glucose	5.5	3.6	3.5
Free fatty acids	0.30	1.15	1.19
Ketone bodies	Negligible	2.9	4.5

9. Following amino acid form an integral part of collagen synthesis:

A. Lysine **B.** Leucine
C. Arginine **D.** Glutamic acid

Ans: A. Lysine

Ref: *Harper's illustrated Biochemistry, 28th edition*

Explanation:

Collagen

- Collagen is a fibrous protein
- Most abundant structural protein
- Accounts for **25%** of the total body proteins
- Found in skin, joints, skeleton, tendons, cartilage, cornea and blood vessels
- Unusual right-handed **triple helix**
- 3 polypeptide chains, an unusual amino acid composition
- **33% glycine, 10% proline, 10% hydroxyproline (Hyp)**
- The sequence **Gly-X-Y-Gly-X-Y** is **repetitive**
- Hydroxylated amino acid (pro, lys) characteristic of collagen
- Synthesized **post- translationally,** a step requiring **vitamin C.**
- **Vitamin C deficiency** symptoms explained by **disturbances** in **collagen biosynthesis.**
- Collagen molecules tend to associate with one another to form larger, more complex cylindrical fibrils (diameter 20-500nm)
- At either end, the individual collagen molecules are **cross-linked via** modified **lysine residues.**
- This gives tensile strength to collagen
- Extent of cross-linking increases with age

PHARMACOLOGY

1. Which of the following has the highest affinity for $5HT_3$ receptors?

A. Dolasetron **B.** Granisetron
C. Ondansetron **D.** Palonosetron

Ans: D. Palonosetron

Ref: *The Pharmacological basis of therapeutics by Good man & Gilman - 12th edition, page no. 1345*

Explanation:

- **Palonosetron** is a **$5HT_3$ antagonist** similar to other antagonists such as ondansetron, dolasetron, granisetron. However palonosetron has the maximal affinity for $5HT_3$ receptors.
- These drugs are administered via **intravenous** route or **oral route**

- **Transdermal granisetron** is also available which can be applied one day before chemotherapy and continued for seven consecutive days.
- All 5 HT_3 antagonists are administered **once daily**.
- They are mainly used in the treatment of
  - **Chemotherapy induced nausea and vomiting**
  - **Nausea secondary to upper abdominal irradiation**
  - **Hyperemesis** of **pregnancy**
  - **Post-operative nausea.**
- Since **palonosetron** has the **maximum half – life (40 hours)** among the $5HT_3$ antagonists, it is also helpful in **delayed emesis**.

2. **Which of the following drugs is found to be effective in both epilepsy and migraine?**

   A. Valproate **B.** Lamotrigine
   C. Vigabatrin **D.** Flunarizine

   Ans: A. Valproate

Ref: *The Pharmacological basis of therapeutics by Good man & Gilman - 12th edition, page no. 597*

Explanation:

- **Sodium valproate** has a beneficial effect in both **migraine** and **epilepsy**.
- It is one of the **first line therapy** in **generalized tonic clonic seizures** and **absence seizures**.
- It also has a beneficial effect in **simple partial seizures, complex partial seizures** and **myoclonic seizures**.
- The drug is used as used as a **prophylactic agent** in patients with **migraine headaches**.
- Some of the other anti-epileptic drugs which are found to be effective in **migraine prophylaxis** include **topiramate, pregabalin** and **gabapentin**.
- Drugs such as **acetazolamide, clonazepam, lamotrigine, oxcarbazepine**, and **vigabatrin** were not more effective than **placebo** in reducing headache frequency according to a Cochrane review.
- **Flunarizine** is a calcium channel blocker which has a beneficial role in **prophylaxis of migraine**. However it has no role in the treatment of epilepsy.
  (See the following table)

Examples of drugs which are effective for migraine prophylaxis

Drug name	Mechanism of action
Propranolol	Beta blocker
Timolol	Beta blocker
Amitriptyline	Tri cyclic antidepressant
Topiramate	Reduces voltage gated sodium currents
Gabapentin	GABA agonist
Pregabalin	GABA agonist
Pizotifen	Serotonin antagonist
Flunarizine	Calcium channel blocker

Ref: *The Pharmacological basis of therapeutics by Good man & Gilman - 12th edition, page no. 1626*

3. **Which of the following is not an example for an NNRTI?**

   A. Efavirenz **B.** Etravirine
   C. Emtricitabine **D.** Delavirdine

   Ans: C. Emtricitabine

Explanation:

- **Nevirapine, efavirenz** and **etravirine** are examples of **non-nucleoside reverse transcriptase inhibitors.(NNRTI)**
- **Emtricitabine** is an example for **nucleoside reverse transcriptase inhibitor.** (**NRTI**)

Classification of anti-retroviral drugs

Class	Examples
Nucleoside reverse transcriptase inhibitors	Zidovudine, lamivudine, didanosine, stavudine, abacavir, tenofovir, emtricitabine,
Non- Nucleoside reverse transcriptase inhibitors	Nevirapine, efavirenz, etravirine, delavirdine
Protease inhibitors	Indinavir, saquinavir, ritonavir, nelfinavir, lopinavir, fosamprenavir, atazanavir, tipranavir, darunavir
Entry inhibitors	Maraviroc, enfuvirtide
Integrase inhibitors	Raltegravir

4. **Heparin treatment is monitored by:**

   A. aPTT **B.** PT
   C. CT **D.** BT

   Ans: A. aPTT

Ref: *The Pharmacological basis of therapeutics by Good man & Gilman - 12th edition, page no. 855-857*

Explanation:

- **Heparin** treatment is monitored using **activated partial thromboplastin time (aPTT)**
- An **aPTT two to three times** the normal **mean aPTT** value generally is therapeutic.
- **Prothrombin time** (International Normalized Ratio) is used to monitor **warfarin therapy**.
- The low molecular weight heparin such as **enoxaparin** and **tinzaparin** and fondaparinux **do not require aPTT** monitoring as with unfractionated heparin. Hence they can be

administered even for out-of –hospital management.

- Another advantage with **LMW heparin** is that they can be given by **subcutaneous injection once or twice daily**.
- **Heparin and fondaparinux** are mainly used in the treatment and **prevention of venous thromboembolism.**
- **Fondaparinux** is a **factor Xa inhibitor**, which also has the same advantages of LMW – subcutaneous injection, **no need of lab monitoring**.
- **Fondaparinux** should not be used in the setting of **angioplasty** as it has a **greater risk of catheter thrombosis**.
- **Anticoagulation** ibn **pregnancy** is best managed with **UFH, LMW heparin and fondaparinux** since they **do not cross placenta to** cause fetal malformations as seen with **warfarin**.
- **Fondaparinux** is least likely to cause **thrombocytopenia** among the anti-coagulants.
- **Heparin** is preferred in **CABG surgery** since **protamine sulfate** can be used to **neutralize** its **effects** following procedure.

5. Which of the following group of drugs is used in the treatment of Kala Azar?

A. Spiramycin
B. Sodium Stibogluconate
C. Praziquantel
D. Niclosamide

Ans: B. Sodium stibogluconate

Ref: *The Pharmacological basis of therapeutics by Good man & Gilman - 12th edition, page no. 1423*

Explanation:

- **Sodium stibogluconate (SSG)** is one of the earliest drugs discovered for the treatment of **Kala-azar**. (Visceral Leishmaniasis).
- However **resistance to SSG** is common in the **Indian population.**
- Other effective drugs for Leishmaniasis include
  - **Liposomal amphotericin B,**
  - **Miltefosine**
  - **Paromomycin.**
- Adverse effects of SSG can cause clinically significant
  - **Pancreatitis**
  - **Arrhythmias**
  - **Hemolytic anemia**
  - **Renal damage**
- The drug is **contra-indicated** in patients with **myocarditis, hepatitis** and **pancreatitis.**
- **Miltefosine** is the **first oral agent** effective in **Visceral Leishmaniasis.**
- The drug should be given for a minimum period **of 28 days** for cure.
- **Nephrotoxicity** and **hepatotoxicity** are rare ADR of miltefosine.
- **Liposomal amphotericin B** is the **drug of choice** in patients with **resistance to SSG.**

6. Anti Helicobacter pylori drugs include all of the following *except:*

A. Amoxicillin	**B.** Clarithromycin
C. Metronidazole	**D.** Sucralfate

Ans: D. Sucralfate

Ref: *The Pharmacological basis of therapeutics by Good man & Gilman - 12th edition, page no. 1320*

Explanation:

- Common eradication regimens *Helicobacter pylori* include **triple therapy** and **quadruple therapy** both of which are given for **14 days.**
- **Triple therapy** – proton pump inhibitor + clarithromycin 500 mg + metronidazole 500 mg or amoxicillin 1 g BD or tetracycline 500mg QID
- **Quadruple therapy** - Proton pump inhibitor twice a day + metronidazole 500 mg three times daily plus bismuth subsalicylate 525 mg + tetracycline 500 mg four times daily
- Quadruple therapy is especially used in areas with high degree of resistane to ***H.pylori***.
- **Alternative regimen** - H_2 receptor antagonist BD plus bismuth subsalicylate 525 mg + metronidazole 250 mg + tetracycline 500 mg QID
- Addition of proton pump inhibitor or H2 antagonist enhances the activity of effectiveness of the antibiotics used against *H.pylori*
- Mucosa associated lymphoid tissue lymphoma of the stomach also requires anti – *H.pylori* eradication regimen.

Sucralfate

- It is not used in any of the *H.pylori* eradication regimens.
- It has a special role in the prevention of **stress induced ulcers.**
- When given in the **rectal route** they may be effective in **radiation proctitis** and **solitary rectal ulcers.**
- Since the drug contains **aluminium**, it should be **avoided** in patients with **renal failure.**

7. Which of the following proton pump inhibitors is known to inhibit CYP2C19?

A. Pantoprazole	**B.** Omeprazole
C. Rabeprazole	**D.** Dexlansoprazole

Ans: B. Omeprazole

Ref: *The Pharmacological basis of therapeutics by Good man & Gilman - 12th edition, page no. 1312*

Explanation:

Omeprazole

- It is the only proton pump inhibitor to inhibit **CYP2C19**.
- As a consequence, it **reduces the clearance of phenytoin, disulfiram, diazepam** and several other drugs metabolized by **CYP2C19**.
- Omeprazole is known to **inhibit the conversion of clopidogrel** into its active metabolite. Thus it can **interfere** with the **efficacy of clopidogrel** in prevention of stent thromboses following coronary stent placement.
- Omeprazole can also **induce the expression of CYP1A2** and hence the metabolism of **imipramine, theophylline, tacrine and several anti-psychotic drugs** is **enhanced.**
- Chronic use of **omeprazole** is known to increase the risk for the development of **bone fractures, increased susceptibility** to **several infections** such as **pneumonia.**
- **Hypergastrinemia** can occur with prolonged use, which can result in **rebound hyper-secretion** of **gastric acid** on **stopping treat-ment.**

8. ACE inhibitors are contraindicated in all the following *except:*

A. Bilateral renal artery stenosis
B. Elderly hypertensive
C. Diabetic microalbuminuria
D. Severe renal failure

Ans: C. Diabetic microalbuminuria

Ref: *Goodman &Gillman's The Pharmacological Basis of Therapeutics, 2011, 12th Edition, McGraw Hill, Burton LL P 735-736*

Explanation:

- ACE inhibitors are **indicated** in **Diabetic nephropathy** because **ACE inhibitors** reduce the **glomerular capillary pressure** by decreasing arterial blood pressure and by dilating renal efferent arterioles
- They also **increase the permeability selectivity** of the **filtering membrane.**
- This will decrease the mesangeal exposure to protenacious factors that may stimulate the mesangeal proliferation and matrix production.
- These two factors are mainly contributing to the diabetic nephropathy
- **Bilateral renal artery stenosis, severe renal failure** are **contraindications** for **ACEI** use because Angiotensin II helps in maintaining adequate glomerular filtration.
- **Elderly hypertensive patient** are more susceptible for the **hypotensive** effect of ACEI.

9. Which of the following is a cardiotoxic anti-cancer drug?

A. Bleomycin　　**B.** Doxorubicin
C. 5 FU　　**D.** Dactinomycin

Ans: B Doxorubicin

Ref: *Goodman &Gillman's The Pharmacological Basis of Therapeutics, 2011, 12th Edition, McGraw Hill, Burton LL P 1712-1718*

Explanation:

- **Cardiomyopathy** is the **most important** long term toxicity of **Doxorubicin**
- In the acute phase, **ST and T wave changes** and **arrhythmias** can be precipitated.
- **Pericarditis- myocardiatis syndrome** following infusion of this drug which either manifests as **CHF** with **pericarditis** and **conduction disturbances.**
- Cumulative toxicity is characterized by **CHF** and **damage** to **myocardial fibrils**
- ***Dexrazoxane*** may reduce **troponin T elevation** and **cardio toxicity**.

Note:

- **Pulmonary toxicity** is the serious adverse reaction of **Bleomycin.**

10. The neurotransmitter secreted by postganglionic sympathetic fibers innervating sweat glands is:

A. Nor epinephrine　　**B.** Epinephrine
C. Acetyl Choline　　**D.** Dopamine

Ans: C. Acetyl choline

Ref: *Katzung 10th ed*

Explanation:

- NE is the neurotransmitter of all postganglionic sympathetic fibers except the ones innervating the sweat glands, where Acetyl choline is the Neuro transmitter.
(See figure on the next page)
- Parasympathetic ganglia are present near the wall of the organ innervated.
- Some sympathetic postganglionic fibers release acetylcholine or dopamine rather than norepinephrine.
- The adrenal medulla, a modified sympathetic ganglion, receives sympathetic preganglionic

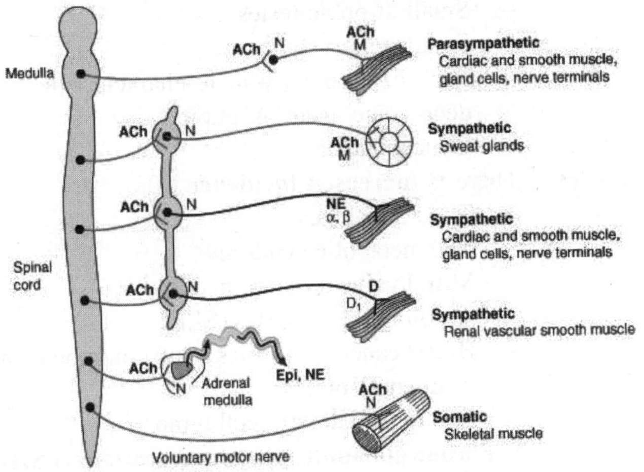

Fig: Schematic diagram comparing some anatomic and neurotransmitter features of autonomic and somatic motor nerves. (ACh, acetylcholine; D, dopamine; Epi, epinephrine; NE, norepinephrine; N, nicotinic receptors; M, muscarinic receptors.)

fibers and releases epinephrine and norepinephrine into the blood.

- The autonomic nervous system lends itself to division on anatomic grounds into two major portions: the **sympathetic (thoracolumbar)** division and the **parasympathetic (craniosacral)** division
- Both divisions originate in nuclei within the central nervous system and give rise to preganglionic efferent fibers that exit from the brain stem or spinal cord and terminate in motor ganglia.
- The sympathetic preganglionic fibers leave the central nervous system through the thoracic and lumbar spinal nerves.
- The parasympathetic preganglionic fibers leave the central nervous system through the cranial nerves (especially the third, seventh, ninth, and tenth) and the third and fourth sacral spinal roots.
- Most of the sympathetic preganglionic fibers terminate in ganglia located in the paravertebral chains that lie on either side of the spinal column.
- The remaining sympathetic preganglionic fibers terminate in prevertebral ganglia, which lie in front of the vertebrae, usually on the surface of the aorta.
- From the ganglia, postganglionic sympathetic fibers run to the tissues innervated. Some preganglionic parasympathetic fibers terminate in parasympathetic ganglia located outside the organs innervated: the ciliary, pterygopalatine, submandibular, otic, and several pelvic ganglia.
- The majority of parasympathetic preganglionic fibers terminate on ganglion cells distributed diffusely or in networks in the walls of the innervated organs.

11. Opiod induced respiratory depression can be reversed with

A. Naloxone **B.** Theophylline
C. Artificial ventillation **D.** Doxapram

Ans: A. Naloxone

Ref: *Goodman &Gillman's The Pharmacological Basis of Therapeutics, 2011, 12th Edition, McGraw Hill, Burton LL P519- 520*

Explanation:

- **Naloxone** is the **treatment of choice** in the **reversal of respiratory depression due to opioids.**
- Naloxone has to be **diluted** and slowly administered **intravenously** to **avoid withdrawal** in opioid dependent patients
- Monitoring of **arousal** and **respiratory function** are essential during this treatment
- Restoration of respiration without naloxone therapy may still results in **death** of the patient due to complication that develop during coma
- **Noncardiogenic pulmonary edema** that develops during **opioid poisoning** can be reversed by **positive pressure ventilation**

12. Which group of drugs potentiates the action of Neuromuscular blockers? (Repeat)

A. Aminoglycosides **B.** Cephalosporins
C. Ampicillin **D.** Penicillin

Ans: A. Aminoglycosides

Ref: *Goodman &Gillman, The pharmacological basis of therapeutics, 12th edition, Pg No. 1514*

Explanation:

- None of the other drugs mentioned have any effect on ACh neurotransmission.
- Potentiating neuromuscular blockers is a class effect exhibited by all **aminoglycoside antibiotics.**
- This is highest with **neomycin** followed by **Kanamycin Amikacin, gentamicin** and **Tobramycin**
- More common with **intrapleural** and **intraperitoneal instillation** of large doses of one of these agents.
- Can also seen with **intravenous** and **intramuscular** route
- This is due to the fact that they **inhibit the release of prejunctional release of ACh** as

well as **reducing the postsynaptic sensitivity to neurotransmitter.**
- Hence aminoglycosides should be used with caution in myasthenia gravis patients

13. Antihelminthic contraindicated in seizure disorder is:

A. DEC **B.** Albendazole
C. Piperazine **D.** Pyrantol Pamoate

Ans: C. Piperazine

Ref: *Essentials of Medical Pharmacology By KD Tripathi 7th edition, Pg.No 708*

Explanation:

- **Piperazine** causes hyperpolarization by GABA agonistic action opening Chloride channels causing **FLACCID PARALYSIS**
- Piperazine high dose can cause **convulsions** and **respiratory failure**
- It is contraindicated in **seizure disorder**
- Other drugs are safely given in seizure disorders.

PATHOLOGY

1. All are true regarding Klinefelter's syndrome *except:*

A. Small Testes
B. Webbing of neck
C. Gynecomastia
D. Increased FSH levels

Ans: B. Webbing of neck

Ref: *Robbins Pathologic Basis of Disease, 8th edition.*

Explanation:

- *Webbing of neck is characteristically seen in Turner's syndrome*

Klinefelter Syndrome

- ***Male hypogonadism*** *that occurs when there are* ***two or more X chromosomes and one or more Y chromosomes.***
- MC genetic disease involving the **sex chromosomes**
- Most common cause of **hypogonadism** in the **male**.
- Incidence **1 in 660** live male births
- It **can rarely be diagnosed before puberty** because the testicular abnormality develop late.
- **Distinctive body habitus -**
  - Increase in length between the soles and the pubic bone → elongated body
  - Eunuchoid body habitus
  - Long legs
  - Small atrophic testes
  - Small penis
  - Lack of secondary male characteristics as deep voice, beard & pubic hair.
  - Gynecomastia
- There is **increased incidence** of
  - Type 2 diabetes
  - The metabolic syndrome
  - Mitral valve prolapse in 50%.
  - Autoimmune diseases (SLE)
  - Breast cancer (**20 times** more common than in **normal males**)
  - Extragonadal germ cell tumors
- ↑↑**Plasma gonadotropin concentrations** (**FSH**) & ↓↓ **testosterone** levels
- ↑↑**Plasma estradiol** levels (Unknown mechanism)
- The ratio of estrogens and testosterone determines the degree of feminization in individual cases.
- **Reduced spermatogenesis** and **male infertility**
- Testicular tubules are totally **atrophied** and replaced by **pink**, **hyaline**, **collagenous ghosts**.
- Sometimes, apparently normal tubules are interspersed with atrophic tubules.
- In some patients all **tubules** are **primitive** and appear **embryonic**, consisting of cords of cells that never developed a lumen or progressed to mature spermatogenesis.
- **Leydig cells** appear **prominent**, as a result of the atrophy and crowding of tubules and elevation of gonadotropin concentrations.
- The classic pattern of Klinefelter syndrome is associated with a **47, XXY karyotype** (90% of cases).
- This complement of chromosomes results from **nondisjunction** during the **meiotic** divisions in one of the parents.
- 15% of patients with Klinefelter syndrome have been found to have a variety of **mosaic patterns**, most of them being **46, XY/47, XXY** (Other patterns are 47, XXY/48, XXXY)

Turner Syndrome

- *Turner syndrome results from complete or partial monosomy of the X chromosome and is characterized primarily by hypogonadism in phenotypic females*
- It is the most common sex chromosome abnormality in females.
- Three types of karyotypic abnormalities are seen in Turner syndrome.
  - Entire X chromosome is absent (57%), resulting in a 45 XO karyotype.

– Structural abnormalities of the X chromosomes (14%)
– Mosaics (29%).

- Examples of karyotypes that mosaic Turner females may have are the following: (1) 45,X/46, XX; (2) 45, X/46, XY; (3) 45, X/47, XXX; or (4) 45, X/46, X, i(X)(q10).
- The mosaics with a Y chromosome–containing population (e.g., **45, X/46, XY karyotype**) may be at risk of developing **Gonadoblastoma**

Classical Features of Turners syndrome

- Present during infancy with **edema of the dorsum of the hand and foot** due to lymph stasis. ***Swelling of the nape of the neck*** (due markedly distended lymphatic channels leading on to **cystic hygroma**)
- Bilateral ***neck webbing***
- **Persistent looseness of skin** on the **back of the neck.**
- *Congenital heart disease* (esp preductal **coarctation of the aorta** and bicuspid aortic valve)
- ***Failure*** *to develop normal* ***secondary sex characteristics.***
- *Turner syndrome is the single most important cause of* ***primary amenorrhea***
- Approximately 50% of patients develop autoantibodies to thyroid gland, and can develop **hypothyroidism**.
- **Glucose intolerance**, **obesity**, and **insulin resistance** in minority of patients

2. **Burkitt's lymphoma is associated with (Repeat)**
   A. t(8, 14)
   B. t(9,22)
   C. t(15,17)
   D. Deletion of 5 chromosome

Ans: A. t(8,14)

Ref: *Robbins Pathologic Basis of Disease, 8th edition, Bone misc tumors chapter*

Explanation:

BURKITT LYMPHOMA

There are three clinical types
(1) African (endemic) Burkitt lymphoma,
(2) Sporadic (nonendemic) Burkitt lymphoma
(3) Aggressive lymphomas asscioated with HIV.
These 3 types are histologically identical

Morphology

- The tumor exhibits a **high mitotic index** and contains numerous **apoptotic cells**, the nuclear remnants of which are phagocytosed by interspersed benign macrophages.
- These phagocytes have abundant clear cytoplasm, creating a characteristic **"starry sky" pattern**.

Immunophenotype

- These are tumors of mature B cells
- It express surface **IgM, CD19, CD20, CD10, and BCL6**, a phenotype consistent with a germinal center B-cell origin.
- Unlike other tumors of germinal center origin, this **does not express** anti-apoptotic protein **BCL2**.

Molecular Pathogenesis

- *All forms of Burkitt lymphoma are associated with translocations of the* ***c-MYC*** *gene on* ***chromosome 8****.*
- The translocation partner is usually the IgH locus [t(8;14)] but may also be the Ig K [t(2;8)] or γ [t(8;22)] light-chain loci.
- *All endemic tumors are latently infected with EBV*, which is also present in about 25% of HIV-associated tumors and 15% to 20% of sporadic cases.

Clinical Features

- **Endemic Burkitt lymphoma** often presents as a mass involving the mandible and shows an unusual predilection for involvement of abdominal viscera, particularly the kidneys, ovaries, and adrenal glands.
- **Sporadic Burkitt lymphoma** most often appears as a mass involving the ileocecum and peritoneum.
- Burkitt lymphoma is very aggressive but responds well to intensive chemotherapy.

3. **Aschoff nodules are characteristically seen in: (Repeat)**
   A. Rheumatic carditis
   B. Infective endocarditis
   C. Viral Myocarditis
   D. Libman-Sacks endocarditis

Ans: A. Rheumatic carditis

Ref: *Robbins Pathologic Basis of Disease, 8th edition, Pg: 529*

Explanation:

Rheumatic Fever (RF)

Morphology

- During acute RF, focal inflammatory lesions are found in various tissues.
- Distinctive lesions occur in the heart, called **Aschoff bodies**, which consist of foci of

lymphocytes (primarily T cells), occasional plasma cells, and

- Plump activated macrophages called **Anitschkow cells (pathognomonic for RF)** with abundant cytoplasm and multiple central round-to ovoid nuclei in which the chromatin is disposed in a central, slender, wavy ribbon (Hence, also known as **"caterpillar cells"**).
- During acute RF, diffuse inflammation and **Aschoff bodies** may be found in any of the three layers of the heart, causing pericarditis, myocarditis, or endocarditis (**pancarditis**).
- Inflammation of the endocardium and the left-sided valves typically results in fibrinoid necrosis within the cusps or along the tendinous cords.
- Overlying these necrotic foci are small (1- to 2-mm) vegetations, called **verrucae**, along the lines of closure.
- These vegetations place RHD within a small group of disorders that are associated with vegetative valve disease, each with its own characteristic morphologic features.
- Subendocardial lesions, perhaps exacerbated by regurgitant jets, may induce irregular thickenings called **MacCallum plaques**, usually in the left atrium.
- The cardinal anatomic changes of the mitral valve in chronic RHD are **leaflet thickening, commissural fusion and shortening, and thickening and fusion of the tendinous cords**.
- In chronic disease the mitral valve is virtually always involved.
- The mitral valve is affected alone in 65% to 70% of cases, and along with the aortic valve in another 25% of cases.
- Tricuspid valve involvement is infrequent, and the pulmonary valve is only rarely affected. Because of the increase in calcific aortic stenosis and the reduced frequency of RHD, rheumatic aortic stenosis now accounts for less than 10% of cases of acquired aortic stenosis.
- Fibrous bridging across the valvular commissures and calcification create "**fish mouth**" or "**buttonhole**" **stenoses.**
- With tight mitral stenosis, the left atrium progressively dilates and may harbor mural thrombi in the appendage or along the wall, either of which can embolize.
- Microscopically, in the mitral leaflets there is organization of the acute inflammation and subsequent diffuse fibrosis and **neovascularization** that obliterate the originally layered and avascular leaflet architecture.

4. **Most common site of gastric cancer is:**

   A. Lesser curvature of stomach
   B. Greater curvature of stomach
   C. Fundus
   D. Antrum

Ans: D. Antrum

Ref: *Robbins Pathologic Basis of Disease, 8th edition.*

Explanation:

*"Most **gastric adenocarcinomas** involve the gastric **antrum**; the lesser curvature is involved more often than the greater curvature" (Ref: Robbins)*

Gastric Adenocarcinoma

- Adenocarcinoma is the most common malignancy of the stomach, comprising over 90% of all gastric cancers.
- Early symptoms are non-specific and resemble those of chronic gastritis, including **dyspepsia**, **dysphagia**, and **nausea**.
- Weight loss, anorexia, altered bowel habits, anemia, and hemorrhage manifests in advanced stages
- As a result, these tumors are often discovered at advanced stages

Morphology

- Most gastric adenocarcinomas involve the gastric antrum
- The lesser curvature is involved more often than the greater curvature
- Gastric tumors are divided into two major types based on morphology
  - Intestinal type
  - Diffusive infiltrative type
- Tumors with **intestinal morphology** tend to form **bulky tumors** composed of **glandular structures** while cancers with a **diffuse infiltrative** growth pattern are more often composed of **signet-ring cells**
- ***Intestinal-type adenocarcinomas*** typically grow along broad cohesive fronts to form either an **exophytic mass** or an **ulcerated tumor**.
- The neoplastic cells often contain **apical mucin vacuoles**, and **abundant mucin** may be present in gland lumens.
- **Diffuse gastric cancer** is generally composed of **discohesive cells** that **do not form glands** but instead have **large mucin vacuoles** that **expand the cytoplasm** and push the **nucleus to the periphery**, creating a **signet-ring cell** morphology.
- **Extracellular mucin release** in either type of gastric cancer can result in formation of large **mucin lakes** that dissect tissue planes.

- A mass may be difficult to appreciate in diffuse gastric cancer, but these infiltrative tumors often evoke a **desmoplastic** reaction that stiffens the gastric wall
- When there are large areas of infitration, diffuse rugal flattening and a rigid, thickened wall may impart a **leather bottle** appearance termed **linitis plastica**
- **Breast** and **lung cancers** that **metastasize** to the **stomach** may also create a **linitis plastica–like appearance.**

Clinical Characteristics

- *The **depth of invasion** and the **extent of nodal and distant metastasis at the time of diagnosis** remain the **most powerful prognostic indicators** for gastric cancer*
- In advanced cases gastric carcinoma may first be detected as metastases to the supraclavicular sentinel lymph node, also called ***Virchow's node.***
- Gastric tumors can also metastasize to the periumbilical region to form a **subcutaneous nodule**, termed a ***Sister Mary Joseph nodule***.
- Local invasion into the duodenum, pancreas, and retroperitoneum is also characteristic.

5. **Zebra bodies seen in:**
   A. Niemann-Pick's disease
   B. Taysach's disease
   C. Pompe's disease
   D. Krabbe's disease

Ans: A. Niemann-Pick's disease

Ref: *Robbins Pathologic Basis of Disease, 8th edition.*

Explanation:

Niemann-Pick Disease

- It is characterized by lysosomal **accumulation of sphingomyelin** due to an inherited deficiency of **sphingomyelinase**
- **Type A**
  - Severe infantile form
  - Extensive neurologic involvement
  - Marked visceral accumulations of sphingomyelin
  - Progressive wasting
  - Early death within the first 3 years of life.
- **Type B**
  - Massive hepatosplenomegaly
  - No central nervous system involvement.
  - They usually survive into adulthood.

Morphology

- Sphingomyelin is a ubiquitous component of cellular (including organellar) membranes, and so the enzyme deficiency blocks degradation of the lipid, resulting in its **progressive accumulation within lysosomes**, particularly within cells of the **mononuclear phagocyte system**.
- Affected cells become **enlarged**, sometimes **to 90 μm** in diameter, due to the distention of lysosomes with **sphingomyelin and cholesterol**.
- **Innumerable small vacuoles** of **relatively uniform size** are created, imparting **foaminess** to the cytoplasm
- In frozen sections of fresh tissue, the **vacuoles stain for fat.**
- Electron microscopy confirms that the vacuoles are engorged secondary lysosomes that often contain **membranous cytoplasmic bodies** resembling **concentric lamellated myelin figures**, sometimes called **"zebra" bodies.**

6. **Which is not a small round cell tumor?**
   A. Osteosarcoma? **B.** Ewing's sarcoma
   C. Neuroblastoma **D.** Wilm's tumor

Ans: A. Osteosarcoma

Ref: *Robbins Pathologic Basis of Disease, 8th edition.*

Explanation:

Small-blue-round-cell tumors

- Aka blue-cell tumor (SRBCT), small-blue-round-cell tumour (SBRCT) or a small-round-cell tumour (SRCT)
- In histopathology, a group of malignant neoplasms have a characteristic similar appearance i.e. consisting of **small round cells** that stain **blue** on routine **H&E** stained sections.
- These tumors are more typically seen in **children** than adults.
- They typically represent **undifferentiated cells.**
- The predominance of blue staining is due the fact that the cells consist predominantly of **nucleus**, thus they have **scant cytoplasm**
- **Tumors that belong to this group are**:
  - Desmoplastic small-round-cell tumour
  - Ewing's Sarcoma/PNET
  - Neuroblastoma
  - Medulloblastoma
  - Rhabdomyosarcoma
  - Carcinoid tumor
  - Small cell lung cancer
  - Wilms' tumour
  - Retinoblastoma
  - Small-cell lymphoma
  - Hepatoblastoma- (Anaplastic form)

Morphology of Osteosarcoma

The tumor cells vary in **size and shape** and frequently have **large hyperchromatic nuclei.**

Bizarre tumor giant cells are common, as are mitoses.

7. **Brown tumor is seen with:**
A. Hyperparathyroidism
B. Hypoparathyroidism
C. Hypothyroidism
D. Hyperthyroidism

Ans: A. Hyperparathyroidism

Ref: *Robbins Pathologic Basis of Disease, 8th edition.*

Explanation:

Primary Hyperparathyroidism

- **Most common** endocrine disorder causing hypercalcemia.
- The frequency of the various parathyroid lesions underlying the hyperfunction is as follows:
  - **Adenoma**: 85% to 95%
  - **Primary hyperplasia** (diffuse or nodular): 5% to 10%
  - **Parathyroid carcinoma**: ~ 1%
- Primary hyperparathyroidism is usually a disease of **adults**
- More common in women than in men by a ratio of nearly **4 : 1.**
- Most common Cause is a **solitary parathyroid adenoma** arising in the **sporadic (nonfamilial) setting**
- Familial syndromes are second commonest cause
- The genetic syndromes associated with familial primary hyperparathyroidism include the following:

Multiple endocrine neoplasia-1 (MEN-1):

- Inactivation of MEN1 gene on chromosome 11q13 (Tumor suppressor gene)

Multiple endocrine neoplasia-2 (MEN-2):

- Activating mutations in the tyrosine kinase receptor, RET, on chromosome 10q.

Familial hypocalciuric hypercalcemia

- Autosomal dominant disorder
- Enhanced parathyroid function due to **decreased sensitivity** to **extracellular calcium.**
- **Inactivating mutations** in the **parathyroid calcium-sensing receptor gene (CASR)** on chromosome 3q

Morphology

Parathyroid adenomas

- These are almost **always solitary**
- The typical parathyroid adenoma averages 0.5 to 5.0 gm; well-circumscribed, soft, tan to reddish-brown nodule; and has a delicate capsule.
- In contrast to primary hyperplasia, the glands outside the adenoma are usually **normal in size** or somewhat **shrunken** because of feedback inhibition by elevated levels of serum calcium.
- Microscopically, parathyroid **adenomas** are mostly composed of ***fairly uniform, polygonal chief cells with small, centrally placed nuclei***
- At least a few nests of larger **oxyphil cells** are present as well;
- Rarely, entire adenomas may be composed of this cell type (**oxyphil adenomas**).

Primary hyperplasia

- It may occur **sporadically** or as a component of **MEN** syndrome.
- Classically **all four glands** are involved
- The combined weight of all glands rarely exceeds 1.0 gm and is often less.
- Microscopically, the most common pattern seen is that of **chief cell hyperplasia**, which may involve the glands in a **diffuse or multinodular** pattern.
- The constituent cells contain **abundant water-clear cells** (**"water-clear cell hyperplasia"**).

Parathyroid carcinomas

- May be **circumscribed lesions** that are difficult to distinguish from adenomas
- These tumors enlarge **one** parathyroid gland and consist of gray-white, irregular masses that sometimes **exceed 10 gm** in weight.
- The cells are usually **uniform** and **resemble normal parathyroid cells.**
- They are arrayed in nodular or trabecular patterns with a dense, fibrous capsule enclosing the mass.
- Diagnosis of carcinoma based on **cytologic detail** is **unreliable**
- **Invasion of surrounding tissues** and **metastasis** are the only reliable criteria.

Morphologic changes in other organs deserving special mention include **skeletal** and **renal lesions.**

Skeletal changes

- Increased numbers of **osteoclasts**, which **erode bone matrix** and b, particularly in the **metaphyses** of **long tubular bones.**
- Bone resorption is accompanied by **increased osteoblastic activity** and the formation of new bony trabeculae.
- In severe cases, the cortex is grossly thinned, and the **marrow** contains increased amounts of **fibrous tissue** accompanied by foci of **hemorrhage** and **cyst formation (osteitis fibrosa cystica)**
- Aggregates of osteoclasts, reactive giant cells, and hemorrhagic debris occasionally form **masses** that may be mistaken for neoplasms (***Brown tumors of hyperparathyroidism***).

- PTH-induced hypercalcemia favors formation of urinary tract stones (**nephrolithiasis**) as well as calcification of the renal interstitium and tubules (**nephrocalcinosis**).
- **Metastatic calcification** secondary to hypercalcemia may also be seen in other sites, including the **stomach**, **lungs**, myocbardium, and **blood vessels.**

Clinical Course

Primary hyperparathyroidism may be:

(1) Asymptomatic and identified after a routine chemistry profile
(2) Associated with the Classic clinical manifestations of primary hyperparathyroidism.

Asymptomatic Hyperparathyroidism

- **Primary hyperparathyroidism** is the most common cause of **asymptomatic hypercalcemia**
- Most common manifestation of **primary hyperparathyroidism** is **hypercalcemia.**
- **Malignancy** is the most frequent cause of clinically apparent hypercalcemia in adults
- In individuals with primary hyperparathyroidism, serum PTH levels are inappropriately elevated for the level of serum calcium, whereas PTH levels are low to undetectable in hypercalcemia caused by of nonparathyroid diseases
- Other laboratory alterations referable to **PTH excess** include **hypophosphatemia** and **increased urinary excretion** of both **calcium** and **phosphate.**
- **Secondary renal disease** may lead to **phosphate retention** with normalization of serum phosphates.

Causes of Hypercalcemia

Raised [PTH]	Decreased [PTH]
Hyperparathyroidism	Hypercalcemia of malignancy
Primary (Adenoma > hyperplasia)	Vitamin D toxicity
Secondary	Immobilization
Tertiary	Thiazide diuretics
Familial hypocalciuric hypercalcemia	Granulomatous disease (sarcoidosis)

Symptomatic Primary Hyperparathyroidism

- The signs and symptoms of hyperparathyroidism reflect the combined effects of **increased PTH** secretion and **hypercalcemia.**
- Classical description of symptoms inPrimary hyperparathyroidism
  - Painful bones
  - Renal stones
  - Abdominal groans
  - Psychic moans

The constellation of symptoms includes:

Bone disease and bone pain secondary to fractures of bones weakened by ***osteoporosis or osteitis fibrosa cystica.***
Nephrolithiasis (renal stones) in ***20%*** of newly diagnosed patients, with attendant pain and ***obstructive uropathy***. ***Chronic renal insufficiency*** and abnormalities in renal function lead to polyuria and secondary polydipsia.
Gastrointestinal disturbances, including constipation, nausea, peptic ulcers, pancreatitis, and gallstones.
Central nervous system alterations, including depression, lethargy, and eventually seizures.
Neuromuscular abnormalities, including weakness and fatigue.
Cardiac manifestations, including ***aortic*** or ***mitral valve calcifications*** (or both).

SECONDARY HYPERPARATHYROIDISM

- It is caused by any condition that gives rise to **chronic hypocalcemia**, which in turn leads to **compensatory overactivity** of the **parathyroid** glands.
- **Causes**
  - ***Renal failure*** *is by far the* ***most common*** *cause of secondary hyperparathyroidism*
  - Inadequate dietary intake of calcium
  - Steatorrhea
  - Vitamin D deficiency
- The etiopathogenesis is complex and not fully understood.
- Chronic renal insufficiency is associated with **decreased phosphate excretion**, which in turn results in **hyperphosphatemia.**
- The **elevated serum phosphate** levels directly **depress serum calcium levels** and thereby **stimulate parathyroid** gland activity.
- In addition, loss of renal substance **reduces** the **availability of α-1-hydroxylase** necessary for the synthesis of the **active form** of **vitamin D,** which in turn **reduces intestinal absorption of calcium** Because **vitamin D** has suppressive effects on **parathyroid growth** and **PTH secretion,** its relative deficiency compounds the **hyperparathyroidism** in renal failure.

8. CD marker of stem cell is:

A. CD 34 **B.** CD 1
C. CD19 **D.** CD 21

Ans: A. CD 34

Ref: *Robbins Pathologic Basis of Disease, 8th edition.*

Explanation:

(See table on the next page)

Some Immune Cell Antigens Detected by Monoclonal Antibodies

Antigen Designation	Normal Cellular Distribution
PRIMARILY T-CELL ASSOCIATED	
CD1	Thymocytes and **Langerhans** cells
CD3	Thymocytes, mature T cells
CD4	Helper T cells, subset of thymocytes
CD5	T cells and a small subset of B cells
CD8	Cytotoxic T cells, subset of thymocytes, and some NK cells
PRIMARILY B-CELL ASSOCIATED	
CD10	Pre-B cells and germinal-center B cells; also called **CALLA**
CD19	Pre-B cells and mature B cells but not plasma cells
CD20	Pre-B cells after CD19 and mature B cells but not plasma cells
CD21	**EBV receptor;** mature B cells and follicular dendritic cells
CD23	Activated mature B cells
CD79a	Marrow pre-B cells and mature B cells
PRIMARILY MONOCYTE- OR MACROPHAGE-ASSOCIATED	
CD11c	Granulocytes, monocytes, and macrophages; also expressed by hairy cell leukemias
CD13	Immature and mature **monocytes** and granulocytes
CD14	**Monocytes**
CD15	Granulocytes; Reed-Sternberg cells and variants
CD33	Myeloid progenitors and **monocytes**
CD64	Mature myeloid cells
PRIMARILY NK-CELL ASSOCIATED	
CD16	NK cells and granulocytes
CD56	NK cells and a subset of T cells
PRIMARILY STEM CELL–AND PROGENITOR CELL–ASSOCIATED	
CD34	**Pluripotent hematopoietic stem cells** and **progenitor cells** of many lineages
ACTIVATION MARKERS	
CD30	**Activated B cells**, **T cells**, and **monocytes**; Reed-Sternberg cells and variants
PRESENT ON ALL LEUKOCYTES	
CD45	All leukocytes; also known as **leukocyte common antigen (LCA)**

9. Infective endarteritis is characteristically seen in:

A. PDA **B.** VSD
C. TOF **D.** Tricuspid atresia

Ans: A. PDA

Ref: *Robbins Pathologic Basis of Disease, 8th edition & Huggon IC, Qureshi SA. Is the prevention of infective endarteritis a valid reason for closure of the patent arterial duct? Eur Heart J. 1997 Mar;18(3):364-6.*

Explanation:

Obliterating endarteritis

- It also called **"obliterating arteritis"** is severe proliferating endarteritis that results in an occlusion of the lumen of the artery.

Causes of Endarteritis

- Patent Ductus arteriosus (PDA)
- Syphilis (All stages, especially the late stages)
- TB Meningitis
- Rheumatoid arthritis
- **Meningovascular neurosyphilis** is a chronic meningitis involving the base of the brain and more variably the cerebral convexities and the spinal leptomeninges. There may be an associated **obliterative endarteritis (Heubner arteritis)**
- **Infective endarteritis (IE)** was a fatal complication and the most common cause of death **(45%)** in patients with **patent ductus arteriosus (PDA),** before the introduction of antibiotic therapy and surgical closure of the ductus.
- In **Rheumatoid arthritis,** segments of small arteries such as **vasa nervorum** and **digital arteries** are obstructed by an **obliterating endarteritis** resulting in **peripheral neuropathy, ulcers,** and **gangrene.** Leukocytoclastic venulitis produces purpura, cutaneous ulcers, and nail bed infarction.
- Florid cases of **TB Meningitis** show well-formed **granulomas,** often with **caseous necrosis** and giant cells. Arteries running through the **subarachnoid space** may show **obliterative endarteritis** with **inflammatory infiltrates** in their walls and marked **intimal thickening.**

10. Negri bodies are found in:

A. Basal ganglia **B.** Hippocampus
C. Spinal cord **D.** Cerebrum

Ans: B. Hippocampus

Ref: *Robbins Pathologic Basis of Disease, 8th edition.*

Explanation:

*"**Negri bodies**, the pathognomonic microscopic finding, are cytoplasmic, round to oval, eosinophilic inclusions that can be found in **pyramidal neurons** of the **hippocampus** and **Purkinje cells** of the **cerebellum**, sites usually **devoid of inflammation**"*

Ref: Robbins.

Rabies

- Rabies is a severe encephalitis transmitted to humans by the bite of a rabid animal, usually a dog or various wild mammals
- Exposure to certain species of **bats**, even **without a bite**, can also lead to rabies.

Morphology

- On macroscopic examination the brain shows intense **edema** and **vascular congestion**.
- On microscopic examination there is
- Widespread neuronal degeneration and an
- Generalised inflammatory reaction that is most severe in the **Brainstem**.
- The **basal ganglia**, **spinal cord**, and **dorsal root ganglia** may also be involved.
- **Negri bodies**, the **pathognomonic microscopic finding**, are **cytoplasmic**, **round** to **oval**, **eosinophilic inclusions** that can be found in **pyramidal neurons** of the **hippocampus** and **Purkinje cells** of the **cerebellum**, sites usually devoid of inflammation.
- The presence of rabies virus can be detected within Negri bodies by **ultrastructural** and **immunohistochemical** examination.

Clinical Features

- The virus enters the CNS by **ascending** along the **peripheral** nerves from the wound site,
- The incubation period (**1 - 3 months**) depends on the distance between the wound and the brain.
- The disease begins with **nonspecific symptoms** of malaise, headache, and fever
- **Local paresthesias** around the wound is Diagnostic.
- In Advanced stages, the affected individual exhibits **extraordinary CNS excitability**
- Even the slightest touch is painful, with violent motor responses progressing to **convulsions**.
- Contracture of the pharyngeal musculature on swallowing produces foaming at the mouth, which may create an aversion to swallowing even water (**hydrophobia**).
- There is **meningismus** and, as the disease progresses, **flaccid paralysis**.
- Periods of alternating **mania** and **stupor** progress to **coma** and **death** from **respiratory center failure**.

11. Juene's syndrome is inherited as: (Repeat)

A. AR **B.** AD
C. XR **D.** XD

Ans: A. AR

Ref: *Robbins Pathologic Basis of Disease, 8th edition.*

Explanation:

(Refer to explanation in 2011 Pediatrics Question)

Jeune syndrome (Familial asphyxiating thoracic dystrophy)

- Autosomal recessive disorder
- Classic manifestations in infancy include
  - ***Dwarfism with short ribs***
  - ***Short limbs***
  - Characteristic ***radiographic changes*** in ribs and pelvis
- Small chests
- Respiratory insufficiency
- Lung hypoplasia (Due to a restricted thoracic cage) Major cause of death in infancy.
- Renal and pancreatic insufficiency (in those who survive newborn period)

Other Clinical Features

- Respiratory distress
- Chest deformity of varying degree
- Short-limbed dwarfism
- Failure to thrive
- Gastroenteritis
- Recurrent rectal prolapse
- Diarrhea
- Congestive cardiac failure
- Puffy face, and
- Ankle swelling

12. All are true regarding Paget's disease *except:*

A. Increased osteolytic activity
B. Increased osteoblastic activity
C. Occurs in young women
D. Increased chances of malignancy

Ans: A. Occurs in young women

Ref: *Robbins Pathologic Basis of Disease, 8th edition, Bone misc tumors chapter Pg:*

Explanation:

Paget Disease (Osteitis Deformans)

This unique skeletal disease can be divided into three phases:

(1) An initial **osteolytic** stage
(2) A mixed **osteoclastic-osteoblastic** stage (Predominance of osteoblastic activity)
(3) A **burnt-out quiescent osteosclerotic** stage

- The net effect is a ***gain in bone mass***, but the newly formed bone is **disordered** and **architecturally abnormal**
- Begins in late adulthood (Mean: 70 years) and increases with age

Pathogenesis

- Autosomal dominant pattern (15 - 40%) .
- Mutations in the ***SQSTM1*** gene (40 -50% of familial Paget disease, and 5% to 10% of non-familial Paget)
- The *SQSTM* mutations enhance **NF-kB** activation by **RANK** signaling, causing **increased osteoclast** activity
- Mutations in ***RANKL*** and ***RANK/OPG*** causes some phenotypic overlap with Paget disease

- **Familial expansile osteolysis**
- **Expansile skeletal hyperphosphatasia**
- **Early-onset Paget disease**
- **Juvenile Paget disease**
- **Syndrome of hereditary inclusion body myopathy**
- **Frontotemporal dementia.**

- **Morphology**
  Paget disease is a focal process that shows remarkable histologic variation over time and from site to site.
- The hallmark is the "**mosaic pattern**" of **lamellar bone.**
- This pattern, which is likened to a **jigsaw puzzle,** is produced by prominent cement lines that anneal haphazardly oriented units of lamellar bone
- In the **initial lytic phase** there are waves of **osteoclastic activity** and **numerous resorption pits.**
- The **osteoclasts** are abnormally large and have many more than the normal 10 to 12 nuclei; sometimes **100 nuclei** are present.
- Osteoclasts persist in the mixed phase, but now many of the bone surfaces are lined by prominent osteoblasts.
- The newly formed bone may be woven or lamellar, but eventually all of it is remodeled into lamellar bone.
- As the **mosaic pattern** unfolds and the cell activity decreases, the periosseous fibrovascular tissue recedes and is replaced by normal marrow.
- Bone is larger than normal and composed of coarsely thickened trabeculae and soft cortices that are porous and lack structural stability.
- These aspects make the bone vulnerable to deformation under stress causing fractures easily.

Clinical Course

- Clinical findings are extremely variable and depend on the extent and site of the disease.
- Most cases are mild and are discovered as an incidental radiographic finding.
- Paget disease is **monostotic** in about **15%** of cases and **polyostotic** in the remainder.
- The **axial skeleton or proximal femur** is involved in up to **80%** of cases.
- Involvement of the **ribs, fibula,** and **small bones** of the **hands** and **feet** is **unusual.**
- **Pain** localized to the affected bone is common.
- It is caused by microfractures or by bone overgrowth that compresses spinal and cranial nerve roots.
- Enlargement of the craniofacial skeleton may produce ***leontiasis ossea***
- Cranium can be so heavy that is difficult for the person to hold the head erect.
- The weakened pagetic bone may lead to **invagination of the skull base *(platybasia)*** and compression of the posterior fossa structures.
- **Weight bearing** causes **anterior bowing** of the **femurs** and **tibiae** and **distorts** the **femoral heads** causing ***severe secondary osteoarthritis.***
- ***Chalkstick-type*** **fractures** is a frequent complication occuring in the long bones of legs.
- **Compression fractures** of the **spine** causes **kyphoses.**
- The **hypervascularity** of pagetic bone warms the overlying skin, and in severe polyostotic disease the increased blood flow acts like an **arteriovenous shunt**, leading to **high-output heart failure** or **exacerbation** of underlying **cardiac disease.**
- A variety of tumor and tumor-like conditions develop in pagetic bone.
- The benign lesions include **giant-cell tumor, giant-cell reparative granuloma,** and **extra-osseous masses of hematopoiesis.**
- The most dreaded complication is **sarcoma,** which occurs **in 0.7% to 0.9%** of all individuals with Paget disease, and in **5% to 10%** of those with **severe polyostotic disease.**
- The sarcomas are usually **osteosarcoma** or **fibrosarcoma,** and they arise in Paget lesions in the long **bones, pelvis, skull** and **spine.**

Investigations & Management

- Pagetic bone is typically enlarged with **thick, coarsened cortices** and **cancellous** bone.
- Active disease has a **wedge-shaped lytic leading edge** that may progress along the length of the bone at a rate of **1 cm per year**
- Many affected individuals have **elevated serum alkaline phosphatase levels** and **increased urinary excretion of hydroxyproline.**
- In the absence of malignant transformation, Paget disease is usually not a serious or life-threatening disease.
- Most affected individuals have mild symptoms that are readily suppressed by **calcitonin** and **bisphosphonates.**

13. CGG repeat sequence is found in:

A. Fragile X syndrome
B. Huntingtons chorea
C. Dentatorubropallidolusyian atrophy
D. Machado Joseph disease

Ans: A. Fragile X syndrome

Ref: *Robbins and Cotran 'Pathologic Basis of Disease' 8th Edition.Elsevier. 2011. Page 168.*

Explanation:

Expansions affecting non-coding regions

Disease	Protein	Repeating Sequence
Fragile X syndrome	FMR-1 protein	CGG
Friedrich ataxia	Frataxin	GAA
Myotonic Dystophy	Myotonic dystrophy protein kinase (MDPK)	CTG

(See the following table)

14. All are oncogenic viruses *except:*

A. Hepatitis C
B. Ebstein Barr virus
C. Human Metapneumovirus
D. Papilloma virus

Ans: C. Human Metapneumovirus

Ref: *Robbins and Cotran 'Pathologic Basis of Disease' 8th Edition.Elsevier. 201. Pg 313.*

Explanation:

Oncogenic RNA Viruses

- Human T-Cell Leukemia Virus Type 1 - T-cell leukemia/lymphoma
- Hepatitis C Virus – Hepatocellular Carcinoma

Oncogenic DNA Viruses

- Human Papillomavirus.
  - Types 1, 2, 4 & 7 – Benign Squamous Papillomas (Warts)
  - Types 16 & 18 - squamous cell Ca of the cervix and anogenital area
- Human herpes virus 8 – Kaposi Sarcoma
- Epstein-Barr Virus
  - The African form of Burkitt lymphoma;
  - B-cell lymphomas in immunosuppressed individuals
  - A subset of Hodgkin lymphoma;
  - Nasopharyngeal carcinoma
  - Gastric carcinomas and rare forms of
  - T cell lymphomas and
  - Natural killer (NK) cell lymphomas.
- Hepatitis B Virus - Hepatocellular Carcinoma
- Merkel cell polyomavirus – Merkel Cell Carcinoma

Oncogenic Bacteria

Helicobacter pylori - gastric adenocarcinomas and gastric lymphomas

15. Which of the following lesion is characteristic of diabetic nephropathy?

A. Hyaline arteriosclerosis
B. Nodular glomerulosclerosis
C. Renal Amyloid deposits
D. Fibrinoid necrosis

Ans: B. Nodular glomerulosclerosis

Ref: *Robbins Pathologic Basis of Disease, 8th edition*

Explanation:

Diabetic Nephropathy

- The term diabetic nephropathy is applied to the conglomerate of lesions that occur in the diabetic kidney.
- Most common lesions involve the **glomeruli** and are associated clinically with three glomerular syndromes:
  - Non-nephrotic proteinuria
  - Nephrotic syndrome
  - Chronic renal failure
- Diabetes also affects the **arterioles** (causing **hyalinizing arteriolar sclerosis**), increases susceptibility to the development of **pyelonephritis** and particularly **papillary necrosis**, and causes a variety of **tubular lesions**.
- The morphologic changes in the glomeruli include
  (1) Capillary basement membrane thickening
  (2) Diffuse mesangial sclerosis
  (3) **Nodular glomerulosclerosis** (**Kimmelstiel-Wilson** lesions).

Expansions non-coding regions

Disease	Protein	Repeating Sequence
Spinobulbar muscular atrophy (Kennedy Disease)	Androgen Receptor	CAG
Huntington Disease	Huntington	CAG
Dentatorubral-pallidoluysian atrophy (Haw River Syndrome)	Atrophin - 1	CAG
Spinocerebellar ataxia type 1	Ataxin-1	CAG
Spinocerebellar ataxia type 2	Ataxin-2	CAG
Spinocerebellar ataxia type 3 (Machado Joseph Disease)	Ataxin-3	CAG
Spinocerebellar ataxia type 6	Alpha 1a-Voltage- dependant calcium channel subunit	CAG
Spinocerebellar ataxia type 7	Ataxin-7	CAG

- The morphology is identical in type 1 and type 2 diabetes
- The **Armanni-Ebstein change** (or **Armanni-Ebstein cells**) consists of deposits of glycogen in the tubular epithelial cells (pars straight of proximal convoluted tubule and loop of Henle).

16. **Superior sulcus tumor of the lungs characteristically present with:**

A. Horner's syndrome	**B.** Breathlessness
C. Hemoptysis	**D.** Pancoast tumor

Ans: D. Pancoast tumor

***Ref:** Robbins Pathologic Basis of Disease, 8th edition*

Explanation:

- Apical lung cancers in the superior pulmonary sulcus tend to invade the neural structures around the trachea, including the cervical sympathetic plexus.
- It produces a group of clinical findings that includes severe ***pain in the distribution of the ulnar nerve*** and ***Horner syndrome*** (enophthalmos, ptosis, miosis, and anhidrosis) on the same side as the lesion.
- Such tumors are also referred to as **Pancoast** tumors.

17. **EBV causes all *except:* (Repeat)**

A. Kaposi sarcoma	**B.** Nasopharyngeal Ca
C. Burkitt lymphoma	**D.** Infecious mononucleosis

Ans: A. Kaposi sarcoma

***Ref:** Robbins Pathologic Basis of Disease, 8th edition*

Explanation:

Diseases associated with Epstein-Barr virus

- Infectious mononucleosis
- Burkitt's lymphoma
- Hodgkin's lymphoma (Mixed cellularity, Lymphocyte rich & Lymphocyte depletion)
- Nasopharyngeal carcinoma
- Multiple sclerosis
- Extranodal NK/T-cell lymphoma
- X-linked lymphoproliferation syndrome (Duncan disease)
- Lymphoepithelioma-like carcinoma of Thymus
- Oral Hairy leukoplakia
  - **Kaposi sarcoma** is associated with Human herpes virus-8 (**HHV-8**) infection.

MICROBIOLOGY

1. **Northern blot is used for identification of: (Repeat)**

A. RNA	**B.** DNA
C. Protein	**D.** Antibodies

Ans: A. RNA

***Ref:** Ananthanarayan R, Paniker CKJ. Textbook of Microbiology. 8th Edition. Hyderabad: Universities Press; 2009. Pg. 69*

Explanation:

- **Southern blotting:**
  The highly sensitive technique for identifying **DNA fragments** by DNA-DNA hybridisation is called Southern blotting, after EM Southern who devised it. This technique has very wide applications in DNA analysis.
- **Northern blotting:**
  An analogous procedure for the analysis of **RNA** has been called northern blotting (as opposed to Southern blotting). Here the RNA mixture is separated by gel electrophoresis, blotted and identified using labelled DNA or RNA probes.
- **Western blotting:**
  A similar technique for the identification of **proteins (antigens)** is called immunoblotting (or, in conformity with other blotting techniques, western blotting). Here the protein antigen mixture is separated by **SDS- PAGE** (sodium dodecylsulfate-polyacrylamide gel electrophoresis), blotted on to nitrocellulose strips and identified by radiolabeled or enzyme-labeled antibodies as probes. E.g. Western blot test for detection of antibodies directed against different antigens of HIV

2. **Non granular fungal disease is:**

A. Cryptococcosis
B. Blastomycosis
C. Candidiasis
D. Paracoccidioidomycosis

Ans: C. Candidiasis

***Ref:** Ananthanarayan R, Paniker CKJ. Textbook of Microbiology. 8th Edition. Hyderabad: Universities Press; 2009. Pg. 607, 610-11*

Explanation:

Blastomycosis

- This is a chronic infection caused by the dimorphic fungus **Blastomyces dermatitidis**
- It is characterised by the formation of **suppurative** and **granulomatous** lesions
- It can affect any part of the body but has a marked predilection for the **lungs and skin.**

Paracoccidioidomycosis

- This is a chronic **granulomatous** disease of the **skin, mucosa, lymph nodes** and **internal organs**

- It is caused by **Paracoccidioides brasiliensis**
- As the disease is confined to South America, it is called **'South American blastomycosis'**.
- **Ulcerative granulomas** of the **buccal** and **nasal mucosa** are a prominent feature of the disease.

Cryptococcosis

- **Cryptococcosis (torulosis)** is a subacute or chronic infection caused by the yeast Cryptococcus neoformans.
- It is a round or ovoid budding cell, 4-20 μm in diameter, with a prominent polysaccharide capsule
- **Pulmonary cryptococcosis** may lead to mild pneumonitis. As no calcification occurs, healed pulmonary lesions are not evident radiologically.
- Dissemination of infection leads to visceral, cutaneous and meningeal disease.
- Visceral forms simulate tuberculosis and cancer clinically.
- Bones and joints may be involved.
- Cutaneous cryptococcosis varies from small ulcers to large granulomas.
- **Cryptococcal meningitis** is the most serious type of infection and can resemble tuberculous or other chronic types of meningitis.

Candidiasis

- Candidosis (candidiasis, moniliasis) is an infection of the skin, mucosa, and rarely of the internal organs
- It is caused by a yeast like fungus, Candida albicans, and occasionally by other Candida species.
- **Cutaneous candidiasis** is an erythematous, scaling or moist lesion with sharply demarcated borders, where papular lesions are most prominent.
- Common mucosal lesions are vaginitis characterised by an acidic discharge and found frequently in pregnancy, and oral thrush found commonly in bottle fed infants and the aged and debilitated. Creamy white patches appear on the tongue or buccal mucosa, that leave a red oozing surface on removal.
- In all forms of candidiasis there is no granuloma formation.

Chronic mucocutaneous candidiasis

- Chronic **mucocutaneous candidiasis** is a form of persistent candidiasis, usually caused by *C. albicans*, of the skin, nails and mucous membranes
- It occurs in patients with various **metabolic disturbances** to **cell-mediated immunity** such as defects in **leukocyte function** or **endocrine disorders** such as **hypoparathyroidism**, **Addison's** disease, **hypothyroidism**, **diabetes**, **dysfunction** of the **thyroid** and **polyglandular autoimmune** disebase.
- The patients are usually **children**.
- *Candida* granuloma is a severe localized form which may occur with or without endocinopathy characterized by marked hyperkeratic granulomatous lesions. Although candidiasis is generally a non-granular infection. This is the only form which is granulomatous.

3. **Phage typing is useful in classification of all *except:***

A. Staphylococcus	**B.** Streptococcus
C. Cholera	**D.** Salmonella

Ans: B. Streptococcus

Ref: *Ananthanarayan R, Paniker CKJ. Textbook of Microbiology. 8th Edition. Hyderabad: Universities Press; 2009. Pg. 199, 205, 293-8, 305*

Explanation:

Staphylococcus

- Staphylococci may be **typed**, based on their susceptibility to **bacteriophages**
- An internationally accepted set of phages is used for typing.
- Staphylococcal phage typing is done by a pattern method.
- The phage type of the strain is expressed by the designations of all the phages that lyse it. Thus, if a strain is lysed only by phages 52 79 and 80, it is called phage type 52/79/80.
- Phage typing is of great importance in epidemiological studies of staphylococcal infections.

Streptococcus

- The Streptococcus are classified on the basis of their **hemolytic** properties as **alpha**, **beta** and **gamma** groups
- Beta hemolytic streptococci were classified by **Lancefield** serologically into groups based on the nature of a **carbohydrate (C) antigen on the cell wall.**
- These are known as **Lancefield groups**, twenty of which have been identified so far and named **A-V (without I and J).**

Vibrio cholerae

- The EI Tor strains are differentiated from Classical strains of Vibrio cholerae based on non-hemolytic nature, negative VP tests, chick cell agglutination, polymyxin sensitivity and **phage susceptibility tests**

Salmonella

- Important pathogens such as S typhi, S paratyphi A and B, and S typhimurium can be further typed for epidemiological purposes by phage susceptibility
- Intraspecies classification of S typhi for epidemiological purposes was made possible by bacteriophage typing, first developed by Craigie and Yen (1937). They found that a bacteriophage acting on the Vi antigen of the typhoid bacillus (Vi phage II) was highly adaptable. The parent phage is called phage A. It could be made specific for a particular strain of typhoid bacillus by serial propagation in the strain.
- **Phage typing** also provides information on the trends and patterns in the epidemiology of typhoid at the local, national and international levels.
- The phage type is stable.

4. **Pinta is caused by:**

A. T pertenue **B.** T pallidum
C. T carateum **D.** Borrelia burgdorferi

Ans: C. T carateum

Ref: *Ananthanarayan R, Paniker CKJ. Textbook of Microbiology. 8th Edition. Hyderabad: Universities Press; 2009. Pg. 371, 378*

Explanation:

- Venereal syphilis is caused by *T pallidum*
- Yaws is caused by *T pertenue*
- Pinta is caused by *T carateum*

Pinta

- Pinta (carate, mal del pinto) is endemic in Central and South America and the neighbouring islands.
- The primary lesion is an extragenital papule, which does not ulcerate but develops into a lichenoid or psoriaform patch.
- Secondary skin lesions are characterised by hyperpigmentation or hypopigmentation Tissues other than skin are seldom affected

5. **Maximum exposure to HIV is seen in:**

A. Intrapartum period **B.** Breastfeeding
C. 1st Trimester **D.** 3rd Trimester

Ans: A. Intrapartum period

Ref: *Ananthanarayan R, Paniker CKJ. Textbook of Microbiology. 8th Edition. Hyderabad: Universities Press; 2009. Pg. 575 & WHO. A review of HIV transmission through breast feeding. 1998*

Explanation:

- About a third to half the number of babies born to infected mothers are infected with
- Transmission of infection from mother to baby can take place before, during or after birth.
- HIV Virus transmission may occur to the fetus in pregnancy as early as the first trimester, but infection is more common during intrapartum period.

Percentage HIV infection acquired by different routes *

	Partially breastfed/ breastfedin fants	Non-breastfed infants
During intrauterine period	20%	33%
During delivery	45-50%	67%
Postpartum, by breastfeeding	30-35%	0

* These rates are observed in the absence of interventions to reduce MTCT

6. **Bacterial adherence to epithelium is mediated through:**

A. Sex pili **B.** Fimbriae
C. Flagella **D.** Mesosomes

Ans: B. Fimbriae

Ref: *Ananthnarayan R, Paniker CKJ. Textbook of Microbiology. 8th Edition. Hyderabad: Universities Press; 2009. Pg. 18-21.*

Explanation:

Fimbriae

- Certain **Gram-negative** bacilli carry very fine, hair-like surface appendages called **fimbriae** or **pili**. They are shorter and thinner than flagella
- Fimbriae can be seen only under the **electron microscope**.
- Fimbriae function as **organs of adhesion**, helping the cells to adhere firmly to particles of various kinds
- Fimbriated bacteria form surface pellicles in liquid media.
- Many fimbriated cells (for example **Escherichia, Klebsiella**) agglutinate red blood cells.
- **Hemagglutination** provides a simple method of detecting the presence of such fimbriae. The hemagglutination is specifically inhibited by D-mannose (mannose sensitive)
- A special type of fimbria is the **sex pili**. They are found on **'male' bacteria** and help in the attachment of those cells to **'female' bacteria**. They do not mediate attachment to epithelium

Flagella

- Flagella are the organs of **locomotion**.
- Flagellum consists of three distinct parts the filament, the hook and the basal

- Flagella are made up of a **protein (flagellin)**
- Flagella are less than 0.02 Jlm in thickness and hence beyond the limit of resolution of the light microscope. They may, in some instances, be seen under dark ground illumination.
- They can be visualised by special staining techniques in which their thickness is increased by mordanting, or by electron microscopy

Mesosomes

- **Mesosomes (chondroids)** are vesicular, convoluted or **multilaminated** structures formed as **invaginations of the plasma membrane** into the cytoplasm.
- They are more prominent in **Gram-positive bacteria**.
- They are the principal **sites of respiratory enzymes** in bacteria and are **analogous to the mitochondria of eukaryotes**.
- Mesosomes are often seen in relation to the nuclear body and the site of synthesis of cross-wall septa, suggesting that they coordinate nuclear and cytoplasmic division during binary fission.

7. **All the following organisms lack capsule *except:***

A. Histoplasma capsulatum
B. Cryptococcus neoformans
C. Candida albicans
D. Coccidioides immitis

Ans: B. Cryptococcus neoformans

Ref: *Ananthnarayan R, Paniker CKJ. Textbook of Microbiology. 8th Edition. Hyderabad: Universities Press; 2009. Pg. 19, 607-12.*

Explanation:

- Some bacteria have a layer of material lying outside the cell wall. When the layer is well organized and not easily washed off, it is called a **capsule**.
- A slime layer is a zone of diffuse, unorganized material that is removed easily.
- **Capsules** and **slime layers** usually are composed of **polysaccharides**, but ***Bacillus anthracis*** has a capsule of **poly-D-glutamic acid.**
- Some bacteria may have both a capsule and a **slime layer** (for example, ***Streptococcus salivarius***).
- Special capsule staining techniques are available, usually employing **copper salts** as mordants. Capsules may be readily demonstrated by **negative staining** in wet films with **India ink.**
- ***Histoplasma capsulatum***:
  - It is dimorphic fungus which causes intracellular infection of the reticuloendothelial system.
  - Blood and marrow smears stained with Giemsa or calcoflour white stain show intracellular 2-4 μm budding yeast cells (within macrophages or histiocytes).
  - It was initially believed to possess a capsule and was named as H. capsulatum.
  - However, it was later found that it does not have a capsule.
- ***Cryptococcus neoformans*** :
  - It is a round or ovoid budding cell, 4-20 μm in diameter, with a prominent polysaccharide capsule.
  - It is a soil saprophyte and is particularly abundant in the feces of pigeons and other birds.
  - The capsule can be demonstrated as a clear halo by India ink.
- ***Candida albicans*** :
  - Candida albicans is an ovoid or spherical budding cell, which produces pseudomycelia both in culture and in tissues.
  - Candida albicans is a pathogenic yeast-like fungus.
- ***Coccidioides immitis*** :
  - The fungus is dimorphic, occurring in the tissue as a yeast and in culture (both at 37°C and at room temperature) as the mycelial form.
  - The tissue form is a spherule, 15-75 μm in diameter, with a thick doubly refractile wall and filled with endospores

8. **Ova with terminal spines is a feature of:**

A. Schistosoma japonicum
B. Schistosoma mansoni
C. Schistosoma haematobium
D. Schistosoma mekongi

Ans: C. Schistosoma haematobium

Ref: *Parija SC. Textbook of Medical Parasitology. 3rd Edition. New Delhi: All India Publishers & Distributors; 2006.*

Explanation:

Identification of Schistosoma spp is based on morphologic features of ova.

- ***S.haematobium***
  - 110 X 170 μ
  - Elongated, oval, yellow browm, non operculated
  - **Terminal spine**

- Eggs are passed in urine

- ***S. mansoni***
  - 114 X 175 μ
  - Yellow – brown
  - Rounded posterior end
  - **Lateral spine**
  - Eggs are passed in faeces
- ***S japonicum***
  - *Smaller*
  - 70- 100μ X 55 – 65 μ
  - **Lateral knob**
  - Eggs are passes in faeces

9. The Tzanck test, which aids in the diagnosis of herpes simplex infection, is a search for:

A. Intracytoplasmic inclusion bodies
B. Koilocytic cells
C. Virus shedding from pustular lesions
D. Multinucleated giant cells

Ans: D. Multinucleated giant cells

Ref: *Jawetz, Melnick, & Adelberg's. Textbook of Medical Microbiology, 25th Edition. 2010. Pg. 456*

Explanation:

- **Tzanck test** is done to demonstrate the multinucleated giant cells in smears of scrapings or swabs of the base of vesicles in patients with herpes simplex infection.
- The multinucleated giant cells are absent in nonherpetic vesicles.

10. A bone marrow transplant recipient becomes febrile and hypoxic and chest films demonstrate diffuse interstitial pneumonia. What is the most likely causative agent?

A. BK virus **B.** Cytomegalovirus
C. Herpes simplex virus **D.** Paramyxovirus

Ans: B. Cytomegalovirus

Ref: *Jawetz, Melnick, & Adelberg's. Text book of Medical Microbiology, 25th Edition. 2010. Pg. 458-462.*

Explanation:

- Immunocompromised patients such as transplant recipients and AIDS patients are prone to severe Cytomegalovirus (CMV) disease such as pneumonitis/ interstitial pneumonia, retinitis, colitis, and encephalopathy.
- Prophylaxis with acyclovir/ganciclovir for all transplant recipients and CMV immunoglobulin for seronegative recipients of graft from seropositive donors should be considered.

11. Chlamydia trachomatis is associated with the following *except:*

A. Endemic trachoma
B. Inclusion conjunctivitis
C. Lymphogranuloma venereum
D. Community acquired pneumonia

Ans: D. Community acquired pneumonia

Ref: *Ananthanarayan, Paniker CJ. Textbook of microbiology. 8th Edition. London: John Wiley & Sons; 2009. Pg. 417.*

Explanation:

- **Chlamydia trachomatis** is not associated with pneumonia.
- The other two species viz, C. pneumoniae and C. psittaci are the causative agents of community acquired pneumonia.

Infections caused by the Chlamydia spp. are listed below:

- ***C. trachomatis***
  - A, B, Ba, C – Endemic blinding trachoma
  - D, E, F, G, H, I, J, K - Urogenital infections, Inclusion conjunctivitis, Infant pneumonia
  - L1, L2, L3 - Lymphogranuloma venereum (LGV)
- ***C. psittaci*** - Pneumonia (psittacosis)
- ***C. pneumoniae*** - **Bronchitis, Sinusitis,** Pneumonia and possibly **Atherosclerosis**

12. Rectal prolapse is associated with:

A. Trichuris trichiura
B. Strongyloides stercoralis
C. Necator americanus
D. Trichinella spiralis

Ans: A. Trichuris trichiura

Ref: *Parija SC. Textbook of Medical Parasitology. 3rd Edition. London: John Wiley & Sons; 2004. Pg 289-291.*

Explanation:

Trichuris trichiura is commonly called as **whipworm.**

Eggs:

- Oval with bipolar plugs
- Bilaterally symmetric & yellow brown
- 35 x 75 um long
- **Floats in saturated solution of salt**

Lifecycle:

- Infection acquired by ingestion of embryonated egg
- **No migratory phase**
- Larvae develop in villi of small intestine

Clinical features:

- Most infections – light and asymptomatic
- Heavy infections – Abdominal pain. Distention, Mucous / bloody diarrhoea

- **Appendicitis**
- **Prolapse of rectum**
- Anemia and eosiniphilia

Diagnosis:
- Demonstration of eggs

Treatment:
- **Mebendazole** – 100 mg twice daily X 3 days

13. All are motile *except:*
A. Klebsiella **B.** E. coli
C. Salmonella **D.** Proteus

Ans: A. Klebsiella

Ref: *Ananthanarayan, Paniker CJ. Textbook of microbiology. 8th Edition. London: John Wiley & Sons; 2009.*

Explanation:

Commonly encountered motile and non-motile bacteria

Motile	Non-motile
Most Enterobacteriaceae except (Shigella and Klebsiella) Eg: Proteus, E. coli, Salmonella	Shigella
Vibrio (darting motility)	Klebsiella
Listeria monocytogenes (tumbling motility)	
Clostridium tetani (stately motility)	
Spirochaetes (Cork-screw motility)	

Types of flagella:
Peritrichous (flagella present all around) – Escherichia coli, Salmonella
Monotrichous (Single polar flagellum) – Vibrio, Pseudomonas
Lophotrichous (tuft of flagella at one pole) – Helicobacter
Amphitrichous (one or more flagella at both poles) - Campylobacter

14. Which of the following is a dimorphic fungus? (Repeat)
A. Rhizopus
B. Sporothrix schenckii
C. Tinea versicolor
D. Microsporum

Ans: B. Sporothrix schenckii

Ref: *Ananthnarayan R, Paniker CKJ. Textbook of Microbiology. 8th Edition. Hyderabad: Universities Press; 2009. Pg. 601-15.*

Explanation:
- Dimorphic fungi can occur as ***filaments or as yeasts***, depending on the conditions of growth.
- In **host tissues or cultures** at **37°C** they occur as **yeasts**, while in the **soil and in cultures** at **22°C** they appear as **moulds**.
- Most fungi causing systemic infections are dimorphic fungi.
- **List of dimorphic fungi**
  – ***Systemic dimorphic fungi***
    ° *Histoplasma capsulatum*
    ° *Blastomyces dermatitidis*
    ° *Coccidiodes immitis*
    ° *Paracoccidiodes brasiliensis*
  – ***Subcutaneous dimorphic fungus*** – *Sporothrix schenckii*
- **Opportunistic fungus** – Penicillium marneffei

FORENSIC MEDICINE

1. Cause of death in a child with sulphuric acid ingestion:
A. Reflex vocal spasm
B. Cardiac arrest
C. Erosive esophageal bleed
D. Pneumomediastinum

Ans: A. Reflex vocal spasm

Ref: *The Essentials of Forensic Medicine and Toxicology by KS Narayan Reddy. 29th edition. 2010. Pg: 475*

Explanation:

Symptoms from swallowing Sulphuric acid
- Breathing difficulty due to throat swelling
- Burns in the mouth and throat
- Drooling
- Fever
- Hypotension
- Severe pain in the mouth and throat
- Dysphonia
- Vomiting, with blood
- Vision loss

Causes of death in sulphuric acid poisoning
a. Circulatory collapse
b. Spasm or edema of glottis
c. Collapse due to perforation of stomach
d. Toxemia
e. Delayed Death due to Pneumonia, secondary infection, renal failure and starvation

2. Entry wound shotgun from 30 to 60 cm is characterised by:
A. Abrasion collar
B. Abrasion rim
C. Tattooing
D. Cruciate shaped wound

Ans: D. Cruciate shaped wound

Ref: *The Essentials of Forensic Medicine and Toxicology by KS Narayan Reddy. 29th edition. 2010. Pg: 195*

Explanation:

SHOTGUN ENTRY WOUNDS

Entry wounds from close range (Upto 1 metre)

Less than 30 cm

- Tissues surrounding the wound are
- Singed by flame
- Blackened by smoke
- Tattooed by unburnt powder granules
- If the powder is smokeless, there may be a greyish or white deposit on the skin around the wound
- The deposit of wound is known as Smudging, fouling or blackening

Between 30 cm and 60 cm

The plastic cup type wad opens up, so that four petals stick out, and a circular entrance wound produced with ***a Maltese cross pattern (Cruciate) or a abrasion encircling it***

Between 60 cm to 90 cm

Produces a single circular aperture 2.5 - 4 cm in diameter, with irregular and lacerated edges

Beyond 90 cm

Air resistance folds back the petals and a single hole of entrance will be produced.

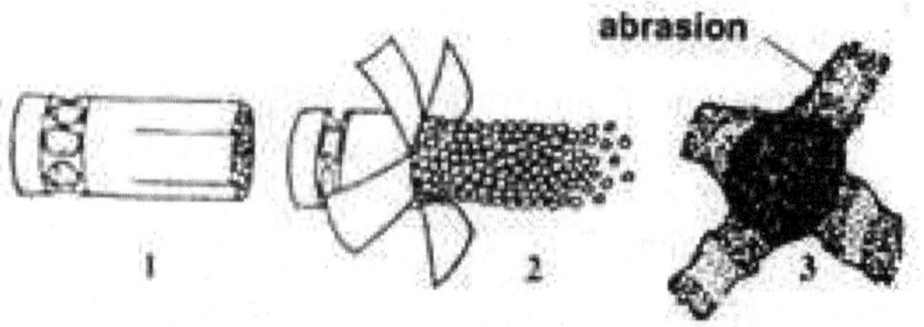

1. Cup not opened
2. Sleeves of cup are opened and are forced backward
3. Cross-like pattern of abrasion around the wound

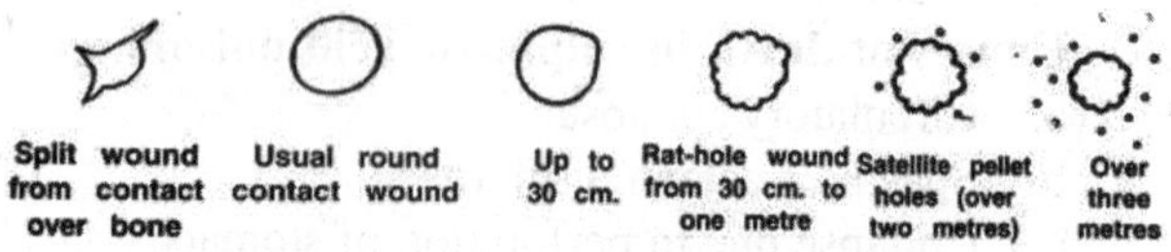

3. Cephalic Index of 80-85 is seen in:

A. Mongols **B.** Chinese
C. European **D.** Negroid

Ans: A. Mongols

Ref: *The Essentials of Forensic Medicine and Toxicology by KS Narayan Reddy. 29th edition. 2010. Pg: 54*

Explanation:

$$\text{Cephalic Index} = \frac{\text{Maximum breadth of skull}}{\text{Maximum length of skull}} \times 100$$

- The length and breadth are measured by calipers between both parietal eminences, between glabella and external occipital protuberance, and not by measuring tape
- The skull of an Indian is Caucasian with a few Negroid characters
- With skull measurements, race can be determined in 85% = 90% of cases

Racial difference in the skull

Race	Type of Skull	Cephalic Index
Pure Aryans Aborigines Negroes	Dolicocephalic (long headed)	**70 - 75**
Europeans Chinese	Mesati-cephalic (Medium headed)	**75 - 80**
Mongolian	Brachy-cephalic (Short headed)	**80 - 85**

4. Medical Negligence is booked under which of the following IPC section?

A. 304 A **B.** 300
C. 375 **D.** 320

Ans: A. 304 A

Ref: *The Essentials of Forensic Medicine and Toxicology by KS Narayan Reddy. 29th edition. 2010. Pg: 34*

Explanation:

Medical Negligence is considered to be criminal negligence if

a. When a doctor shows gross absence of skill or care during treatment resulting in serious injury to or death of a patient
b. When a doctor performs an illegal act
c. When an assaulted person dies, the defence may attribute the death to the negligence or undue interference in the treatment of the deceased by the doctor.

Section 304-A IPC deals with Criminal Negligence

"Whosoever causes the death of any person by doing any rash or negligent act not amounting to culpable homicide shll be punished with imprisonment upto 2 years or with fine or with both"

(See tables on the next page)

5. Man commits rape even if he has sex with his wife when she is less than:

A. 15 years **B.** 16 years
C. 14 years **D.** 13 years

Ans: A. 15 years

Ref: *The Essentials of Forensic Medicine and Toxicology by KS Narayan Reddy. 29th edition. 2010. Pg: 359*

Explanation:

Section 375 in The Indian Penal Code, 1860 defines RAPE

Difference between Civil and Criminal Negligence

Trait	Civil Negligence	Criminal Negligence
Offence	No specific or clear violation of law needs to be proved	Must have specifically violated a particular criminal law in question
Negligence	Simple absence of care & skill	Gross negligence, inattention or lack of competency
Conduct of Physician	It is compared to a generally accepted simple standard of professional conduct	Not compared to a single test
Consent for act	Good defence; cannot recover damages	Not a defence; can be prosecuted
Trial by	Civil Court	Criminal Court
Evidence	Strong evidence is sufficient	Guilt should be proved beyond doubt
Punishment	Liable to pay damages	Imprisonment

Other important sections to remember

Murder	Section 300 IPC
Culpable homicide amounting to murder	Sec 299 IPC
Culpable homicide not amounting to murder	Sec 304 IPC
Rash or Negligent homicide	Sec 304-A IPC
Injury	Sec 44 IPC
Punishment of Murder by imprisonment & fine	Sec 302 IPC
Punishment of Murder by life convict (death sentence)	Sec 303 IPC
Attempt to commit suicide	Sec 309 IPC
Dowry Death	Sec 304 - B IPC
Rape - Definiton	Sec 375 IPC
Punishment for rape	Sec 376 IPC
Unnatural sexual offence	Sec 377 IPC
Criminal abortion	Sec 312 IPC

Definition of grevious injury comes under section 320 of Indian Penal Code (IPC)

375. Rape— A man is said to commit "rape" who, has sexual intercourse with a woman under circumstances falling under any of the six following descriptions:

a. Against her will.
b. Without her consent.
c. With her consent, when her consent has been obtained by putting her or any person in whom she is interested in fear of death or of hurt.
d. With her consent, when the man knows that he is not her husband, and that her consent is given because she believes that he is another man to whom she is or believes herself to be lawfully married.
e. With her consent, when, at the time of giving such consent, by reason of unsoundness of mind or intoxication or the administration by him personally or through another of any stupefying or unwholesome substance, she is unable to understand the nature and consequences of that to which she gives consent.
f. With or without her consent, when she is under sixteen years of age.

What constitutes Rape?

Penetration is sufficient to constitute the sexual intercourse necessary to the offence of rape.

Exception: Sexual intercourse by a man with his **own wife**, the wife not being **under 15 years** of age, is not rape.

PSM

1. When there is an extreme value, best indicator of average to be used is:

A. Median **B.** Mean
C. Mode **D.** Standard deviation

Ans: A. Median

Ref: *Text book of preventive and social medicine, K. Park, 22nd edition page no 790*

Explanation:

- When there is an **extreme value**, **mean** will be **affected** greater extent, than **median**. So **median** is the best indicator.
- **Mode** is better used for **discrete variables** and **not better** measure of **average**.
- **Standard deviation** is a measure of **dispersion**.

2. **Pearl Index is: (Repeat)**
   A. Failure rate per 100 women years of exposure
   B. Success rate per 100 women years of exposure
   C. Failure rate per 1000 women years of exposure
   D. Success rate per 1000 women years of exposure

Ans: A. Failure rate per 100 women years of exposure

Ref: *Text book of preventive and social medicine, K. Park, 22nd edition page no 471*

Explanation:

$$\text{Pearl index} = \frac{\text{Number of accidental pregnancies} \times 12 \times 100}{\text{Number of months of exposure}}$$

(Number of women × Number of months)

- Pearl index is used for measuring contraceptive effectiveness. Lower the value higher is the effectiveness, higher the value poorer the effectiveness.
- **Pearl index of various contraceptives** used are
  - Calendar Method - **9 / 100 HWY (9%)**
  - BBT Method - **1 - 2 / 100 HWY (1-2%)**
  - Cervical mucus Method - **3 / 100 HWY (3%)**
  - Symptothermal Method - **2 / 100 HWY (2%)**
  - Foam tablets- **0.5%**
  - Condoms- **12%**
  - Condoms correctly used- **3%**
  - IUCD- **1-2%**
  - OCP- **0.1%**

3. **The most important index of screening test for a patient:**
   A. Positive predictive value
   B. Negative predictive value
   C. Sensitivity
   D. Specificity

Ans: A. Positve predictive value

Ref: *Text book of preventive and social medicine, K. Park, 22nd edition page no 131*

Explanation:

- **Sensitivity and specificity** are measure of **validity of test.**
- **Sensitivity** is ability of test to detect true positive. In other words, it is Probability of being test positive when disease present.
- **Specificity** of screening test is ability of test to eliminate true negative. In other words Probability of being test negative when disease absent.
- **Sensitivity and specificity** are **inversely proportional.**
- **Positive predictive value** probability of person being actually positive when tested positive. This gives information to patient information that if he/she positive, what is the percentage chance that he/she is really positive.
- **Negative predictive value** is probability of person being actually negative when test gives negative. This gives information to patient information that if he/she is negative, what is the percentage chance that he/she is really negative.

PPV and **NPV** are **directly proportional** to **prevalence** of **disease** in the community

(See the following table)

- **Sensitivity** = a/a+c
- **Specificity** = d/d+b
- **Positive Predictive Value**=a/a+b
- **Negative Predictive Value**=d/c+d

4. **Normal water fluoride level in mg/L:**
   A. 0.5-0.8 **B.** 1.5-2.0
   C. 0.05-0.08 **D.** 5-8

Ans: A. 0.5 - 0.8

Ref: *Textbook of preventive and social medicine, K. Park, 22nd edition page no 579*

Explanation:

- Normal flouride level is **0.5 to 0.8 mg/l**.
- Increased level causes **dental** and **skeletal flurosis**
- Moderate amounts lead to **dental effects**
- Long-term ingestion of large amounts can lead to potentially severe skeletal problems
- **Low** levels of **fluoride intake** help to prevent **dental caries**
- The dental effects of fluorosis develop much earlier than the skeletal effects in people exposed to large amounts of fluoride

(See tables on the next page)

	Gold standard disease positive	Gold standard disease negative	
Test positive	A (true positive)	B (false positive)	Total test positive
Test negative	C (false negative)	D (true negative)	Total test negative
	Total diseased (a+c)	Total normal (B+D)	Total population (A+B+C+D)

	Dental flurosis	Skeletal flurosis
Water Level of fluorine	High >2mg/l	Very high (3-6mg/l or more)
Duration	Early	Late
Onset of symptoms	During early age for 1-2 years	For lifetime exposure
Timing	when the teeth are forming under the gums (<8 years age)	
Symptoms	Staining and pitting of the teeth, enamel damage	Stiffness and pain in the joints, bone structure may change and ligaments may calcify, impairment in muscle activity and pain

- Acute high-level exposure to fluoride causes immediate effects of abdominal pain, excessive saliva, nausea and vomiting. Seizures and muscle spasms may also occur.

Control:

- Removal of excessive fluoride from drinking-water is difficult and expensive.
- The preferred option is to find a supply of safe drinking-water with safe fluoride levels.
- Where access to safe water is already limited, de-fluoridation is the solution

Different de-fluoridation techniques: Use of bone charcoal, contact precipitation, use of Nalgonda (aluminum sulfate used) or activated alumina.

- Only water for drinking and cooking purposes should be treated as all methods produce sludge with very high concentration of fluoride.

5. A screening test for Ca Breast has sensitivity of 90% and specificity of 90%. What is the chance that a patient with Ca breast remains undetected for two consecutive years?

A. 1/10 **B.** 2/10
C. 1/100 **D.** 2/100

Ans: A. 1/10

Ref: *Text book of preventive and social medicine, K. Park, 22nd edition page no 131*

Explanation:

- Sensitivity = a/a+c
- Specificity = d/d+b *(See the following table)*

Sensitivity = a/a+c=0.9
a/10=0.9
a=9
Specificity = d/d+b= 0.9
d/90=0.9
d= 81

- Chance that a patient with Ca breast remains undetected is nothing but false negative rate and that remains same irrespective of time period (so, no need to multiply by 2)
- False negative rate = false negative/diseased= 1/10=0.1
- False positive rate = false positive /normal =9/90= 0.1 or 1/10
- **False positive rate = 1- specificity = b/b+d**
- **False negative rate = 1-sensitivity = c/a+c**

6. Most common sources of lead to cause increased blood level is from:

A. Inhalation **B.** Ingestion of food
C. Ingestion of Water **D.** Cuteneous

Ans: A. Inhalation

Ref: *Text book of preventive and social medicine, K Park, 22 nd edition, page no 752*

Explanation:

- Lead poisoning is both Occuaptional hazard and Envronmental health hazard
- Highest source of environmental (non-occupational) exposure is **gasoline**
- Normal total body level of lead **150-400 mg**, in **blood 25µg/dl**
- **More than 70µg/dl** in blood is associated with clinical symptoms

Diagnositic modality	Value
CPU in urine	>150 µg/L
ALA in urine	>5mg/L
Lead in urine	>0.8mg/L
Lead in blood	>70µg/dl

	Gold standard disease positive	Gold standard disease negative	
Test positive	A (true positive) 9	B (false positive) 9	Total test positive
Test negative	C (false negative) 1	d (true negative) 81	Total test negative
	Total diseased (a+c) 10	Total normal (B+D) 90	Total population (A+B+C+D) 100

7. **The term family size in demographic parlance means:**

   A. The total number of children women has borne at a point of time
   B. The total number of children of couples
   C. The total number of children by women borne in a female between 15- 45 yrs
   D. The total number of members in the family

Ans: C. The total number of children by women borne in a female between 15- 45 yrs

Ref: *Text book of preventive and social medicine, K Park, 22nd edition, page no 450*

Explanation:

- **Completed family size** is the **total no. of children** by **women** borne in a female **between 15- 45 yrs.**
- This is approximately equivalent to **TFR**.
- **TFR= average number children a woman would have**, if she were to **pass through her reproductive years bearing children at the same rates as the women now in each age group**.
- India TFR is **2.5** in (**2012 SRS report, GOI**)
- This is calculated by adding up the **ASFRs** for the different age groups and multiplying the sum by the class - interval on which the age groups have been formed; e.g. if we have made the age groups **as 15-19, 20-24 years** and so on (thus the class interval being 5 years), the ASFRs would be summed up and multiplied by 5 to get the TFR.
- **Target** as per **National Population Policy-2000** is **2.1**

8. **Test used to study the ordinal data of two independent groups which are not distributed normally:**

   A. Student T test
   B. Paired T Test
   C. Wilocoxon's signed rank test
   D. Mann Whitney U test

Ans: D. Mann Whitney U test

Ref: *Text book of community medicine, AFMC, page no 275*

Explanation: *(See the following table)*

9. **Which of the following is true about Cohort study?**

   A. Incidence can be calculated
   B. It is from effect to cause
   C. It is inexpensive
   D. Shorter time than case control

Ans: A. Incidence can be calculated

Ref: *Text book of preventive and social medicine, K Park, 22nd edition, page no 72*

Explanation:

Cohort study

- It is an important study design to measure **incidence**.
- It is followed from **exposure to outcome** (**cause to effect**), unlike case control study (effect to cause)
- It involves follow up of a **cohort** (group with common character, birth cohort, cohort joining service in particular year etc.)
- During follow up **exposure** and **outcome** is **measured** at **periodic intervals**

		Outcome					
		Continuous	*Discrete*	*Numerical Ordinal*	*Dichotomous*	*Polycho-tomous Nominal*	*Polychotomous Ordinal*
Exposure	Continuous	Pearson Correlation & Regression	Pearson Correlation & Regression	Spearman Rank correlation	't' test	ANOVA	ANOVA
	Discrete	- do -	- do -	- do -	- do -	- do -	- do -
	Numerical Ordinal	Spearman Rank correlation	Spearman Rank correlation	Spearman Rank correlation	Mann Whitney U test	Kruskal Wallis test	Kruskal Wallis test
	Dichotomous	't' test	't' test	Mann Whitney U test	Chi square for 2x2 table	Chi square for r x c table	Chi square for linear trend in proportions
	Polychotomous Nominal	ANOVA	ANOVA	Kruskal Wallis	Chi square for r x c table	Chi square for r x c table	Chi square for r x c table
	Polychotomous Ordinal	ANOVA	ANOVA	Kruskal Wallis	Chi square for linear trend in proportions	- do -	- do -

- Generally followed for **long time**, until outcome occurs
- Thus, it involves **high cost**
- Measures **relative risk, attributable risk, population attributable risk** as strength of association

10. Which of the following diseases is not included in international health regulations

A. Plague **B.** Yellow fever
C. Cholera **D.** Polio

Ans: D. Polio

***Ref*:** *Text book of preventive and social medicine, K Park, 22nd edition, page no 112 & International Health Regulation 2005, 2nd edition by WHO*

Explanation:

- International health regulations, mentioned quarantinable diseases **yellow fever, plague** and **cholera**.
- Earlier six diseases were there which were reduced to three in 1981.
- Now a days in **2005**, many more diseases are to be kept under **surveillance**.
- A case of the following diseases is unusual or unexpected and may have serious public health impact, and thus shall be notified, like
  - **Smallpox**
  - **Poliomyelitis** due to wild-type poliovirus
  - **Human influenza** caused by a new subtype
  - Severe acute respiratory syndrome (**SARS**).

And

- An event involving the following diseases shall always lead to utilization of the algorithm, because they have demonstrated the ability to cause serious public health impact and to spread rapidly internationally:
  - **Cholera**
  - **Pneumonic plague**
  - **Yellow fever**
  - **Viral haemorrhagic fevers** (Ebola, Lassa, Marburg)
  - **West Nile fever**
  - Other diseases that are of special national or regional concern, e.g. dengue fever, Rift Valley fever, and **meningococcal disease.**

11. The size of sand particle in slow sand filter is:

A. 0.1 -0.2 mm **B.** 0.2-0.3 mm
C. 0.3-0.4 mm **D.** 0.4-0.5 mm

Ans: B. 0.2-0.3 mm

***Ref*:** *Text book of preventive and social medicine, K Park, 22nd edition, page no 662*

Explanation:

- Smaller the sand size, better is the filtration, and slower is the filtration
- Rapid filtration doesn't need preliminary storage
- **Backwashing** is required for **rapid sand filtration**
- **Rapid** is **costly**
- **Zoogeal layer/ vital layer** is with **slow filter**, this **bacteriologically** better.
  (See the following table)

12. Which of the following is used to destroy algae in water?

A. Copper sulphate **B.** Potassium permanganate
C. Hypochlorite **D.** Bleaching powder

Ans: A. Copper sulphate

***Ref*:** *1. Text book of preventve and social medicine, K Park, 22 nd edition, page No 676*
2. http://www.cdc.gov/nceh/publications/books/housing/cha14.htm

Explanation:

- **Copper sulphate** or **Copper ion system** is used to **destroy algae in water**, specially in maintaining **swimming pool sanitation.**
- Other aspects of swimming pool sanitation are
- **Chlorine level: 1 ppm**

Comparison of Rapid and Slow Sand Filters

	Rapid Sand filter	Slow Sand filter
Space	Occupies very little space	Occupies large area
Rate of filtration	200 m.g.a.d	2-3 m.g.a.d
Effect size of sand	0.4-0.7 mm	0.2 -0.3 mm
Preliminary treatment	Chemical coagulation and sedimentation	Plain sedimentation
Washing	By back-washing	By scraping the sand bed
Operation	Highly skilled	Less skilled
Loss of head allowed	6-8 feet (2-2.5 m)	4 feet (1.5m)
Removal of turbidity	Good	Good
Removal of colour	Good	Good
Removal of bacteria	98-99%	99.9-99.99%

- **Replacement of water: 15% everyday** (to remove organic matter, ammonia, alubuminoid matter)
- Space: **2.2sq m** (24 sq feet) per **person**
- **pH :7.4-7.8**
- Bacteriological quality : **near to drinking water**

Note:

- If **sodium bromide** is there in options, it would be the best answer.

13. **Validity of a screening test includes all *except:***
A. Sensitivity B. Specificity
C. Repeatability D. Accuracy

Ans: C. Repeatability

Ref: *Textbook of preventive and social medicine, K Park, 22nd edition, page no 130*

Explanation:

- **Repeatability** - Test must give consistent results when repeated more than once on the same individual or material, under the same conditions. It is also called **reproducibility, reliability**.
- **Validity** includes **sensitivity, specificity**, and **accuracy**.
- **Accuracy** = (true positive + true negative)/Total

14. **Vector of Japanese Encephalitis in South India is**
A. Culex tritaneorhyncus B. Anopheles
C. Aedes D. Mansonoides

Ans: A. Culex tritaneorhyncus

Ref: *Park's textbook of preventive and social medicine,20th edition, page no:684 & 676*

Explanation:

Major vector borne diseases

Anopheles mosquito	**Malaria; filaria (not in India)**
Culex mosquito	**Bancroftian filariasis;** Japanese encephalitis; **West Nile fever; Viral arthritis (epidemic/polyarthritis)**
Aedes mosquito	Yellow fever **(not in India),** Dengue; **Dengue haemorrhagic fever; Chikungunya fever; Chikungunya haemorrhagic fever; Rift valley fever; Filaria (not in India)**
Mansonoides mosquito	Malayan (Brugian) filariasis Chikungunya fever
Phlebotomus (sandfly)	Leishmaniasis, kala azar
Xenopsylla cheopis (Flea)	Bubonic plague
Tsetse fly	Sleeping sickness
Reduviid bugs	Chagas' disease
Cyclops	Dracontiasis, Fish tape worm
Flea	Endemic/Murine Typhus
Louse	Epidemic typhus, Trench fever
Mite	Scrub typhus, Rickettsial pox

ENT

1. **Mastoid tip develops by:**
A. 1yr B. 2 yr
C. 3 yr D. 4yr

Ans: B. 2 yr

Ref: *Diseases of the Ear Nose and Throat by PL Dhingra 5th edn .2010 Page 411*

Explanation:

- Mastoid tip develops by **2 years** of age
- Surgical importance: Since mastoid tip is not developed in less than 2 years, the facial nerve lies superficial and is at a risk of injury while making the **post aural incision** for **mastoidectomy**.
- Therefore the **post aural incision** should be made more **slanting inferiorly** to **prevent damage to the facial nerve** in children **less than 2 years**.

2. **Advantage of flexible bronchoscopy is:**
A. Can be done in awake patient
B. Can examine the sub segmental bronchi
C. Can be used in jaw and neck abnormalities
D. All of the above

Ans: D. All of the above

Ref: *Diseases of the Ear Nose and Throat by PL Dhingra 5th edn .2010Page 435*

Explanation:

- **Flexible bronchoscopy** is done using a flexible fibre optic bronchoscope
- It provides **better illumination** and **magnification** than the rigid bronchoscope
- Can be done **under topical anaesthesia** in an **awake patient** and is especially useful for **bedside examination** of **critically ill patients**
- More useful adults and limited utility in children because of the problem in ventilation
- Can be used for taking **biopsy**, **suctioning** of **secretions** or **mucus plugs** and **removing small foreign bodies**

3. **Deafness is seen with: (Repeat)**
A. Essential hypertension
B. Congenital QT syndrome
C. Marfan syndrome
D. Turners syndrome

Ans: B. Congenital QT syndrome

Ref: *Diseases of the Ear Nose and Throat by PL Dhingra.5th edn .2010Page 129*

Explanation:

Congenital deafness associated syndromes

Jervell and Lange-Nielsons syndrome
- Autosomal recessive
- Repeated syncopal attacks
- Congenital sensorineural hearing loss
- Prolonged QT in ECG

Alports syndrome
- Autosomal dominant or X linked
- Delayed onset of sensorineural hearing loss
- Hereditary progressive glomerulonephritis
- Corneal dystrophy

Pendred syndrome
- Autosomal recessive
- Congenital SNHL
- Goitre

Usher syndrome
- Autosomal recessive
- Delayed onset of SNHL
- Retinitis pigmentosa
- Night blindness

Treacher Collin syndrome and **Aperts syndrome** are associated with **conductive hearing loss**

4. **Acoustic neuroma commonly involves**
   A. Superior vestibular nerve
   B. Inferior vestibular nerve
   C. Facial nerve
   D. Cochlear nerve

Ans: ? B > A

Ref: *Logan Turner page 339 & Diseases of the Ear Nose and Throat by PL Dhingra .5th edn 2010Page 124-126*

Explanation:

Acoustic neuroma
- They are the **most common tumours of cerebellopontine angle** and account for around **80%** of the cases
- They constitute **10%** of all brain tumours
- Most commonly arises from the **superior vestibular nerve**
- Though textbooks mention superior vestibular nerve, recent research indicates clearly that Inferior vestibular nerve is the commonest to be involved. ***Ref:*** *Komatsuzaki A, Tsunoda A. Nerve origin of the acoustic neuroma.J Laryngol Otol. 2001 May;115(5):376-9*
- Can compress **V, VII, IX, X, XI** and rarely **III, IV, VI cranial nerves**
- **Depending** on the size they can be classified as
  - Small - up to 1.5 cm
  - Medium – up to 4cm
  - Large > 4 cm
- Generally have a **delayed presentation**
- Most commonly present with **unilateral progressive sensorineural hearing loss** and **tinnitus**
- Vestibular symptoms are very rare
- **Earliest cranial nerve** to be involved is **Vth CN**
- Other symptoms are due to brainstem and cerebellar compression like ataxia
- Late features are due to raised intracranial pressure like headache, nausea, vomiting
- **Investigations** include
  - PTA - shows SNHL with Higher frequency more affected than the lower ones
  - Poor speech discrimination score
  - Absent recruitment on SISI and ABLB tests
  - Acoustic reflex decay
  - Vestibular testing shows decreased caloric–response
  - MRI with Gandolinium contrast is the gold standard test
  - BERA delay of >0.2ms in wave V between both the ears is significant
  - CT scan – even size of 0.5cm tumour can be detected
- **Treatment** is with
  - Surgery via various approaches like middle cranial fossa, translabrynthine
  - Radiotherapy either conventional or with Gamma knife using a Cobalt-60 source

5. **All take part in anastomosis in little's area *except:* (Repeat)**
   A. Post ethmoid artery
   B. Anterior ethmoid artery
   C. Sphenopalatine artery
   D. Greater palatine artery

Ans: A. Post ethmoid artery

Ref: *Diseases of the Ear Nose and Throat by PL Dhingra 5th edn .2010.page190*

Explanation:
- Kiesselbach's plexus is situated in the Little's area which is the anterior inferior part of the septum
- Anterior ethmoidal, septal branch of superior labial, greater palatine and sphenopalatine arteries for the plexus *(See figure on the next page)*

6. **Test for malingering of hearing loss:**
   A. Tympanometry **B.** Lombard test
   C. ABC test **D.** Gringe test

Ans: B. Lombard test

Ref: *Clinical audio-vestibulometry by Anirban biswas 1st edn page 69 Diseases of the Ear Nose and Throat by PL Dhingra. 5th edn. 2010. Page 42*

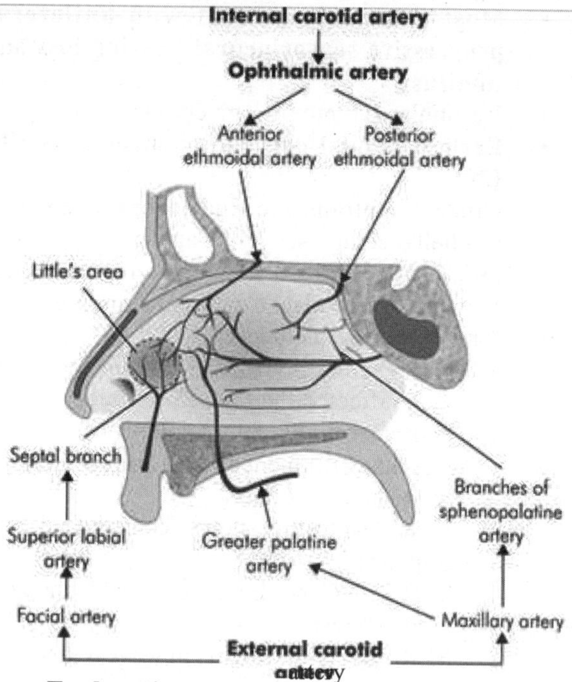

Explanation:

- In **Lombard's voice reflex test** the patient is asked to read and slowly a masking noise is induced into his ear.
- Normal patient will increase his vocal intensity in presence of background noise but a malingering patient will keep reading in the same intensity

Other tests for malingering are

a. Brainstem evoked response audiometry
b. Electrocochleography
c. Acoustic reflex threshold (not tympanometry)
d. Stenger test
e. Delayed auditory feedback test

ABC – **Absolute bone conduction test** – Patients bone conduction is compared with the examiners (assuming that the examiners hearing is normal)

7. **Cottel's test is used to test the patency of the nares in:**

A. Atrophic rhinitis
B. Rhinosporidiosis
C. Deviated nasal septum
D. Hypertrophied inferior turbinate

Ans: C. Deviated nasal symptom

Ref: *Diseases of the Ear Nose and Throat by PL Dhingra 5th edn .2010.Page 164-165*

Explanation:

- In this test the cheek is pulled laterally and subjective improvement in the airway is assessed
- If there is relief in nasal obstruction then the test is positive and indicates an abnormality in the vestibular component of the nasal valve.

8. **In a patient with hypertrophied adenoids the voice abnormality that is seen is:**

A. Rhinolalia clausa **B.** Rhinolalia aperta
C. Hot potato voice **D.** Muffled voice

Ans: A. Rhinolalia clausa

Ref: *Diseases of the Ear Nose and Throat by PL Dhingra 5th edn .2010.Page 334*

Explanation:

Rhinolalia clausa

- It is due to **blockage** of **nasal cavity or nasopharynx**
- Causes include
  - Common cold
  - Nasal allergy
  - Nasal polyps
  - Nasal growth
  - Adenoids
  - Nasal mass

Rhinolalia Aperta

- Due to failure of nasopharynx to cut off from Oropharynx or abnormal connection between the nasal cavity and oral cavity
- Causes include
  - Velopharyngeal insufficiency
  - Sub mucus palate
  - Cleft palate
  - Paralysis of soft palate
  - Oroantral fistula

Note: Hot potato voice muffled and **thick speech** seen in **peritonsillar abscess**

9. **Abductor of the vocal cord is: (Repeat)**

A. Lateral cricoarytenoid
B. Cricothyroid
C. Posterior cricoarytenoid
D. Interarytenoid

Ans: C. Posterior cricoarytenoid

Ref: *Diseases of the Ear Nose and Throat by PL Dhingra 5th edn .2010.Page 300*

Explanation:

Muscles of the larynx are divided into intrinsic and extrinsic groups

Intrinsic muscles of the larynx are

Those acting on the vocal cord

a. *Abductors* – Posterior cricoarytenoid
b. *Adductors* – Lateral cricoarytenoid
   Interarytenoid
   Thyroarytenoid
c. *Tensors* – External – Cricothyroid
   Internal – Vocalis

Those acting on the laryngeal inlet

Opening the inlet - Thyroepiglottis (Part of thyroarytenoid)

Closing the inlet -

Interarytenoid (oblique part)

Aryepiglottic (posterior oblique part of interarytenoid)

Extrinsic muscles of the larynx

Elevators

- Primary–Stylopharyngeus, Salphingopharyngeus, Palatopharyngeus & Thyrohyoid
- Secondary – Mylohyoid, Stylohyoid, Digastric, Geniohyoid

Depressors

- Sternohyoid, sternothyroid, omohyoid

10. **Carhart's notch in otosclerosis is observed at: (Repeat)**

A. 1000 HZ	**B.** 2000 HZ
C. 3000 HZ	**D.** 4000 HZ

Ans: B. 2000HZ

Ref: *Diseases of the Ear Nose and Throat by PL Dhingra 5th edn .2010.pg 97-100*

Explanation:

Carhart's notch

- Carhart's notch is classically seen as a dip centered around **2 kHz** range of bone conduction curve audiometery.
- This feature is seen in patients with **otosclerosis.**
- This notch will disappear after a succesful stapedotomy
- There is also effective improvement in the patient's level of hearing at 2 KHz frequency levels.

11. **One of the following abscesses occur in sternocleidomastoid sheath in relation to mastoid infections:**

A. Bezold's abscess	**B.** Meatal abscess
C. Luc's abscess	**D.** Citelli's abscess

Ans: A. Bezold's abscess

Ref: *Diseases of the Ear Nose and Throat by PL Dhingra 5th edn .2010.pg87*

Explanation:

Bezold's abscess

It is an extra cranial complication of **CSOM – attico antral type**

- Pus breaks through the **mastoid tip** and extends along the **sternocleidomastoid** to present as a **neck abscess**
- Other abscess are

1. **Post aural abscess:**
   Most common
   Displaces the pinna forwards, outwards and downwards
2. **Meatal abscess:**
   Luc's abscess
   Pus breaks into the bony osseous external auditory meatus.
3. **Citelle's abscess:**
   Pus tracks along the digastric muscle and presents in the digastric triangle.
4. **Zygomatic abscess:**
   Presents at the root of zygoma.
   Swelling seen in front and above the pinna.

OPHTHALMOLOGY

1. **Tear drop sign: (Repeat)**

A. # floor of orbit
B. Retinoblastoma
C. Dry eyes
D. Congenital nasolacrimal duct obstruction

Ans : A. # floor of the orbit

Ref: *Basak Essentials of ophthalmology 5th edition, pg no 421; kanski 7th edition clinical ophthalmology, pg no 873- 874*

Explanation:

Blow out fracture of orbit:

- Caused by a sudden increase in the orbital pressure by an impacting object of size > **5cm** like tennis ball or fist.
- The fracture usually involves the floor **of the orbit**, along the thin bone covering the infra orbital canal.

Two types:

- ***Pure Blow Out*** fracture **does not involve the orbital rim** or the other bones
- ***Impure Form*** involves other bones

Symptoms:

- **Diplopia** – due to the entrapment of muscle into the fracture , intraorbital hemorrhage or injury to the muscle itself
- **Double Diplopia** - Diplopia in both upgaze & downgaze due to entrapment of both Inferior rectus (Depression) & inferior oblique (Elevation)
- Periocular ecchymosis & edema
- Enophthalmos
- Infraorbital nerve anaesthesia

Investigations: X-ray (**WATER'S view**) - **'*Tear Drop Sign'*** because of the protruding orbital tissue from the floor if the orbit into the maxillary antrum.

Management:

- Conservative management with antibiotics & anti inflammatory drugs
- Orbital floor repair with bone graft, silicone plate within 2 weeks
- Indications:
  - Fracture involving > one third of the floor
  - Persisting diplopia
  - Enophthalmos > 2mm

Blow-In Fracture:

- Sudden rise of pressure in the **maxillary antrum** due to trauma to the face with subsequent **elevation of bone fragments into the orbit.**

2. **Pupillary reflex begins at:**

A. Intra uterine life	**B.** 3 months of age
C. 6 months of age	**D.** 4 months of age

Ans: A. Intra uterine life

Ref: *AK Khurana comprehensive ophthalmology* 5th *edition pg no 11.*

Explanation:

- **Pupillary reflex** is present in the neonatal period. So it should have developed in the intra uterine life.
- **Fixation reflex** – 2- 4 months of age.
- **Macula** – develops by 4-6 months.
- **Fusional reflexes** (stereopsis & accommodation) - develops between 4-6 months.
- Cornea attains normal adult diameter(11mm) by 2 years of age.
- Lens grows throughout life.

3. **Muscle of iris are derived from: (Repeat)**

A. Neuro ectoderm	**B.** Endoderm
C. Mesoderm	**D.** Mesencephalon

Ans: A. Neuroectoderm

Ref: *Parson* 21st *edition diseases of the eye. pg.no. 5*

Explanation: *(See the following table)*

These are the only muscles which originate from the neuroectoderm.

4. **Hazy media can be examined with:**

A. Indirect ophthalmoscopy
B. Direct ophthalmoscopy
C. Distant direct
D. Fluorescein angiography

Ans: A. Indirect ophthalmoscopy

Ref: *Basak essentials of ophthalmology* 5th *edition; pg no 87*

Explanation: *(See table on the next page)*

5. **Symblepharon is caused by:**

A. Diphtheria
B. Gonococci
C. Chlamydia
D. Opthalmia neonatorum

Ans: A. Diphtheria

Ref: *Basak Diseases of the eye* 5th *edition, pg no 118-119*

Explanation:

SYMBLEPHARON:

- Adhesion between the bulbar & the palpebral conjunctiva.

ETIOLOGY:

- Any condition which produces raw surfaces on the opposing areas of the bulbar & palpebral conjunctiva will lead to adhesion during the healing process.
  - Chemical burns mostly alkali
  - **Thermal burns**
  - **Membranous conjunctivitis** [corynebacterium dihtheriae, pneumococcus, streptococcus]
  - **Ocular pemphigoid**
  - **Stevens Johnson syndrome**
  - Post operative
  - **Trachoma**

PPREVENTION: Sweeping a glass rod with antibiotic eye ointment around the upper & lower fornices, scleral contact shell fitting

TREATMENT:

- Small band – Just excision
- Extensive – excision with conjunctival autograft, buccal mucous membrane graft, amniotic membrane graft

SURFACE ECTODERM	NEURAL ECTODERM	MESODERM	NEURAL CREST
▪ Conjunctival epithelium ▪ Corneal epithelium ▪ Lens ▪ Tarsal gland ▪ Lacrimal gland	▪ Iris epithelium ▪ Ciliary epithelium ▪ Sphincter pupillae ▪ Dilator pupillae ▪ Part of vitreous retina ▪ RPE ▪ Optic nerve	▪ Extraocular muscle ▪ Corneal stroma ▪ Sclera ▪ Iris stroma ▪ Choroid ▪ Vessels ▪ Part of vitreous	▪ Corneal endothelium ▪ Trabecular meshwork endothelium ▪ Ciliary muscle ▪ Part of vitreous ▪ Uveal melanocytes ▪ Meningeal sheaths of optic nerve ▪ Ciliary ganglion

	Direct ophthalmoscopy	Indirect ophthalmoscopy
Magnification	About **15 times**	**5 times** when a +13D condensing lens is used
Diameter of the field of observation\view	**Smaller** (about 10° in diameter)	**Wider** (about 37° in diameter)
Brightness	There is relatively low brightness	There is relatively greater brightness
Structures seen	**Central retina** only	**Peripheral retina** seen *(by using a scleral depressor in addition to the indirect ophthalmoscopy itself)*
Image of the fundus that is seen	Virtual & erect image	Real & inverted image
Stereopsis	Image formed is not stereoscopic	Binocular indirect ophthalmoscopy provides better stereopsis
Retina anterior to the equator	Not well seen (seen with difficulty)	Seen better
Scleral indentation	Difficult	Can be easily done in binocular indirect ophthalmoscopy
Visualization in hazy media	Poor	Better

6. **Iridectomy is a treatment option in:**
A. Pigmentary glaucoma
B. Angle closure
C. Psuedoexfoliative glaucoma
D. Open glaucoma

Ans: B. Angle closure glaucoma

Ref: *Basak Diseases of the eye 5th edition, pg no 455*

Explanation:

IRIDECTOMY:
Abcision of a portion of the iris usually done in the upper part where it is covered by the upper lid [Prevents diplopia, glare].

Types of iridectomy:
- Peripheral Button Hole Iridectomy.

Indications:
1. Angle closure glaucoma.
2. As a part of trabeculectomy operation.
3. In Intracapsular cataract extraction
4. In penetrating keratoplasty

To prevent **Pupillary Block Glaucoma**
- Complete Iridectomy
- Optical Iridectomy- Done in cases of **Central corneal opacity, axial congenital cataract**

IRIDOTOMY: Section of the iris without abscising any portion of it.

Indications:
- To create artificial pupil
- Laser iridotomy – PACG & post operative papillary block glaucoma
- 4 point iridotomy – to prevent glaucoma in iris bombe.

7. **Ring Scotoma is seen in:**
A. Retinitis pigmentosa
B. End stage of glaucoma
C. CRAO with cilioretinal artery sparing
D. CRVO

Ans: A. Retinitis pigmentosa

Ref: *Basak Diseases of the eye 5th edition, pg no 283*

Explanation:

RING SCOTOMA:
Annular scotoma
- A ring shaped area is not seen.
- The central & peripheral area is seen.
- A circular scotoma surrounding the centre of the field of vision.

Causes
- Double arcuate scotoma in glaucoma
- High myopia
- Aphakia with spectacle correction
- Retinitis pigmentosa
- Panretinal photocoagulation.

Tunnel/Tubular Vision: Only central vision remains clear.

Causes:
- Retinitis pigmentosa [late stage]
- High myopia
- CRAO with cilioretinal artery sparing
- End stage glaucoma.

8. **To assess the refraction state of eye, the investigation done is:**
A. USG - Bscan **B.** Retinoscopy
C. Binoculoscopy **D.** Opthalmoscopy

Ans: B. Retinoscopy

Ref: Basak Diseases of the eye 5th edition, pg no 83,529,530, 532

Explanation:

- **Retinoscopy** – to assess the **refractive status** of the eye.
- **USG B- scan** – similar to ultrasonography to visualize the **globe & orbit** (2 dimensional picture).
- **Binoculoscopy** – to assess the **binocular single vision** [**stereoacuity**].
- **Ophthalmoscopy** – to examine the posterior segment [fundus] of the eye.
- **Gonioscopy** – to visualise the **anterior chamber angle**
- **Tonometry** – to **measure the IOP**.
- **Keratometry** – to measure the **radius of curvature of cornea**.
- **Pachymetry** – to measure the **thickness of cornea**.
- **Specular microscopy** – to **visualize the corneal endothelium**.
- **Corneal topography** –to **analyse** the **anterior surface of the cornea**.

9. **Cherry red spot in retina is a feature of:**
   A. Infantile Gaucher's disease
   B. Niemann Pick disease
   C. Fabry's disease
   D. CRVO

Ans: B. Niemann Pick disease

Ref:Kanski 7th edition Clinical ophthalmology, pg no 683-684

Explanation:

Causes of cherry red spot:

- Central retinal artery occlusion
- Blunt injury – Berlin's edeme or commotion retinae
- Quinine toxicity
- Macular hole
- Gangliosidosis
- Mucolipidosis
- Tay Sachs disease
- Sandhoff disease
- Niemann Pick disease
- Faber disease

Mechanism of Cherry red spot

- The **fovea** is the **thinnest** part of the **retina** & is **devoid of ganglion cell layer**.
- The following mechanisms causes cherry red spot
  - When the retina becomes **opaque** due to **edema** (CRAO)
  - Injury to the **photoreceptors (Commotion retina)**
  - Due to **intracellular accumulation of glycolipids & phospholipids** in the **ganglion cell**
- The fovea remains **transparent** & transmits the **underlying choroid.**
- This appears as **cherry red spot.**

10. **Preganglionic and post ganglionic Horner's syndrome are differentiated by application of:**
    A. Atropine
    B. Pilocarpine
    C. Timolol
    D. Hydroxy amphetamine

Ans: D. Hydroxy amphetamine

Ref: Kanski 7th edition clinical ophthalmology;812-814

Explanation:

HORNER'S SYNDROME – Sympathetic paralysis

Components:

- Minimal ptosis (due to **MULLER'S muscle paralysis**)
- Miosis
- Anhydrosis
- Not apparent enophthalmous ; because of ptosis the eye looks smaller
- Loss of ciliospinal reflex

(See table on the next page)

Sympathetic pathway:

- First Order Neuron [central] → From the posterior hypothalamus to the ciliospinal centre of Budge (C8 – T2)
- Second Order Neuron [Preganglionic] → from the ciliospinal centre to the superior cervical ganglion in the neck
- Third Order Neuron [Postganglionic] → from the superior cervical ganglion talong the internal carotid artery to the eye

Causes:

- **Central** – Brain stem disease [tumor, vascular, demyelination]
- **Preganglionic** – Pancoast tumor, carotid & aortic aneurysm & dissection, neck lesions like tumor, surgery
- **Postganglionic** – Migrainous neuralgia, internal carotid artery dissection, nasopharyngeal tumor, otitis media, cavernous sinus mass

Pharmacological tests:

- To differentiate between Preganglionic & Postganglionic lesion

Features	Horner's	Adie's pupil	Argyl Robertson pupil
Size	Small	Dilated	Small, irreg
Laterality	Mostly unilateral Bil: cervical spine inj & diabetic neuropathy	Mostly unilateral	Bil,symmetrical
Light reflex	+	Absent/ sluggish[vermiform movements]	Absent
Accommodation reflex	+	Reacts slowly to near, redilation is also slow[TONIC pupil]	Present
Asstd		Holmes Adie syndrome – diminished deep tendon reflexes	Dorsal midbrain syndrome
Pharmacological tests	Cocaine- no dilatation	0.125% pilocarpine – constriction	Cocaine – dilatation

Hydroxy amphetamine1% → potentiates the release of NA from the postganglionic nerve ending

In preganglionic lesion & in normal eyes, neurone is intact & NA is released → pupil will dilate.

To differentiate between normal eye and Horner's syndrome:

- **Cocaine Test:** it inhibits the reuptake of NA released at the nerve endings
  Normal pupil → dilate
  Horner's pupil → no NA released from the nerve ending → no dilatation
- **Adrenaline Test 0.1%**, Apraclonidine 0.5 % TEST: sympathethetic agonist
  Horner's pupil will dilate due to denervation hypersensitivity

11. Axial proptosis is caused by:

A. Blow out fracture of the orbit
B. Maxillary tumor invading the orbit
C. Frontal mucocele
D. Optic glioma

Ans: D. Optic glioma

Ref: *Basak Essentials of ophthalmology 5th edition pg no 361 & 371; Parson's Diseases of the eye 22nd edition pg no 472*

Explanation:

- **Proptosis**: passive protrusion of the eyeball , seen in space occupying lesion in the orbit & hence usually unilateral
- **Exophthalmos** : active or dynamic protrusion of the eyeball seen in thyroid eye disease, usually bilateral.
- **Axial proptosis**
  - The eye is being pushed directly forwards.
  - Most commonly seen in intraconal lesions like
    - Optic nerve glioma
    - Optic nerve sheath meningioma
    - Cavernous hemangioma
    - AV malformations.
  - Thyroid exophthalmous is also axial.
  - The eye can be displaced from its central location, opposite to the site of the space occupying lesion

12. Which of the following is used for treatment of myopia?

A. Nd YAG laser **B.** Excimer laser
C. Argon laser **D.** Hormium laser

Ans: B. Excimer laser

Ref: *BASAK essentials of ophthalmology, 5 th edition,pg no 7o; kanski clinical ophthalomolgy 6th edition; page no 320 -321*

Explanation:

- **Myopia** can be corrected by **LASIK**.
- **Excimer** laser causes photoablation

Laser insitu keratomileusis (LASIK)

- The curvature of cornea is altered using laser energy, thereby correcting refractive error.
- For myopia, the cornea is flattened. In hypermetropia, it becomes more curved.

Indication:

- Myopia upto 6-8 D
- Hypermetropia upto 4 D
- Astigmatism upto 5D
- **To prevent corneal ectasia** , the residual bed of 250 micron of cornea should be left.
- **Procedure**: Lamellar corneal flap is raised by microkeratome. Excimer laser photoablation of the corneal bed. Flap repositioned.
- **Complications**:
  - Flap – Button holing, Amputation, Irregular flap
  - Dry eyes, Dislocation or Wrinkling of flap, Sub epithelial haze
  - Epithelial in growth

- Diffuse lamellar keratitis [**Sands of Sahara**],
- Bacterial keratitis especially due to Mycoplasma

MEDICINE

1. **Features of 'Brainstem death' are all *except:***
   A. No respiration for 15secs after disconnecting from ventilator
   B. Absent pupillary response
   C. Absent DTR
   D. Isoelectric EEG

Ans: C. Absent DTR

Ref: Harrison's Principles of Internal Medicine 18th edition

Explanation:

Brain Death

- This is a state of cessation of cerebral function with preservation of cardiac activity and maintenance of somatic function by artificial means.
- It is the only type of brain damage recognized as equivalent to death.
- Several sets of criteria have been advanced for the diagnosis of brain death and it is essential to adhere to those standards endorsed by the local medical community.
- They contain **three essential elements**:
  - Widespread cortical destruction that is reflected by deep coma and **unresponsiveness** to **all forms of stimulation**
  - Global brainstem damage demonstrated by **absent pupillary light reaction** and by the **loss of oculovestibular and corneal reflexes**
  - Destruction of the **medulla**, manifested by **complete apnea**.
- The **heart rate** is **invariant** and unresponsive to **atropine**.
- **Diabetes insipidus** is often present but may only develop hours or days after the other clinical signs of brain death.
- The **pupils** are usually **midsized** but may be enlarged
- **Loss of deep tendon reflexes** is **not required** because the **spinal cord remains functional**.
- **Babinski signs** are generally **absent** and the toe response is often **flexor**.
- Demonstration that **apnea** is due to **irreversible medullary damage** requires that the **Pco2** be **high enough** to **stimulate respiration** during a test of spontaneous breathing.
- **Apnea testing** can be done safely by the use of diffusion oxygenation prior to removing the ventilator. This is accomplished by **preoxygenation** with **100%** oxygen, which is then sustained during the test by oxygen administered through a tracheal cannula. co2 tension increases 0.3–0.4 kPa/min (2–3 mmHg/min) during apnea. At the end of a period of observation, typically several minutes, **arterial Pco2** should be **at least >6.6–8.0 kPa (50–60 mmHg)** for the test to be valid.
- **Apnea** is confirmed if no respiratory effort has been observed in the presence of a sufficiently elevated Pco2.
- An **isoelectric EEG** may be used as a confirmatory test for total cerebral damage.
- Radionuclide brain scanning, cerebral angiography, or transcranial Doppler measurements may also be included to demonstrate the absence of CBF but they have not been extensively correlated with pathologic changes.
- The possibility of profound **drug-induced** or **hypothermic depression** of the nervous system should be **excluded**, and some period of observation, usually **6–24 hours**, is desirable, during which the clinical signs of **brain death** are **sustained**.
- It is advisable to delay clinical testing for at least **24 hours** if a cardiac arrest has caused brain death or if the inciting disease is not known.

2. **All are true regarding Pulmonary embolism *except:* (Repeat)**
   A. T wave inversion V1 to V4
   B. Sinus bradycardia
   C. Right ventricular strain
   D. S1Q3TS sign

Ans: B. Sinus bradycardia

Ref: Harrison's Principles of Internal Medicine 18th edition pg 2170

Explanation:

Pulmonary embolism

Predisposing factors for pulmonary embolism are:

- **Prothrombotic states:** Mutant factor V Leiden, deficiency of antithrombin, protein C & S, hyperhomocysteinemia, APLA, OC pills, pregnancy, cancer, surgery, trauma, bed-ridden patient, long-air travel, COPD

- **Pathophysiology**:
  - Hypoxemia, increased alveolar-arterial gradient, increased pulmonary vascular & airway resistance
  - Impaired gas exchange, alveolar hyperventilation, decreased pulmonary compliance
- **Symptoms:** massive VTE- sudden hypotension, moderate: RV hypokinesia on ECHO
  - Pleuritic chest pain- small, peripheral infarction,
  - Unexplained breathlessness- MC symptom, tachypnea –MC sign
  - Non thrombotic PE- fat, air, amniotic fluid,cement, hair, talc, cotton
- **Tests:**
  - D-Dimer assay- sensitive 'rule out' test
  - False positive inMI, pneumonia, sepsis, cancer, pregnancy, post-op state
  - ABG- low pO2 & pCO2, high A-a gradient
  - S.troponin, heart- type fatty acid binding protein, BNP, NT-pro BNP} due to RV microinfarction
- **ECG:**
  - Sinus tachycardia
  - Acute right axis deviation
  - RBBB
  - S1Q3TS sign
  - T-wave inversion in V1-V4
- **CXR:**
  - **Hampton's sign**-peripheral wedge shaped density above diaphragm,
  - **Westermark's sign** – focal oligemia,
  - **Palla's sign**- enlarged right pulmonary artery
- **ECHO- Mc-Connel's sign**- Hypokinesia of RV free wall, normal RV apex
- **Multidetector**-row spiral CT- Very sensitive, non invasive test
- **Pulmonary angiography** — **Gold standard** Test (Most specific)
- **Treatment**:
  - UFH/ LMWH/Fondaparinux/ Warfarin
  - Novel anticoagulants- DTI-Argatroban, lepirudin, bivalirudin; Factor Xa inhibitor-Rivaroxaban
  - Fibrinolysis with t-PA dissolves thrombus, prevents serotonin release, prevents recurrence of PE by lysing source of thrombus
  - Embolectomy
- **Prevention**:
  - High risk surgery, total hip replacement, medical illness, long-term bed ridden patient
  - Mini-UFH/LMWH/fondaprinux/IPC/rivaroxaban/dalteparin
  - For 4-5 wks
  - IVC filters

3. Man coughed and developed sudden severe headache and fainting. The most probable diagnosis is:

A. Subarachnoid hemorrhage
B. Migraine
C. Cluster Headache
D. Posterior fossa tumor

Ans: A. Subarachnoid hemorrhage

Ref: Harrison's Principles of Internal Medicine 18th edition

Explanation:

Subarachnoid Hemorrhage

- Excluding **head trauma**, the most common cause of SAH is rupture of a saccular aneurysm.
- Other causes include bleeding from a **vascular malformation** (arteriovenous malformation or dural arterial-venous fistula)

Saccular ("Berry") Aneurysm

- 2% of adults harbor intracranial aneurysms
- The three most common locations are the
  - **Terminal internal carotid artery**
  - **Middle cerebral artery (MCA) bifurcation**
  - **Top of the basilar artery**.
- **Mycotic aneurysms** are usually located **distal to the first bifurcation of major arteries** of the **circle of Willis**.
- Most result from infected emboli due to **bacterial endocarditis** causing septic degeneration of arteries and subsequent dilation and rupture.

Pathophysiology

- Saccular aneurysms occur at the **bifurcations** of the **large- to medium-sized** intracranial arteries
- Rupture is into the subarachnoid space in the basal cisterns and often into the parenchyma of the adjacent brain.
- Approximately 85% of aneurysms occur in the anterior circulation, mostly on the circle of Willis.
- About 20% of patients have multiple aneurysms, many at mirror sites bilaterally.

Clinical Manifestations

- Most unruptured intracranial aneurysms are completely asymptomatic.
- At the moment of aneurysmal rupture with major SAH, the **ICP** suddenly **rises**.
- This may account for the sudden **transient loss of consciousness** that occurs in nearly half of patients.

- Sudden loss of consciousness may be preceded by a brief moment of **excruciating headache,** but most patients first complain of headache upon regaining consciousness.
- Severe headache associated with **exertion** is the presenting complaint. The patient often calls the headache **"the worst headache of my life"**; however, the most important characteristic is **sudden onset**.
- The headache is usually **generalized**, often with **neck stiffness**, and vomiting is common.
- **Sudden headache** in the **absence of focal neurologic symptoms** is the **hallmark** of **aneurysmal** rupture.
- Focal deficits can occur rarely.
- **Anterior communicating artery** or **MCA bifurcation** aneurysms may bleed enough to produce mass effect. The deficits that result can include **hemiparesis**, **aphasia**, and **abulia**.
- **A third cranial nerve palsy**, particularly when associated with pupillary dilation, loss of ipsilateral (but retained contralateral) light reflex, and focal pain above or behind the eye, may occur with an expanding aneurysm at the junction of the posterior communicating artery and the internal carotid artery.
- A **sixth nerve palsy** may indicate an aneurysm in the cavernous sinus, and visual field defects can occur with an expanding supraclinoid carotid or anterior cerebral artery aneurysm.
- **Occipital** and **posterior cervical pain** may signal a **posterior inferior cerebellar artery** or **anterior inferior cerebellar artery** aneurysm.
- **Pain in or behind the eye** and in the low temple can occur with an **expanding MCA aneurysm.**

4. **Urine turns dark on standing in: (Repeat)**

A. Alkaptonuria
B. Maple syrup urine disease
C. Phenyl ketonuria
D. Acute intermittent porphyria

Ans: A. Alkaptonuria

Ref: *Harrison's Principles of Internal Medicine 18th edition & Harper's illustrated Biochemistry, 28th edition, Chapter 29, pp 254)*

Explanation:

Alkaptonuria

- Due to deficiency in ***homogentisic acid oxidase***
- Results in the accumulation of ***homogentisic acid***
- The illness has three characteristic symptoms:
  - **Homogentisicaciduria** (the patient's urine contains elevated levels of **homogentisic acid**, which is oxidized to a **dark pigment** on **standing,**
  - Large joint arthritis
  - Black **ochronotic** pigmentation of cartilage and collagenous tissue (**Oochronsis**)
- **Diets low in protein**—especially in phenylalanine and tyrosine—help reduce the levels of homogentisic acid, and decrease the amount of pigment deposited in body tissues.
- Although alkaptonuria is not life-threatening, the associated arthritis may be severely crippling.

5. **H. influenzae causes hydrocephalus due to:**

A. Gliosis
B. Fibrosis
C. Adhesion of subarachnoid villi
D. ?

Ans: ??

Ref: *Internet Article International Federation For Hydrocephalus And Spina Bifida . Post infectious hydrocephalus*

Explanation:

Sorry, Couldn't find the answer.

Post infectious hydrocephalus

"Meningitis cause inflammation and destruction of the ependymal lining of the ventricles and inflammatory exudates and scarring which may obstruct the aqueduct, the outlets of the IVth ventricle, or the basal subarachnoid spaces around the IVth ventricle."

This statement is in general for all postinfectious hydrocephalus.

I am not sure whether H. influenza has some different mechanism to cause hydrocephalus.

6. **Roth spots are seen in:**

A. Infective endocarditis
B. Central retinal vein occlusion
C. Retintits pigmentosa
D. Diabetic retinopathy

Ans: A. Infective endocarditis

Ref: *Harrison's Principles of Internal Medicine 18th edition*

Explanation:

- Roth's spots are **retinal hemorrhages** with **white or pale centers** composed of **coagulated fibrin**.
- They are typically seen using an ophthalmoscope or slit lamp exam.

- They are usually caused by immune complex mediated vasculitis often resulting from **bacterial endocarditis.**

Roth's spots may also be seen in

- Leukemia
- Diabetes
- Subacute bacterial endocarditis
- Pernicious anemia
- Ischemic events
- HIV retinopathy

Manifestations of Infective Endocarditis

HISTORY

- Prior congenital or rheumatic heart disease
- Preceding dental, urinary tract, or intestinal procedure
- Intravenous drug use
- Central venous catheter
- Prosthetic heart valve

SYMPTOMS

- Fever
- Chills
- Chest and abdominal pain
- Arthralgia, myalgia
- Dyspnea
- Malaise, weakness
- Night sweats
- Weight loss
- CNS manifestations (stroke, seizures, headache)

SIGNS

- Elevated temperature
- Tachycardia
- **Embolic phenomena** (Roth spots, petechiae, splinter nail bed hemorrhages, Osler nodes, CNS or ocular lesions)
- **Janeway lesions** (painless small erythematous or hemorrhagic lesions on the palms and soles)
- New or changing murmur
- Splenomegaly
- Arthritis
- Heart failure
- Arrhythmias
- Metastatic infection (arthritis, meningitis, mycotic arterial aneurysm, pericarditis, abscesses, septic pulmonary emboli)
- Clubbing

LABORATORY

- Positive blood culture
- Elevated erythrocyte sedimentation rate
- Elevated C-reactive protein
- Anemia
- Leukocytosis
- Hypergammaglobulinemia
- Hypocomplementemia
- Cryoglobulinemia
- Rheumatoid factor
- Hematuria
- Renal failure: azotemia, high creatinine (glomerulonephritis)
- Chest radiograph: bilateral infiltrates, nodules, pleural effusions
- Echocardiographic evidence of valve vegetations, prosthetic valve dysfunction or leak, myocardial abscess, new-onset valve insufficiency

7. **In type 1 DM all true *except:***

A. Decreased Gluconeogenesis
B. Increased Glycogenolysis
C. Increased Lipolysis
D. Increased Ketogenesis

Ans: A. Decreased Gluconeogenesis

Ref: Harrison's Principles of Internal Medicine 18th edition & Nelson

Explanation:

Pathophysiology of Type 1 DM

- Insulin performs a critical role in the storage and retrieval of cellular fuel.
- Its secretion in response to feeding is exquisitely modulated by the interplay of neural, hormonal, and substrate-related mechanisms to permit controlled disposition of ingested foodstuff as energy for immediate or future use.
- Insulin levels must be lowered to then mobilize stored energy during the fasted state.
- Thus, in normal metabolism, there are regular swings between the postprandial, high-insulin anabolic state and the fasted, low-insulin catabolic state that affect liver, muscle, and adipose tissue.
- **T1DM is a progressive low-insulin catabolic state** in which feeding does not reverse but rather exaggerates these catabolic processes.
- With moderate **insulinopenia**, glucose **utilization by muscle** and **fat decreases** and **postprandial hyperglycemia** appears.
- At even lower insulin levels, the liver produces excessive glucose via **glycogenolysis** and **gluconeogenesis**, and **fasting hyperglycemia begins**.
- Hyperglycemia produces an **osmotic diuresis (glycosuria)** when the renal threshold is **exceeded (180 mg/dL; 10 mmol/L).**
- The resulting loss of calories and electrolytes, as well as the persistent dehydration, produce a

physiologic stress with **hypersecretion of stress hormones (epinephrine, cortisol, growth hormone**, and **glucagon**).

- These hormones, in turn, contribute to the metabolic decompensation by further **impairing insulin secretion** (epinephrine), by **antagonizing its action** (epinephrine, cortisol, growth hormone), and by **promoting glycogenolysis, gluconeogenesis, lipolysis, and ketogenesis** (glucagon, epinephrine, growth hormone, and cortisol) while **decreasing glucose utilization** and **glucose clearance** (epinephrine, growth hormone, cortisol).
- The combination of insulin deficiency and elevated plasma values of the counter-regulatory hormones is also responsible for **accelerated lipolysis** and **impaired lipid synthesis**, with resulting **increased plasma concentrations of total lipids, cholesterol, triglycerides**, and **free fatty acids.**
- The hormonal interplay of insulin deficiency and glucagon excess shunts the free fatty acids into **ketone body formation**; the rate of formation of these ketone bodies, principally â-hydroxybutyrate and acetoacetate, **exceeds the capacity for peripheral utilization** and renal excretion.
- Accumulation of these **keto acids** results in **metabolic acidosis** (diabetic ketoacidosis, DKA) and compensatory **rapid deep breathing** in an attempt to excrete excess CO2 (Kussmaul respiration)
- **Acetone**, formed by nonenzymatic conversion of acetoacetate, is responsible for the characteristic **fruity odor** of the breath.

8. **Pulses bisferiens is seen in:**

A. AR **B.** AS
C. MR **D.** MS

Ans: A. AR

Ref: Harrison's Principles of Internal Medicine 18th edition

Explanation:

Abnormal Pulses

Anacrotic Pulse

- This is slow rising pulse of smaller amplitude seen in conditions like aortic stenosis
- Anacrotic means upbeating; refers to exaggerated anacrotic notch seenin AS

Double beating Pulses

- Occurs when there are two palpable arterial pulses per cardiac cycle

A. Bisferiens Pulse

- Two positive peaks during systole
- Felt best in carotid arteries
- Seen in Severe AR, Combined AR and AS, HOCM & in high output states

B. Bifid Pulse

- Commonly recorded than palpated
- The initial spike is followed by a mid systolic pulse collapse and then by late systolic impulse
- Seen in Hypertrophic cardiomyopathy

C. Dicrotic Pulse

- Second palpable component is a diastolic reflection wave.
- The detectable delay between two palpable peaks is much longer than in bisferiens pulse

Pulsus Alternans

- Strong and weak beat occuring alternatively
- Seen in left ventricular dysfunction

Pulsus Paradoxus

- Marked and exaggerated inspiratory fall in systolic BP
- It is seen in
- Pericardial tamponade
- Constrictive pericarditis
- Emphysema
- Asthma
- Severe CHF

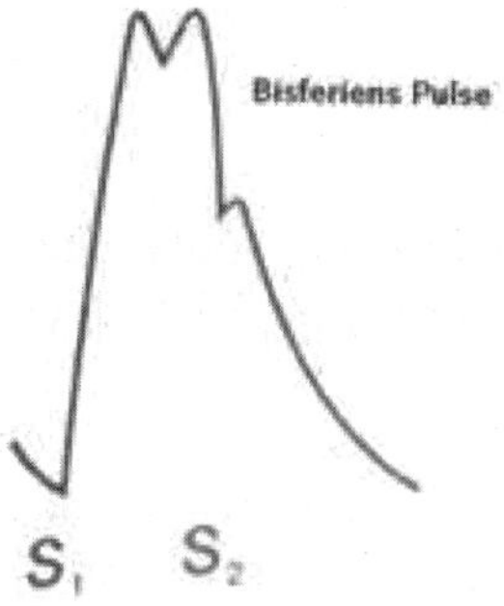

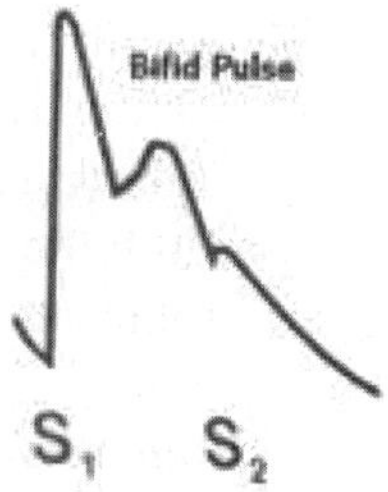

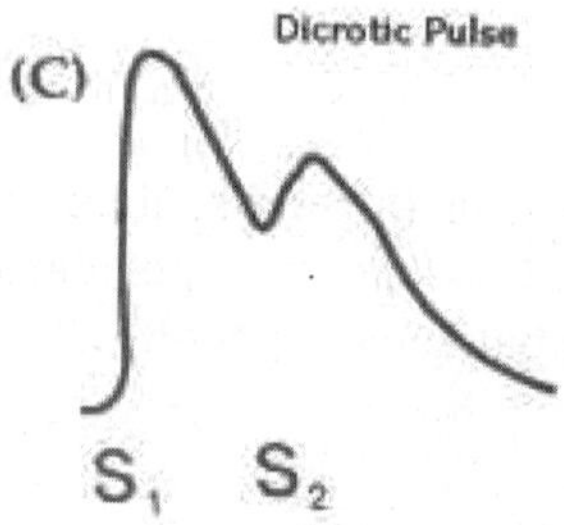

9. **All the following commonly cause nephrotic syndrome *except:***

A. Tuberculosis **B.** HIV
C. Malaria **D.** Hepatitis C

Ans: A. Tuberculosis

Ref: *Harrison's Principles of Internal Medicine 18th edition & Nelson textbook of Pediatrics, 19th edition.*

Explanation:

Focal Segmental Glomerulosclerosis

- Secondary focal segmental glomerulosclerosis
  - **Viruses**: HIV/Hepatitis B/Parvovirus
  - **Hypertensive nephropathy**
- Reflux nephropathy
- Cholesterol emboli
- **Drugs**: Heroin/ Analgesics/ Pamidronate
- Oligomeganephronia
- Renal dysgenesis
- Alport's syndrome
- Sickle cell disease
- Lymphoma
- Radiation nephritis
- Fabry's disease

Membranous Glomerulonephritis

Secondary membranous glomerulonephritis

Infection:

- Hepatitis B and C
- Syphilis
- Malaria
- Schistosomiasis
- Leprosy
- Filariasis

Cancer:

- Breast
- Colon
- Lung
- Stomach
- Kidney
- Esophagus
- Neuroblastoma

Drugs:

- Gold
- Mercury
- Penicillamine
- Nonsteroidal anti-inflammatory agents
- Probenecid

Autoimmune diseases:

- Systemic lupus erythematosus
- Rheumatoid arthritis
- Primary biliary cirrhosis
- Hashimoto's thyroiditis

Other systemic diseases:

- Fanconi's syndrome
- Sickle cell anemia
- Diabetes
- Sarcoidosis

Secondary Cause of Childhood Nephrotic Syndrome

Infections

- *Hepatitis B, C*
- *HIV-1*
- *Malaria*
- *Syphilis*
- *Toxoplasmosis*

10. In Hyperthyroidism increased cardiac output is due to all the following *except*::

A. Increased afterload

B. Increased ventricular contractility

C. Decreased total peripheral resistance

D. Peripheral vasodilatation

Ans: A. Increased afterload

Ref: *Harrison's Principles of Internal Medicine 18th edition & DeGroot WJ, Leonard JJ. Hyperthyroidism as a high cardiac output state. Am Heart J. 1970 Feb;79(2):265-75.*

Explanation:

- Hyperthyroidism is the **most common cause** of **hyperkinetic circulatory disease.**
- Thyroid hormone probably produces this high output state by inducing **vasodilatation** of the **circulatory beds supplying muscle and skin.**
- This hormone induced effect **lowers the total peripheral resistance** which increases cardiac output.
- The heart responds to the **low peripheral resistance** by **accelerating the heart rate** and **augmenting stroke volume.**
- Thyroid hormone **enhances ventricular contractility**.
- These cardiac responses are generated by a direct effect of thyroid hormone on the cardiovascular system and are essentially independent of autonomic influence.

11. Interleukin involved in asthma:

A. IL 5 **B.** IL-1

C. IL-2 **D.** INF-alpha

Ans: A. IL-5

Ref: *Harrison's Principles of Internal Medicine 18th edition & Nelson Textbook of Pediatrics, 19th ed.*

Explanation:

Pathogenesis of Bronchial asthma

- Airflow obstruction in asthma is the result of numerous pathologic processes.
- In the small airways, airflow is regulated by smooth muscle encircling the airways lumens; bronchoconstriction of these bronchiolar muscular bands restricts or blocks airflow.

- A cellular inflammatory infiltrate and exudates distinguished by **eosinophils**, but also including **other inflammatory cell types (neutrophils, monocytes, lymphocytes**, mast cells, basophils), can fill and obstruct the airways and induce **epithelial damage** and **desquamation** into the **airways lumen**.
- Helper T lymphocytes and other immune cells that produce **proallergic, proinflammatory** cytokines **(IL-4, IL-5, IL-13)**, and **chemokines (eotaxin)** mediate this inflammatory process.
- Pathogenic immune responses and inflammation may also result from a breach in normal immune regulatory processes (such as regulatory T lymphocytes that produce **IL-10** and transforming growth factor **[TGF]-β)** that dampen effector immunity and inflammation when they are no longer needed.
- Hypersensitivity or susceptibility to a variety of provocative exposures or triggers can lead to various processes that contribute to airflow obstruction
  - Airways inflammation
  - Bronchial hyperresponsiveness
  - Airway edema
  - Basement membrane thickening
  - Subepithelial collagen deposition
  - Smooth muscle
  - Mucous gland hypertrophy
  - Mucus hypersecretion

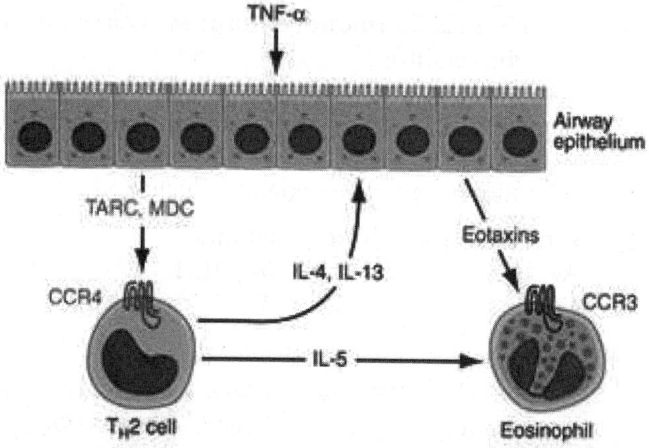

12. **Monoclonal Antibody used in Asthma is:**
A. Omalizumab **B.** Trastuzumab
C. Muromonab **D.** Alemtuzumab

Ans: A. Omalizumab

Ref: Harrison's Principles of Internal Medicine 18th edition

Explanation:

Omalizumab (Anti-IgE antibody)

- It is a blocking antibody that neutralizes circulating IgE without binding to cell-bound IgE and, thus, inhibits IgE-mediated reactions.
- This treatment has been shown to reduce the number of exacerbations in patients with severe **asthma** and may **improve asthma control**.
- However, the treatment is **very expensive** and is only suitable for highly selected patients who are not controlled on maximal doses of inhaler therapy and have a circulating IgE within a specified range.
- **Omalizumab** is usually given as a **subcutaneous** injection every **2–4 weeks** and appears not to have significant side effects, although **anaphylaxis** is very occasionally seen.

13. **A 22-year-old female presented with fever, cough for 6 months, chest X-ray shows mediastinal widening and blood tests revealed Increased ACE levels. That is the most probable diagnosis:**
A. Sarcoidosis **B.** Tuberculosis
C. Churg Strauss syndrome **D.** Lymphoma

Ans: A. Sarcoidosis

Ref: Harrison's Principles of Internal Medicine 18th edition & Nelson Textbook of Pediatrics, 19th ed.

Explanation:

- Raised ACE levels points towards Sarcoidosis. The given history is also compatible with pulmonary tuberculosis, but serum ACE levels will be normal.

Sarcoidosis

- It is a multisystem granulomatous disease and lesions may occur anywhere in the body.
- The clinical manifestations depend on the extent and degree of granulomatous inflammation and are extremely variable.
- **Children** may present with **nonspecific symptoms**, such as **fever**, **weight loss**, and general **malaise**.
- In adults and older children, **pulmonary involvement** is most frequent, with **infiltration** of the **thoracic lymph nodes** and **lung parenchyma**.
- **Isolated bilateral hilar adenopathy** on chest radiograph is the most common finding, but **parenchymal infiltrates** and **miliary nodules** may also be seen
- Patients with lung involvement are commonly found to have **restrictive changes** on pulmonary function testing.
- **Extrathoracic lymphadenopathy** and **infiltration** of the **liver**, **spleen**, and **bone**

marrow leading on to isolated **hepatomegaly** and **splenomegaly**
- **Cutaneous disease**, such as **plaques, nodules, erythema nodosum** in acute disease, or lupus **pernio** in chronic sarcoidosis
- **Red-brown to purple maculopapular lesions** <1 cm on the **face, neck, upper back**, and **extremities** are the most common skin finding
- **Ocular involvement** is frequent, **anterior** or **posterior uveitis, conjunctival granulomas, eyelid inflammation**, and **orbital** or **lacrimal gland infiltration**.
- The **arthritis** in sarcoidosis can be confused with JRA
- **Central nervous system (CNS) involvement** is rare in childhood but may manifest as seizures, **cranial nerve involvement, intracranial mass lesions**, and **hypothalamic dysfunction**.
- **Kidney disease** also occurs infrequently in children but typically manifests as renal insufficiency, proteinuria, transient pyuria, or microscopic hematuria as a result of either early monocellular infiltration or granuloma formation in kidney tissue.
- Only a small fraction of children have **hypercalcemia or hypercalciuria**, which is therefore an infrequent cause of kidney disease.
- **Sarcoid granulomas** can also infiltrate the **heart** and lead to **cardiac arrhythmias** and **sudden death**.
- In contrast to the variable clinical presentation of sarcoidosis in older children, early-onset sarcoidosis classically manifests as the triad uveitis, arthritis, and rash.
- Pulmonary disease and lymphadenopathy are less common.
- The **arthritis** is **polyarticular** and **symmetric**, with large **boggy effusions**.
- The **rash** is **diffuse, erythematous, papular**
- **Noncaseating granulomas** are demonstrated with biopsy of the skin or joint synovium

Laboratory Findings
- There is no single laboratory test diagnostic of sarcoidosis.
- **Anemia, leukopenia**, and **eosinophilia** may be seen.
- **Hypergammaglobulinemia** and elevations in **acute-phase reactants (ESR & CRP)**
- **Hypercalcemia** and/or **hypercalciuria**
- **Angiotensin-converting enzyme (ACE)** is produced by the epithelioid cells of the granuloma, and its serum value may be **elevated**, but this finding **lacks diagnostic sensitivity and specificity**.
- Fluorodeoxyglucose F18 positron emission tomography (**18FDG PET**) can help identify **nonpulmonary sites** for a diagnostic biopsy.
- A **positive gallium scan** can support the diagnosis if increased activity is noted in the **parotids** and **lacrimal** glands (**panda sign**) or in the right **paratracheal and left hilar area (lambda sign)**.

14. All the following are causes of hyperthermia *except:*

A. Hypothyroidism
B. Cerebral hemorrhage
C. Succinyl Choline
D. Pheochromocytoma

Ans: A. Hypothyroidism

Ref: *Harrison's principles of Internal Medicine. 18th edition. 2012. Chapter 16. Pg.143*

Causes of Hyperthermia

Heat Stroke
Exertional: Exercise in higher than normal heat and humidity
Nonexertional: Anticholinergics, antiparkinsonian drugs; diuretics; phenothiazines
Drug-Induced Hyperthermia
Amphetamines, cocaine, phencyclidine (PCP), lysergic acid diethylamide (LSD), salicylates, lithium, anticholinergics
Neuroleptic Malignant Syndrome
Phenothiazines; butyrophenones, haloperidol and bromperidol; fluoxetine; loxapine; tricyclic dibenzodiazepines; metoclopramide; domperidone; thiothixene; molindone.
Serotonin Syndrome
Selective serotonin reuptake inhibitors (SSRIs), monoamine oxidase inhibitors (MAOIs), tricyclic antidepressants
Malignant Hyperthermia
Inhalational anesthetics, succinylcholine
Endocrinopathy
Thyrotoxicosis, pheochromocytoma
Central Nervous System Damage
Cerebral hemorrhage, status epilepticus, hypothalamic injury

15. All the following are characteristic feature of Cluster headache *except:*

A. Periodic pain
B. Conjunctival injection
C. Bilateral photophobia
D. No response to oral sumatriptan

Ans: C. Bilateral photophobia

Ref: *Harrison's principles of Internal Medicine. 18th edition. 2012. Chapter 14. Pg.112*

Explanation:

CLUSTER HEADACHE

- The pain is deep, usually retroorbital, excruciating in intensity, nonfluctuating, and explosive in quality.
- A core feature of cluster headache is **Periodicity**. At least one of the daily attacks of pain recurs at about the same hour each day for the duration of a cluster bout.
- The typical cluster headache patient has daily bouts of one to two attacks of relatively short-duration unilateral pain for 8 to 10 weeks a year; this is usually followed by a pain-free interval that averages a little less than 1 year.
- Patients are generally **perfectly well between episodes.**
- Onset is nocturnal in about 50% of patients, and men are affected three times more often than women.
- Patients with cluster headache tend to move about during attacks, pacing, rocking, or rubbing their head for relief. This is in sharp contrast to patients with migraine, who prefer to remain motionless during attacks.
- Cluster headache is associated with ipsilateral symptoms of cranial parasympathetic autonomic activation: **conjunctival injection or lacrimation, rhinorrhea or nasal congestion**, or cranial sympathetic dysfunction such as **ptosis.**
- The sympathetic deficit is peripheral and likely to be due to parasympathetic activation with injury to ascending sympathetic fibers surrounding a dilated carotid artery as it passes into the cranial cavity.
- When present, **photophobia** and **phonophobia** are far more likely to be unilateral and on the same side of the pain, rather than **bilateral, as is seen in migraine**.
- Cluster headache is likely to be a disorder involving central pacemaker neurons in the region of the posterior hypothalamus

Treatment:

Acute Attack Treatment

- Oxygen inhalation.
- Sumatriptan 6 mg SC is rapid in onset and will usually shorten an attack to 10–15 min
- Sumatriptan (20 mg) and zolmitriptan (5 mg) nasal sprays
- **Oral sumatriptan is not effective** for prevention or for **acute treatment** of cluster headache.

Preventive Treatments

(See the following table)

Neurostimulation Therapy

- Indicated when medical therapies fail
- Deep-brain stimulation of the region of the posterior hypothalamic gray matter has proven successful in a substantial proportion of patients.

16. Loss of gastric acidity increases the risk of infection due to:

A. Salmonella species **B.** Staph aureus
C. Giardiasis **D.** Candida

Ans: A. Salmonella species

Ref: *Harrison's principles of Internal Medicine. 18th edition. 2012. Chapter 153/Chapter 119 (Table 119-1)*

Explanation: *(See table on the next page)*

17. Which of the following drug decreases the clearance of Theophylline?

A. Rifampicin **B.** Smoking
C. Phenobarbitone **D.** Cimetidine

Ans: D. Cimetidine

Ref: *Harrison's principles of Internal Medicine. 18th edition. 2012. Chapter 254 (Table 254-4)*

Explanation:

Factors Affecting Clearance of Theophylline

Increased Clearance

- Enzyme induction (rifampicin, phenobarbitone, ethanol)
- Smoking (tobacco, marijuana)
- High-protein, low-carbohydrate diet
- Barbecued meat
- Childhood

Decreased Clearance

- Enzyme inhibition (cimetidine, erythromycin, ciprofloxacin, allopurinol, zileuton, zafirlukast)

Preventive Management of Cluster Headache

Short-Term Prevention	Long-Term Prevention
Episodic Cluster Headache	**Episodic Cluster Headache & Prolonged Chronic Cluster Headache**
Prednisone 1 mg/kg up to 60 mg qd, tapering over 21 days	Verapamil 160–960 mg/d
	Lithium 400–800 mg/d
Methysergide 3–12 mg/d	Methysergide 3–12 mg/d
Verapamil 160–960 mg/d	Topiramate[a] 100–400 mg/d
Greater occipital nerve injection	Gabapentin[a] 1200–3600 mg/d
	Melatonin[c] 9–12 mg/d

Host Defect	Disease or Therapy Associated With Defect	Common Etiologic Agent of Infection
Nonspecific Immunity		
Impaired cough	Rib fracture, neuromuscular dysfunction	Bacteria causing pneumonia, aerobic and anaerobic oral flora
Loss of gastric acidity	Achlorhydria, histamine blockade	*Salmonella* spp., enteric pathogens
Loss of cutaneous integrity	Penetrating trauma, athlete's foot	*Staphylococcus* spp., *Streptococcus* spp.
	Burn	*Pseudomonas aeruginosa*
	IV catheter	*Staphylococcus* spp., *Streptococcus* spp., gram-negative rods, coagulase-negative staphylococci
Implantable device	Heart valve	*Streptococcus* spp., coagulase-negative staphylococci, *Staphylococcus aureus*
	Artificial joint	*Staphylococcus* spp., *Streptococcus* spp., gram-negative rods
Loss of normal bacterial flora	Antibiotic use	*Clostridium difficile*, *Candida* spp.
Impaired clearance		
Poor drainage	Urinary tract infection	*Escherichia coli*
Abnormal secretions	Cystic fibrosis	Chronic pulmonary infection with *P. aeruginosa*

- Congestive heart failure
- Liver disease
- Pneumonia
- Viral infection and vaccination
- High carbohydrate diet
- Old age

18. Stage 5 chronic kidney disease is diagnosed when GFR falls below:

A. 5 mL/min per 1.73 m2
B. 10 mL/min per 1.73 m2
C. 15 mL/min per 1.73 m2
D. 20 mL/min per 1.73 m2

Ans: C. 15 mL/min per 1.73 m2

Ref: *Harrison's principles of Internal Medicine. 18th edition. 2012. Chapter 44. Pg.334 (Table 52-1)*

Explanation:

ESRD is Stage 5 CKD

Classification of Chronic Kidney Disease (CKD)

Stage	GFR, mL/min per 1.73 m^2
0	>90[a]
1	90[b]
2	60–89
3	30–59
4	15–29
5	<15 (ESRD)

19. The most common class of lupus nephritis is:

A. Class 2
B. Class 3
C. Class 4
D. Class 5

Ans: C. Class 4

Ref: *Harrison's Principles of Internal Medicine. 18th edition. 2012. Chapter 283*

Explanation:

- Class 4 (Diffuse nephritis) lupus nephritis is the **MOST COMMON** type and carries the WORST PROGNOSIS *(See table on the next page)*

Lupus Nephritis

- Lupus nephritis is a common and serious complication of systemic lupus erythematosus (SLE).
- 30 – 50% percent of patients will have clinical manifestations of renal disease at the time of diagnosis.
- Lupus nephritis results from the deposition of circulating immune complexes, which activate the complement cascade leading to complement-mediated damage, leukocyte infiltration, activation of procoagulant factors, and release of various cytokines. In situ immune complex formation following glomerular binding of nuclear antigens, particularly necrotic nucleosomes, also plays a role in renal injury.
- The presence of antiphospholipid antibodies may also trigger a thrombotic microangiopathy in a minority of patients.
- The most common clinical sign of renal disease is proteinuria, but hematuria, hypertension, varying degrees of renal failure, and active urine sediment with red blood cell casts can all be present.

Classification for Lupus Nephritis

Class I	Minimal mesangial	Normal histology with mesangial deposits
Class II	Mesangial proliferation	Mesangialhypercellularity with expansion of the mesangial matrix
Class III	Focal nephritis	Focal endocapillary ± extracapillary proliferation with focal subendothelial immune deposits and mild mesangial expansion
Class IV	Diffuse nephritis	Diffuse endocapillary ± extracapillary proliferation with diffuse subendothelial immune deposits and mesangial alterations
Class V	Membranous nephritis	Thickened basement membranes with diffuse subepithelial immune deposits; may occur with class III or IV lesions and is sometimes called mixed membranous and proliferative nephritis
Class VI	Sclerotic nephritis	Global sclerosis of nearly all glomerular capillaries

- Although significant renal pathology can be found on biopsy even in the absence of major abnormalities in the urinalysis, most nephrologists do not biopsy patients until the urinalysis is convincingly abnormal.
- The extrarenal manifestations of lupus are important in establishing a firm diagnosis of systemic lupus because, while serologic abnormalities are common in lupus nephritis, they are not diagnostic.
- Anti-dsDNA antibodies that fix complement correlate best with the presence of renal disease.
- Hypocomplementemia is common in patients with acute lupus nephritis (70–90%) and declining complement levels may herald a flare.
- **Class I** nephritis describes normal glomerular histology by any technique or normal light microscopy with minimal mesangial deposits on immunofluorescent or electron microscopy.
- **Class II** designates mesangial immune complexes with *mesangial proliferation.* Both class I and II lesions are typically associated with minimal renal manifestation and normal renal function; nephrotic syndrome is rare. Patients with lesions limited to the renal mesangium have an excellent prognosis and generally do not need therapy for their lupus nephritis.
- **Class III** describes focal lesions with proliferation or scarring, often involving only a segment of the glomerulus. Hypertension, an active urinary sediment, and proteinuria are common with nephrotic-range proteinuria in 25–33% of patients. Elevated serum creatinine is present in 25% of patients
- **Class IV** describes global, diffuse proliferative lesions involving the vast majority of glomeruli. Have high anti-DNA antibody titers, low serum complement, hematuria, red blood cell casts, proteinuria, hypertension, and decreased renal function; 50% of patients have nephrotic-range proteinuria. Patients with crescents on biopsy often have a rapidly progressive decline in renal function. Without treatment, this aggressive lesion has the worst renal prognosis.
- The **class V** lesion describes subepithelial immune deposits producing a membranous pattern; a subcategory of class V lesions is associated with proliferative lesions and is sometimes called mixed membranous and proliferative disease.

20. Non-erosive arthritis is characteristic of:

A. SLE **B.** Psoriasis
C. RA **D.** Gout

Ans: A. SLE

Ref: *Harrison's Principles of Internal Medicine, 18th edition, pg 2728*

Explanation:

- **SLE** causes **non erosive polyarthritis** of the hands, wrist & knees.
- Can cause avascular necrosis of joints increased by steroid use.
- **Psoriasis, RA & gout** cause **erosive arthritis.**

Psoriatic arthritis (PsA):

- DIP involved, nail changes (pitting, ridging, onycholysis, yellow discoloration, hyperkeratosis) dactylitis
- Asymmetrical oligoarthritis
- Symmetrical polyarthritis
- ***Arthritis mutilans*** with destruction and telescoping of digits
- ***CASPAR criteria*** used to diagnose PsA
- Treatment: Anti-TNF-α- infliximab, etanercept, adalimumab, golimumab
- Anti T cell- Alefacept
- ***Newer agent- Ustekinumab***
- Methotrexate, sulfasalazine, leflunomide

Rheumatoid Arthritis (RA):
- MCP, PIP, &MTP involved
- Juxta-articular osteopenia- earliest radiological finding
- ACR & EULAR revised criteria used to diagnose RA
- Treatment: Anti TNF- α- Infliximab, Etanercept, adalimumab, golimumab, certolizumab
- Abatacept, anakinra, rituximab, tocilizumab

Gouty arthritis:
- Acute, monoarthritis, 1st MTP involved
- Precipitated by diet, trauma, surgery, alcohol, stress
- Joint aspirate for needle shaped MSU crystals, birefringent with negative elongation, TC 2-60 thousand
- S.uric acid can be low /normal during attack
- Acute attack-NSAIDS, Colchicine, steroids, anakinra
- Hypouricemic drugs- Allopurinol, febuxostat, Rasburicase, pegloticase

21. All are indications for dialysis in a case of acute renal failure *except:*

A. Uremia B. Hyponatremia
C. Hyperkalemia D. Metabolic acidosis

Ans: B. Hyponatremia

Ref: *Harrison's principles of Internal Medicine. 18th edition. 2012. Chapter 279.*

Explanation:

Indications for Dialysis in ARF
- Volume overload,
- Hyperkalemia,
- Metabolic acidosis,
- In some toxic ingestions
- Severe complications of uremia (asterixis, pericardial rub or effusion, encephalopathy, uremic bleeding).

22. Candida albicans infection seen in:

A. Chronic granulomatous disease
B. Lazy leukocyte syndrome
C. Myeloperoxidase deficiency
D. Chediak - higashi syndrome

Ans: C. Myeloperoxidase deficiency

Ref: *Harrison's Principles of Internal Medicine, 18ed. Pg & Nelson*

Explanation:

Chediak-Higashi Syndrome
- Autosomal recessive disorder
- Increased susceptibility to infection due to ***defective degranulation of neutrophils***
- Mild bleeding diathesis
- Partial ***oculocutaneous albinism***,
- Progressive peripheral neuropathy
- Hemophagocytic lymphohistiocytosis
- Pigmentary dilution involving the hair, skin, and ocular fundus results from pathologic aggregation of melanosomes.
- Neurologic deficits are associated with a ***failure of decussation*** of the ***optic*** and ***auditory*** nerves.
- Defects in neutrophil chemotaxis, degranulation, and bactericidal activity.
- **Giant granules** in the **neutrophils**
- ***LYST*** **(for lysosomal traffic regulator)**, the gene mutated in CHS, is located at chromosome **1q2-q44.**

Clinical Manifestations
- Light skin and silvery hair
- Solar sensitivity and photophobia
- ***Rotary nystagmus.***
- The infections involve **mucous membranes, skin,** and **respiratory tract.**
- Increased susceptibility to ***gram-positive bacteria, gram-negative bacteria and fungi***
- ***Staph aureus*** being the **most common** offending organism.
- The neuropathy may be **sensory or motor** in type, and **ataxia** may be a prominent feature.
- ***Prolonged bleeding times*** with ***normal platelet counts***, resulting from impaired platelet aggregation associated with a deficiency of the dense granules containing adenosine diphosphate and serotonin.
- Natural killer cell function of large granular lymphocytes is also impaired.
- The **most life-threatening complication** of CHS is the development of an accelerated phase characterized by pancytopenia, high fever, and **lymphohistiocytic infiltration** of liver, spleen, and lymph nodes.
- The onset of the accelerated phase is related to the inability of these patients to contain and **control Epstein-Barr virus** infection, leading to features of **hemophagocytic lymphohistiocytosis (HLH).**
- The diagnosis of CHS is established by finding **large inclusions** in all **nucleated blood cells.** These can be seen on Wright-stained blood films and are accentuated by a peroxidase stain.
- **High-dose ascorbic acid (Vitamin C)** (200 mg/day for infants, 2,000 mg/day for adults) improves the clinical status of some children in the stable phase.

Myeloperoxidase Deficiency

- Autosomal recessive disorder of oxidative metabolism
- **Most common inherited disorder** of phagocytes,
- **MPO** is a **green heme protein** located in the **azurophilic lysosomes** of **neutrophils** and **monocytes**
- It is the basis for the greenish tinge to pus accumulated at a site of infection.
- MPO deficiency is caused by a ***missense mutation in the MPO gene*** that results in an MPO precursor that does not incorporate heme.
- Partial or complete MPO deficiency leads to diminished production of **hypochlorous acid** (HOCl) and HOCl-derived chloramines.
- The deficiency in HOCl leads to early depression of **gram-positive** and **gram-negative** bacterial rates of killing in vitro that normalizes after 1 hr incubation.

Clinical Manifestations

- MPO deficiency is usually **clinically silent**.
- **Disseminated candidiasis**, usually in conjunction with **diabetes mellitus**.
- Can develop in **acute myelogenous leukemia** and in **myelodysplastic syndromes.**
- Deficiency of neutrophil and monocyte MPO can be identified by histochemical analysis.
- There is **no specific therapy**.
- Aggressive treatment disseminated candidal infections.
- The prognosis is usually excellent.

Chronic Granulomatous Disease (CGD)

- Basic pathology is a defect in the generation of microbicidal oxygen metabolites.
- Neutrophils & Monocytes are unable to kill **catalase-positive microorganisms.** But they are capable of normal chemotaxis, ingestion, and degranulation.
- Caused by 4 genes, 1 X-linked and 3 autosomal recessive in inheritance.
- The CGD **phagocytic vacuoles** lack **microbicidal reactive oxygen species** and remain **acidic**, so bacteria are not killed or digested properly

Clinical Manifestations

- Recurrent pneumonia, lymphadenitis, hepatic or other abscesses, osteomyelitis, family history of recurrent infections, or any infection with an unusual catalase-positive organism requires evaluation.
- The most common pathogen is ***S. aureus***, although any catalase-positive microorganism may be involved.
- ***List of Catalase Positive Organisms***:
  - Staphylococcus
  - Pseudomonas
  - Aspergillus
  - Candida
  - Enterobacteriaceae
- Other organisms frequently causing infections include ***Serratia marcescens, Burkholderia cepacia, Aspergillus, Candida albicans, Nocardia***, and ***Salmonella***.
- Increased susceptibility to **mycobacterium** including the **BCG vaccine**.
- Anemia of chronic disease
- Poor growth
- Lymphadenopathy
- Hepatosplenomegaly
- Chronic purulent dermatitis
- Restrictive lung disease
- Gingivitis
- Hydronephrosis
- Pyloric outlet narrowing
- ***Perirectal abscesses*** and ***recurrent skin infections***, including folliculitis, ***cutaneous granulomas***, and ***discoid lupus erythematosus***
- **Granuloma formation** and inflammatory processes are a hallmark of CGD

Laboratory Findings

- The diagnosis is most often made by performing **flow cytometry** using dihydrorhodamine 123 (DHR) to measure oxidant production through its increased fluorescence when oxidized by H_2O_2.
- The **nitroblue tetrazolium (NBT) dye test** is frequently cited in the literature is obsolete

Treatment

- HSCT is the only known **cure** for CGD.
- Prophylaxis with daily oral Cotrimoxazole and an antifungal drug, such as itraconazole
- **Interferon-γ (IFN-γ)** 50 ?g/m^2 3 times/wk reduces the number of hospitalizations and serious infections. The mechanism of action of IFN- γ therapy in CGD is unknown.
- **Itraconazole** (200 mg/day for patients >50 kg and 100 mg/day for patients <50 kg and ≤ 5 yr of age) administered prophylactically reduces the frequency of fungal infections.
- **Corticosteroids** are tried in antral and urethral obstruction & severe granulomatous colitis.

23. A female patient presents with amenorrhea, galactorrhea and bitemporal hemianopia. Most likely diagnosis is: (Repeat)

A. Cushing's disease
B. Empty sella syndrome

C. Prolactinoma
D. Hypothyroidism

Ans: C. Prolactinoma

Ref: *Harrison's Principles of Internal Medicine, 18ed*

Explanation:

PROLACTINOMA

The symptoms due to a **prolactinoma** are broadly divided into those that are caused by increased **prolactin levels** or **mass effect.**

A. Those that are caused by **increased prolactin** levels are:
- **Amenorrhea**
- **Galactorrhea** (infrequent in men)
- Loss of **axillary and pubic hair**
- **Hypogonadism, gynecomastia, erectile dysfunction** (in males)

B. Those that are caused by **mass effect** are:
- **Bitemporal hemianopsia** (due to pressure on optic chiasm)
- Vertigo
- Nausea, vomiting

24. Exaggerated physiological splitting of S2 seen in:

A. VSD **B.** Severe AS
C. RBBB **D.** ASD

Ans: C. RBBB

Ref: *Hutchison's clinical methods, 22nd ed.*

Explanation:

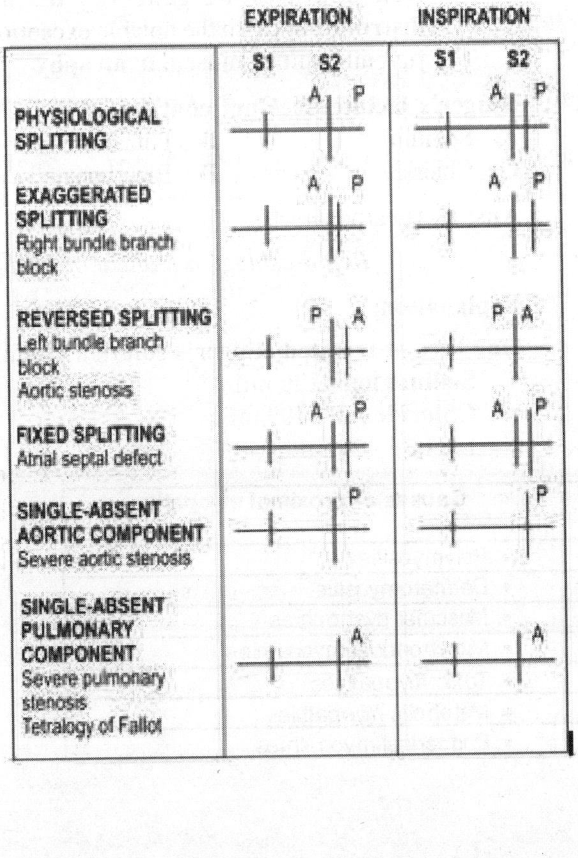

25. Inorganic lead toxicity does not cause:

A. Wrist drop **B.** Insomnia
C. Anemia **D.** Blue line

Ref: *Harrison's 18th edition*

Ans: B. Insomnia

Explanation:

Lead Toxicity

- Lead is in general a **CNS depressant**, hence causes **lethargy** and **not insomnia**. All other options are characteristic features of inorganic lead toxicity
- There are two principal mechanisms of lead toxicity.
  - First, **lead complexes** with important functional chemical groups including –COOH, –NH2, and –SH and so **disrupts the function of enzymes** and other biologically important molecules.
  - Secondly, lead substitutes for **divalent ions, particularly calcium**, with the potential for widespread chemical interactions both at cell **membranes** and within **intracellular organelles**.
- Lead depresses the enzymes responsible for haem synthesis and shortens erythrocyte lifespan leading to a ***microcytic or normocytic hypochromic anaemia.***
- For example, **lead blocks** the **conversion of δ-aminolaevulinic acid** to **porphobilinogen** leading to an **increase in δ-aminolaevulinic acid** in blood and urine.
- Lead also **inhibits ferrochelatase**, which results in an **elevated free erythrocyte protoporphyrin (FEP)** concentration.
- There is a concomitant **increase in urinary coproporphyrins and FEP**, commonly assayed as zinc protoporphyrin.
- ***Basophilic stippling*** of erythrocytes is due to nuclear remnants that persist due to inhibition of erythrocyte 5′ nucleotidase by lead.
- Mild intoxication may result in no more than ***lethargy*** and occasional abdominal discomfort, whereas ***abdominal pain*** (which is usually diffuse but may be colicky), vomiting, constipation, and encephalopathy develop in more severe cases. ***Encephalopathy*** (seizures, mania, delirium, coma) is more common in children than in adults. Classically, lead poisoning results in ***foot drop***, attributable to primary motor peripheral neuropathy; ***wrist drop*** occurs only as a late sign.

- Renal effects include reversible ***renal tubular dysfunction*** causing **glycosuria**, **amino-aciduria**, and **phosphaturia** and **irreversible interstitial fibrosis** with **progressive renal insufficiency** leading to hypertension.
- ***A bluish discoloration of the gum margins (blue line)*** due to deposition of lead sulphide is observed occasionally.

26. Which of the following causes distal myopathy:

A. Myotonic dystrophy
B. Duchenne Muscular Dystrophy
C. Becker Muscular Dystrophy
D. Polymyositits

Ans: A. Myotonic dystrophy

Ref: *Harrison's Principles of Internal Medicine, 18th ed, pg 3499,3500*

Explanation:*(See the following table)*

Myotonic Dystrophy:

- Facial muscle (hatchet face), neck,palatal, pharyngeal, distal muscle of hands and feet weakness
- Frontal baldness
- Myotonia of thenar muscle, tongue, wrist extensor
- Cardiac conduction defects, cataract, insulin resistance
- Myotonia treated with phenytoin/mexilitine

Drug induced proximal weakness

- Amiodarone
- Chloroquine
- HCQ
- Colchicine
- Lipid lowering drugs
- Glucocorticoids
- Zidovudine
- Alcohol
- Amphetamine
- d-Penicillamine
- Clofibratte
- Vincristine

Endocrine causes:

- Hypo/hyperthyroidism
- Hyper/hypoparathyroidism
- Cushing's syndrome
- Osteomalacia
- Renal osteodystrophy
- Adrenal insufficiency
- Conn's syndrome
- Acromegaly
- DM

Channelopathies:

1. Malignant hyperthermia- Calcium channel
2. Hypokalemic periodic paralysis- Calcium & sodium channel
3. Hyperkalemic periodic paralysis- Sodium channel
4. Paramyotonia congenita-Sodium channel
5. Myotonia congenital (Thompson's disease)- Chloride channel
6. Anderson-Tawil syndrome- Potassium channel
   - Mitochondrial myopathies: MERFF, MELAS,CPEO, MNGIE, Kearns-Sayre syndrome
   - Disorders of carbohydrate & lipid metabolism: Mc Ardle disease, CPT deficiency
   - In general, **myopathies** follow a **proximal distribution of weakness** and **muscle wasting** (with the notable exception of **myotonic muscular dystrophy**)
   - **Neuropathies** are generally **distal in distribution** (with the notable exception of **juvenile spinal muscular atrophy**

27. Ringer's lactate does not contain:

A. Sodium
B. Potassium
C. Chloride
D. Bicarbonate

Ans: D. Bicarbonate

Ref: *Washington Manual of Medicine*

Explanation:

One litre of lactated Ringer's solution contains:

- **Sodium** ion - 130 mEq
- **Chloride** ion - 109 mEq
- **Lactate** - 28 mEq

Cause of distal myopathies	Causes of proximal myopathy
• Myotonic dystrophy	• Polymyositis
• Welander's myopathy	• Dermatomyositis
• Tibial(Udd's) muscular dystrophy	• Muscular dystrophies
• Markesbery-Griggs distal myopathy	• Mitochondrial myopathies
• Laing's, Nonaka's	• Toxic myopathies
• Miyoshi's distal myopathy	• Metabolic myopathies
• Myofibrillar myopathy	• Endocrinal myopathies

- **Potassium** ion - 4 mEq
- **Calcium** ion - 3 mEq
- Lactated Ringer's has an osmolarity of **273 mOsm**/L.

SURGERY

1. **Allen's test is used to diagnose: (Repeat)**
   A. Thoracic outlet syndrome
   B. Palmar arch insufficiency
   C. Superior vena cava syndrome
   D. Coarctation of aorta

Ans: B. Palmar arch insufficiency

Ref: Bailey and Love's Short Practice of Surgery 25th Edition

Explanation:

Allen's test

- It is a test for the ***patency of the radial artery*** after insertion of an indwelling monitoring catheter. The patient's hand is formed into a fist and the ulnar artery is compressed
- Compression continues while the fist is opened.
- If blood perfusion through the radial artery is adequate, the hand should flush and resume its normal pinkish coloration.

Adson's test

- It is the loss of the radial pulse in the arm by rotating head to the ipsilateral side with extended neck following deep inspiration.
- It is seen in ***thoracic outlet syndrome (TOS)***

2. **Desmoid Tumor is associated with: (Repeat)**
   A. Colonic polyps **B.** Pancreatic Cancer
   C. Ovarian cancer **D.** Gastric cancer

Ans: A. Colonic polyps

Ref: Sabiston Textbook of Surgery, 19th Edition, Pg: 1095.

Explanation:

*"Desmoid tumours are commonly associated with **familial adenomatous polyposis (FAP)**, in which **colonic polyps** are the most common feature"*

Desmoid Tumour

- Desmoid tumor, also known as **fibromatosis or aggressive fibromatosis**,
- It is an uncommon neoplasm that occurs sporadically or as part of an inherited syndrome assc with
  - **Familial adenomatous polyposis** (FAP)
  - **Gardner's syndrome**, an autosomal dominant syndrome of ***GI adenomatous polyps*** or ***adenocarcinoma***, ***osteomas***, and ***skin and soft tissue tumors***.

Pathophysiology

- Arise from fibroaponeurotic tissue and
- Lack metastatic potential,
- Locally aggressive and invasive, with a high propensity for recurrence.
- Associated with Oral contraceptive use
- Estrogen receptors are present within the tumor; suggest a regulatory role for estrogen in this disease.

Classification

Desmoid tumors are typically classified by location

1. ***Extra-abdominal or extremity desmoids*** (i.e., those tumors occurring in the proximal extremities or limb girdle)
2. ***Abdominal wall tumors***
3. ***Intra-abdominal desmoids***, which involve the mesentery, pelvis, or bowel wall.

Clinical features

- Majority of desmoid tumors are **sporadic**,.
- Typically in **young women** during **pregnancy** or **within a year of childbirth.**
- Typically present as a **slowly growing** mass
- Usually present with an asymptomatic mass or with symptoms related to mass effect from the tumor.
- Often a temporal association between the discovery of the tumor and an antecedent history of abdominal trauma or operation.

Investigations

- ***Imaging (CT or MRI)*** is necessary to delineate the extent of tumor involvement fully
- No need to perform staging for metastatic disease.
- ***Biopsy*** is required to establish the diagnosis.
- ***Core needle biopsy or incisional biopsy*** will demonstrate a tumor composed of bundles of spindle cells and an abundant fibrous stroma.
- **Immunohistochemistry** can help clarify difficult diagnoses
- Typically stain **positive for β-catenin, actin, and vimentin** and **stain negative for cytokeratin and S-100**

Management

Surgery

- **Surgery** is the treatment of choice.
- Resection of the tumor with a wide margin of normal tissue is the optimal treatment.
- Often, the extent of this resection will require abdominal wall reconstruction with local tissue flaps or mesh prostheses.

Radiation

- Abdominal wall desmoids are responsive to radiation therapy, although the treatment effect is slow and may be progressive over several years

Radiotherapy as primary treatment

- Radiotherapy alone is an acceptable treatment option for patients with ***unresectable desmoid tumors*** or tumors for which resection will be associated with high morbidity risks or major functional loss.

Adjuvant Radiotherapy

- Adjuvant radiation therapy is **controversial**, with most centers reserving this modality for **patients with positive margins, or close margins**

Neoadjuvant radiotherapy

- The use of neoadjuvant radiation therapy is **less well accepted** than adjuvant radiation therapy because of the slow response times, **often 1 year or more**, with the potential for making subsequent abdominal wall reconstruction more difficult, and few studies demonstrating a clear benefit.

Adjuvant medical Therapy

1. ***Tamoxifen***
2. NSAIDS particularly Indomethacin and Sulindac
3. ***Imatinib***- A tyrosine kinase inhibitor
4. ***Chemotherapy***- Methotrexate with vinblastine, doxorubicin-based therapy, and ifosfamide-based regimens.
5. For **desmoids with rapid growth**, medical oncologists may recommend therapies typically used for sarcomas, such as **doxorubicin and dacarbazine**

3. Which of the following type of lipoma is prone to develop Intussusception?

A. Submucous lipoma **B.** Subserosal lipoma
C. Intramural lipoma **D.** Serosal lipoma

Ref: Bailey & Love's *Short Practice of Surgery 25th Edition Chapter 66 | Intestinal Obstruction Pages1191-12 & Donald A. Antonioli, " Gastrointestinal Autonomic Nerve Tumors, expanding the spectrum of gastrointestinal stromal tumors," Arch Pathol Lab Med; 1989; 113; 831-833.*

Ans: A. Submucosal lipoma

Explanation:

Intussusception

- **Invagination of an intestinal segment** (the **intussusceptum**) into the next distal part of the intestine forms a sheath around it (the **intussuscipiens**) producing a form of intestinal obstruction called 'intussusception'.
- The **most common cause** is **hypertrophy of the Peyer's patches** in the **terminal ileum** from an antecedent viral infection.
- The hypertrophied lymphatic patch becomes drawn into the lumen of the terminal ileum and is moved progressively into the ascending and transverse colon.
- Other predisposing factors include
  - Polyps
  - Meckel's diverticulum
  - Benign tumors like lipoma
  - Leiomyoma
  - Malignant tumors such as lymphoma which may act as lead points for intussusception.
- **GI lipomas**, most common in the **ileum**, are single **intramural** lesion, **submucosal** in location and usually small.
- One portion of the gut becomes invaginated within an immediately adjacent segment; almost invariably, it is the proximal into the distal.
- The condition is encountered most **commonly in children**, with a peak incidence **between 5 and 10 months of age.**
- About **90%** of cases are **idiopathic** but an associated upper respiratory tract infection or gastroenteritis may precede the condition.
- It is believed that **hyperplasia of Peyer's patches** in the **terminal ileum**.
- Weaning, loss of passively acquired maternal immunity and common viral pathogens have all been implicated in the pathogenesis of intussusception in infancy.

Children Pathological lead points

- Meckel's diverticulum
- Polyp
- duplication,
- Henoch–Schönlein purpura
- Appendix

Adult cases lead point

- A polyp (e.g. Peutz–Jeghers syndrome)
- A submucosal lipoma
- other tumours

Pathology

An intussusception is composed of three parts:

- The entering or inner tube (intussusceptum)
- The returning or middle tube;
- The sheath or outer tube (intussuscipiens).
  - The part that advances is the apex, the mass is the intussusception and the neck is the junction of the entering layer with the mass.
  - An intussusception is an example of a strangulating obstruction as the blood supply of the inner layer is usually impaired.

– The degree of ischaemia is dependent on the tightness of the invagination, which is usually greatest as it passes through the ileocaecal valve.

Intussusception may be **anatomically deûned** according to the site and extent of invagination.

- In most **children,** the intussusception is **ileocolic**
- In **adults, colocolic** intussusception is common

Intussusception

- Most common in children
- Primary or secondary to intestinal pathology, e.g. polyp

Meckel's diverticulum

- Ileocolic is the commonest variety
- Can lead to an ischaemic segment
- Radiological reduction is indicated in most cases
- The remainder require surgery

4. **Circumcisscion not done in: (Repeat)**

A. Paraphimosis **B.** Balanophosthitis
C. Hypospadias **D.** Ca Penis

Ans: C. Hypospadias

Ref: *Bailey and Love's Short Practice of Surgery 25th Edition*

Explanation:

"Most of the procedures for hypospadias make use of ***prepuceal skin*** *and so* ***circumcision should be avoided*** *until repair is done" (Ref: Bailey)*

Contraindications for Circumcision

- In infants with certain genital structure abnormalities
- Misplaced urethral opening (as in hypospadias and epispadias)
- Curvature of the head of the penis (chordee)
- Ambiguous genitalia
- This is because the **foreskin** may be **needed** for **reconstructive surgery.**

Circumcision is also avoided in

- Premature infants
- Clinically unstable infants
- Undiagnosed bleeding conditions

5. **Characteristic radiological finding in Frontal mucocoele is:**

A. Loss of scalloping
B. Thickening of wall of sinus
C. Heterogenous opacification
D. Patchy osteolysis

Ans: D. Patchy osteolysis

Ref: *Aggarwal SK et al. Frontal sinus mucocele with orbital complications: Management by varied surgical approaches. Asian J Neurosurg. 2012 Jul-Sep; 7(3): 135-140.*

Explanation:

- There are three criteria for **CT diagnosis** of a mucocoele:
  - Homogeneous isodense mass
  - Clearly defined margin
  - Patchy osteolysis around the mass
- **Erosion** of the **sinus** wall with **marginal sclerosis** is also an indicative finding
- In MRI, mucocoeles tend to be fairly bright on T1W images compared to the brain and iso-hyperintense on T2W images (Pathognomonic MRI finding)

6. **Which of the following causes Adynamic intestinal obstruction?**

A. Gall stones **B.** Bands
C. Intussusception **D.** Paralytic ileus

Ans: D. Paralytic ileus

Ref: *The Washington Manual of Surgery, 6th edition, Bailey and Love's Short Practice of Surgery 25th Edition & Schwartz's Principles of Surgery, 9th Edition*

Explanation:

Intestinal obstruction

- **Defn**: Lack of transit of intestinal contents
- Classification according to pathology

Dynamic: Where peristalsis is working against a mechanical obstruction

Adynamic: Where there is absence of peristalsis without obstruction

- Absent peristalsis (eg: Paralytic ileus)
- Non-propulsive form (ef: Mesenteric vascular occlusion, Pseudo-obstruction)

Causes of Dynamic Intestinal Obstruction

Intraluminal causes

- Impacted stools
- Foreign bodies
- Bezoars
- Gall stones
- Ascariasis
- Meconium ileus

Intramural causes

- Atresia
- Inflammatory stricture – TB, Crohn's disease
- Malignant stricture – Ca Colon, GIST

Extramural causes

- Intraperitoneal bands and adhesions
- Hernia
- Volvulus
- Intussusception

7. **True about hypospadias: (Repeat)**
   A. Associated with chordee
   B. Associated with undescended testis in 50% cases
   C. Due to failure of fusion of posterior wall of urethra
   D. Circumcision should be done immediately

Ans: A. Associated with chordee

***Ref:** Bailey and Love's Short Practice of Surgery 25th Edition*

Explanation:

*"Up to **10%** of boys with hypospadias have at least one undescended testis"*

Hypospadias

- 1 in 350 male births
- **Most common** congenital malformation of the urethra.
- The external meatus opens on the underside of the penis or the perineum
- The inferior aspect of the prepuce is poorly developed (***'hooded prepuce')***.
- Hypospadias is classified according to position of the meatus.

Glandular hypospadias

- **Most common** type
- Does not usually require treatment.
- The normal site of the external meatus is marked by a blind pit, although it occasionally connects by a channel to the ectopic opening on the underside of the glans.

Coronal hypospadias

- The meatus is placed at the junction of the underside of the glans and the body of the penis.

Penile and penoscrotal hypospadias

- The opening is on the underside of the penile shaft

Perineal hypospadias

- This is the most severe abnormality.
- The scrotum is split and the urethra opens between its two halves.
- There may be testicular maldescent which may make it difficult to determine the sex of the child.
  - The more severe varieties of hypospadias represent an absence of the urethra and corpus spongiosum distal to the ectopic opening.
  - The absent structures are represented by a ***fibrous cord*** which deforms the penis in a downward direction (***chordee***).
  - The more distant the opening from its normal position, the more pronounced the bowing.

Treatment

- Glandular hypospadias does not need treatment unless the meatus is stenosed, in which case a ***meatotomy*** is performed.
- Surgery is indicated for other forms of hypospadias to ***improve sexual function*** and for ***cosmetic reasons***.
- Most of these procedures make use of ***prepuceal skin*** and so ***circumcision should be avoided*** until the hypospadias has been repaired.

8. **Hernia least prone for strangulation is:**
   A. Femoral hernia
   B. Umbilical hernia
   C. Indirect inguinal hernia
   D. Direct inguinal hernia

Ans: B. Umbilical hernia or **D.** Direct inguinal hernia

***Ref:** Sabiston Textbook of Surgery, 19th Edition, Pg: 31, 1135. & Bailey & Love's Short Practice of Surgery, 25th Edition, 979. & Washington manual of Surgery, 6th ed.*

Explanation:

"As the neck of the sac is wide, direct inguinal hernias do not often strangulate." (Bailey)
"In Umbilical hernia, Obstruction or strangulation below the age of 3 years is extremely uncommon." (Bailey)

Incidence of Strangulation (Ref: Washington)

- **Inguinal** hernia - **10%**
- **Femoral** hernia - **25%**

I could not get the incidence for other 2 types.

Femoral hernia

- A femoral hernia occurs through the femoral canal, which is bounded superiorly by the iliopubic tract, inferiorly by Cooper's ligament, laterally by the femoral vein, and medially by the junction of the iliopubic tract and **Cooper's ligament (lacunar ligament).**
- Recurrence of femoral hernia after operation is **only 2%.**
- There are three approaches to femoral hernia repair.
- **The low operation (Lockwood)**
  The sac is dissected out below the inguinal ligament via a groin crease incision.
- **The high (McEvedy) operation**
  Classically, a vertical incision is made over the femoral canal and continued upwards above the inguinal ligament.
- **Lotheissen's operation (Inguinal Approach)**
  The inguinal canal is opened as for ***inguinal herniorrhaphy***.

Indirect and Direct Inguinal Hernia

	Indirect Inguinal Hernia	Direct Inguinal Hernia
Age	Any age	Common in elderly
Herniation	Protusion through deep inguinal ring	Through posterior wall of inguinal canal
Shape	Pyriform in shape	Round Shape
Descent to Scrotum	Oblique and downward into the scrotum	Directly forwards; Usually does not reach the bottom of scrotum
Neck	Narrow	Wide
Sac	Lateral to inferior epigastric artery	Medial to inferior epigastric artery
Zieman's test	Cough impulse on index finger	Cough impulse on middle finger
Invagination test	Tip of the finger	Pulp of the finger
Ring occlusion test	Does not bulge	Bulge medial to occluding finger
Coverings from outside to inside	Skin External spermatic fascia Cremasteric fascia Internal spermatic fascia Extraperitoneal tissue	Skin External spermatic fascia Conjoint tendon Fascia transversalis Extraperitoneal tissue
Strangulation & obstruction	Common	Uncommon
Laterality	Unilateral	Bilateral
Sac	Should be opened during surgery	Need not be opened unless strangulation is present

9. **Ramsteads operation is done in:**
   A. Congenital hypertrophic pyloric stenosis
   B. Achlasia cardia
   C. Diffuse esophageal spasm
   D. Ca Esophagus

Ans: A. Congenital hypertrophic pyloric stenosis

Ref: *Sabiston textbook of surgery,19th Edition 1841*

Explanation:

Congenital Hypertrophic Pyloric Stenosis

EtioPathology

- One of the **most common GI surgical disorders** in **early infancy**
- Most common between the ages of **2 and 8 weeks**.
- **Boys** are affected four times as often as girls,
- **First-born male** infants being at highest risk.
- Hypertrophy of the circular muscle of the pylorus results in constriction and obstruction of the gastric outlet, leading to **nonbilious & projectile emesis**
- Emesis leads to Loss of hydrochloric acid with the onset of hypokalemic hypochloremic metabolic alkalosis, and dehydration.
- Exact cause for HPS remains unknown, a lack of nitric oxide synthase in pyloric tissue has been implicated.

Clinical Presentation

- Progressively worsening nonbilious emesis.
- With time, the emesis becomes more frequent, forceful, and projectile in nature.
- Occasionally, visible gastric peristalsis may be observed as a wave of contractions from the left upper quadrant to the epigastrium.
- Shortly after emesis, infants usually crave additional feedings.
- Palpation of the **pyloric tumor (olive-shaped)** in the epigastrium or right upper quadrant by an experienced examiner is pathognomonic for the diagnosis. If the olive is palpated, no additional diagnostic testing is necessary.

Investigations

Abdominal Radiograph;

- Upper abdominal gas bubble in the stomach.

Ultrasound

- A persistent **pyloric muscle thickness more than 3 to 4 mm** or a **pyloric length more than 15 to 18 mm** in the presence of functional gastric outlet obstruction is diagnostic. When the olive is nonpalpable, the diagnosis of HPS can be made by ultrasound

Upper GI Contrast

- With equivocal clinical history, an upper GI contrast study is useful to evaluate for other causes of vomiting.

Treatment:

Surgical Management

- The treatment of HPS is pyloromyotomy **(Ramstedt procedure)**
- Incising through thickened pyloric musculature while preserving the underlying mucosa
- Right upper quadrant or periumbilical incision is used

- Laparoscopic pyloromyotomy has better cosmesis, with similar outcomes to those of the open technique.

Perioperative management:

- Before surgery, it is important that the infant be fully rehydrated with IV fluids to establish an adequate urine output and correct electrolyte disturbances such as metabolic alkalosis.
- Because the infant with underlying metabolic alkalosis will compensate with respiratory acidosis, postoperative apnea may occur. Thus, the serum HCO3 level needs to be normalized before surgery.
- Postoperatively, infants are usually allowed to resume enteral feedings.
- Complications include **incomplete myotomy**, **mucosal perforation**, and **wound** infection

10. Best invesigation in hirschsprung disease:

A. Rectal biopsy **B.** Rectal manometry
C. Invertogram **D.** Clinical examination

Ans: A. Rectal biopsy

Ref: *Sabiston Textbook of Surgery, 19th edition. Page 1849*

Explanation:

Hirschsprung disease (HD)

- **Absence of ganglion cells** in the **myenteric (Auerbach)** and **submucosal (Meissner) plexus**
- 1 in 5000 live births, M:F 4:1
- Neurogenic parasympathetic abnormality
- Muscular spasm of **distal colon** and **internal anal sphincter** - functional obstruction - abnormal bowel is contracted distal segment and the normal bowel is the proximal dilated portion
- **Aganglionosis** begins at **anorectal line**
- **Rectosigmoid** - **80%**; **splenic or transverse** colon **17%**; **entire colon 8%**
- **Transition zone:** Area between dilated and contracted segments - ganglion cells begin to appear, in reduced numbers
- 3-5% have Down syndrome
- Risk for HD is greater with family history
- Abnormal locus on the chromosome 10 identified; associated with the RET oncogene
- >90% present with progressive abdominal distention, bilious vomiting and failure to pass meconium within first 24 hours of life
- Diarrhea may develop due toenterocolitis
- ***Enterocolitis*** *is the* ***most common*** *cause of* ***death*** *in patients with uncorrected HD* - Diarrhea alternating with obstipation, abdominal distention, fever, hematochezia, and peritonitis.

Diagnosis:

- Initial diagnostic step in a newborn: distal bowel obstruction is a barium enema.
- Normal barium enema: Rectum is wider than sigmoid colon
- HD: spasm of distal rectum - smaller caliber compared to proximal sigmoid
- Identification of **transition zone** may be helpful in diagnosis of HD
- Failure to evacuate instilled contrast completely after 24 hours
- Exclude other causes of constipation in the newborn - meconium plug and small left colon syndrome, atresia
- **Manometry**: Failure of the internal sphincter to relax when the rectum is distended with a balloon
- ***Rectal biopsy: gold standard***
  - Newborn period - Bedside with special suction rectal biopsy instrument
  - Obtain biopsy specimen from at least 2 cm above the dentate line to avoid sampling the normal transition from ganglionated bowel to paucity or absence of ganglia in the region of the internal sphincter
  - Older children: full-thickness biopsy under general anesthesia (thicker rectal mucosa is not amenable to suction biopsy)
  - ***Features:***
    - Absent ganglia
    - Hypertrophied nerve trunks
    - Robust immunostaining for acetylcholin-esterase (AChE)
    - Loss of calretininimmunostaining-superior to AChEin evaluation of suction rectal biopsies

Surgical Management

- Traditionally: *Leveling colostomy*, confirmation of transition zone by frozen section evaluation of multiple seromuscular biopsies
- Diverting colostomy (end or loop) in the region of normal ganglionated bowel

Definitive surgical options:

- **Swenson procedure**: Aganglionic bowel removed down to the level of the internal sphincters;coloanal anastomosis
- **Duhamel procedure**: Aganglionic rectal stump left in place and ganglionated normal colon is pulled behind the stump
- **Soave technique:** Endorectal mucosal dissection within aganglionic distal rectum; Normally ganglionated colon then pulled through the remnant muscular cuff;coloanal anastomosis

- Nowadays, performed in newborn period as a primary procedure without an initial colostomy
- **Constipation** is the most frequent postoperative problem; others - soiling, incontinence, and enterocolitis

11. The most common site of involvement in Angiodysplasia of colon is:

A. Caecum B. Transverse colon
C. Rectum D. Descending colon

Ans: A. Caecum

Ref: *Robbins Pathologic Basis of Disease, 8th ed.*

Explanation:

Angiodysplasia of Colon

- It is characterized by ***malformed submucosal*** and ***mucosal blood vessels.***
- It occurs most often in the **cecum** or **right** colon
- It usually after the **sixth decade** of life.
- It accounts for **20%** of major episodes of lower intestinal bleeding
- The pathogenesis of angiodysplasia remains undefined but has been attributed to mechanical and congenital factors.
- Normal distention and contraction may intermittently occlude the submucosal veins that penetrate through the muscularis propria and can lead to focal dilation and tortuosity of overlying submucosal and mucosal vessels.
- Because the **cecum** has the **largest diameter** of any colonic segment, it develops the greatest wall tension.
- It is associated with aortic stenosis and Meckel diverticulum
- Lesions of angiodysplasia are **ectatic nests of tortuous veins, venules,** and **capillaries.**
- The vascular channels may be separated from the intestinal lumen by only the vascular wall and a layer of attenuated epithelial cells
- Even limited injury may therefore result in significant hemorrhage.

12. Most common posterior mediastinal tumor is:

A. Neurofibroma B. Thymoma
C. Germ cell Tumors D. Aortic aneursym

Ans: A. Neruofibroma

Ref: *Robbins Pathologic basis of Disease, 8th ed.*

Explanation:

Mediastinal Tumors

Anterior (front) mediastinum

- ***Germ cell Tumors*** - The majority of germ cell neoplasms (60 to 70%) are benign and are found in both males and females.
- ***Lymphoma*** – Malignant tumors that include both Hodgkin's disease and non Hodgkin's lymphoma.
- ***Thymoma and thymic cyst*** - The most common cause of a thymic mass, the majority of thymomas are benign lesions that are contained within a fibrous capsule. However, about 30% of these may be more aggressive and become invasive through the fibrous capsule.
- ***Mediastinal Thyroid mass*** – Usually a benign growth, such as a goiter, these can occasionally be cancerous.

Middle mediastinum

- ***Bronchogenic cyst*** – A benign growth with respiratory origins.
- ***Mediastinal Lymphadenopathy*** – An enlargement of the lymph nodes.
- ***Pericardial cyst*** – A benign growth that results from an "out-pouching" of the pericardium (the heart's lining).
- ***Mediastinal Thyroid mass*** – Usually a benign growth, such as a goiter. These types of tumors can occasionally be cancerous.
- ***Tracheal tumors*** – These include tracheal neoplasms and non-euplastic masses, such as tracheobronchopathia osteochondroplastica (benign tumors).
- ***Vascular abnormalities*** including aortic aneurysm and aortic dissection.

Posterior (back) mediastinum

- ***Extramedullary haematopoiesis*** – A rare cause of masses that form from bone marrow expansion and are associated with severe anemia.
- ***Mediastinal Lymphadenopathy***– An enlargement of the lymph nodes.
- ***Mediastinal Neuroenteric cyst***– A rare growth, which involves both neural and gastrointestinal elements.
- ***Mediastinal Neurogenic neoplasm***– The **most common** cause of posterior mediastinal tumors, these are classified as nerve sheath neoplasms, ganglion cell neoplasms, and paraganglionic cell neoplasms. Approximately 70% of neurogenic neoplasms are benign.
- ***Oesophageal abnormalities*** including achalasia oesophageal, oesophageal neoplasm and hiatal hernia.
- ***Paravertebral abnormalities*** including infectious, malignant and traumatic abnormalities of the thoracic spine.
- ***Mediastinal Thyroid mass***– Usually a benign growth, such as a goiter, which can occasionally be cancerous. Vascular abnormalities – Includes aortic aneurysms.

13. **False regarding thyroglossal fistula:**
A. Congenital
B. Midline location
C. Moves with tongue protrusion
D. Rx is Sistrunk operation

Ans: A. Congenital

Ref: *Bailey & Love's Short Practice of Surgery, 25th Edition 729 A Textbook on Surgical Short cases-S,Das. 2nd edition 142*

Explanation:

Embryology of thyroglossal cyst

- The thyroid gland **descends** early in **fetal life** from the base of the tongue towards its position in the lower neck with the isthmus lying over the second and third tracheal rings.
- At the time of its descent, the **hyoid bone** has **not been formed** and the track of the descent of the thyroid gland is variable, passing in front, through or behind the eventual position of the hyoid bone
- **Thyroglossal duct cysts** represent a **persistence of this track** and may therefore be found any where in or adjacent to the midline from the tongue base to the thyroid isthmus.
- Rarely, a **thyroglossal cyst** may contain the **only functioning thyroid tissue** in the body

Thyroglossal Fistula

Aetiology

Thyroglossal fistula is **never congenital**. It is usually due to

1. Bursting of infected thyroglossal cyst
2. Incision of infected thyroglossal cyst due to misdiagnosis as abscess
3. Incomplete excision of thyroglossal cyst

Clinical Features

- 15-40 years of age
- History of mucus discharge with recurrent episodes of inflammation
- History of thyroglossal cyst which was excised incompletely/incised
- Usually in the midline - suprahyoid, subhyoid or in front of thyroid cartilage
- Fistulous opening is covered with hood of skin and gets pulled up on protrusion of tongue – *Characteristic feature*

Treatment

Sistrunk's operation

- Excision of the whole thyroglossal tract,which involves removal of the body of the hyoid bone and the suprahyoid tract through the tongue base to the vallecula at the site of the primitive foramen caecum, together with a core of tissue on either side.

ORTHOPEDICS

1. **A footballer complains of sudden giving away of knee off late which could be due to:**
A. Medial collateral ligament tear
B. Anterior cruciate ligament tear
C. Medial meniscal tear
D. Posterior cruciate ligament tear.

Ans: B. Anterior cruciate ligament tear

Ref: *System of Orthopaedics and Fractures, 9th edition, pg. 875-881http://orthopedics.about.com/od aclinjury/psymptoms.htm*

Explanation:

- Giving way is a feature of instability.
- An **ACL tear** most often occurs during **sports** or **athletic** events.
- About **80% of ACL tears** occur **without contact** with another athlete.
- The most typical story is an athlete suddenly **changing direction** (**cutting or pivoting**) and feeling their **knee give out** from under their body.
- Patient who suffer an ACL tear usually report hearing a "**pop**" at the time of the injury. Even if the pop is not heard, usually patients will feel the **sudden shift** in the joint.
- The **ACL** is **critical** to the **stability of the knee joint**, and when an ACL tear occurs, the joint is usually **unstable**.
- **Locking** is **not a feature** of **instability** and always **suggests a meniscal tear.**
- In the **less common posterior cruciate insufficiency**, symptoms are **mild** unless the **arcuate ligament complex** also is **torn** or **stretched**; instability is sometimes felt only on climbing stairs.
- A **solitary MCL injury**, if sufficiently **severe**, can be shown to cause the knee joint to **'open' on the medial side** when the joint is flexed to **30 degrees** a valgus stress is applied, but if this is still detectable when the knee is extended, then it is likely the expansions of the semi-membranosus tendon, capsule and ACL are also damaged. At **30 degrees of flexion**, the **MCL** is the **primary stabilizer.**

2. **A 30 yrs. man with radio dense mass around elbow, with a clear zone between the mass and humerus. What is the probable diagnosis?**

A. Paraosteal osteosarcoma
B. Periosteal osteosarcoma
C. Myositis ossificans
D. Tumour calcinosis.

Ans: **A.** Paraosteal osteosarcoma

***Ref**: Apleys System of Orthopaedics and Fractures, 9th edition, pg. 210, 720-1.http://www.orthobullets.com pathology/8077/tumoral-calcinosis*

Explanation:

PAROSTEAL OSTEOSARCOMA

- It is a low-grade sarcoma situated on the **surface of one of the tubular** bones, usually at the distal **femoral** or **proximal tibial metaphysis** or **proximal humeral metaphysis.**
- The patient is a young adult who presents with a **slowly enlarging mass** near the bone end.
- X-ray shows a **dense bony mass** on the **surface of the bone** or **encircling** it; the cortex is not eroded and usually a thin gap remains between cortex and tumour.
- CT and MRI will show the boundary between tumour and surrounding soft tissues.
- Although the lesion is outside the bone, it **does not spread** into the adjacent muscle compartment until fairly late.
- Staging, therefore, often defines it as a **low grade intracompartmental tumour** (stage IA).
- The described clinical fits this best.

PERIOSTEAL OSTEOSARCOMA

- It is a rare tumour is quite distinct from parosteal osteosarcoma.
- It is more like an **intramedullary osteosarcoma**, but situated on the **surface of the bone.**
- It occurs in **young adults** and causes **local pain** and **swelling.**
- X-ray shows a **superficial defect of the cortex,** but CT and MRI may reveal a larger soft-tissue mass. The appearances sometimes suggest a **periosteal chondroma** and the diagnosis may not be certain until a **biopsy** is performed.
- Histologically this is a **true osteosarcoma,** but characteristically the sections show a **prominent cartilaginous element.**

Myositis Ossificans

- **Heterotopic ossification** in the muscles sometimes occurs after an **injury, articularly dislocation** of the elbow or a **blow to the brachialis, deltoid** or **quadriceps.**
- It is thought to be due to **muscle damage,** but it also occurs without a **local injury** in **unconscious or paraplegic** patients.
- It also occurs in **hip injuries,** after **hip surgeries (THR)** and **burns** patients.
- There may be a history of **native massage treatment** with **passive manipulation.**
- Soon after the injury, the patient (usually a fit young man) complains of **pain**; there is **local swelling** and **soft-tissue tenderness.**
- **X-ray is normal** but a **bone scan** may **show increased activity.**
- Over the next 2–3 weeks the pain gradually subsides, but **joint movement is limited;** X-ray may show **fluffy calcification in the soft tissues.**
- By 8 weeks the **bony mass** is **easily palpable** and is clearly defined in the X-ray.
- Above scenario is not falling into this choice.

Tumoral calcinosis

- It is a rare and poorly understood entity characterized by **calcium salt deposits** in the **extra-capsular soft tissues.**
- More common in **females** and **African-Americans.**
- Onset is usually in **childhood** or **early adolescence.**
- Typically occurs around **joints,** primarily the **hip shoulder** and **elbows.**
- Pathophysiology – is **unknown.**
- There is evidence suggesting an inborn abnormality of **phosphorus metabolism.**
- Associated conditions - **calcinosis of renal failure,** radiographically similar appearance to **tumoral calcinosis,** but not as strongly associated with hip and shoulder distribution.
- Renal aetiology differentiates it from tumoral calcinosis.
- Associated with **hyperphosphatemia, chronic renal failure,** and **long term dialysis**
- Symptoms - **mass or swelling typically** around **joints, pain** secondary to compression of normal, surrounding structures, palpable mass around joint

Imaging

- **Radiographs - circular or oval, well-demarcated masses** of **calcium** around joints, direct involvement of the bones or joints is rare.
- CT may demonstrate **fluid-fluid levels** within some of these masses
- MRI may demonstrate **fluid-fluid levels** within some of these masses.
- Bone scan may reveal **intense uptake in the calcific masses.**

3. Spondylolysis means:

A. Defect of pars interarticularis
B. Degenerative changes of the spine
C. Arthritic changes in facetal joints
D. Fracture of vertebral body.

Ans: A. Defect of pars interarticularis

***Ref:** Apley's Orthopedics, 9th ed.*

Explanation:

Spondylolysis

- It is a defect of a vertebra.
- More specifically it is defined as **a defect in the pars interarticularis of the vertebral arch.**

'Spondylolisthesis'

- It means **forward translation of one segment** of the **spine** upon another.
- The shift is nearly always between **L4 and L5,** or **between L5 and the sacrum.**

Basically there are **six types** of spondylolisthesis:

A. Dysplastic (20 per cent)
- The superior sacral facets are congenitally defective; slow but inexorable forward slip leads to severe displacement.
- Associated anomalies (usually **spina bifida occulta**) are common.

B. Lytic or isthmic (50 per cent) in this,
- The most common variety
- There are **defects** in the **pars interarticularis (spondylolysis),** or repeated breaking and healing may lead to elongation of the pars.
- The defect is usually present by the age of 7, but the slip may appear only some years later.
- An acquired factor probably supervenes to produce what is essentially an ununited stress fracture.
- The condition is more common than usual in those whose spines are subjected to extraordinary stresses (e.g. competitive gymnasts and weight-lifters).

C. Degenerative (25 per cent)
- Degenerative changes in the facet joints and the discs permit forward slip (nearly always at L4/5 and mainly in women of middle age) despite intact laminae.
- Many of these patients have generalized osteoarthritis and pyrophosphate crystal arthropathy.

D. Post-traumatic
- Unusual fractures may result in destabilization of the lumbar spine.

E. Pathological
- Bone destruction (e.g. due to tuberculosis or neoplasm) may lead to vertebral slipping.

F. Postoperative (iatropathic)
- Excessive operative removal of bone in decompression operations results in progressive spondylolisthesis.

4. Rigid flat foot is not seen in:

A. Athlete's foot
B. Rheumatoid arthritis
C. Peroneal spasm
D. Congenital tarsal coalition.

Ans: A. Athlete's foot

***Ref:** Apley's System of Orthopaedics and Fractures 9th edition – p596 -599 Rapini, Ronald P.; Bolognia, Jean L.; Jorizzo, Joseph L. (2007). Dermatology: 2-Volume Set. St. Louis: Mosby. p. 1135.*

Explanation:

Rigid flatfoot

- It is characterized by the restriction of subtalar joint motion.
- The arch remains flat when the foot is dangling in the air, while the individual is seated, as well as during toe-standing and the toe-raising test.
- This type of flatfoot can occasionally cause pain and disability.

Causes of rigid flatfoot in children

a. Congenital vertical talus
b. Congenital tarsal coalition
c. Peroneal spastic flatfoot without coalition
d. Iatrogenic or post-traumatic flatfoot
e. Skewfoot
f. Neuro-muscular abnormalities – spastic CP, muscular dystrophies
g. Genetic syndromes
h. Collagen disorders

Causes of rigid flatfoot in adults

a. Posterior tibial tendon dysfunction
b. Arthritis – rheumatoid arthritis causing peroneal spasm, tarsal tuberculosis
c. Traumatic – midfoot tarsal fracture dislocations
d. Neuropathic or charcot foot
e. Muscle imbalance due to neurological disorders.
f. Among elderly who are sedentary and obese

Athlete's foot

- Also known as ringworm of the footand tinea pedis
- It is a fungal infection of the skin that causes scaling, flaking, and itch of affected areas, and in severe cases, swelling and amputation of the foot.
- It is caused by fungi in the genus Trichophyton.

- The disease is typically transmitted in moist communal areas where people walk barefoot, such as showers or bathhouses, and requires a warm moist environment, such as the inside of a shoe, in order to incubate.

5. **What is the diagnostic radiological finding in skeletal fluorosis?**
   A. Interroseous membrane ossification
   B. Sub-periosteal cortical resorption of the middle phalanges
   C. Osteosclerosis of vertebral body
   D. Ossification of ligaments of knee joint

   Ans: B. Sub-periosteal cortical resorption of the middle phalanges

   Ref: *http://radiopaedia.org/articles/fluorosis & Apley's System of Orthopaedics and Fractures, 9th edition, p141.*

   Explanation:

   - **Radiological features seen in Skeletal Fluorosis**

   a. Increased bone density – **osteosclerosis**
   b. Osteopaenia/osteoporosis
   c. Trabecular blurring or haziness
   e. Compact bone thickening
   e. Periosteal bone formation
   f. **Ossification** of the attachments of **tendons, ligaments, and muscles**
   g. **Interosseous membrane calcification** - peculiar to this condition but a late finding
   h. Ossification of the **posterior longitudinal ligament**

   - Involvement of the **axial skeleton** is **characteristic**, and changes are most marked in the spine, pelvis and ribs.
   - In early fluorosis, the first changes are bone **deposition and thickening** at the junctions of **trabeculae**. This is seen as **sandlike, granular, or particle like bone structure** on **radiographs.**
   - In more advanced fluorosis, the trabeculae are more generally **thickened** because of **new bone formation on the trabecular surface**. At this stage, radiographs show thickening and condensation of trabeculae, with **coarse reticulum or woven bone striations.**
   - If the trabeculae are fused, focal round densities are seen in the medullary bone.
   - **Osteopenia** (less common) also may occur in fluorosis - especially in **younger patients** at an earlier stage.
   - **Sub-periosteal cortical resorption** of the **middle phalanges** is the **classical** and almost **pathognomic feature** which should always be sought in **primary hyperparathyroidism**.
   - Other features being **osteoporosis** (sometimes including vertebral collapse) and areas of **cortical erosion**, non-specific features such as **renal calculi, nephrocalcinosis** and **chondrocalcinosis.**

6. **Which of the following childhood disorders is a common differential diagnosis of osteomyelitis?**
   A. Chondrosarcoma **B.** Ewing's sarcoma
   C. Osteosarcoma **D.** Synoviosarcoma

   Ans: B. Ewing's sarcoma

   Ref: *Apley's System of Orthopaedics and Fractures, 9th edition, p 212-213*

   Explanation:

   Ewing's sarcoma

   - It is believed to arise from **endothelial cells** in the **bone marrow.**
   - It occurs most commonly between the ages **of 10 and 20 years.**
   - It is located in the **diaphysis** of **long tubular bones - tibia, fibula** or **clavicle.**
   - The patient presents with **pain** – often throbbing in character – and **swelling.**
   - Generalized illness and **pyrexia**, together with a **warm, tender swelling** and a **raised ESR, may suggest a diagnosis of osteomyelitis.**
   - X-rays usually show an area of **bone destruction** which, unlike that in osteosarcoma, is predominantly in the mid-diaphysis.
   - **New bone formation** may extend along the shaft and sometimes it appears as fusiform layers of bone around the lesion – the socalled **'onion-peel'** effect.
   - Often the tumour extends into the surrounding soft tissues, with radiating streaks of ossification and reactive periosteal bone at the proximal and distal margins. These features (the **'sunray' appearance and Codman's triangles**) are usually associated with osteosarcoma, but they are just as common in Ewing's sarcoma.
   - CT and MRI reveal the **large extraosseous component.**
   - **Radioisotope** scans may show multiple areas of activity in the skeleton.
   - **The condition which should be excluded as rapidly as possible is bone infection.**
   - On biopsy the essential step is to recognize this as a malignant round-cell tumour, distinct from osteosarcoma.
   - Other round-cell tumours that may resemble Ewing's are **reticulum-cell sarcoma** and **metastatic neuroblastoma.**

7. **After closed reduction of supracondylar fracture of humerus, flexion greater than 90 degree causes disappearance of radial pulse. The next line of management is:**

A. Conservative
B. Exploration for arterial rupture
C. Reduce the flexion till the pulse is restored and immobilise in that position
D. Open reduction & internal fixation

Ans: C. Reduce the flexion till the pulse is restored and immobilise in that position

Ref: *Watson-Jones Fractures and joint Injuries, 7th edition, pg. 524-526*

Explanation:

- **Closed reduction** of the **posterior displacement** of the supracondylar fracture of the humerus is **stable** only with the **elbow flexed to about 30 degrees** above the **right angle** (the hand coming to lie on the opposite shoulder.
- The **forearm is placed in pronation** to release the **tension** of the **flexor-pronator muscle group**.
- Vascular obstruction can occur from positioning a swollen elbow into gross flexion.
- If the reduction is lost on check X-Ray then it is wiser to treat the fracture in either **skeletal or skin traction (Dunlop Traction).**

8. **Osteochondroma is a disease of:**

A. Metaphysis **B.** Diaphysis
C. Epiphysis **D.** Periosteum

Ans: A. Metaphysis

Ref: *Apley's System of Orthopaedics and Fractures, 9th edition, pg. 199-200*

Explanation:

Osteochondroma

- It is one of the commonest 'tumours' of bone.
- It is a **developmental lesion** which starts as a **small overgrowth** of **cartilage** at the edge of the **physeal plate** and develops by **endochondral ossification** into a bony protuberance still covered by the cap of cartilage.
- **Most common** sites are the **fast-growing ends of long bones** and the **crest of the ilium**.
- In long bones, growth leaves the **bump** stranded further down the **metaphysis.**
- At the **end of the normal growth period** for that bone it **stops enlarging.**
- Any further enlargement after the end of the growth period is suggestive of **malignant transformation.**
- X-ray appearance is **pathognomonic.**
- There is a **well-defined exostosis** emerging from the **metaphysis**, its base co-extensive with the parent bone.
- It looks smaller than it feels because the **cartilage cap** is usually **invisible on X-ray**; however, large lesions undergo cartilage degeneration and calcification and then the X-ray shows the bony exostosis surrounded by clouds of calcified material.
- **Multiple lesions** may develop as part of a heritable disorder – **hereditary multiple exostoses** – in which there are also features of abnormal bone growth resulting in characteristic deformities.
- The incidence of malignant transformation is difficult to assess because troublesome lesions are so often removed before they show histological features of malignancy.
- Figures usually quoted are **1 per cent** for **solitary lesions** and **6 per cent for multiple.**
- **Features suggestive of malignant change are:**
  (1) ***Enlargement*** of the cartilage cap in successive examinations.
  (2) A ***bulky cartilage cap*** (more than 1 cm in thickness).
  (3) Irregularly scattered flecks of ***calcification*** within the cartilage cap.
  (4) Spread into the surrounding soft tissues.
- MRI may be needed to reveal these changes.

9. **Open reduction & internal fixation does all *except:***

A. Consolidation **B.** Stability
C. Better function **D.** Better alignment

Ans: A. Consolidation

Ref: *Apley's System of Orthopaedics and Fractures, 9th edition, Pg. 692, 701.*

Explanation:

- **Consolidation** is a **stage in fracture healing** which is **different from union** in that union is incomplete repair; the ensheathing callus is calcified.
- Clinically the fracture site is still a little tender and, though the bone moves in one piece (and in that sense is united), attempted angulation is painful.
- X-Rays show the **fracture line** still **clearly visible**, with fluffy callus around it.
- Repair is incomplete and it is not safe to subject the unprotected bone to stress.

- But **consolidation is complete repair**; the **calcified callus is ossified**.
- Clinically the fracture **site is not tender**, no movement can be obtained and attempted angulation is painless.
- X-rays show the **fracture line to be almost obliterated** and crossed by bone trabeculae, with well-defined callus around it.
- **Repair is complete** and **further protection is unnecessary**.
- **Stability**, **better function** and **alignment** are advantages conferred by the technique of **open reduction and internal fixation** in fractures that cannot be treated by close reduction (fracture neck of femur), are unstable and liable to cause functional derangement if treated by closed methods.

10. **Most sensitive test to detect anterior cruciate ligament injury in the setting of acute knee injury is:**

A. Lachman's test
B. Pivot shift test
C. Anterior drawer test
D. Apley's grinding test

Ans: A. Lachman's test

Ref: *"Lachman Test". Wheeless' Textbook of Orthopaedics. 8th ed.*

Explantion:

Lachman's test

- This is a variant of the anterior drawer test, in which the examination is carried out with the knee in 15 deg of flexion, and external rotation (relaxes IT band).
- This is more sensitive and useful in an acute situation.
- The Anterior drawer test is usually not possible in an acute injury due to pain.
- The **pivot-shift test, anterior drawer test and the Lachman test** are used during the clinical examination of suspected **anterior cruciate ligament** (ACL) injury.
- The ACL can also be visualized using a magnetic resonance imaging scan (MRI scan).
- An ACL tear can present with a popping sound heard after impact, swelling after a couple of hours, severe pain when bending the knee, and buckling or locking of the knee during movement.

11. **Fracture subluxation of the volar or dorsal rim of the distal radius is termed as:**

A. Galeazzi # **B.** Barton's #
C. Smith # **D.** Chauffeur's #

Ans: B. Barton's #

Ref: *Wheeless' Textbook of Orthopaedics, 8th ed.*

Explantion:

- Fracture dislocation or subluxation in which the rim of distal radius, dorsally or ventrally is displaced with the hand and carpus is called as **Barton's Fracture.**
- **Smith fracture** - Extra-articular palmar displaced distal radius fracture. (volar angulation of fracture is referred to as "Garden Spade" deformity (reversed Colles Fracture).
- **Galeazzi fracture** – fracture of radial shaft at the junction of middle and distal third associated with dislocation of distal radio ulnar joint.
- **Chauffeur's fracture** is a type of fracture of the forearm, specifically the radial styloid process. The injury is typically caused by compression of the scaphoid bone of the hand against the styloid process of the distal radius.

12. **Most common cause of punched out lesions in phalanges is:**

A. Enchondroma **B.** Chondrosarcoma
C. Anerysmal bone cyst **D.** Multiple myeloma

Ans: A. Enchondroma

Ref: *www.radiologyassistant.nl*

Explantion:

- **Enchondroma** is a benign cartilage tumor.
- Frequently it is a coincidental finding.In the phalanges of the hand it frequently presents with a fracture.
- It is the most common lesion in the phalanges, i.e. a well-defined lytic lesion in the hand is almost always an enchondroma.

Features that favor the diagnosis of a low-grade chondrosarcoma:

a. Higher age
b. Size > 5 cm
c. Activity on bone scan
d. Fast enhancement on dynamic contrast enhanced MR series
e. Endosteal scalloping of the cortical bone

13. **Most common site of clavicle fracture is:**

A. Junction of middle and outer 1/3
B. Middle 1/3
C. Medial 1/3
D. Lateral 1/3

Ans: A. Junction of middle and outer 1/3

Ref: *Practical fracture treatment by Ronald McRae 4th edition, p 116.*

Explanation:

Site of Clavicular #

- Clavicular fractures are commonest at the junction of the **middle** and **outer 1/3**
- It is also common throughout the **middle 1/3** and to a lesser extent, the outer 1/3 where the incidence is 18%.
- Fractures at the **medial 1/3** or **medial end** are **uncommon.**

OBS AND GYNE

1. **All are symptoms of molar pregnancy *except:***
   A. Amenorrhea
   B. Symptoms of Hypothyroidism
   C. Abnormal vaginal bleeding
   D. Expulsion of grape like vesicles

   Ans: B. Symptoms of Hypothyroidism

   Ref: *Shaw's textbook, of gynaecology 15th ed. Pg 253*

   Explanation: *(See the following table)*

   CLASSIC CLINICAL FEATURES OF COMPLETE MOLE

   - Amenorrhoea of 8- 12 weeks
   - Abnormal vaginal bleeding
   - Lower abdominal pain
   - **Hyperemesis gravidarum**
   - **Features of early onset preeclampsia** (< 20 weeks)
   - Uterine Ht > POG
   - Absence of fetal parts and fhr
   - Expulsion of grape like vesicles
   - Theca lutein cyst of ovaries
   - **Symptoms of Hyperthyroidism (High HCG can mimic TSH)**
   - Serum HCG > 100000 miu/ml
   - **USG : Snow storm appearance**

2. **Engaging diameter in fully extended head:**
   A. Submento bregmatic
   B. Suboccipito bregmatic
   C. Mento vertical
   D. Suboccipito frontal

   Ans: A. Submento bregmatic

   Ref: *DC Dutta's Textbook of Obstetrics, 7th edn p 85*

   Explanation

Presentation	Engaging diameter
Complete flexion vertex	Suboccipito bregmatic
Deflexed head	Suboccipito frontal / occipito frontal
Face	Submento bregmatic
Brow	Mento vertical

3. **Choice of contraception in recently delivered lactating mother: (Repeat)**
   A. Safe period **B.** OCP
   C. IUCD **D.** Depot provera

   Ans: D. Depot provera

   Ref: *Williams Obstetrics 23rd edition pg.652 table 30-4*

   Explanation:

   In the above options, appropriate choice would be depot provera.

   CONTRACEPTIVE PRESCRIPTION

   - **Conventional contraceptives can be safely prescribed during the entire reproductive period.**
   - Advice on the usage of pill or IUCD during different phases of reproductive life

   1. **Post partum**
   - ***Contraception for lactating women***
     - **Progestin only pill** to be started at **2-3 weeks postpartum (best choice)**
     - Depot **medroxyprogesterone acetate** initiated at **6 weeks postpartum**
     - **Hormonal implants** inserted at **6 weeks postpartum**
     - **Levonorgestrel IUCD** inserted at **6 weeks postpartum**
     - **POP** contains LNG 75 microgm taken from day of cycle at same time every day-failure rate 0.5-2 per HMY
     - **Depot provera** dose 150mg every 3 months within 5th day of cycle, administered i.m - failure rate 0-0.3per HWY

	PARTIAL MOLE	COMPLETE MOLE
Fetus, Fetal vessels, Placenta	Present	Absent
Karyotype	69 XXY (triploid)	46 XX
Hydropic changes	Focal	Marked
Malignant potential	Rare	15-20%
USG:	Focal cystic spaces in placenta Fetus and placenta are seen Transverse diameter of uterus increases	Snowstorm appearance

- **NORPLANT** contains 75 microgm LNG, releases 50microgm/day for 3 yrs- failure rate 0.1 per HWY
- **LNG-IUD** contains 58 mg LNG releases 20 microgm/day

- *Non lactating*
  - Contraception started as early as **3 weeks** following delivery
  - **OCPs /IUCD/ DMPA** inj./ **Implanon**

2. **Adolescent girls**
   - LD OCPs – most effective
   - Alternatives – DMPA, Norplant
3. **Newly married**
   - OCPs – most effective
4. **Post abortal**
   - Started immediately following abortion
   - OCPs / IUCD
5. **Women at risk of STDs**
   - Need dual protection against pregnancy and STDs
   - Condom with spermicides/ condom with any other contraceptive method
6. **Women using enzyme inducers**
   - **High dose** OCPs, if prescribed/ IUCD/ DMPA inj.

4. Deep transverse arrest occurs in which type of pelvis? (Repeat)

A. Platypelloid **B.** Gynecoid
C. Android **D.** Anthropoid

Ans: C. Android pelvis

Ref: Williams obstetrics 23rd ed pg.480, Dutta textbook of obstetrics 5th ed pg 346

Explanation:

DEEP TRANSVERSE ARREST

- Arrest in occipito transverse position may be due to **incomplete anterior rotation of oblique occipito posterior position**
- **Causes:**
  - Pelvic architecture abnormality
  - Android pelvis
  - Deflexion of head
  - Weak uterine contractions
  - Laxity of pelvic floor
- **Management:**
  1. Caesarean section if big baby or inadequate pelvis
  2. If pelvis adequate, ventouse delivery, manual rotation and forceps application, forceps rotation and delivery
  - **Kielland forceps** for **rotation**
  - **Simpson and Mclane forceps** for **head delivery**

5. Clue cells are seen in: (Repeat)

A. Gardenella vaginitis
B. Trichomoniasis
C. Moniliasis
D. Pelvic inflammatory diseases

Ans: A. Gardenella vaginits

Ref: Dutta gynae pg156

Explanation:

GARDNERELLA VAGINOSIS

- Alteration in normal vaginal flora
- **Decrease in number of lactobacilli in vaginal discharge** - lactobacilli reduce pH and release hydrogen peroxide toxic to other bacteria
- 100 fold increase in anerobic bacteria
- **Hemophilus vaginalis, Gardnerella, Mobiluncus and Mycoplasma hominis**—cause
- Vaginal discharge without discharge
- White , milky non-viscous discharge, **pH** of discharge more than **4.5**
- **Whiff Test - Fishy odour** when vaginal discharge is mixed with 10% KOH - due to release of amino metabolites from various organisms
- Presence of **Clue Cells** - epithelial cells with granular cytoplasm caused by gram negative bacilli adhering on the surface
- Wet smear, gram stain and culture are investigations
- Treatment—
  - Metronidazole 500mg bd for 7 days
  - Ampicillin 500mg or cephalosporin 500mg bd for 7 days
  - Tetracycline 500mg 4 times a day
  - Doxycycline 100mg bd
  - Sulphafurazole 1g 4 times daily for 10-14 days
  - Clindamycin 300mg daily for 7 days
  - Clindamycin 2%cream locally
  - Ornidazole 500mg vaginal tablet for 7 days
  - **Lacteal** is protein free acidifying lactate gel neutralises vaginal ph 5ml applied for 7 days

AMSEL CRITERIA for diagnosing Bacterial Vagninosis

- Thin, white, yellow, homogeneous discharge
- Clue cells on microscopy
- pH of vaginal fluid >4.5
- Release of a fishy odor on adding alkali—10% potassium hydroxide (KOH) solution.
- **At least three of the four criteria** should be present for a confirmed diagnosis.

6. IUD of choice in menorrhagia: (Repeat)

A. Lippe loop
B. Cu-T 375
C. Cu-T 200
D. Levonorgestrel IUCD

Ans: D. Levonorgestrel IUCD

Ref: *Shaw's Textbook of Gynaecology 15th Edition Pg: 230*

Explanation:

- Levonorgestrel IUCD is progesterone impregnated IUCD and is recommended to control bleeding in menorrhagia.

Other non contraceptive benefits of LNG IUCD:

- DUB
- Endometrial hyperplasia

Intrauterine contraceptive devices (IUCD)

Biologically inert devices : Lippe's loop

Copper containing devices : Copper T

Hormonal IUCDS : Progestasert, Levonova, MIRENA

Hormonal IUCDs

Progestasert

- ***38mg*** of **Progesterone**
- Releases 65micrograms/day
- Effective for **1 year**
- 40% reduction in Menorrhagia
- 40% reduction in Dysmenorrhea

Levonova

- ***60 mg*** of **Levonorgestrel**
- Releases 20 micrograms/day
- Increased chances of **ectopic pregnancy**
- Safe during lactation
- Effective for **5 years**

MIRENA

- ***52 mg*** of **levonorgestrel**
- Releases 25 micrograms/day
- Does not suppress ovulation
- Acts on endometrium and cervical mucus
- Used in DUB, Endometrial hyperplasia, HRT
- Effective for **5 years**

7. **Most common site for fibroids in uterus is:**

A. Subserous **B.** Intramural
C. Subserous **D.** Cervical

Ans: B. Intramural

Ref: *Shaw's Textbook of Gynaecology 15th Edition Pg 352.*

Explanation:

Uterine Fibroids

- Fibroids are the **most common** benign solid tumours in **females**
- Most common tumour of uterus.
- Fibroids are **estrogen dependent** for growth
- **Progesterone inhibits** their **growth.**
- **GnRH shrinks size** of **fibroid**
- **Increases in size** during **pregnancy** and **OCP intake**
- **Decreases** in size after **menopause**
- The presence of **myoma** causes **hyperplasia** of the **myometrial wall.**
- The cavity of the uterus is often distorted and enlarged.
- The **endometrium** tends to be **thicker** due to **endometrial hyperplasia.**
- The ovaries at times are **enlarged**, cystic and hyperaemic with evidence of **salpingo-oophoritis** in about **15%** cases.
- Distribution of fibroid in the body of uterus:
  a. **Intramural** **75%**
  b. **Submucus** **15%**
  c. **Subserous** **10%**
- Most **common site** is **body of uterus**
- A typical myoma is a well-circumscribed tumour with a **pseudocapsule**
- The vessels which supply blood to the tumour lie in the capsule and send radial branches into the tumour. Because of this arrangement of blood supply, the **central portion of the tumour** receives the **least blood supply**, and **degeneration** is noticeable early and most often in this part of the tumour. On the other hand, **calcification begins at the periphery** and spreads inwards along the vessels.
- Microscopically, the tumour consists of **bundles of plain muscle cells,** separated by varying amount of fibrous strands. Areas of embryonic muscle tissue may be present in a myoma.
- The endometrium tends to be thicker due to **endometrial hyperplasia.** The ovaries at times are enlarged, cystic and hyperaemic with evidence of **salpingo-oophoritis in about 15%** cases.

Points to be Remembered in Fibroid

- Most common complication of fibroid during **pregnancy– Red degeneration**
- Incidence of **sarcomatous** change in fibroid – **0.5%**
- Most common presenting symptom is **menorrhagia**
- **Metrorrhagia** is caused by – **sub mucus fibroid**
- Most common **degeneration** – **Hyaline** degeneration.
- Recurrent pregnancy loss is associated with **submucous fibroid**
- **Polycythemia** in **myoma** is due to **extramedullary erythropoisis** within the substance of **myoma**

- **Danazole, GnRH** and **RU 486 reduces** the size **of fibroids**

8. **All are True regarding adenomyosis *except:***
   A. Occurs in parous woman around 40 yrs
   B. Menorrhagia
   C. Uterus symmetrically enlarged
   D. Uterus not tender on palpation

   Ans: D. Uterus not tender on palpation

   Ref: *474 Shaw's Textbook of Gynaecology 15th Edition.*

Explanation:

Adenomyosis
- Common in women aged 40 yrs & above.
- Often co-exists with **fibroid, endometriosis** and **endometrial cancer.**
- Uterus is **symmetrically enlarged** to **not more than 14 wk size.**
- Histology – Islands of **endometrial glands** surrounded by stroma seen in the **myometrial** tissue beyond the **endomyometrial junction.**
- The distance b/w basal endometrium and the endometrial gland should be > 2.5 mm.
- Common complaint-**Menorrhagia** & **Progressive dysmenorrhoea.**
- Clinical examination reveals symmetrical enlargement of uterus & tender uterus.
- Treatment is localized excision, hysterectomy.
- Medical treatment includes **danazol, GnRH, Mirena IUCD.**

9. **Which is the most common complication during vaginal delivery in diabetic women?**
   A. Uterine inertia
   B. Shoulder dystocia
   C. Obstructed labour
   D. Post partum haemorrhage

   Ans: B. Shoulder dystocia

   Ref: *Current diagnosis & treatment – Obstetrics and Gynaecology 10th edition pg 316.*

Explanation:
- **Shoulder dystocia** is the **most common** complication encountered in diabetic women during vaginal delivery, especially when the baby is **macrosomic.**
- Uterine **inertia** and **PPH** can occur if **hydramnios** is present.

Maternal complications of DM
- Abortion
- Preterm labour
- Pre eclampsia
- Polyhydramnios

Fetal complications of DM
- Hydramnios
- Big baby
- Shoulder dystocia
- Fetal macrosomia
- Sacral agenesis
- Anencephaly and microcephaly
- VSD

Neonatal complications
- Hypoglycemia
- ARDS
- Hyperbilirubinemia
- Polycythemia
- Hypocalcemia

10. **Polyhydramnios is seen in all *except:***
    A. Diabetes mellitus
    B. Anencephaly
    C. Trachea- esophageal fistula
    D. Renal agenesis

    Ans: D. Renal agenesis

    Ref: *Ian Donald; Practical Obstetric Problems 6th ed. Pg 366, D.C.Dutta's Textbook of Obstetrics, 7th ed. pg. 211,215.*

Explanation:
- The main source for amniotic fluid is **fetal urine.**
- So, when there are no kidneys, there is no urine.
- So, it results in oligohydramnios.
- Hence, D (Renal agenesis) is the answer.

Causes for Hydramnios

Fetal malformations

CNS defects -
- Anencephaly
- Spina bifida
- Hydrocephalus

Cardiac defects
- VSD
- ASD
- Pulmonary stenosis

Craniofacial
- Cleft lip
- Cleft palate
- Choanal atresia

Thorax
- Diaphragmatic hernia

Gastrointestinal
- Oesophageal atresia
- Tracheo-esophageal fistula

Maternal causes
- Diabetes
- Multiple pregnancy.

11. **Sher's classification is done in cases of:**
 A. Uterine prolapse B. Puerperal sepsis
 C. Abruption D. Placenta praevia

 Ans: C. Abruption

Ref: Practical guide to high risk pregnancy & Delivery: Fernando Arias 3rd ed. Pg 344.

Explanation:

Sher's Classification is for Abruptio Placenta

Grade I	• Mild Retro-Placental Clot of Vol. < 150 ml
Grade II	• Classical features of abruption are present. • Fetus is alive. • Most of them have abnormal FHR pattern. • Perinatal mortality is high. • Retro-Placental Clot - 150-500 ml
Grade III	• Features of Gr II with fetal demise • A - Presence of coagulopathy • B - Absence of coagulopathy

12. **Shortest fetal skull diameter is**
 A. Bimastoid B. Submentovertical
 C. Submentobregmatic D. Occipito-frontal

 Ans: A. Bimastoid

Ref: Dutta textbook of obstetrics 5th ed pg85

Explanation: *(See the following figure and table)*

13. **Modified biophysical profile includes:**
 A. Fetal tone and breathing

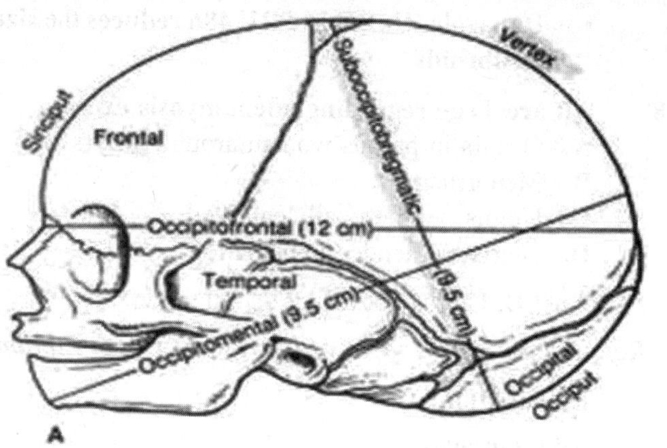

 B. Fetal movements and tone
 C. NST and AFI
 D. AFI

 Ans: C. NST & AFI

Ref: Dutta's Text Book of Obstetrics, 7th edition. Pg 109.

Explanation:

(See table on the next page)

- Normal score = **2 Abnormal = 0**
- **Total score = 10**
- But the disadvantage with biophysical profile is it takes **half an hour for each patient.**
- Hence, **modified biophysical score** is designed. It includes **AFI and NST.**
- Modified BPP is considered abnormal if NST is non reactive and/ or AFI<5.

Diameters of the Fetal Skill

FETAL SKULL DIAMETER	BORDERS	LENGTH
Suboccipito-bregmatic	From **nape of neck** to **center of bregma**	9.5 cm
Suboccipito-frontal	From **nape of neck** to **anterior fontanelle** or center of sinciput	10cm
Occipito-frontal	From **occipital eminence** to **root of nose**	11.5cm
Mentovertical	From **midpoint of chin** to **highest point of sagittal suture**	14cm
Submentovertical	From **junction of floor of the mouth and neck** to **highest point of sagittal suture**	11.5cm
Submentobregmatic	From **junction of mouth** and **neck to center of bregma**	9.5cm
Biparietal	Extends **between two parietal eminences**	9.5cm
Super sub-parietal	From a point placed **below one parietal eminence** to a point placed above the **other parietal eminence on opposite side**	8.5cm
Bitemporal	Distance **between two anterior ends of coronal suture**	8cm
Bimastoid	Distance between **tips of mastoid processes**	7.5cm

Biophysical Profile (Manning) Scoring includes

PARAMETERS	MINIMAL CRITERIA	SCORE
NST	Reactive pattern	2
Fetal breathing movements	≥1 episode lasting >30 sec	2
Gross body movement	≥ 3 discrete body/ limb movements	2
Fetal muscle tone	≥ 1 episode of extension of limb or trunk with return to flexion	2
Amniotic fluid	≥ 1 pocket measuring 2 cm in two perpendicular planes	2

PEDIATRICS

1. **Koplik spot is located:**

A. Opposite to first molar **B.** Opposite to premolar
C. Opposite to incisor **D.** Opposite to canine

Ans: B. Opposite to premolar

Ref: *Nelson's Textbook of Pediatrics. 19th Edition*

Explanation:

Koplik spots

- These lesions represent the **enanthem** and are the **pathognomonic sign of measles**, appearing **1 to 4 days prior** to the onset of the **rash**.
- They first appear as **discrete red lesions** with **bluish white spots** in the **center** on the inner aspects of the cheeks at the level of the **premolars**.
- They may spread to involve the **lips, hard palate,** and **gingiva**.
- They also may occur in **conjunctival folds** and in the **vaginal mucosa**.
- Koplik spots have been reported in **50-70%** of measles cases.

2. **Grasp reflex begins at: (Repeat 2011)**

A. 24 weeks **B.** 28 weeks
C. 32 weeks **D.** 36 weeks

Ans: B. 28 weeks

Ref: *Fanaroff and Martin's Neonatal-Perinatal Medicine, Diseases of the Fetus and Infant, Eighth Edition & Fenichel GM: Neonatal Neurology, 2nd ed. New York, Churchill Livingstone, 1985.*

Explanation:

Developmental reflexes

- These reflexes appear at specific ages of gestation to become fully developed and strong in the healthy full-term infant
- The **sucking** and **rooting** reflexes do not develop until **33 to 36 weeks'** gestational age.
- The **palmar** and **plantar** grasp responses become **apparent** at approximately **28 weeks** and are strong by **36 weeks'** gestation.
- The Moro reflex makes its appearance at **24 to 26 weeks'** gestation and evolves through **38 weeks,** at which age the **entire abduction-adduction response** is present.
(See the following table)

3. **Cystic fibrosis is associated with:**

A. Meconium ileus
B. Short bowel syndrome
C. Hirschprung disease
D. Congenital pyrolic stenosis

Ans: A. Meconium ileus

Neurologic Maturation of the Fetus and Newborn

FUNCTION	26 WEEKS	30 WEEKS	34 WEEKS	38 WEEKS
Resting posture	Flexion of arms; Flexion or extension of legs	Flexion of arms; Flexion or extension of legs	Flexion of all limbs	Flexion of all limbs
Arousal	Unable to maintain	Maintain briefly	Remain awake	Remain awake
Rooting	Absent	Long latency	Present	Present
Sucking	Absent	Long latency	Weak	Vigorous
Pupillary reflex	Absent	Variable	Present	Present
Traction	No response	No response	Head lag	Mild head lag
Moro	No response	Extension; no adduction	Adduction variable	Complete
Withdrawal	Absent	Withdrawal only	Crossed extension	Crossed extension

***Ref:** Nelson's Textbook of Pediatrics. 19th Edition & Harrison's 18th edn, pg 2149*

Explanation:

- In 15-20% of newborn infants with Cystic fibrosis CF, the **ileum** is completely obstructed by **meconium** (meconium ileus).
- The frequency is **greater (≈30%)** among siblings born subsequent to a child with meconium ileus and is particularly striking in monozygotic twins
- Abdominal distention, emesis, and **failure to pass meconium** appear in the 1st **24-48** hr of life
- Abdominal radiographs show **dilated loops** of **bowel** with **air-fluid levels** and, frequently, a collection of granular, **"ground-glass" material** in the lower central abdomen.
- Rarely, **meconium peritonitis** results from intrauterine **rupture** of the bowel wall and can be detected radiographically as the presence of **peritoneal or scrotal calcifications.**
- **Meconium plug syndrome** occurs with increased frequency in infants with CF but is less specific than meconium ileus.
- **Ileal obstruction with fecal material** (**distal intestinal obstruction syndrome** [**DIOS**]) occurs in older patients, causing **cramping abdominal** pain and **abdominal distention.**

Cystic fibrosis

- Autosomal Recessive
- Mutation in **CFTR** (cysic fibrosis transmembrane conductance regulator) gene
- Clinical Features
  - **Bronchiectasis**
  - Exocrine pancreatic insufficiency
  - Intestinal dysfunction
  - Abnormal sweat gland function
  - Urogenital dysfunction
- CF airway **epithelia** exhibit **abnormal Cl- secretion & Na+ absorption**
- Predisposes to infections. **Staph.aureus, Pseud.aeruginosa**. Others are **H.influenz, Alcaligenes, Burkholderia, Proteus**, E.coli, **Klebsiella, Aspergillus**
- Lack of CFTR Cl- channel in the apical membrane of pancreas, **failure to secrete NaHCO3 & water, destruction** of the **pancreas**
- In the sweat glands, inability to absorb Cl- from the sweat leads to **high Cl- concentrations** in **sweat** measured after iontophoresis of cholinergic agents
- Spirometry: ↑ RV/TLC, & ↓ FVC & ↓ FEV1
- **CXR**- hyperinflation, brochiectasis, **right upper lobe (Earliest** involved)
- Clubbing, pneumothorax, hemoptysis, corpulmonale
- **GIT: Meconium ileus**, DIOS, protein & fat malabsorption, diabetes later
- **GUT:** late onset puberty, azoospermia, female infertility

Treatment

- Gene therapy of CFTR gene
- Clearance of secretions with hypertonic saline, antibiotics
- Recombinant human DNAse to degrade DNA in sputum
- **Pancreatic enzyme replacement**, Vit E & K, Insulin
- **Megalodiatrizoate enema** for acute intestinal obstruction
- **Urodeoxycholic** acid for cholestatic liver disease
- Predisposed to **renal stones** and **osteoporosis**

4. Amount of fluid to be given to 8 month baby weighing 10 kg with severe dehydration: (Repeat)

A. 100 ml **B.** 800 ml
C. 400 ml **D.** 1000 ml

Ans: D. 1000 ml

***Ref:** Nelson's Textbook of Pediatrics. 19th Edition & OP GHAI, Textbook of Pediatrics; 7th edition, page: 267*

Explanation:

According to WHO guidelines for management of severe dehydration 100ml/kg of intravenous fluid should be given.

AGE	FIRST GIVE	THEN GIVE
<12 months	30 ml/kg in 1 hour	70ml/kg in 5 hours
12months upto 5 years	30ml/kg in 30 minutes	70 ml/kg in 2 ½ hours

- The best IV fluid solution is Ringer's lactate. If it is not available 0 .9% NaCl or half normal saline can be used.
- Total fluid to be given is 100 ml/kg
- 10 × 100 = **1000 ml**

5. All are true regarding Hypereosinophilic syndrome in children *except:*

A. Eosinophilia of > 1500 cells/microliter
B. Persistent eosinophilia for 6 months
C. Absence of any specific organ involvement
D. Corticosteroids are first line therapy

Ans: C. Absence of any specific organ involvement

***Ref:** Nelson Textbook of Pediatrics, 19th edition. Pg 740.*

Explanation:

Hypereosinophilic Syndrome (IHS)

- The idiopathic hypereosinophilic syndrome is a leukoproliferative disease characterized by **sustained overproduction of eosinophils**.
- The three diagnostic criteria for this disorder are
  1. Eosinophilia >1,500 cells/µL persisting for **>6 mo**
  2. Absence of another diagnosis to explain the eosinophilia
  3. Signs and symptoms of **organ involvement**.
- **Eosinophilic leukemia** may be distinguished from IHS by demonstrating a **clonal F1P1L1-PDGFRA fusion gene** resulting from a **cryptic deletion** of part of the **long arm of chromosome 4**.
- **Loeffler endocarditis**, most serious and life-threatening complication causing cardiac failure due to **endomyocardial thrombosis and fibrosis**.
- Other organ systems that can be involved can include the skin, liver, spleen, gastrointestinal tract, brain, and lungs.
- Therapy is aimed at **suppressing eosino**philia and is initiated with **corticosteroids**.
- **Imatinib mesylate**, an inhibitor of BCR-ABL, c-kit, and PDGF tyrosine kinases has antileukemic activity and has been effective in patients without elevated IL-5 levels.
- **Hydroxyurea** or **α-interferon** may be beneficial in patients unresponsive to corticosteroids.
- The underlying causes of hypereosinophilic syndrome remains **unknown**.
- For patients with prominent organ involvement who fail to respond to therapy, the mortality **is ≈ 75% after 3 yr.**
- Many patients in the past categorized as having the idiopathic hypereosinophilic syndrome had **eosinophilic leukemia**.

6. **All are causes of eosinophilia *except:***

   A. Allergic Rhinitis
   B. Trichinosis
   C. Corticosteroid therapy
   D. Rhematoid arthritis

   Ans: C. Corticosteroid therapy

Ref: *Nelson Textbook of Pediatrics, 19th edition. Pg 740.*

Explanation:

Corticosteroid therapy causes eosinopenia.

Causes of Eosinophilia

Allergic Disorders
- Allergic rhinitis
- Asthma
- Acute and chronic urticaria
- Hypersensitivity drug reactions

Infectious Diseases
- Tissue-Invasive Helminth Infections Trichinosis
  – *Toxocariasis*
  – *Strongyloidosis*
  – *Ascariasis*
  – *Filariasis*
- Pneumocystis carinii
- Toxoplasmosis
- Amebiasis
- Malaria
- Bronchopulmonary aspergillosis
- Scabies

Malignant Disorders
- Brain tumors
- Hodgkin disease and T-cell lymphoma
- Myeloproliferative disorders

Gastrointestinal Disorders
- Inflammatory bowel disease
- Eosinophilic gastroenteritis
- Chronic active hepatitis

Rheumatologic Disease
- Rheumatoid arthritis
- Eosinophilic fascitis

Immunodeficiency Disease
- Hyper-IgE syndrome
- Wiskott-Aldrich syndrome
- Löffler syndrome
- Eosinophilic leukemia
- Hypersensitivity pneumonia

Miscellaneous
- Thrombocytopenia with absent radii
- Vasculitis
- Histiocytosis with cutaneous involvement

7. **Children can reach for objects by:**

   A. 4 months **B.** 6 months
   C. 8 months **D.** 10 months

   Ans: A. 4 months

Ref: *Nelson Textbook of Pediatrics, 19th edition. Pg 27.*

Explanation:

(See table on the next page)

8. **Which of the following symptoms of rheumatic fever can be the only isolated manifestation?**

   A. Carditis **B.** Arthritis
   C. Chorea **D.** Subcutaneous nodules

   Ans: C. Chorea

Fine motor milestones

Milestone	Average age of attainment (in months)	Developmental implications
Grasps rattle	3.5	Object use
Reaches for objects	4	Visuomotor coordination
Palmar grasp gone	4	Voluntary release
Transfers object hand to hand	5.5	Comparison of objects
Thumb-finger grasp	8	Able to explore small objects
Turns pages of book	12	Increasing autonomy during book time
Scribbles	13	Visuomotor coordination
Builds tower of 2 cubes	15	Uses objects in combination
Builds tower of 6 cubes	22	Requires visual, gross, and fine motor coordination

Ref: *Nelson's Textbook of Pediatrics. 19th Edition*

Explanation:

Clinical Features of Rheumatic Fever

Migratory Polyarthritis

- Arthritis occurs in about **75%** of patients
- Involves ***larger joints***, particularly the knees, ankles, wrists, and elbows.
- Involvement of the spine, small joints of the hands and feet, or hips is uncommon.
- Affected joints are **Hot**, **red**, **swollen**, and exquisitely **tender**
- The joint involvement is **migratory** in nature
- Severe arthritis can persist for several weeks in untreated patients.
- A dramatic response to even small doses of **salicylates** is a characteristic feature
- Absence of such a response to salicylates should suggest an alternative diagnosis.
- Rheumatic arthritis is typically ***not deforming*** and ***disappears completely*** without any permanent changes
- Synovial fluid in acute rheumatic fever usually has ***10,000-100,000*** white blood cells/mm^3 with a predominance of **neutrophils**, a protein level of about **4 g/dL**, a **normal glucose** level, and forms a **good mucin clot**.
- Frequently, arthritis is the **earliest manifestation** of acute rheumatic fever and may correlate temporally with peak antistreptococcal antibody titers.
- *There is often an inverse relationship between the severity of arthritis and the severity of cardiac involvement.*

Carditis

- Carditis occurs in about **50-60%** cases.
- **Pancarditis** (active inflammation of myocardium, pericardium, and endocardium)
- **Endocarditis** (valvulitis) is a **universal finding**
- Presence of pericarditis or myocarditis is variable
- Isolated mitral valvular disease or combined aortic and mitral valvular disease
- Isolated aortic or right-sided valvular involvement is uncommon.
- Acute rheumatic carditis usually presents as tachycardia and cardiac murmurs, with or without evidence of myocardial or pericardial involvement.
- Moderate to severe rheumatic carditis can result in cardiomegaly and congestive heart failure with hepatomegaly and peripheral and pulmonary edema.
- Echocardiographic findings include **pericardial effusion**, **decreased ventricular contractility**, and **aortic and/or mitral regurgitation**.
- The major consequence of acute rheumatic carditis is chronic, **progressive valvular disease**, particularly valvular stenosis.

Chorea

- Occurs in **10-15%** of patients
- Presents as an isolated, subtle, neurologic behavior disorder.
- Symptoms include
  - Emotional lability
  - Incoordination
  - Poor school performance
  - Uncontrollable movements
  - Facial grimacing
  - Symptoms exacerbated by stress and disappearing with sleep
- The latent period from acute GAS infection to chorea is usually longer than for arthritis or carditis and can be months.
- Onset can be insidious, with symptoms being present for several months before recognition.
- Clinical maneuvers to elicit features of chorea include

- Demonstration of **milkmaid's grip** (irregular contractions of the muscles of the hands while squeezing the examiner's fingers)
- ***Spooning and pronation*** of the hands when the patient's arms are extended
- ***Wormian darting movements*** of the ***tongue*** upon ***protrusion***
- Examination of ***handwriting*** to evaluate ***fine motor*** movements.

• Chorea does not cause permanent neurologic sequelae.

Erythema Marginatum

• Very rare (<3% cases)
• Characteristic rash of acute rheumatic fever.
• ***Erythematous, Serpiginous, macular lesions*** with pale centers that are not pruritic
• It occurs primarily on the ***trunk and extremities***, but ***not on*** the ***face***
• It is accentuated on warming the skin.

Subcutaneous Nodules

• Very rare (de1% cases)
• Firm nodules of 1 cm in diameter along the ***extensor surfaces of tendons*** near ***bony prominences***.
• Assc with severe cardiac involvement

Minor Manifestations

• The 2 clinical minor manifestations are
  - **Arthralgia** (in the absence of polyarthritis as a major criterion) and
  - **Fever** (typically temperature ee102F and occurring early in the course of illness).
• The 2 laboratory minor manifestations are
  - Elevated acute-phase reactants (**CRP & ESR**)
  - **Prolonged PR** interval on ECG (**1st degree heart block**).
• Prolonged P-R interval alone does not constitute evidence of carditis or predict long-term cardiac sequelae.

Essential criteria (Evidence of recent Group A Streptococcus Infection)

• An absolute requirement for the diagnosis is supporting evidence of a recent GAS infection.
• Acute rheumatic fever typically develops **2-4 wk** after an acute episode of GAS **pharyngitis**
• Elevated or increasing serum antistreptococcal antibody titers.
• A slide agglutination test (Streptozyme)
• Single **antibody ASLO** (antistreptolysin O), is elevated in **80-85%** of patients
• Elevation of any **3 antibodies (antistreptolysin O, anti-DNase B, antihyaluronidase)** is seen in **95-100%** cases

9. **Which of the following is a risk factor for developing Type 1 Diabetes mellitus?**

A. Male Gender **B.** Old age
C. Gestational diabetes **D.** HLA DR3

Ans: D. HLA DR3

Ref: *Nelson's Textbook of Pediatrics. 19th Edition*

Explanation:

Pathophysiology and Risk factors for Type 1 Diabetes mellitus

• Type 1 DM is the culmination of ***lymphocytic infiltration*** and ***destruction of insulin-secreting beta cells*** of the islets of Langerhans in the pancreas.
• As beta-cell mass declines, insulin secretion decreases until the available insulin no longer is adequate to maintain normal blood glucose levels.
• After 80-90% of the beta cells are destroyed, hyperglycemia develops and diabetes may be diagnosed.
• **Autoimmunity** – Major determinant
• **Viral infection** may stimulate the production of ***antibodies against a viral protein*** that trigger an autoimmune response against antigenically similar beta cell molecules.
• Approx 85% of type 1 DM patients have circulating islet cell antibodies, and the majority also have detectable ***anti-insulin antibodies*** before receiving insulin therapy.
• The most commonly found ***islet cell antibodies*** are directed against ***glutamic acid decarboxylase (GAD)***, an enzyme found within pancreatic beta cells.
• The prevalence is increased in other autoimmune diseases, such as
  - Graves disease
  - Hashimoto thyroiditis
  - Addison disease
• Polymorphisms of the ***class II human leukocyte antigen (HLA***) genes that encode **DR** and **DQ** are the major genetic determinants
• Approximately **95%** of patients with type 1 DM have either ***HLA-DR3 or HLA-DR4***.
• **HLA-DQs** are also considered **specific markers** of **type 1 DM susceptibility**.
• Some haplotypes (e.g, **HLA-DR2**) confer **strong protection** against type 1 DM

10. **False about Hartnup's disease: (Repeat)**

A. Defect in neutral aminoacid transport
B. Mental retardation is the common presentation
C. Most children are asymptomatic
D. Photosensitivity

Ans: B. Mental retardation is the common presentation

***Ref:** Nelson's Textbook of Pediatrics. 19th Edition, Page:*

Explanation:

Hartnup disease

- It is a rare inborn error of metabolism with **autosomal recessive** inheritance.
- Neutral amino acids, including **tryptophan**, are not transported across the brush border epithelium of the intestine and kidneys,
- This results in deficiency of synthesis of **nicotinamide**
- It causes a **photo-induced pellagra-like syndrome**.
- Increased urinary **monoamine monocarboxylic amino acids.**
- **Cutaneous signs** precede neurologic manifestations
- Eczematous, occasionally vesiculobullous eruption noted on the face and extremities in a **glove-and-stocking photodistribution**.
- **Hyperpigmentation** and **hyperkeratosis** may supervene and are intensified by further exposure to sunlight.
- Episodic flares may be precipitated by febrile illness, sun exposure, emotional stress, and poor nutrition.
- Emotional instability and **episodic cerebellar ataxia**.
- Neurologic symptoms are fully **reversible**.
- Administration of **nicotinamide** and protection from sunlight improves both cutaneous and neurologic manifestations.

SKIN

1. **Not a fungal infection is:**

A. Mycoses fungoides **B.** Tinea nigra Palmaris
C. White Piedra **D.** Black Piedra

Ans: A. Mycoses fungoides

***Ref:** Rook's Dermatology, 8th ed.*

Explanation:

Mycosis Fungoides/Sézary Syndrome

- Mycosis fungoides and Sézary syndrome are different manifestations of a **tumor of CD4+ helper T cells**
- Clinically, the cutaneous lesions of mycosis fungoides typically progress through three somewhat distinct stages, an inflammatory **premycotic phase,** a **plaque phase**, and a **tumor phase**
- Histologically, the **epidermis and upper dermis** are **infiltrated by neoplastic T cells**, which often have a **cerebriform appearance** due to marked **infolding of the nuclear membrane**.
- Sézary syndrome is a variant in which skin involvement is manifested as a **generalized exfoliative erythroderma**.
- In contrast to mycosis fungoides, the skin lesions **rarely proceed to tumefaction**, and there is an associated **leukemia of "Sézary" cells** with characteristic **cerebriform nuclei**.
- The tumor cells express the **adhesion molecule CLA** and the chemokine receptors **CCR4** and **CCR10**
- Transformation to **aggressive T-cell lymphoma** occurs occasionally as a terminal event.

FUNGAL INFECTIONS

Natural defence against fungi

- Fatty acid content of the skin
- pH of the skin, mucosal surfaces and body fluids
- Epidermal turnover
- Normal flora

Predisposing factors

- Tropical climate, Manual labour population
- Low socioeconomic status, Profuse sweating
- Friction with clothes, synthetic innerwear
- Malnourishment, Immunosuppressed patients

HIV, Congenital Immunodeficiencies, patients on corticosteroids, immunosuppressive drugs, Diabetes

Fungal Infections: Classification

- Superficial cutaneous:
- Surface infections eg. P.versicolor, Dermatophytosis, Candidiasis, T.nigra, Piedra
- Subcutaneous:
  Mycetoma, Chromoblastomycosis, Sporotrichosis
- Systemic (opportunistic infection)

Histoplasmosis, Candidiasis

Of these categories, Dermatophytosis, P.versicolor, Candidiasis are common in daily practice

Pityriasis versicolor

- Etiologic agent: ***Malassezia furfur***

Clinical Features:

- Multiple, discrete, discoloured, macules.
- Fawn, brown, grey or hypopigmented
- Pinhead sized to large sheets of discolouration
- Seborrheic areas, upper half of body: trunk, arms, neck, abdomen.
- Scratch sign positive
- Wood's Lamp examination: **Yellow fluoroscence**

- KOH preparation: **Spaghetti and meatball appearance**

Coarse mycelium, fragmented to short filaments 2-5 micron wide and up to 2-5 micron long, together with spherical, thick-walled yeasts 2-8 micron in diameter, arranged in grape like fashion.

Treatment

Topical:

- Ketoconazole, Clotrimazole, Miconazole, Bifonazole, Oxiconazole, Butenafine,Terbinafine, Selenium sulfide, Sodium thiosulphate

Oral:

- Fluconamg 400mg single dose
- Ketoconazole 200mg OD x 14days
- Griseofulvin is NOT effective.
- Hypopigmentation will take weeks to fade
- Scaling will disappear soon

Pityrosporum folliculitis

- **Etiology:** ***Malassezia furfur***
- **Age group:** Teenagers or young adult males
- **Clinical features:** Itchy papules and pustules, scattered on the shoulders and back.
- **Treatment:** Oral Itraconazole, Ketaconazole, Fluconazole or topical Ketoconazole shampoo.

Tinea nigra palmaris

- **Etiology:** ***Exophiala werneckii***
- **Clinical features:** Asymptomatic superficial infection of palms; deeply pigmented, brown or black macular, non-scaly patches, resembling a silver nitrate stain.
- **Treatment:** Topical Econazole, Ketoconazole, Benzoic acid compound, Thiabendazole 2% in 90% DMSO or 10% Thiabendazole suspension.

Black piedra

- **Etiology:** ***Piedraia hortae***
- **Clinical features:** Hard, dark, multiple superficial nodules; firmly adherent black, gritty, hard nodules on hairs of scalp, beard, moustache or pubic area, hair may fracture easily.
- **Treatment:**
  Shaving or cutting the hair.
  Terbinafine, Benzoic acid compound ointment, 1:2000 solution of mercury perchloride

White piedra

- **Etiology:** ***Trichosporon beigelii***
- **Clinical features:**
  Soft, white, grey or brown superficial nodules on hairs of the beard, moustache, pubic areas. Hair shaft weakened and breaks.
- **Treatment:** Shaving or cutting the hair. Responses to topical antifungals, azoles and allyamines have been reported but are unpredictable.

Dermatophytosis

Mycology:

- Three genera:
  Microsporum, Trichophyton, Epidermophyton
- Thrive on dead, keratinized tissue - within the stratum corneum of the epidermis, within and around the fully keratinized hair shaft, and in the nail plate and keratinized nail bed.

Tinea capitis

Endothrix and Ectothrix

Most common - trichophyton violaceum

Varieties:

- Non inflammatory
- Gray patch
- Black dot
- Seborrheic dermatitis
- Inflammatory
- Favus
- Kerion, agminate folliculitis

Non inflammatory Tinea capitis:

Black dot/Grey patch

- Breakage of hair gives rise to 'black dots'
- Patchy alopecia, often circular, numerous broken-off hairs, dull grey
- Wood's lamp examination: green fluorescence (occasional non-fluorescent cases)

Tinea capitis: Kerion, agminate folliculitis

- Inflammatory variety
- Microsporum,Trichophyton verrucosum, Trichophyton mentagrophytes
- Painful, inflammatory boggy swelling with purulent discharge.
- Hairs may be matted, easily pluckable
- Lymphadenopathy
- Co-infection with bacteria is common
- May heal with scarring alopecia

Tinea capitis: Favus

- Inflammatory variety
- Kashmir
- Trichophyton schonleinii
- Yellowish, cup-shaped crusts develop around a hair with the hair projecting centrally.
- Extensive patchy hair loss with cicatricial alopecia

Tinea faciei

- Erythematous scaly patches on the face
- Annular or circinate lesions and induration
- Itching, burning and exacerbation after sun exposure
- Seen often in immunocompromised adults

Tinea barbae

- Ringworm of the beard and moustache areas
- Invasion of coarse hairs

- Disease of the adult male
- Highly inflammatory, pustular folliculitis
- Hairs of the beard or moustache are surrounded by inflammatory papulopustules, usually with oozing or crusting, easily pluckable
- Persist several months

Tinea corporis

- Lesions of the trunk and limbs, excluding ringworm of the specialized sites such as the scalp, feet and groins etc.
- The fungus enters the stratum corneum and spreads centrifugally. Central clearing results once the fungi are eliminated.
- A second wave of centrifugal spread from the original site may occur with the formation of concentric erythematous inflammatory rings.

Classical lesion:

- Annular patch or plaque with erythematous papulovesicles and scaling at the periphery with central clearing resembling the effects of ring worm.
- Polycyclic appearance in advanced infection due to incomplete fusion of multiple lesions
- Sites: waist, under breasts, abdomen, thighs etc.

Tinea cruris

- Itching
- Erythematous plaques, curved with well demarcated margins extending from the groin down the thighs.
- Scaling is variable, and occasionally may mask the inflammatory changes.
- Vesiculation is rare

Tinea mannum

Two varieties:

- Non inflammatory: Dry, scaly, mildly itchy
- Inflammatory: Vesicular, itchy

Tinea pedis

- Wearing of shoes and the resultant maceration
- Adult males commonest, children rarely
- Peeling, maceration and fissuring affecting the lateral toe clefts, and sometimes spreading to involve the undersurface of the toes.

Varieties:

- Interdigital type
- Papulosquammous ('moccasin foot')
- Vesiculo-bullous

Tinea Unguium

Dirty, dull, dry, pitted, ridged, split, discoloured, thick, uneven, nails with subungual hyperkeratosis Different types described depending on the site of nail involvement and its depth.

- Distal and lateral onychomycoses
- Proximal subungual onychomycoses
- White superficial onychomycoses
- Total dystrophic onychomycoses

Treatment: Ringworm

- Topical: Bifonazole, Ketoconazole Oxiconazole, Clotrimazole, Miconazole, Butenafine, Terbinafine.
- Vehicle: Lotions, creams, powders, gels are available.

CANDIDIASIS

- **Causative organism:**
  Candida albicans, Candida tropicalis, Candida pseudotropicalis
- **Sites of affection:**
  - Mucous membrane
  - Skin
  - Nails

Candidiasis : Mucosal

- Oral thrush:
  Creamy, curd-like, white pseudomembrane, on erythematous base
- Sites:
  - Immunocompetent patient: cheeks, gums or the palate.
  - Immunocompromised patients: affection of tongue with extension to pharynx or oesophagus; ulcerative lesions may occur.
- Angular cheilitis (angular stomatitis / perleche): Soreness at the angles of the mouth
- Vulvovaginitis (vulvovaginal thrush): Itching and soreness with a thick, creamy white discharge
- Balanoposthitis:
  - Tiny papules on the glans penis after intercourse, evolve as white pustules or vesicles and rupture.
  - Radial fissures on glans penis in diabetics. Vulvovaginitis in conjugal partner

Candidiasis - Flexural

- Intertrigo: (Flexural candidiasis):
  Erythema and maceration in the folds; axilla, groins and webspaces.
- Napkin rash:
  Pustules, with an irregular border and satellite lesions

Candidiasis: Nail

- Chronic Paronychia:
  - Swelling of the nail fold with pain and discharge of pus.
  - Chronic, recurrent.
  - Superadded bacterial infection
- Onychomycosis:
  - Destruction of nail plate.

Treatment of candidiasis

- Treat predisposing factors like poor hygiene, diabetes, AIDS, conjugal infection

- Topical:
  Clotrimazole, Miconazole, Ketoconazole, Ciclopirox olamine
- Oral:
  Ketoconazole 200mg, Itraconazole 100-200mg and Fluconazole 150mg

2. **Dermatitis herpeteformis is associated with:**
   A. Gluten senstive enteropathy
   B. Celiac disease
   C. Protein losing enteropathy
   D. Whipple's disease

Ans: A. Gluten sensitive enteropathy

Ref: *Robbins Pathologic basis of disease, 8th ed*

Explanation:

DERMATITIS HERPETIFORMIS (DH)

Epidemiology
- Age-**20 to 40** yrs , **M=F,** Whites > Blacks/Asians

Etiology
- Genetics: **HLA B8, DRw17 and DQw2**
- External factors: **Gluten containing diet** like **wheat**, **barley**, **oats** and **rye**
- Antigen: Gut epithelial antigen that cross reacts with skin
- Antibodies: **IgA directed** against **gliadin** and autoantigens like **reticulin** and **endomysium**

Pathogenesis
- Gluten or its fragments are taken up by antigen presenting cells like lymphocytes
- Activation of cytokines and inflammatory cells
- Plasma cells release IgA2 directed against **gliadin**
- Cross-reacts with autoantigens of skin and gut like reticulin, endomyosium

Clinical Features
- Intensely pruritic
- Most vesicles have been scratched away
- Chronic recurrent grouped **papulo vesicles** , **symmetrically**
- Most common on **extensor surfaces, back of neck, and sacrum, buttocks,**
- Associated with **gluten-sensitive enteropathy**

Diagnosis
- **Tzanck smear**: plenty of **neutrophils**
- Histopathology: Neutrophilic **microabscesses** at the tips of dermal papilla with **sub-epidermal** vesicle
- Immunopathology:
  Clinically normal skin on forearm or **buttock** shows granular **IgA deposits in** the **dermal papilla.**

Treatment
- Strict **gluten free diet**
- **Systemic steroids** not the mainstay of therapy
- **Dapsone** 100-200 mg/day
- **Sulphapyridine** 1.5 g/ day
- **Tetracycline with nicotinamide**
- **Colchicine** when the above drugs are contraindicated

3. **Vesicular lesion is seen in:**

A. Primary syphilis	**B.** Secondary syphilis
C. Tertiary syphilis	**D.** Congenital syphilis

Ans: D. Congenital syphilis

Ref: *Nelson's Textbook of Pediatrics. 19th Edition, Page: 1017, Thappa, Essentials in dermatology, 1st ed.*

Explanation:

"Vesicular lesions in an adult are never due to secondary syphilis"

Primary Syphilis
- Painless chancre (Primary Chancre / Hunterian Chancre / Hard Chancre)
- Typical chancre is round or oval ulcer, 1 -2 cm across, has indurated margin, clear base and without any exudate
- Moderate enlargement of inguinal lymph nodes
- Nontender, nonsuppurative, firm, shotty (***Indolent bubo***)
- Relapse of primary syphilis extremely rare (***Chancre Redux)***

Secondary Syphilis
- Lesions are due to hematogeneous dissemination of treponomes
- Flu like symptoms - malaise, loss of appetite, fever, headache, stiff neck, myalgia & arthralgia
- Skin manifestation are termed as **'Syphilids'**, are asymptomatic, polymorphous, variegate, bilateral and symmetrical
- Evanescent macular rash involving entire trunk, extremities and palms & soles
- Papular lesions demonstrate **OLLENDORF SIGN**
- Even nodules may appear; They may be pustular bu **NEVER VESICULAR**
- **Condlylomata lata:** The moist, smooth surfaced warty intertriginous plaques (MOST INFECT-IOUS LESION)
- Generalised lymphadenopathy: especially epitrochelear lymph nodes
- **'Moth eaten alopecia'** in scalp

Tertiary Syphilis
- Gummatous: Non tender, pink to dusky red nodules or plaques that vary in size
- Cardiovascular and Neurosyphilis

Congenital Syphilis

Early manifestations
- Hepatosplenomegaly, jaundice, and elevated liver enzymes are common.

- Histologically, liver involvement includes bile stasis, fibrosis, and extramedullary hematopoiesis.
- Lymphadenopathy tends to be diffuse and resolve spontaneously, although shotty nodes can persist.
- Coombs-negative hemolytic anemia
- Thrombocytopenia associated with platelet trapping in an enlarged spleen.
- Characteristic osteochondritis and periostitis and a mucocutaneous rash manifesting with ***erythematous maculopapular*** or ***vesiculobullous*** lesions followed by ***desquamation*** involving ***hands and feet*** .
- Furuncle of barlow
- Mucous patches, persistent rhinitis (snuffles), and ***condylomatous*** lesions contain abundant spirochetes and are highly infectious.
- Blood and moist open lesions from infants with congenital syphilis and children with acquired primary or secondary syphilis are infectious until 24 hours of appropriate treatment.
- Bone involvement is common. Roentgenographic abnormalities include
  - **Wimberger's lines** (metaphyseal demineralization - medial aspect of proximal tibia)
  - Multiple sites of osteochondritis at the wrists, elbows, ankles, and knees, and
  - Periostitis of the long bones and rarely the skull.
  - ***Sawtooth metaphysis***
- The osteochondritis is painful, often resulting in irritability and refusal to move the involved extremity (**pseudoparalysis of Parrot**).
- Central nervous system (CNS) abnormalities, failure to thrive, chorioretinitis, nephritis, and nephrotic syndrome may also be seen.
- Manifestations of renal involvement include hypertension, hematuria, proteinuria, ***hypoproteinemia***, ***hypercholesterolemia***, and ***hypocomplementemia***, probably related to glomerular deposition of circulating immune complexes.
- Less common clinical manifestations of early congenital syphilis include gastroenteritis, peritonitis, pancreatitis, pneumonia, eye involvement (glaucoma and chorioretinitis), nonimmune hydrops, and testicular masses.

Late manifestations (children >2 years of age)

- These result primarily from **chronic granulomatous inflammation** of bone, teeth, and CNS and are summarized in Table 210-1.
- Skeletal changes are due to persistent or recurrent **periostitis** and associated thickening of the involved bone.
- Dental abnormalities such as **Hutchinson teeth**, repeated caries and tooth destruction.
- Saddle nose is a depression of the nasal root and may be associated with a perforated nasal septum.
- Other late manifestations of congenital syphilis can manifest as hypersensitivity phenomena. These include unilateral or bilateral **interstitial keratitis** and the **Clutton** joint. Other common ocular manifestations include choroiditis, retinitis, vascular occlusion, and optic atrophy.
- **Soft tissue gummas** (identical to those of acquired disease) and paroxysmal cold hemoglobinuria are rare hypersensitivity phenomena.

  (See table on the next page)

4. In chronic folliculitis the treatment of choice is

A. Topical antibiotics **B.** Systemic antibiotics
C. Both A and C **D.** Surgery

Ans: C. Both A and C

Ref: *DM. Thappa, Essentials in Dermatology. 1st ed. pg 28. & Prasad P, Anandhi V, Jaya M. Chronic folliculitis - A clinico-epidemiological study. Indian J Dermatol Venereol Leprol 1997;63:304-6*

Explanation:

Folliculitis (Hot Tub Rash)

Pyoderma affecting the hair follicles

Classified according to the depth of invasion

Superficial Folliculitis (aka Follicular or ***Bockhart's*** impetigo)

A small fragile dome shaped pustule occurs at the infundibulum of hair follicle

Common location: ***Scalps in children***; ***Beard area***, ***axilla***, ***extremities*** and ***buttocks*** in adults

Deep Folliculitis

Sycosis barbae is a deep folliculitis with perifollicular inflammation occurring in the beard areas.

Lupoid sycosis is a deep chronic form of sycosis barbae associated with ***SCARRING (Circinate lesion)***

Furuncle or Boil

- It is a deep seated inflammatory nodule that develops about a hair follicle
- Arise in hair bearing areas, regions subjected to friction, occlusion and perspiration

Carbuncle

- Cluster of furuncles
- More extensive and deeper, communicating, infiltrated lesion

Late Manifestations of Congenital Syphilis

SYMPTOM/SIGN	DESCRIPTION/COMMENTS
Olympian brow	Bony prominence of the forehead due to persistent or recurrent periostitis
Clavicular or Higouménaki sign	Unilateral or bilateral thickening of the sternoclavicular third of the clavicle
Saber shins	Anterior bowing of the midportion of the tibia
Scaphoid scapula	Convexity along the medial border of the scapula
Hutchinson teeth	Peg-shaped upper central incisors; they erupt during 6th yr of life with abnormal enamel, resulting in a notch along the biting surface
Mulberry molars	Abnormal 1st lower (6 yr) molars characterized by small biting surface and excessive number of cusps
Saddle nose	Depression of the nasal root, a result of syphilitic rhinitis destroying adjacent bone and cartilage
Rhagades	Linear scars that extend in a spoke-like pattern from previous mucocutaneous fissures of the mouth, anus, and genitalia
Juvenile paresis	Latent meningovascular infection; it is rare and typically occurs during adolescence with behavioral changes, focal seizures, or loss of intellectual function
Juvenile tabes	Rare spinal cord involvement and cardiovascular involvement with aortitis
Hutchinson triad	Hutchinson teeth, interstitial keratitis, and 8th nerve deafness
Clutton joint	Unilateral or bilateral painless joint swelling (usually involving knees) due to synovitis with sterile synovial fluid; spontaneous remission usually occurs after several wk
Interstitial keratitis	Manifests with intense photophobia and lacrimation, followed within weeks or months by corneal opacification and complete blindness.
Eighth nerve deafness	May be unilateral or bilateral, appears at any age, manifests initially as vertigo and high-tone hearing loss, and progresses to permanent deafness

- Seen when suppuration occurs in inelastic skin
- Seen in Nape of neck, back or thighs
- Associated with Diabetes Mellitus

Organisms causing Folliculitis

- ***Staph aureus*** (MC organism)
- Pseuduomonas (Hot tub folliculitis)
- Klebsiella
- Gram negative folliculitis (following prolonged acne treatment)
- Fungal pityrosporum folliculitis - currently known as Malassezia folliculitis
- Herpetic folliculitis - Herpes simplex virus

Non-infectious Folliculitis

- **Pseudofolliculitis barbae** - When hair curves back into the skin and causes inflammation.
- **Eosinophilic folliculitis** may appear in persons with impaired immune systems.
- **Folliculitis decalvans or tufted folliculitis** usually affects scalp. Several hairs arise from the same hair follicle. Scarring and permanent hair loss may follow. The cause is unknown.
- **Folliculitis keloidalis** scarring on the nape of the neck, most common among males of curly hair.
- **Oil folliculitis** is inflammation of hair follicles due to exposure to various oils and typically occurs on forearms or thighs. It is common in refinery workers, road workers, mechanics, sheep shearers. Even c may cause it.

Chronic Folliculitis

- Chronic folliculitis is a chronic infection of hair follicles
- Predominantly seen on the legs.
- Common among Asians and Africans, especially young adult males in India.
- The inflammatory changes are confined to the ostium or slightly below it and heals without scar formation.
- Apart from coagulase positive Staphylococcus aureus, physical or chemical injury may also precipitate this condition.
- It involves the **legs, thighs, forearms and arms**.

- Combination therapy with **antiseptic lotions, long term systemic antibiotics, topical antibiotics** and **avoidance of risk factors are essential** in controlling the disease.

5. Condyloma accuminatum is produced by which type of papilloma virus?

A. HPV 6, 16 **B.** HPV 6, 11
C. HPV 16, 18 **D.** HPV 11, 18

Ans: B. HPV 6, 11

Ref: *Rook's dermatology, 8th ed & Internet sources*

Explanation:

HPV associated condition	HPV types
Common warts	2, 7
Plantar warts	1, 2, 4, 63
Flat warts	3, 10, 8
Anogenital warts (Condyloma accuminatum)	6, 11, 42, 44
Anal lesions	6, 16, 18, 31, 53, 58
Genital cancers	16, 18, 31, 45
Focal epithelial hyperplasia (oral)	13, 32
Oral papillomas	6, 7, 11, 16, 32
Oropharyngeal cancer	16
Verrucous cyst	60
Laryngeal papillomatosis	6,11

6. Herald patch is seen in:

A. Pityriasis rosea **B.** lichen planus
C. DLE **D.** Reiter syndrome

Ans: A. Pityriasis rosea

Ref: *Rook's Dermatology, 8th ed.*

Explanation:

PITYRIASIS ROSEA

- **Gibert disease, Six week disease**
- Viral-**HHV6, 7**
- Drugs - **Metronidazole, Captopril, Gold**
- Initial lesion-**herald patch** -1-2 cms oval plaque in trunk with **collarette of scales** inside the border (**Hanging curtain sign**)
- 2weeks later – multiple small similar lesions appear which will be arranged in **christmas tree or fir tree pattern**
- Self limiting

REITER'S SYNDROME

- Triad of **urethritis, arthrzitis, and conjuctivitis**

Cutaneous eruption:

- Limpet like scales
- **Circinate balanitis**
- Shallow **painless ulcers** of **palate, tongue and glans**
- **Keratoderma blennorrhagica-Palms and soles**
- **HLA B 27** in **80%** of cases
- Prior episode of **urogenital or gastrointestinal infection** with microorganisms like
  - Chlamydia trachomatis
  - Ureaplasma urealyticum
  - Shigella
  - Salmonella
  - Neisseria gonorrhoea
  - Yersinia
- Treatment - **Methotrexate**

7. A 20 year old woman with past history of enteric fever 4 months back presents with diffuse hair loss for 1 month. The likely cause is:

A. Androgenic alopecia **B.** Telogen effuvium
C. Anageneffuvium **D.** Alopecia areata

Ans : B. Telogen effluvium

Ref: *Disorders of hair and nails. In: Thappa DM, editor. Essentials in Dermatology, 2nd edn., NewDelhi: Jaypee brothers medical publishers (P) Ltd 2009;189-97.*

Explanation:

- **Telogen effluvium (Diffuse)**
  - Hair follicles enter telogen phase and shed 6-10 weeks
  - Occurs after a precipitating event like parturition, high fever, surgery, stress and drugs like OCP, beta blockers, ACE
- **Alopecia areata (Patchy)**
  - Autoimmune disorder
  - Exclamation mark hairs (broken short hairs with proximal tapering) which are dystrophic anagen hairs are characteristic – Patchy hair loss
- **Androgenetic alopecia (Diffuse)**
  - Terminal to vellus hair transformation
  - Frontal hairline recession and thinning over vertex in males
  - Diffuse thinning more so in vertex in females
- **Anagen effluvium (Diffuse)**
  - Abrupt cessation of hair growth in anagen phase and shed due to
  - Cytotoxic drugs like cyclophosphamide, doxorubicin, nitrosureas, heparin, warfarin, vitamin A, INH.

ANESTHESIA

1. Which is non invasive positive pressure ventilation?

A. CPAP **B.** SIMV
C. CMV **D.** IMV

Ans : A. CPAP

Ref : Medscape Emedicine

Explanation :

Noninvasive ventilation (NIV)

- It refers to the administration of ventilatory support without using an invasive artificial airway (endotracheal tube or tracheostomy tube).
- It is divided into two types

Non-invasive Positive pressure ventilation

- Positive-pressure ventilation delivered through a mask has become the predominant method of providing noninvasive ventilatory support

Non invasive Negative pressure ventilation

- Negative-pressure ventilators provide ventilatory support using a device that encases the thoracic cage starting from the neck, and devices range from a whole-body tank to a cuirass shell.
- The general principal is the same with a vacuum device, which lowers the pressure surrounding the thorax, creating subatmospheric pressure and thereby passively expanding the chest wall with diaphragmatic descent, all leading to lung inflation.
- Exhalation occurs with passive recoil of the chest wall.

Non-invasive Positive Pressure Ventilation Patient Interfaces

- Nasal masks and
- Orofacial masks
- Full face masks
- Mouthpieces
- Nasal pillows
- Helmets.

Modes of ventilation

- **CPAP**
- **BiPAP**
- **PAV**
- Most patients who are provided noninvasive ventilation are provided support with pressure ventilation, with **continuous positive airway pressure (CPAP),** which is the most basic level of support. CPAP may be especially useful in patients with congestive heart failure or obstructive sleep apnea.
- **Bilevel positive airway pressure (BiPAP)** is probably the most common mode of support and requires provision of inspiratory positive airway pressure (IPAP) and expiratory positive airway pressure (EPAP). The difference between IPAP and EPAP is a reflection of the amount of pressure support ventilation provided to the patient, and EPAP is synonymous with positive end-expiratory pressure (PEEP).
- Some noninvasive ventilation is provided using **proportional-assist ventilation (PAV)**, which provides flow and volume assistance with each breath.

2. Anesthetic drug of choice in asthmatic: (Repeat)

A. Ketamine **B.** Propofol
C. Etomidate **D.** Propofol

Ans: B. Ketamine

Ref: Miller's Anesthesia, 7th ed. & Ajay Yadav

Explanation:

Ketamine

- Causes **Dissociative anesthesia**
- Phencyclidine derivative
- **NMDA receptor agonist**
- **Anesthetic Properties**
  - Onset of Action: 30 – 60 seconds
  - Early regain of consciousness after 15 – 20 min due to **Redistribution**
  - Elimination half life: 2-3 hours
  - **Strong analgesic property**
  - Metabolised in **Liver** and products exreted in **urine**
  - Not a muscle relaxant
- Primary site of action – **Thalamo-neo-cortical projections**

Cardiovascular System

- Increases arterial BP,
- Increases heart rate &
- Increases cardiac output
- IV agent of choice in **SHOCK**

Respiratory System

- **Potent Bronchodilator**
- Good induction agent for asthmatics
- **Upper airway reflexes remain largely intact**
- Increases salivatory & Tracheo bronchial secretions
- Using glycopyrollate or atropine becomes necessary

Central Nervous System

- **Increases Intracranial pressure** and can precipitate **seizures**
- **Emergence reactions:**
  - These are seen at emergence
  - Vivid dreaming
  - Illusions
  - Extracorporeal experiences like floating
  - Excitement
  - Confusión
  - Euphoria
  - Fear

- **Hallucinations:**
  - Auditory and Visual hallucinations (Most common side effect of Ketamine)
  - Treated with Benzodiazepine

Other Systems

- **Eye**
  - Increase intraocular tensión
  - Pupils dilate moderately
  - Nystagmus
- **GIT**
  - Increases intragastric pressure
  - Salivary secretions increased
- **Muscluar**
  - Increases muscle tone
  - Increased non-puposeful movements

Dose

- Can be given IV, IM, oral, Rectal and intrathecal route
- IV – 2mg/kg
- IM- 5-10mg/kg

Advantages

- **Induction Agent of Choice in**
  - Asthmatics
  - Shock ***(HYPOTENSION)***
  - Children (Now Sevoflurance is DOC)
  - Constrictive pericarditis
  - Cardiac tamponade
- Can be used as **SOLE** agent
- Can be used safely at remote places and in inexperienced hands since does not depress heart or respiration
- Preferred agent when patient is in ***FULL STOMACH*** (Preserves laryngo- pharyngeal reflexes)

Contraindicated in

- Head injury
- ICSOL
- Eye injury
- Opthal pathology
- Ischemic heart disease
- Vascular aneurysm
- Psychiatric diseases
- Drug addicts
- Hypertensives

3. **Neuromuscular blocker of choice in real failure:**

A. Atracurium B. Pancuronium
C. Rocuronium D. Tubocurare

Ans: A. Atracurium

Ref: *Ajay Yadav's Short Textbook of Anaesthesia, 1st ed. Pg 89.*

Explanation:

Atracurium

- It has a unique method of degradation
- Its metabolism is independent of hepatic and renal functions
- It undergoes **HOFFMAN DEGREDATION** (95%) and **ester hydrolysis** (5%) in plasma
- **Systemic effects.**
- CVS: Can cause hypotension because of histamine release
- Resp: Can cause Bronchospasm due to histamine release
- CNS: At higher doses, its metabolic product **Laudanosine** can precipitate convulsions
- Allergic reactions from pruritic rash to angioedema can occur
- **Uses**
- **Atracurium** is **relaxant of choice** in
  - Hepatic failure
  - Renal failure
  - Myasthenia gravis

4. **Hoffman's elimination is seen with:**

A. Atracurium B. Pancuronium
C. Suxamethonium D. Rocuronium

Ans: A. Atracurium

Ref: Miller text book of Anaesthesia. 6th edition.

Explanation

Atracurium

- **Atracurium and cisatracurium** (stereoisomer of atracurium) are the only two drugs metabolized by **Hoffman elimination**
- Atracurium is a **short acting non-depolarizing neuromuscular blocker**
- Atracurium is metabolized by **Non-specific esterases & Hoffman's elimination, independent of renal and hepatic metabolism**
- Hence **Drug of choice in hepatic and renal failure**

Hoffman's elimination

- It is the **spontaneous non-enzymatic chemical breakdown** at physiologic PH and temperature
- Hoffman's elimination of atracurium gives a metabolite called **laudanosine** which can precipitate **seizures**
- It **triggers the release of histamine** leading to **hypotension, tachycardia & bronchospasm**
- Dosage – 0.5mg/kg *(See table on the next page)*

5. **Anaesthetic agent which can cause massive hepatic necrosis?**

A. Halothane B. Isoflurane
C. Methoxyflurane D. N 2 O

Ans: A. Halothane

	Atracurium	Cisatracurium (stereoisomer of Atracurium)
Potency	Less	More
Non specific ester hydrolysis	Yes	No
Hoffman elimination	Yes	Yes
Metabolite - Laudanosine		
Quantity produced	More	Less
CNS toxicity seizures	Yes	No
Histamine release	Yes	No

Ref: Miller text book of Anaesthesia. 6th edition.

Explanation

Halothane- Effects of Halothane

- **CVS**: Myocardial depression, hypotension
- **RS**: respiratory depression & apnea
- **Hepatic: Halothane hepatitis**
- **Centrilobular necrosis** can occur rarely because of an **immune mediated mechanism** triggered by the **metabolite of halothane** called **trifluroacetic acid**
- Halothane administered in frequent intervals leads to hepatic dysfunction in the post-operative period

Nitrous oxide

- **Nitrous oxide can diffuse into cavities faster than air**, hence dangerous in intestinal obstruction, pneumothorax and air embolism
- Prolonged exposure can cause **megaloblastic anemia and neurological deficiencies**
- Avoided in pregnancy because of possible **teratogenic effects**

Methoxyflurane

- Methoxyflurane leads to **high output renal failure**

6. **Ventilator breath dyssynchrony is maximum with which mode of ventilation?**

A. CMV **B.** CPAP
C. SIMV **D.** PSV

Ans: A. CMV

Ref: Miller text book of Anaesthesia. 6th edition.

Explanation

CMV – Controlled mandatory ventilation

- Here all the breaths are delivered by the ventilator. Hence suitable for patients who are not breathing.
- If patients on this mode start breathing, there will be stacking of patient & ventilator breaths causing dyssynchrony
- This mode is commonly used to ventilate the paralyzed patients during general anesthesia

CPAP- Continuous positive airway pressure

- Here the patient breathes spontaneously and their breaths are only supported by positive pressure by the ventilator thus decreasing the work of breathing

SIMV – Synchronized intermittent mandatory ventilation

- Here the ventilator synchronizes its mandatory breaths with the patient efforts

PSV – Pressure support ventilation

- Here the ventilator supports the patient's spontaneous breaths.

7. **Anesthetic not impairing CNS activity is:**

A. Isoflurane **B.** Enflurane
C. Ketamine **D.** Desflurane

Ans: A. Isoflurane

Ref: Miller text book of Anaesthesia. 6th edition.

Explanation:

Isoflurane

- Raise in intracranial pressure is minimal with isoflurane when compared with other inhalational agents and this rise can be reversed with hyperventilation
- It also decreases brain oxygen consumption.
- These properties make isoflurane the ***agent of choice*** for ***neurosurgical procedures***

Other characteristics of Isoflurane

- Pungent ethereal odor, so induction is not smooth
- Not a good analgesic
- Moderate muscle relaxation
- **Cardiovascular Effects**
  - **Hypotension is maximum** with isoflurane (Agent of choice for controlled hypotension)
  - It does not depress myocardium
  - Does not cause bradycardia and baroreceptor reflex is preserved
  - It increases coronary blood flow to non-ischemic area which in patients with myocardial ischemia can cause **CORONARY STEAL**
- Respiratory system effects
  - Respiratory depression is relatively less
  - It blunts ventilatory response to hypercarbia and hypoxia

- Isoflurane is agent of choice for **Cardiac patients** and **Neurosurgery**

RADIODIAGNOSIS

1. Investigation of choice for pulmonary embolism is: (Repeat)

A. CT angiography
B. Contrast enhanced MRI
C. Pulmonary angiography
D. Echocardiography

Ans: A. CT angiography

Ref: *Harrison's Principles of internal medicine. 18th edition.*

Explanation:

*"Computed tomography of the chest with intravenous contrast is the **principal imaging test** for the diagnosis of PE" (Ref: Harrison)*

- **CT angiography** is the **investigatin of choice** for the diagnosis of **Pulomary Embolism**
- Multidetector-row spiral CT acquires all chest images with 1 mm of resolution during a short breath hold.
- Sixth-order branches can be visualized with resolution superior to that of conventional invasive contrast pulmonary angiography.
- The CT scan also obtains excellent images of the RV and LV and can be used for risk stratification along with its use as a diagnostic tool.
- In patients with PE, **RV enlargement** on chest CT indicates an increased likelihood of death within the next 30 days compared with PE patients who have normal RV size on chest CT.
- When imaging is continued below the chest to the knee, pelvic and proximal **leg DVT** also can be diagnosed by CT scanning.

2. Best investigation to see calcification is:

A. CT **B.** MRI
C. X-ray **D.** USG

Ans: A. CT ?

Ref: *Harrison's Principles of internal medicine. 18th edition.*

Explanation:

- **CT** is the best technique to detect **pericardial calcification**; however, overpenetrated films, conventional tomography, fluoroscopy, and MRI may be helpful.
- Plain radiographs have **poor sensitivity** for detection of coronary calcification and have a reported accuracy as low as 42%
- **High-quality mammography** is the best diagnostic tool for the **identification of breast calcifications.**

3. In chest radiograph, the right border of mediastinum is formed by all *except:*

A. SVC
B. Right atrium
C. Right Ventricle
D. Right brachiocephalic vein

Ans: C. Right Ventricle

Ref: *Cardiac X-rays by V. Chockalingam & A. Chockalingam. 1st edition. Elsevier. 2008. Page10*

Explanation:

In PA view

The right cardiac border is formed above by

- Superior vena cava
- Right atrium
- Sometimes Small portion of Ascending aorta (which contributes to right cardiac border between superior vena cava and right atrium , especially above 40 years)
- Rarely Inferior Vena cava (which forms a shadow at right costophrenic angle in 10 % patients)

The left cardiac border is formed from above by

- Aortic knuckle
- Pulmonary bay
- Small portion of left atrial appendage
- Left ventricle

Also note

- Aortic knuckle corresponds to the junction of arch and descending aorta
- Pulmonary bay is concave and the most constricted portion of cardiac shadow known as cardiac waist. It is occupied by main pulmonary artery and proximal left pulmonary artery.
- Left ventricle forms major portion of left cardiac border. It is smooth and convex.
- Right ventricle does not form border in postero-anterior view.

In lateral view

Anterior border is formed from above downwards by

- Ascending aorta
- Pulmonary artery
- Right ventricle

Normally there is 3 - 5 mm clear retrosternal space

Posterior border is formed by the following structures

- Pulmonary artery
- Left atrium
- Left ventricle from above downwards

4. **In a child with coarcation of aorta, all the following are seen in plain chest radiograph *except:***
   A. Rib notching
   B. Three sign
   C. 'E' Sign or 'Reverse Three sign'
   D. Prominent ascending aorta

Ans: C. 'E' Sign or 'Reverse Three sign'

Ref: *Cardiac X-rays by V. Chockalingam & A. Chockalingam. 1st edition. Elsevier. 2008. Page 99.*

Explanation:

'E' Sign or 'Reverse Three sign' is feature of coarctation, but seen in barium swallow, not in plain chest radiograph.

Features of Coarctation of Aorta

- Left ventricular configuration
- Prominent ascending aorta due to hypertension and bucuspid aortic valve
- **'Three sign':** The upper convexity is due to pre-stenotic dilatation and the lower convexity is due to post-stenotic dilatation. The mid portion represents the coarcted segment
- **'E' Sign or 'Reverse Three sign':** Seen in barium swallow due above aortic shadows
- **Rib notching:** Bilateral rib notching is seen between the third and eighth posterior ribs along its lower border usually after the age of 9 years.
- **Unilateral rib notching**: A feature of coarctation, if it involves the origin of the left subclavian artery also.

Differential diagnosis for rib-notching

- Rib notching is also seen in the following conditions
- Chronic superior vena cava obstruction
- Chronic inferior vena cava obstruction
- Aortoarteritis in rare occasion
- Intercostal neurofibromatosis
- Intercostal arteriovenous malformations
- Post Blalock-Tausig shunt

PSYCHIATRY

1. **Neuroleptic malignant syndrome is treated with:**
   A. Dantrolene B. Corticosteroids
   C. Diazepam D. Hemodialysis

Ans: A. Dantrolene

Ref: *A Short Textbook of Psychiatry by Niraj Ahuja, 7th edition. 2011. JAYPEE.*

Explanation:

NEUROLEPTIC MALIGNANT SYNDROME

- It is a life-threatening neurological disorder most often caused by an adverse reaction to neuroleptic or antipsychotic drugs.
- NMS typically consists of muscle rigidity, fever, autonomic instability and cognitive changes such as delirium, and is associated with elevated plasma creatine phosphokinase

Presentation: Fairly rare & potentially **life-threatening** condition

- Increased body temperature >38°C
- Confused or altered consciousness
- Diaphoresis "sweat shock"
- Rigid muscles
- Autonomic imbalance
- Muscular rigidity, Hyperthermia, autonomic instability & Delirium
- Associated with high dosages of high-potency APMs

Diagnosis: Increased CPK levels

Treatment

- Discontinuation of the medication
- Physiologic supportive measures (ICU)
- ***Dantrolene*** or ***Bromocriptine*** may be used

2. **Impulsivity, angry outbursts, unstable relationships, deliberate self harm & suicidal tendencies are characteristic of:**
   A. Narcissitic personality disorder
   B. Schizoid personality
   C. Borderline personality
   D. Schizotypal PD

Ans: C. Borderline personality

Ref: *A short textbook of Psychiatry by Niraj Ahuja*

Explanation:

Personality disorders (PD)

Cluster A (Odd & Eccentric)

a. ***Paranoid PD***
- Excessive sensitiveness to setbacks & rebuffs
- Tendency to bear grudges persistently
- Suspiciousness
- Combative and tenacious sense of personal rights
- Excessive self-importance
- Preoccupation with unsubstantiated 'conspiratorial' claims

b. ***Schizoid PD***

- Emotional coldness, detachment
- Limited capacity to express feelings
- Apparent indifference to either praise or criticism
- Preference for solitary activities
- Lack of of close friends & relationships

c. ***Schizotypal PD***
- Inappropriate or constricted affect
- Odd, eccentric or peculiar behaviour or appearance
- Poor rapport & Social withdrawal
- Odd beliefs or magical thinking
- Suspiciouness & paranoid ideas

Cluster B (Dramatic, emotional & Erratic)

d. ***Anti-social PD***
- Callous unconcern for the feelings for others
- Disregard for social norms, rules and obligations
- Incapacity to maintain relationships
- Low tolerance to frustration, aggression & violence

e. ***Histrionic PD***
- Self-dramatization, exaggerated expression of emotions
- Easily influenced by others
- Shallow & Labile affectivity
- Attention seeking
- Excessive importance to physical appearance

f. ***Narcissistic PD***
- Inflated self importance & ideas of grandiosity
- Preoccupation with fantasies of unlimited success
- Attention seeking, dramatic behaviour, needs constant praise
- Lack of empathy, exploitative behaviour
- Shaky self-esteem & inferiority

g. ***Borderline PD***
- Significant disturbance of identity of self
- Unstable & intense interpersonal relationships
- Impulsivity, angry outbursts
- Deliberate self harm & suicidal tendencies

Cluster C (Anxious & Fearful)

h. ***Avoidant PD***
- Persistent feelings of tension & apprehension
- Belief that one is unappealing & inferior to others
- Unwillingness to become involved with people
- Restrictions in lifestyle
- Avoidance of social activities

i. ***Dependent PD***
- Allowing others to make important decisions in one's life
- Subordination & undue compliance
- Exaggerated fears of inability to care for oneself
- Limited capacity to make everyday decisions

j. ***Obsessive compulsive (Anankastic) PD***
- Feelings of excessive doubt & Caution
- Preoccupation with details, rules, lists, order organisation or schedule
- Perfectionism that interferes with task completion
- Rigidity & stubbornness

3. True regarding Delirium are all *except:*

A. Acute onset
B. Sleep disturbance
C. Myoclonus
D. Normal consciousness

Ans: D. Normal consciousness

Ref: *A Short Textbook of Psychiatry by Niraj Ahuja, 7th edition. 2011. Jaypee. Page 22.*

Explanation:

Clouding of consciousness is a characteristic of Delirium

DELIRIUM

- Most commen organic disorder seen in clinical practice
- Delirium is characterized by the following
  - Acute onset
  - Clouding of consciousness
  - Disorientation
  - Decreased attention span
  - Distractibility
  - Marked perceptual disturbances
  - Insomnia at night with daytime drowsiness
  - Worsening of symptoms in evening and night (**Sun downing)**
  - Impairment of registration and retention of new memories
  - Psychomotor disturbances – agitation & retardation
  - **Autonomic dysfunction**
  - Speech disturbances – slurring of speech, incoherence, dysarthria
  - **Fleeting delusions**
  - **Motor symptoms** – asterixis, mutifocal myoclonus, carphologia, floccillation (Picking movements at coversheets & clothes)

- **Occupational delirium** (elaborate pantomimes as if continuing the usual occupation in a hospital bed)

4. **Contraindication for electroconvulsive therapy:**

   A. 1st trimester Pregnancy **B.** Elderly
   C. Raised ICT **D.** Catatonia

   Ans: C. Raised ICT

   ***Ref**: A Short Textbook of Psychiatry by Niraj Ahuja, 7th edition. 2011. Jaypee. (Ref: Miller LJ. Use of electroconvulsive therapy during pregnancy. Hosp Community Psychiatry 1994: 45 (5): 444–50*

Explanation:

ECT is generally considered safe during pregnancy. *"ECT is generally accepted to be relatively **safe** during all trimesters of **pregnancy**, particularly when compared to pharmacological treatments" (Miller LJ article)*

Electroconvulsive Therapy (ECT)

- Induction of a grand mal seizure lasting for atleast 15 seconds using an electrical pulse through brain under general anesthesia
- Exact mechanism of action is not known

Indications:

- Depression refractory to adequate drug therapy
- High suicide risk
- Medical risk in addition to depression (dehydration, electrolytes, pregnancy)
- Previous good response to ECT
- Familial response to ECT
- Elderly
- Psychotic depression
- Catatonic features
- Marked vegetative features
- Acute schizophrenia
- Mania unresponsive to medications

Side effects:

- Risk of anesthesia
- Memory loss (may be retrograde and/or anterograde
- Tends to resolve by 6 to 9 months, permanent impairment controversial), headaches,
- Myalgias

Contraindications: Increased intracranial pressure

5. **Wernicke's encephalopathy occurs due to the deficiency of: (Repeat)**

   A. Thiamine **B.** Riboflavin
   C. Folate **D.** Vitamin B12

   Ans: A. Thiamine

   ***Ref:** Synopsis of psychiatry, Kaplan & Sadock, 10th edition.p.400.*

Explanation:

Wernicke's encephalopathy

- It is a condition which is **acute in onset** (cf. Korsakoff psychosis is **insidious**)
- It is characterized by the triad

1. **Confusion** (delirium tremens)
2. **Ataxia** (in-coordination of movements)
3. **Nystagmus** (due to **ophthalmoplegia** and / or vestibular dysfunction). [CAN- the Mnemonic]

- Chronic alcohol intake depletes **thiamine** (Vitamin B1) by various mechanisms.
- During acute intoxication, such deficiency results in degeneration of paraventricular regions of brain (**mammillary bodies, thalamus** and **hypothalamus**).
- The treatment is **'THIAMINE'** IV **250-500 mg/** day as slow infusion for first five days, followed by oral route (100 mg tds) for at least 15 days.
- It is **reversible** if treated early.
- Otherwise, the condition progresses into "**Korsakoff's psychosis**", which is characterized by **amnesia** (both **anterograde & retrograde**) [declarative memory deficit], **confabulation** (to fill up the gaps in memory), **apathy** & **lack of insight**.
- Less than 20% only respond to thiamine and often need as long as two years to show moderate improvement.

Other neuropsychiatric disorders due to alcohol are:

- Cerebellar degeneration,
- Central Pontine Myelinosis &
- Corpus callosum demyelination (Marchiafava-Bignami disease).

Riboflavin deficiency

- Mucositis (Chelitis, Stomatitis, Glossitis)
- Dermatitis (Seborrheic)
- Normochromic, normocytic anemia.

Folate deficiency - Depression.

Vitamin B12

- Depression & Psychosis (both folate and Vit.B12 cause mental disorders either directly or by increasing homocysteine levels in brain).

JIPMER-2007

ANATOMY

1. **Bulbourethral glands in males develops from:**
   A. Urogenital sinus **B.** Mesonephric duct
   C. Paromesonephric duct **D.** Phallus

   Ans: A. Urogenital sinus

   Ref: *Grays Anatomy 40th edition pg: 1305*

   Explanation: *(See the following table)*

2. **True regarding trigeminal nerve:**
   A. Supplies muscles of mastication
   B. Sensation of neck
   C. Mandibular division of trigeminal nerve supply angle of mandible
   D. Mandibular division of trigeminal nerve pass through foramen rotundum

   Ans: A. Supplies muscles of mastication

   Ref:*Grays Anatomy 40th edition pg: 535*

   Explanation:

   - **The mandibular nerve** is the largest trigeminal division and is a mixed nerve.
   - **Sensory supply**
     – Teeth and gums of the mandible
     – Skin in the temporal region
     – Part of the auricle – including the external meatus and tympanic membrane
     – Lower lip
     – Lower part of the face
     – Mucosa of the anterior two-thirds (presulcal part) of the tongue
     – Mucosa of the floor of the oral cavity

Embryology of Reproductive System

Gonad	MALES (Testis)	FEMALES (Ovary)
Gubernacular cord	Gubernaculum testis	Ovarian and round ligaments
Mesonephros (Wolffian body)	Appendix of epididymis (?)	Appendices vesiculosae (?)
	Efferent ductules	Epoöphoron
	Lobules of epididymis	
	Paradidymis	Paroöphoron
	Aberrant ductules	
Mesonephric duct (Wolffian duct)	Duct of epididymis	Duct of epoöphoron (Gartner's duct)
	Vas deferens	
	Ejaculatory duct	
	Part of bladder and prostatic urethra	Part of bladder and urethra
Paramesonephric duct (Müllerian)	Appendix of testis	Uterine tube
		Uterus
	Prostatic utricle	Vagina
Allantoic duct	Urachus	Urachus
Cloaca:		
Dorsal part	Rectum and upper part of anal canal	Rectum and upper part of anal canal
Ventral part	Most of bladder	Most of bladder and urethra
	Part of prostatic urethra	
Urogenital sinus	Prostatic urethra distal to utricle	
	Bulbo-urethral glands	Greater vestibular glands
	Rest of urethra to glans	Vestibule
Genital folds	Ventral penis	Labia minora
Genital tubercle	Penis	Clitoris
	Urethra in glans	
Genital ridge	Testis	Ovary
Genital swelling	Scrotum	Labia majora

- **Motor Supply** - The muscles of **mastication.**
- The ***large sensory root*** emerges from the lateral part of the trigeminal ganglion and exits the cranial cavity through the ***foramen ovale.***
- The ***small motor root*** passes under the ganglion and through the ***foramen ovale*** to unite with the sensory root just outside the skull.
- The mandibular nerve immediately passes between tensor velipalatini, which is medial, and lateral pterygoid, which is lateral, and gives off a meningeal branch and the nerve to medial pterygoid from its medial side.
- The nerve then divides into a ***small anterior*** and ***large posterior*** trunk.
- The ***anterior division*** gives off branches to the ***four main muscles of mastication*** and a ***buccal branch*** which is ***sensory*** to the ***cheek***.
- The ***posterior division*** gives off three main sensory branches, the ***auriculotemporal***, ***lingual*** and ***inferior alveolar nerves***, and ***motor*** fibres to supply ***mylohyoid***and the ***anterior belly of digastric***.

3. **Angle formed by the shaft and the neck of the femur is ___ degrees.**

A. 115 **B.** 125
C. 135 **D.** 145

Ans: B. 125

Ref: *Grays Anatomy 40th Ed pg .1349*

Explanation:

Femoral Neck Angle:

- Neck extends inferolaterally from head to meet shaft of femur at angle of about **125 deg**
- Angle varies with **age, stature, & width of pelvis**, being less in adult, in persons with short limbs, and in women
- When this angle **is > 135 deg - Coxa valga**
- When < 120 deg - **Coxa vara**
- Femoral neck is not parallel to frontal plane or plane of femur
- Head is located anterior to midline of shaft of femur and is thus said to be anteverted
(See the following figure)

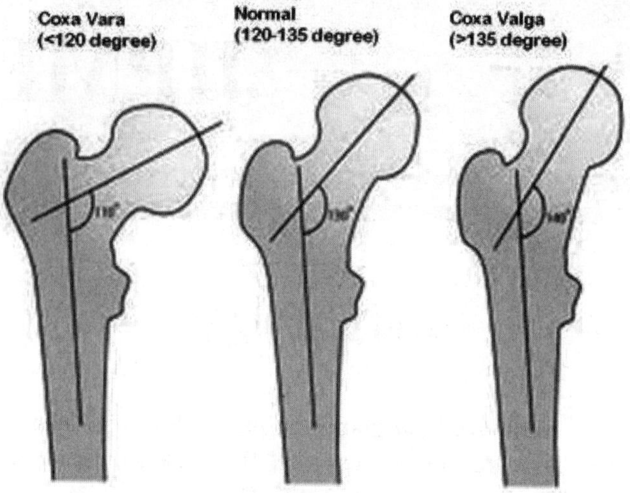

4. **All the following are Secondary lymphoid organs *except:***

A. Spleen **B.** Lymph node
C. Bone marrow **D.** MALT

Ans: C. Bone marrow

Ref: *Grays Anatomy 40th Ed pg .127*

Explanation:

Organs of the Immune System:

- The immune system is made up of many different organs and tissues dispersed throughout the body.
- **PRIMARY lymphoid organs** are the sites of **lymphocyte birth, maturation**, in an Antigen independent fashion.
- **SECONDARY lymphoid organs** are the sites of mature lymphocyte selection and expansion in an Antigen dependent fashion.

Primary Lymphoid Tissues:

- Generate and/or mature and educate cells of the immune system
- Maturation and central selection
- Diversity created in an Antigen independent fashion

Bone Marrow—————— B cells
Thymus—————— T cells

Secondary Lymphoid Tissues:

- Site where mature, immunocompetent lymphocytes are exposed to Antigen
- Ag is collected and brought to tissue and lymphocytes are exposed to Antigen.
  - **Lymph nodes**— Antigen from intracellular tissue fluids
  - **Spleen** ——— blood-borne Antigen
  - **MALT** ——— Antigen from mucosal surfaces. Includes Peyer's patches, tonsils, and adenoids

5. **Internal anal sphincter is formed by:**

A. Puborectalis
B. Circular muscle fibres
C. Longitudinal muscle fibres
D. Deep peroneal muscle

Ref: *Grays Anatomy 40th edition*

Ans: C. Longitudinal muscle fibres

Explanation:

Internal anal sphincter

- The internal anal sphincter is a **well-defined ring** of **obliquely orientated smooth muscle** fibres that is continuous with the circular muscle of the rectum, and which terminates at the junction of the superficial and subcutaneous components of the external sphincter.
- Its thickness varies between **1.5 and 3.5 mm**, depending upon the height within the anal canal and whether the canal is distended.
- It is usually **thinner in females** and becomes thicker with age.
- It may also be **thickened** in disease processes such as **rectal prolapse** and **chronic constipation.**
- The lower portion of the sphincter is **crossed by fibres** from the conjoint longitudinal coat which passes into the submucosa of the lower canal.

External anal sphincter

- The external anal sphincter is an **oval tube-shaped complex** of striated muscle, composed mainly of type 1 (slow twitch) skeletal muscle fibres, which are well suited to prolonged contraction.
- Endoanal ultrasound and magnetic resonance imaging reveal that the uppermost fibres blend with the **lowest fibres** of **puborectalis.**
- In the **upper third** some of these upper fibres decussate anteriorly into the **superficial transverse perineal muscles** and **posteriorly** some fibres are attached to the **anococcygeal raphe.**
- The majority of the fibres of the middle third of the external anal sphincter surround the lower part of the internal sphincter.
- The **middle third** is attached **anteriorly** to the **perineal body** and **posteriorly** to the **coccyx** via the **anococcygeal ligament**: some fibres from each side of the sphincter decussate in these areas to form a commissure in the anterior and posterior midline.
- The fibres of the lower third lie below the level of the internal anal sphincter and are separated from the lowest anal epithelium by submucosa.

6. **Tongue is protruded by which of the following muscle: (Repeat)**

A. Hyoglossus **B.** Palatoglossus
C. Myelohyoid **D.** Genioglossus

Ans: D. Genioglossus

Ref: Grays Anatomy 40th Ed pg.499

Explanation:

- **Genioglossus** is a **extrinsic muscle** of the tongue
- It forms the bulk of the tongue muscle and **traversed by intrinsic muscles of tongue**
- It arises from a **short tendon** attached to the **superior genial tubercle** behind the **mandibular symphysis**
- From this point it fans out backwards and upwards .
- It is also called as **safety muscle of the tongue** due to it **prevents the fall back of the tongue**
- Vascular supply -Genioglossus is supplied by the **sublingual branch** of the **lingual artery** and the submental branch of the facial artery.
- Innervation - Genioglossus is innervated by the **hypoglossal nerve.**
- Actions
  1. Brings about the **forward traction** of the tongue to **protrude its apex** from the mouth.
  2. Acting bilaterally, the two muscles depress the central part of the tongue, making it concave from side to side.
  3. Acting **unilaterally**, the tongue **diverges to the opposite side.**

7. **Which of the following joint is a syndesmosis? (Repeat)**

A. Superior Tibiofibular joint
B. Inferior tibiofibular joint
C. Talocalcaneal joint
D. Calcaneocuboid joint

Ans: B. Inferior tibiofibular joint

Ref: Grays Anatomy 40th Ed Pg 101

Explanation:

Syndesmosis

- It is a type of ***fibrous*** joint.
- It may be represented by an ***interosseous ligament.***
- Such ligament persist throughout life
- ***Slight movement*** is possible
- Example :
  - Inferior tibio fibular joint
  - Interosseous membranes of the forearm and leg
  - Ligament flava

Function

- Responsible for integrity of ankle mortis

Physical Exam

- Test to identify a syndesmosis injury include
- External rotation test
- Squeeze test

Imaging

- AP and mortise ankle radiographs
- Used to evaluate the tibiofibular clear space and tibiofibular overlap
- ***Tibiofibular clear space*** shoulde be < ***5 mm***
- ***Tibiofibular overlap*** for AP view > ***10 mm***
- ***Weight bearing mortise view*** is most accurate for diagnosis

Clinical conditions

- High ankle sprain & syndesmosis injury
- Ankle fracture

8. **All of the following are features of flat type of pelvis *except:* (Repeat)**
   A. Narrow subpubic angle
   B. Short concave sacrum
   C. Divergent side walls
   D. Wide sciatic notch

Ans: A. Narrow subpubic angle

Ref: Grays Anatomy 40th Ed pg.1329

Explanation:

- All pelvic measurements display individual variation and the values quoted are means from limited surveys.
- Sexual and racial differences also occur.
- Many attempts to classify human pelves, especially female.
- The four most common terms used today are gynaecoid, anthropoid, platypelloid and android.

Gynaecoid

- The gynaecoid pelvis is the traditional Western female pelvis with a heart-shaped brim and the range of measurements quoted above.

Anthropoid pelvis

- An anthropoid pelvis has a larger midcavity and a wide anteroposterior inlet which is oval in shape
- It is more common in women of African origin and may be associated with a 'high assimilation' pelvis where there is an additional lumbar vertebra.

Platypelloid pelvis

- A platypelloid pelvis is flat and oval from side to side at the brim
- it is a contracted pelvis that is rarely seen nowadays, having previously been associated with rickets.

Android pelvis

- An android pelvis has a triangular brim and is the shape of a male pelvis.

9. **A lesion involving the C8 nerve root will affect:**
   A. Extensors of fingers and wrist
   B. Flexors of fingers and wrist
   C. Small muscles of hand
   D. None of above

Ans: B. Flexors of fingers and wrist

Ref: Grays Anatomy 40th Ed pg.791

Explanation:

Lateral cord

- Lateral pectoral - C5, 6, 7
- Musculocutaneous - C5, 6 7
- Lateral root of median - C(5), 6, 7

Medial cord

- Medial pectoral - C8, T1
- Medial cutaneous of forearm - C8, T1
- Medial cutaneous of arm - C8, T1
- Ulnar - C(7), 8, T1
- Medial root of median - C8, T1

Posterior cord

- Upper subscapular - C5, 6
- Thoracodorsal - C6, 7,8
- Lower subscapular - C5, 6
- Axillary - C5, 6
- Radial - C5, 6, 7, 8, (T1)

Klumpke's paralysis

- Upward traction on the arm, e.g. in a forcible breech delivery, may tear the lowest root, T1, which provides the segmental supply to the intrinsic muscles of the hand.
- The hand assumes a **clawed appearance** reflecting the unopposed action of the long flexors and extensors of the fingers
- There is **sensory loss along the medial aspect of the forearm** and there is often an associated **Horner's syndrome** (ptosis and constriction of the pupil) which occurs as a result of traction on the cervical sympathetic chain.

Malignant infiltration of the brachial plexus

- It may result from extension of an apical lung carcinoma (Pancoast tumour) or from metastatic spread, often from carcinoma of the breast.
- There is slowly progressive weakness which usually starts in the small muscles of the hand (T1) and spreads to involve the finger flexors (C8).

- This is usually a painful condition, and the pain may be severe.
- There is sensory loss on the medial aspect of the forearm (T1) extending into the medial side of the hand and to the little finger (C8).

Thoracic outlet syndrome

- The lower trunk of the brachial plexus **(C8, T1),** together with the subclavian artery, may be angulated over a cervical rib
- Patients may present with **vascular symptoms** as a result of **kinking of the subclavian artery** and they may present with **neurological deficit**

Cervical ribs

- Cervical ribs are quite common and are rarely associated with symptoms.
- There is a slow insidious onset of wasting of the small muscles of the hand, which often starts on the lateral side with involvement of the thenar eminence and first dorsal interosseous.
- There is **pain** and **paraesthesiae** in the medial aspect of the forearm extending to the little finger, and this is often aggravated by carrying shopping or suitcases.
- A **bruit may be heard over the subclavian artery**, and the **radial pulse may be easily obliterated** by movements of the arm, particularly with the arm extended and abducted at the shoulder.

10. Dorsal scapular nerve supplies:

A. Levator scapulae and rhomboids
B. Supraspinatus and infra spinatus
C. Lattismus dorsi
D. Serratus anterior

Ans: A. Levator scapulae and rhomboids

Ref: Grays Anatomy 40th Ed pg 791

Explanation:

Dorsal scapular nerve

- It is also called as **nerve to rhomboids**
- It araises from the **root C5**
- It pierces **scalenus medius**, passes **behind levator scapulae**, which it **occasionally supplies**, and runs with the deep branch of the **dorsal scapular artery** to the rhomboids, which it supplies.

11. Long head of biceps atttached to:

A. Coracoid process
B. Supraglenoid tubercle
C. Acromion process
D. Bicipital groove

Ans: B. Supraglenoid tubercle

Ref: Grays Anatomy 40th Ed

Explanation:

- Biceps brachii has two head-long head & short head
- **Long head** orginate from **supraglenoid tubercle**
- **Short head** orginate from **coracoid process**
- **Biceps tendon** inserted into the **radial tuberosity**
- The muscle is innervated by **musculo cutaneous nerve**
- The action of the muscles are **flexion** and **supinator**

12. All the following muscles are innervated by oculomotor nerve *except:*

A. Superior rectus **B.** Inferior rectus
C. Superior oblique **D.** Medial rectus

Ans: C. Superior oblique

Ref: Grays Anatomy 40th Ed Pg 655

Explanation:

- Remember: **LR6 & SO4**
- **Lateral rectus** supplied by **6th** Cranial nerve - **Abducens** nerve
- **Superior oblique** supplied by **4th** cranial nerve - **Trochlear** nerve
- **All other extraocular muscles** are supplied by **Oculomotor nerve**
- Oculomotor Nerve also supplies **Levator palpebrae superioris** (muscle that elevates the upper eyelid)

13. With foot off the ground and knee flexed, medial rotation of tibia is brought about by

A. Popliteus **B.** Gastrocnemius
C. Vastus medialis **D.** Adductor magnus

Ans: A. Popliteus

Ref: Grays Anatomy 40th Ed pg 1393

Explanation:

- **Popliteus** rotates the **tibia medially** on the **femur** or, **when the tibia is fixed,** rotates the **femur laterally on the tibia.**
- It is usually regarded as the muscle that **'unlocks'** the joint at the beginning of flexion of the fully extended knee: electromyography supports this view.
- Its connection with the **arcuate popliteal ligament**, fibrous capsule and lateral meniscus has led to the suggestion that popliteus may

retract the posterior horn of the lateral meniscus during lateral rotation of the femur and flexion of the knee joint, thus protecting the meniscus from being crushed between the femur and the tibia during these movements.

- The muscle is markedly active in crouching, perhaps to provide stability as the tibia rotates internally during flexion of the knee.
- However, the main function is likely to be provision of dynamic stability to the posterolateral part of the knee by preventing excessive external rotation of the tibia, partly by its direct action, but more significantly by tensing the popliteofibular ligament.

Testing

- Popliteus plays a part in **medially rotating the leg** when the knee is **flexed** and **non-weightbearing**, but its individual actions cannot be isolated clinically.
- Damage to the **popliteus complex** of ligament and tendon is manifest as **excessive external rotation of the tibia** on the **femur at 90°** and **especially at 30° of knee flexion.**, reflecting the function of the popliteus complex as a 'static tether'.

14. Which is not a branch of facial nerve?

A. Chorda tympani
B. Lingual nerve
C. Greater superficial petrosal nerve
D. Branch to stylohyoid muscle

Ans: B. Lingual nerve

Ref: *Grays Anatomy 40th Ed*

Explanation:

- **Lingual nerve** arises from **mandibular branch** of **trigeminal nerve**

Braches of Facial Nerve

A. Intra cranial branches

- **Greater petrosal nerve** –
- **Nerve to stapedius** -
- **Chorda tympani**
  - Submandibular gland
  - Sublingual gland
  - Special sensory taste fibers for the anterior 2/3 of the tongue.

B. Extra cranial branches

Distal to stylomastoid foramen, the following nerves branch off the facial nerve:

- **Posterior auricular nerve** -
- Branch to **Posterior belly of Digastric muscle** and **Stylohyoid muscle**
- **Five major facial branches** (in **parotid** gland)
  - **Temporal** branch of the facial nerve
  - **Zygomatic** branch of the facial nerve
  - **Buccal** branch of the facial nerve
  - **Marginal mandibular** branch of the facial nerve
  - **Cervical** branch of the facial nerve

PHYSIOLOGY

1. In plasma, carbon-di-oxide is mainly transported as: (Repeat)

A. Dissolved CO_2
B. HCO_3^-
C. Carboxy haemoglobin
D. Carbamino haemoglobin

Ans: B. HCO_3^-

Ref: *Pal GK. Transport of gases in blood. In: Textbook of medical physiology. Ahuja publishing house. 2007; 91: 733.*

Explanation:

Carbon Dioxide Transport in Blood

1. HCO_3^- in plasma and in RBCs – 70%
2. Formation of carbamino compounds with plasma protein (23%)
3. Dissolved form (7%)

2. Hardy-Weinberg law is used to predict inheritance of which of the following type (Repeat)

A. Autosomal dominant **B.** Autosomal recessive
C. X-linked dominant **D.** X-linked recessive

Ans: ?

Ref: *Internet Sources*

Explanation:

Hardy–Weinberg Principle

- Also known as the Hardy–Weinberg equilibrium, model, theorem, or law
- It states that allele and genotype frequencies in a population will remain constant from generation to generation in the absence of other evolutionary influences.
- These influences include:
  - Non-random mating
  - Mutation
  - Selection
  - Genetic drift
  - Gene flow
  - Meiotic drive.
- Since one or more of these influences are typically present in real populations, the Hardy–

Weinberg principle describes an ideal condition against which the effects of these influences can be analyzed.

3. Blood flow changes are least during exercise in:

A. Brain **B.** Heart
C. Skin **D.** Kidney

Ans: A. Brain

Ref: *Pal GK. Physiology of Exercise and sports science. In: Textbook of medical physiology. Ahuja publishing house. 2007; 140: 1019.*

Explanation:

Redistribution of blood during exercise

Organ	Blood flow during exercise
Visceral	↓ 80%
Cutaneous	↓, later increased
Cerebral	No change
Coronary	↑ 4-5 fold (symp Vd, local metabolites)
To adipose tissue	↑ 4 fold

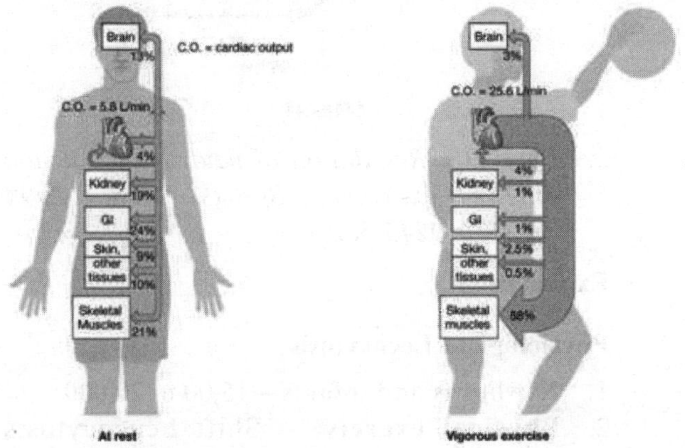

4. The main fuel used by brain, during starvation is: (Repeat)

A. Free fatty acids **B.** Amino acids
C. Glucose **D.** Ketone body

Ans: D. Ketone body

Ref: *Guyton & Hall. Dietary Balances; Regulation of Feeding; Obesity and Starvation; Vitamins and Minerals. In: Textbook of Medical Physiology.12th ed. Philadelphia: Saunders Elsevier; 2012. p 852*

Explanation:

- The **ketone bodies**, like **glucose**, can cross the **blood-brain barrier** and can be used by the brain cells for energy.
- About **two thirds of the brain's energy**, during **starvation**, is derived from **ketone bodies**(esp. **beta-hydroxybutyrate**)

5. Which of the following sensations is not converging on thalamus?

A. Smell **B.** Fine touch
C. Hearing **D.** Vision

Ans: ? None of the above

Ref:

1. *Guyton & Hall. The Chemical Senses-Taste and Smell. In: Textbook of Medical Physiology.12th ed. Philadelphia: Saunders Elsevier; 2012. p 651.*
2. *Kandel ER, Schwartz JH, Jessell TM. Smell and Taste: The Chemical Senses. In: Principles of Neural Science, 4th ed. New York: McGraw-Hill; 2000. p 632-633.*
3. *W F Ganong. Cutaneous, deep & visceral sensation. In: Review of Medical Physiology. 21st ed. California: McGraw-Hill Companies; 2003. p. 141.*
4. *Kandel ER, Schwartz JH, Jessell TM. Smell and Taste: The Chemical Senses. In: Principles of Neural Science, 4th ed. New York: McGraw-Hill; 2000. p 641.*
5. *W F Ganong. Central and Peripheral Neurophysiology: Hearing & Equilibrium. In: Review of Medical Physiology. 24th ed. California: McGraw-Hill Companies; 2012. p. 208.*
6. *W F Ganong. Central and Peripheral Neurophysiology: Vision. In: Review of Medical Physiology. 24th ed. California: McGraw-Hill Companies; 2012. p. 189.*

Explanation:

- A ***newer olfactory pathway that passes through the thalamus***, passing to the dorsomedial thalamic nucleus and then to the lateroposterior quadrant of the orbitofrontale cortex, has been found
- On the basis of studies in monkeys, this newer system probably helps in the conscious analysis of odor.
  (See figures on the next page)

6. Neutrophils increase in number after exercise due to:

A. Increased colony stimulating factor levels
B. Reduction in ECF
C. Demargination
D. Epithelial destruction

Ans: C. Demargination

Ref:

1. *Pal GK. Total Leucocyte count. In: Practical physiology. 2nd ed. Hyderabad. Orient Longman Private Limited. 2005; 9: 58.*

Olfactory pathway

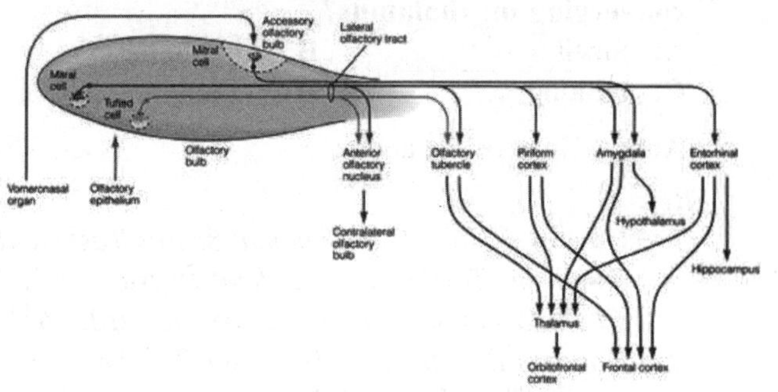

Pathway for hearing

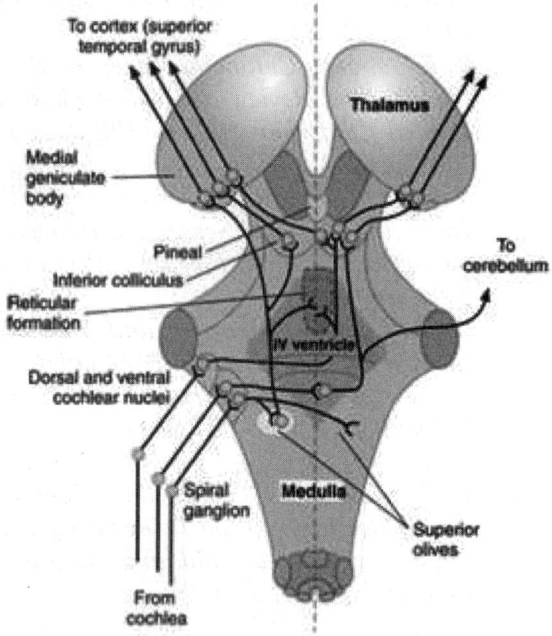

Visual pathway

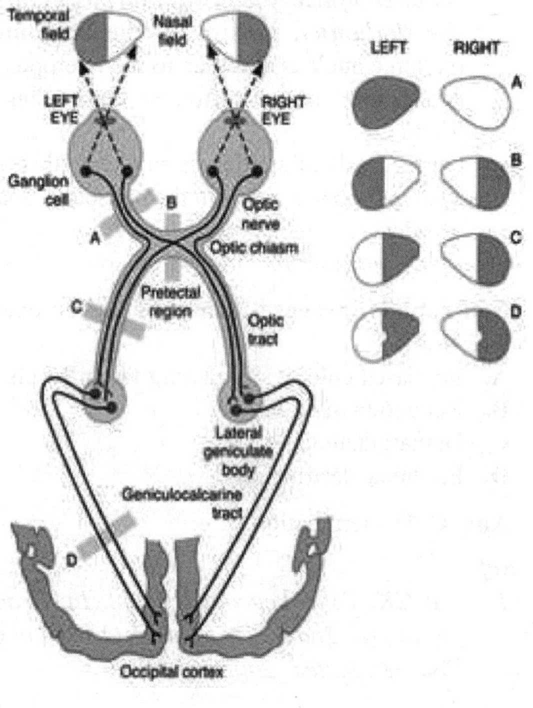

Ascending sensory pathway

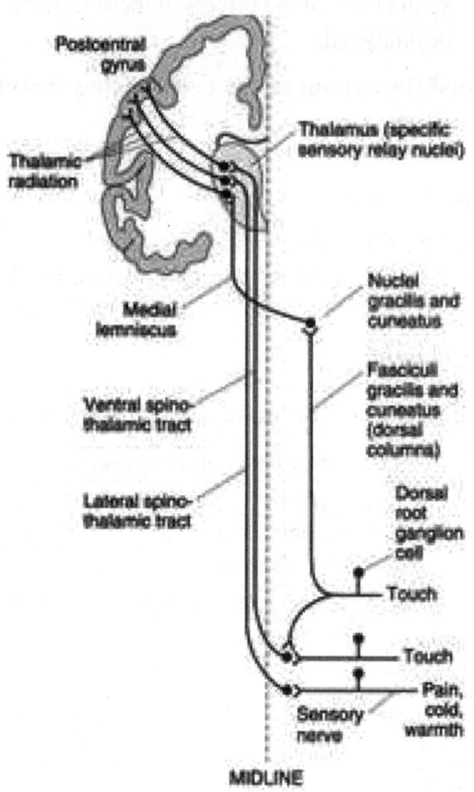

2. *Pyne DB. Regulation of neutrophil function during exercise. Sports Med. 1994 Apr;17(4):245-58.*

Explanation:

Physiological Lecocytosis

1. **Newborns and infants** – 15,00 to 20,000
2. **Physical exercise** – Shift Leucocytosis (leucocytes are shifted from their margination pool into the general circulation pool). It does not occur due to increased formation of cells
   - Increase in the number of circulating neutrophils with exercise is a result of demargination of cells from endothelial tissues (mediated by ***catecholamines***) and bone marrow (mediated by ***cortisol***), or as part of the phagocytic and inflammatory response to exercise-induced tissue damage
3. After food intake – As body metabolism increases following food intake, body temperature increases and circulation improves
4. Increased environmental temperature
5. Pregnancy
6. Parturition
7. Pain, nausea, vomiting
8. Menstruation
9. Emotion, anxiety

10. Pepsin is activated by: (Repeat)
A. HCL **B.** Enterokinase
C. Uropepsinogen **D.** Tripsinogen

Ans: A. HCL

Ref: *Pal GK. Gastric function tests; Pathophysiology of peptic ulcer. In: Textbook of medical physiology. Ahuja publishing house. 2011; 94: 754-55.*

Explanation:

Refer 2011 Physiology question explanation

- **Pepsinogen** is secreted from **Chief or peptic** cells
- Type I pepsinogen – fundus and body
- Type II pepsinogen – throughout stomach
- Pepsinogen is converted into pepsin by **HCl**
- **Hcl** is secreted by Parietal and Oxyntic cells
- Pepsin acts best at pH of 2-4

11. Brunner's glands are seen in:
A. Duodenum **B.** Stomach
C. Esophagus **D.** Colon

Ans: A. Duodenum

Ref: *Guyton & Hall. Textbook of Medical Physiology.12th Edn.Chapter 64. Secretory Functions of the Alimentary Tract. Page 786.*

Explanation:

Brunner's glands

- They are ***compound mucous*** glands.
- They are located in the ***wall of the first few centimeters of the duodenum***, mainly between the ***pylorus of the stomach and the papilla of Vater***, where pancreatic secretion and bile empty into the duodenum.
- Brunner's glands are stimulated by ***tactile or irritating stimuli*** on the duodenal mucosa, ***vagal stimulation*** & ***secretin***. They are ***inhibited by sympathetic stimulation***
- Mucus secreted by Brunner's glands ***protects the duodenal wall*** from digestion by the highly acidic gastric juice.

12. Pneumotaxic centre is situated in:
A. Medulla
B. Pons
C. Midbrain
D. Reticular activating system

Ans: B. Pons

Ref: *Guyton & Hall. Respiratory Center. In: Textbook of Medical Physiology.12th ed. Philadelphia: Saunders Elsevier; 2012. p 506.*

Explanation:

Pneumotaxic center

- Located dorsally in the ***nucleus parabrachialis*** of the ***upper pons***
- Transmits signals to the ***inspiratory area***
- Control the "***switch-off***" point of the inspiratory ramp (control the duration of the filling phase of the lung cycle
- When the signal is strong, inspiration lasts for 0.5 second, when the pneumotaxic signal is weak, inspiration continues for 5 or more seconds
- Secondary effect - Increases the rate of breathing (limitation of inspiration also shortens expiration; ie strong signal can increase upto 30 to 40 breaths / minute; weak pneumotaxic signal may reduce the rate to only 3 to 5 breaths per minute)

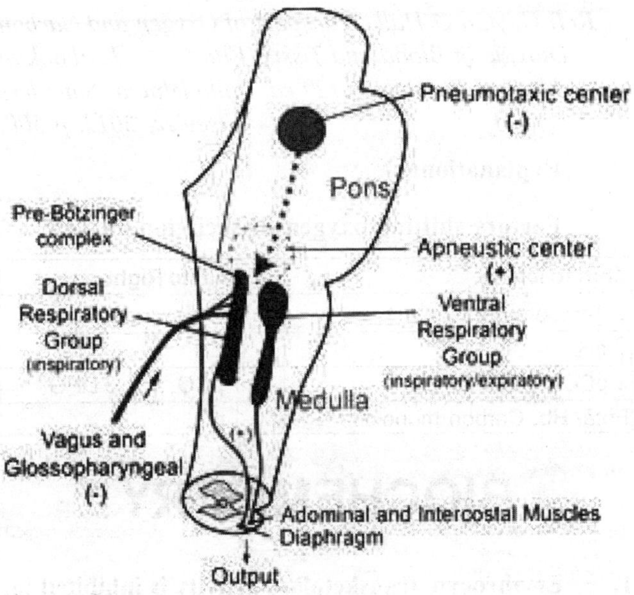

13. A 5-year-old obese boy has persistent food-seeking and aggressive behavior. A hypothalamic nuclei lesion is being suspected. What is the probable site of the lesion?
A. Lateral
B. Supraoptic
C. Suprachiasmatic
D. Ventromedial

Ans: D. Ventromedial

Ref: *Guyton & Hall. Behavioral and Motivational Mechanisms of the Brain-The Limbic System and the Hypothalamus. In: Textbook of Medical Physiology.12th ed. Philadelphia: Saunders Elsevier; 2012. p 716.*

Explanation:

- Area associated with hunger is the ***lateral hypothalamic*** area. ***Damage*** to this area ***on both sides of the hypothalamus*** causes the animal ***to lose desire for food***, sometimes causing lethal starvation.
- ***Satiety center*** **(ventromedial nuclei)** opposes the desire for food. When it is stimulated electrically, an animal stops eating suddenly and shows complete indifference to food
- If it is destroyed bilaterally, the animal cannot be satiated; instead, it has a voracious appetite, resulting in tremendous obesity

14. **All the following factors shift the oxygen dissociation curve to the right *except:***

A. ↑ CO2 **B.** ↑ temperature
C. ↑ 2, 3 DPG **D.** ↑ pH

Ans: D. ↑ pH

Ref: *Guyton & Hall. Transport of Oxygen and Carbon Dioxide in Blood and Tissue Fluids. In: Textbook of Medical Physiology.12th ed. Philadelphia: Saunders Elsevier; 2012. p 500.*

Explanation:

Factors shifting oxygen dissociation curve

Shift to left	Shift to Right
↓ Temperature	↑ Temparature
↑ pH	↓ pH
↓ pCO_2 ↓ 2, 3 DPG	↑ pCO_2 ↑ 2, 3 DPG
Fetal Hb, Carbon monoxide	↓ pO_2

BIOCHEMISTRY

1. **Erythrocyte transketolase activity is inhibited in:**

A. Pellagra **B.** Beri-beri
C. Scurvy **D.** Rickets

Ans: B. Beri-beri

Ref: *Harper's illustrated Biochemistry,28th edition,Chapter 44,pp-473 & Chapter 21, p-181*

Explanation:

BERI BERI

Beri beri is due to the deficiency of Thiamine (Vitamin B1) which manifests as below:

- **Wet BeriBeri** – Edema, Palpitation & Dyspnea (CVS Manifestation)
- **Dry BeriBeri** –Muscle wasting& peripheral neuritis (CNS manifestation)
- **Cerebral BeriBeri** (Wernicke – Korsakoff syndrome) - Seen in chronic alcoholics
  - **Initial stage** - Psychosis (mental confusion, impaired cognitive abilities)
  - **Later stage** - Encephalopathy – Ophthalmoplegia, Nystagmus, cerebellar ataxia

Biochemical Investigations

- ↓ Blood B1, ↓ RBC Transketolase activity
- ↑ Blood Pyruvate, Lactate & α- Ketoglutarate

Biochemical basis of these findings

- Coenzyme of vitamin B1–Thiamin pyrophosphate (TPP)
- TPP is required for 2 types of reactions
  - **Oxidative decarboxylation** reactions (Pyruvate → Acetyl CoA, α Ketoglutarate → Succinyl CoA)
  - Reactions catalyzed by **Transketolase**
- In Beri beri, both the above reactions are inhibited,resulting in accumulation of pyruvate which is converted to lactate, ↑ in α-Ketoglutarate levels and ↓ RBC transketolase levels.

2. **Oasthouse syndrome is due to malabsorption of:**

A. Methionine **B.** Valine
C. Cysteine **D.** Tryptophan

Ans: A. Methionine

Ref: *C. Hooft, D. Carton, J. Snoeck et al.Helvetica paediatricaacta, Basel, 1968, 23: 334-349.*

Explanation:

Methionine malabsorption syndrome (Oasthouse syndrome)

- A rare inherited disorder characterized by **impaired absorption of methionine** and other amino acids.
- The methionine that is not absorbed is **converted** by an **intestinal bacteria** into an **acid** which gives the **urine a distinctive odor**.
- Clinical features
  - Mental retardation
  - Diarrhea
  - Convulsions
  - Rapid breathing
- Unabsorbed methionine is converted by colonic bacteria to **α-hydroxybutyric acid.**
- This gives the urine a characteristic odor similar to that of **dried malt** or an **oasthouse (a building for drying hops).**
- High level of **alpha-hydroxybutyric acid in the urine** is found.

3. **In glycolysis ATP is produced by the following enzyme:**
A. Hexokinase
B. Phosphoglycerate kinase
C. Encolase
D. Phosphohexoseisomerase

Ans: B. Phosphoglycerate kinase

Ref: *Harper's illustrated Biochemistry,28th edition,Chapter 18,pp 151*

Explanation

GLYCOLYSIS: (Embden - Meyerhof Pathway)

- Definition: Partial oxidation of Glucose to give **pyruvate** (under aerobic) or **lactate** (under anaerobic conditions)

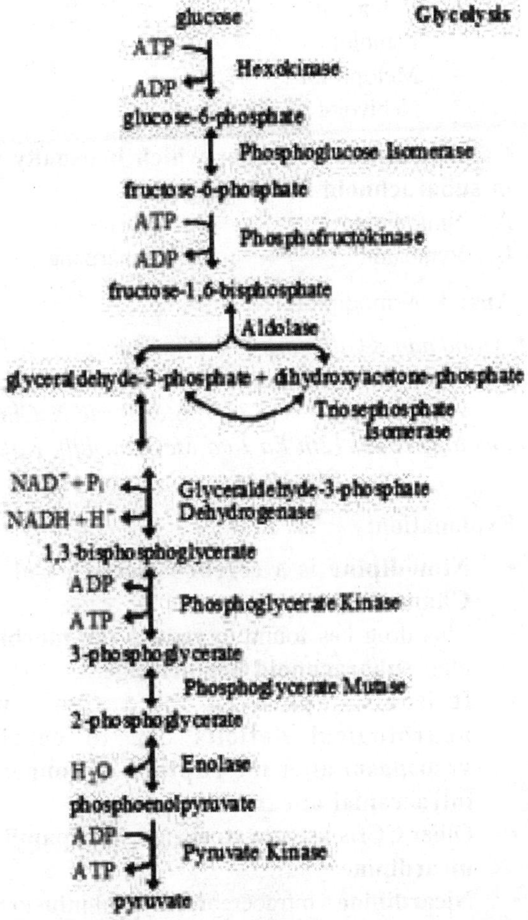

4. **McArdles disease is due to the deficiency of:**
A. Glucose 1 phosphatase
B. Glucose 1, 6 diphosphatase
C. Glucose 6 phosphatase
D. Myophosphorylase

Ans: D. Myophosphorylase

Reference:*Harper's illustrated Biochemistry,28th edition,Chapter 19,pp 160*

Explanation:

McArdles disease

- Type V Glycogen storage disease
- Deficiency: muscle phosphorylase/myophosphorylase
- Premature chain termination, incorrect folding etc can cause loss of catalytic activity
- Skeletal muscle is affected
- Exercise-induced muscular pain, cramps, progressive weakness, myoglobinuria
- No increase in blood lactate after exercise

Glycogen storage disorders

Disorder	Affected Tissue	Enzyme defect
Type 0	Liver	Glycogen synthase
Type I; Von Gierke's	Liver, kidney, intestine	Glucose-6-phosphatase
Type II; Pompe's	All	Lysosomal alpha glucosidase
Type III; Forbe's	Liver, muscle, heart	Glycogen debranching enzyme
Type IV; Anderson's	Liver	Branching enzyme
Type V; Mc Ardle's	Muscles	muscle phosphorylase
Type VI; Her's	Liver	Liver phosphorylase
Type VII; Tauri's	Skeletal muscle, RBC	Muscle and Liver PFK

5. **Reactive oxygen intermediates are released by:**
A. NADPH oxidase
B. Superoxidedismutase
C. Catalase
D. Glutathione peroxidase

Ans: A. NADPH oxidase

Ref: *Harper's illustrated Biochemistry,28th edition,Chapter 52,pp-606*

Explanation:

- **Neutrophils** and **phagocytic cells** engulf bacteria and exhibit a **rapid increase O2** consumption and production of a large amount of **reactive oxygen species (superoxide anions).**
- This is called **respiratory** burst.
- **NADPH oxidase** of electron transport is responsible for it.
- Genetic **deficiency** of **NADPH oxidase** → **Chronic Granulomatous Disease**

6. **All are bile acids *except:* (Repeat)**
A. Lithocholic acid
B. Taurocholic acid

C. Deoxycholic acid
D. Chenodeoxycholic acid

Ans: B. Taurocholic acid

Ref: *Harper's Illustrated Biochemistry,28th edition*

Explanation:

- Bile acids are the ***end products*** of ***cholesterol metabolism***.
- Primary bile acids are synthesized in the hepatocytes directly from cholesterol.
- The most abundant ***primary bile acids*** *are* ***Cholic*** *and* ***Chenodeoxycholic*** *acids.*
- Primary bile acids are transformed by colonic bacteria into *secondary bile acids* in intestine.
  - Deconjugation
  - Dehydroxylation
    - *Deoxycholic acid*
    - *Lithocholic acid*
- This conjugation process makes the bile acids more water soluble
- These are then secreted into gall bladder since bile contains plenty of Na^+, K^+
- The bile acids form **"BILE SALTS"** when they get conjugated with ***glycine/taurine***

7. **Stability of alpha helix is affected by which amino acid? (Repeat)**

A. Tryptophan **B.** Proline
C. Glutamate **D.** Valine

Ans: B. Proline

Ref: *Harper's illustrated biochemistry,28th edition, chapter 5,pp32.*

Explanation:

- The stability of **alpha helix** is arises from **hydrogen bonds** between **oxygen** of **peptide bond carbonyl** and **hydrogen** of **peptide bond** nitrogen of fourth residue down the polypeptide chain.
- **Van der waals interactions** in the core of the structure provides thermodynamic driving force for the formation of helix.
- Since peptide bond nitrogen of **proline** lacks hydrogen atom to contribute to hydrogen bond, proline can only be stably accommodated within the first turn of helix. If present elsewhere disrupts the conformation of the helix.

PHARMACOLOGY

1. **Which of the following is the most beta-1 selective antagonist?**

A. Acebutolol **B.** Atenolol
C. Metoprolol **D.** Bisoprolol

Ans: D. Bisoprolol

Ref: *Goodman &Gillman's The Pharmacological Basis of Therapeutics, 2011, 12th Edition, McGraw Hill, Burton LL P 328*

Explanation:

- **Bisoprolol** is highly selective **beta-1 selective antagonist** among the given drugs
- However **nebivolol** has **higher beta-1 selective** antagonist than **bisoprolol**
- **Beta-1 selective antagonist** include
  - Acebutolol
  - Atenolol
  - Betaxolol
  - Bisoprolol
  - Celiprolol
  - Esmolol
  - Metoprolol
  - Nebivolol

2. **Calcium channel blocker which is usually used in subarachnoid hemorrhage is:**

A. Nimodipine **B.** Diltiazem
C. Verapamil **D.** Flunarizine

Ans: A Nimodipine

Ref: *Goodman &Gillman's The Pharmacological Basis of Therapeutics, 2011, 12th Edition, McGraw Hill, Burton LL P 735-736 & Basic & Clinical Pharmacology,2012, 12th Ed,Tata McGraw hill, Katzung BG, Masters SB, Trevor AJ, P 204.*

Explanation:

- **Nimodipine** is a **cerebroselective Calcium Channel Blocker.**
- This drug has found to **reduce the morbidity** after **subarachnoid hemorrhage.**
- It is also **approved** for **patients with neurological deficits** due to **cerebral vasospasm** after the **rupture of congenital intracranial aneurysm**
- Other CCBs used in **stroke** are **verapamil** and **nicardipine**
- **Nicardipine** - intracerebral arterial infusion has found to **prevent cerebral vasospasm** associated with **stroke**

3. **Drug induced cirrhosis is not seen with:**

A. Methotrexate **B.** Phenobarbitone
C. Valproic acid **D.** Amiadarone

Ans: B. Phenobarbitone

Ref: *Semin Liver Dis 2002; 22(2): 185-194 & Morphologic Alterations in Patients with Alpha-*

Methyldopa-induced Liver Damage after Short- and Long-term Exposure Scandanavian Journal Of Gastroenetrology, 1981, Vol. 16, No. 7, Pages 853-863

Explanation:

- **Drugs most commonly known to cause cirrhosis**
  - Amiodarone
  - Methotrexate
  - Vitamin A
  - Valproic acid.
- **Autoimmune hepatitis** that may lead to **cirrhosis** are
  - Fibrates
  - Statins
  - Alpha and beta interferon
  - Tumor necrosis factor antagonists
- **Vanishing bile duct syndrome** which may lead to cirrhosis is associated with
  - Nonsteroidal antiinflammatory agents
  - Sulfonamides
  - Macrolide
  - Fluoroquinolone antibiotics
  - The penicillins, amoxicillin/clavulanate
  - Tricyclic antidepressants
  - Antifungal agents
- **Other drugs implicated in cirrhosis of liver**
  - Perhexiline maleate
  - Amiodarone
  - Tamoxifen
  - Estrogens
  - Corticosteroids
  - Calcium channel blockers

4. **Which of the following is not used in the prophylaxis of febrile seizures?**

A. Sodium valproate	**B.** Carbamazepine
C. Phenobarbitone	**D.** Diazepam

Ans: B. Carbamezapine

Ref: *NP Rosman, NP et al . A controlled trial of diazepam administered during febrile illnesses to prevent recurrence of febrile seizures NEJM, Vol 329, 1993 79-84 & Nelson Textbook of Pediatrics, 19th ed.*

Explanation:

- Drugs that can be used for prophylaxis of febrile seizures are **Phenobarbitone, Primidone diazepam** and **Sodium Valproate.**
- However currently only **oral diazepam** is preferred during febrile episodes to reduce the risk of recurrent febrile seizures
- Intravenous **benzodiazepines, phenobarbital, phenytoin,** or **valproate** may be needed in the case of **febrile status epilepticus.**
- If the parents are very anxious concerning their child's seizures, **intermittent oral diazepam** can be given during febrile illnesses (0.33 mg/kg every 8 hr during fever) to help reduce the risk of seizures in children known to have had febrile seizures with previous illnesses.
- Intermittent oral **nitrazepam, clobazam,** and **clonazepam** (0.1 mg/kg/day) have also been used. Other therapies have included **intermittent diazepam prophylaxis** (0.5 mg/kg administered as a rectal suppository every 8 hr), **phenobarbital** (4-5 mg/kg/day in 1 or 2 divided doses), and **valproate** (20-30 mg/kg/day in 2 or 3 divided doses).

5. **Which of the following drugs will not cause hypothyroidism?**

A. Ethambutol	**B.** Lithium
C. Amiodarone	**D.** Pyrazinamide

Ans: D Pyrazinamide

Ref: *Basic & Clinical Pharmacology,2012, 12th Ed, Tata McGraw hill, Katzung BG,Masters SB, Trevor AJ, P 243, 516 & Naveen Chhabra et al Analysis of thyroid function tests in patients of multidrug resistance tuberculosis undergoing treatment.* ***J Pharmacol Pharmacotherapy. 2011*** *Oct-Dec; 2(4): 282–285.*

Explanation:

- **Amiodarone**, contains large amounts of **inorganic iodine**
- It can cause **hypothyroidism** as well as **hyperthyroidism**
- Hypothyroidism is due to **blockade of peripheral conversion of T4 to T3**
- **Lithium** cause **reversible and nonprogressive hypothyroidism**
- **Ethambutol** when used in combination with **PAS**, has found to cause **hypothyroididsm** even though it is inconclusive.

6. **Atropine is added with diphenoxylate to:**
   - **A.** Increase effect
   - **B.** Decrease side effects
   - **C.** Decrease abuse potential
   - **D.** Enhance absorption

Ans: C. Decrease abuse potential

Ref: *Basic & Clinical Pharmacology, 2012, 12th Ed, Tata McGraw hill, Katzung BG,Masters SB, Trevor AJ,P 1095*

Explanation:

- **Diphenoxylate** is an **opioid agonist without any analgesic property.**

- It has **Antimotility** action hence it is used in **non-infective diarrhoea**
- It can cause **drug dependence** since it has **CNS effects**
- **Atropine** in small doses (0.025 mg) is added with **diphenoxylate** 2.5 mg to discourage overdose since this may cause atropine side effects which unpleasant

7. **Monitoring of drug level is not required with:**

   A. Lithium **B.** L-Dopa
   C. Digoxin **D.** Phenytoin

   Ans: B. L-Dopa

Ref: Goodman &Gillman's The Pharmacological Basis of Therapeutics, 2011, 12th Edition, McGraw Hill, Burton LL P 447, 803,592

Explanation:

- Except **L- dopa** all other drugs are having a **narrow safety margin** hence monitoring of these drugs are essential
- **Digoxin** : 0.5-1ng/mL
- **Phenytoin** : Total- 10-20mcg/mL (free concentration of 0.75-1.25 mcg/Ml)
- **Lithium** : 0.6-1.5 mEq /L

8. **Carbamazepine toxicity is precipitated by:**

   A. Erythromycin **B.** Vitamin K
   C. Theophyllin **D.** Phenytoin

   Ans: A. Erythromycin

Ref: Goodman &Gillman's The Pharmacological Basis of Therapeutics, 2011, 12th Edition, McGraw Hill, Burton LL P 597

Explanation:

Carbamazepine Toxicity

- **Cimetidine**, **Erythromycin**, **Fluoxatine**, **isoniazid** and **propoxyphene** may **inhibit** the **metabolism** of **Carbamezapine** and lead to **toxicity**
- This is characterized by
  - Hyperirritability
  - Stupor
  - Convulsions
  - Respiratory depression
  - Coma
- Toxicity can be presented as **drowsiness, vertigo, ataxia, diplopia, blurred** vision and increase in **seizure** frequency
- **Hematological toxicity** can manifest as **agranulocytosis** and **aplastic anemia**
- **Sodium Valproate** will induce the metabolism of **Carbamezapine**

9. **The drug of choice for management of infantile spasm is:**

   A. Phenytoin **B.** Valproate
   C. ACTH **D.** Diazepam

   Ans: C. ACTH

Ref. Essentials of Medical Pharmacology by K.D.Tripathi p.411-12

Explanation:

Drugs of choice in epilepsy

Type of seizure	First choice drugs
Generalised tonic-clonic /simple partial with or without generalization	Carbamazepine,Phenytoin
Complex partial with orwithout generalization	Carbamazepine,Valproate, Phenytoin
Absence	Valproate
Myoclonic	Valproate
Atonic	Valproate
Febrile seizures	Diazepam (rectal)
Status epilepticus	Diazepam (I.V.) Lorazepam (I.V.)
Infantile spasm	ACTH (Drug of choice) Also, Vigabatrin

10. **All are true about Buspirone *except:***

    A. Not a Benzodiazepine
    B. Is an anti anxiety drug
    C. Used as sedative hypnotic
    D. Used as anti depressant

    Ans: C. Used as sedative hypnotic

Ref: Katzung 11th p 374

Explanation:

Buspirone

- **Buspirone** is a **non benzodiazepine arylpiperazine** used as **anxiolytic** and **antidepressants**.
- **Gepirone** and **ipsapirone** are other drugs in this group.
- It **does not interact** with **GABA-A receptors** or **display the sedative** and **anticonvulsant** properties of **benzodiazepines**.
- It may exert its **anxiolytic** effects by acting as a **partial agonist at brain 5-HT1-A receptors**, but it also has affinity for **brain dopamine D2 receptors**.
- The drug is used in **generalized anxiety states** but is **less effective in panic disorders**.
- **Adverse Effects**
  - Nonspecific chest pain
  - Tachycardia

- Palpitations
- Dizziness
- Nervousness
- Tinnitus
- Gastrointestinal distress
- Paresthesias
- ***Dose-dependent pupillary constriction***

11. Which is a characteristic adverse effect of chronic amiodarone therapy?

A. Corneal deposition **B.** Cataract
C. Glaucoma **D.** Retinal pigmentation

Ans: A. Corneal deposition

Ref: *GG 12th 834-837*

Explanation:

Amiodarone – Adverse effects

- The most serious adverse effect during chronic amiodarone therapy is **pulmonary fibrosis,** which can be **rapidly progressive and fatal.**
- With low doses (200 mg/day) used in **atrial fibrillation, pulmonary toxicity** is unusual.
- Supportive measures and corticosteroids may be used to treat pulmonary toxicity.
- Other adverse effects during long-term therapy include
  - Corneal microdeposits (which often are asymptomatic),
  - Hepatic dysfunction,
  - Neuromuscular symptoms (most commonly **peripheral neuropathy** or **proximal muscle weakness)**
  - Photosensitivity
  - Hypo- or hyperthyroidism.
- Despite the marked **QT prolongation** and **bradycardia** typical of chronic amiodarone therapy, **torsades de pointes** and other drug-induced **tachyarrhythmias** are not unusual.

12. Drug of choice for treatment of gastrointestinal stromal tumors is:

A. Rituximab **B.** Imatinib mesylate
C. Anagrelide **D.** Denileukin diftitox

Ans: B. Imatinib mesylate

Ref: *Goodman & Gillman, The pharmacological basis of therapeutics, 12th edition, Pg No. 1732-1734.*

Explanation:

Imatinib mesylate is used in the treatment of (**Approved indications**)

- **Chronic** phase of **CML**
- **GIST**- Gastrointestinal Stromal tumor
- **Chronic Myelomonocytic leukemia**
- **Hypereosinophilic** syndrome
- **Dermatofibrosarcoma protruberance**
- **Progressive plexiform neurofibromatosis**

It is also tried in (Experimental and Not approved for routine use)

- Systemic Mastocytosis
- Pulmonary hypertension
- Alzheimer's disease
- Lowering or reversing opioid tolerance
- Desmoid tumor

PATHOLOGY

1. Histological scoring of chronic hepatitis does not include:

A. Periportal inflammation
B. Portal fibrosis
C. Bridging necrosis
D. Cholestasis

Ans: D. Cholestasis

Ref: *Robbins Pathologic Basis of Disease, 8th edition*

Explanation:

Histologic Features of Chronic Hepatitis.

The histologic features of chronic hepatitis range from exceedingly mild to severe

In Mild Hepatitis

- Inflammation is limited to portal tracts and
- Lymphocytes, macrophages, occasional plasma cells infiltrate
- Liver architecture is usually well preserved,
- Smoldering hepatocyte apoptosis throughout the lobule
- In ***chronic HCV infection***, Lymphoid aggregates and bile duct reactive changes in the portal tracts, and focal mild to moderate macrovesicular steatosis.
- The steatosis is more prevalent and prominent in HCV genotype 3 infections.

Moderate to Severe Hepatitis

- Interface hepatitis and bridging necrosis between portal tracts and portal tracts-to-terminal hepatic veins
- Progressive liver damage.
- The ***hallmark*** of chronic liver damage is the ***deposition of fibrous tissue***.
- At first, only portal tracts show increased fibrosis followed by periportal septal fibrosis, followed by linking of fibrous septa (bridging fibrosis),
- Continued loss of hepatocytes and fibrosis results in cirrhosis.

- It is characterized by irregularly sized nodules separated by variable but mostly broad scars (post-necrotic cirrhosis)

Causes of Chronic hepatitis

- Viral hepatitis,
- **Autoimmune hepatitis**,
- Hepatotoxins (carbon tetrachloride, mushroom poisoning),
- Drugs (acetaminophen, α-methyldopa)
- Alcohol

In about 20% of cases the inciting cause of the cirrhosis cannot be determined, and these are labeled as ***cryptogenic cirrhosis***.

2. **Pulmonary surfactant is synthesized by:**
   A. Type I pneumocytes
   B. Type II pneumocytes
   C. Clara cells
   D. Endothelium

Ans: A. Type II Pneumocytes

Ref: *Robbins Pathologic Basis of Disease, 8th edition*

Explanation:

- Surfactant is produced by **type II alveolar cells**
- **Type II pneumocytes** also called alveolar type II cells, **great alveolar cells** or **septal cells** are granular and roughly cuboidal in shape.
- Type II pneumocytes are typically found at the **alveolar-septal** junction.
- Although they comprise **60%** of the alveolar lining cells, because of their shape they cover a much smaller surface area than type I cells (**<5%**).
- Type II cells start to develop at about **24 weeks** of gestation, secreting small amounts of surfactant. However, adequate amounts of surfactant are not secreted until about **35 weeks** of gestation - this is the main reason for increased incidence rates of Infant respiratory distress syndrome, which drastically reduces at ages above 35 weeks gestation.
- Type II cells are responsible for the production and secretion of surfactant (the majority of which are **dipalmitoylphosphatidylcholine**), a group of phospholipids that reduce the alveolar surface tension.
- Surfactant phospholipids are stored in Type II pneumocytes in **lamellar bodies**, which are specialized vesicles.
- Release of surfactant in lamellar bodies occurs from an infant's first breath onwards.
- Type II pneumocytes can replicate in the alveoli and will replicate to replace damaged Type I pneumocytes.
- **MUC1**, a human gene associated with type II pneumocytes, has been identified as a marker in lung cancer

Clara cells

- These are ***dome-shaped cells*** with short ***microvilli*** found in the small airways (***bronchioles***) of the lungs.
- Clara cells are found in the **ciliated simple epithelium**.
- These cells may secrete **glycosaminoglycans** to protect the **bronchiole lining**.
- Bronchiolar cells gradually increase in number as the number of goblet cells decrease.

3. **Regarding DIC all the following features are correct *except:***
   A. Increased fibrin degradation products
   B. Decreased platelets
   C. Increased fibrinogen levels
   D. Prolonged Thrombin time (TT)

Ans: C. Increased fibrinogen

Ref: *Robbins Pathologic Basis of Disease, 8th edition*

Explanation:

- Fibrinogen levels are decreased in DIC

Disseminated Intravascular Coagulation (DIC)

- DIC is a thrombohemorrhagic disorder characterized by the ***excessive activation of coagulation***, which leads to the formation of ***thrombi in the microvasculature*** of the body.
- Due to thrombotic diathesis there is ***consumption of platelets, fibrin***, and ***coagulation*** factors and, secondarily, ***activation of fibrinolysis***.
- DIC can present with signs and symptoms relating to the tissue hypoxia and infarction caused by the myriad microthrombi
- Can also present with hemorrhage caused by the depletion of factors required for hemostasis and the activation of fibrinolytic mechanisms

Etiology and Pathogenesis

- It is a coagulopathy that occurs in the course of a variety of clinical conditions.
- Clotting can be initiated by either of two pathways:

(1) The ***extrinsic pathway***, which is triggered by the release of ***tissue factor ("tissue thromboplastin")***

(2) The ***intrinsic pathway***, which involves the ***activation of factor XII by surface contact*** with collagen or other negatively charged substances.

- Both pathways, through a series of steps, result in the generation of thrombin, which in turn converts fibrinogen to fibrin.
- When Thrombin interacts with normal vessels, it is converted to an anticoagulant through binding to thrombomodulin, a protein found on the surface of endothelial cells.
- The thrombin-thrombomodulin complex ***activates protein C***, which is an important inhibitor of two procoagulants, ***factor V*** and ***factor VIII***.
- DIC results from pathologic activation of the **extrinsic and/or intrinsic pathways** of coagulation or the impairment of clot-inhibiting mechanisms.
- DIC is most likely to be associated with **obstetric** complications, **malignant neoplasms**, **sepsis**, and **major trauma**.
- Among cancers, **acute promyelocytic leukemia** and **adenocarcinomas of the lung**, **pancreas**, **colon**, and stomach are most frequently associated with DIC.
- Widespread deposition of fibrin within the microcirculation leads to Ischemia & **microangiopathic hemolytic anemia**
- **Consumption of platelets** and **clotting factors** and the activation of **plasminogen** leads to a **hemorrhagic diathesis**.
- **Plasmin not only cleaves fibrin**, but it also **digests factors V and VIII**, thereby reducing their concentration further.
- **Fibrin degradation products** resulting from **fibrinolysis** inhibit **platelet aggregation**, **fibrin polymerization**, and **thrombin**.
- All of these derangements contribute to the hemostatic failure seen in DIC.

Morphology

- **Thrombi** are most often found in the **brain, heart, lungs, kidneys, adrenals, spleen, and liver**, in decreasing order of frequency.
- Affected **kidneys** may have **small thrombi** in the glomeruli that evoke only reactive swelling of endothelial cells or, in severe cases, **microinfarcts** or even bilateral renal cortical necrosis.
- Numerous **fibrin thrombi** may be found in alveolar capillaries, sometimes associated with pulmonary edema and fibrin exudation, creating "**hyaline membranes**" reminiscent of acute respiratory distress syndrome.
- In the central nervous system, fibrin thrombi can cause **microinfarcts**, occasionally complicated by simultaneous **hemorrhage**, which can sometimes lead to variable neurologic signs and symptoms.
- In meningococcemia, fibrin thrombi within the microcirculation of the adrenal cortex are the probable basis for the massive adrenal hemorrhages seen in ***Waterhouse-Friderichsen syndrome***
- ***Sheehan postpartum pituitary necrosis*** is a form of DIC complicating labor and delivery.

Clinical Features

- Microangiopathic hemolytic anemia
- Dyspnea,
- Cyanosis
- Respiratory failure
- Convulsions
- Coma;
- Oliguria and acute renal failure
- Sudden or progressive circulatory failure
- Shock

Lab findings in DIC (All coagulation parameters are deranged)

- Decreased fibrinogen levels
- Decreased platelets
- Prolonged PT (Prothrombin time)
- Prolonged aPTT (Activated partial thromboplastin time)
- Prolonged TT (Thrombin time)
- Increased Fibrin degradation products.
- Increased D-dimer levels

4. **Which is false regarding von meyenberg complexes?**

A. Bile duct microhamartomas
B. Dilated bile ducts
C. Free of pigmented material
D. Premalignant

Ans: D. Premalignant

Ref: *Robbins and Cotran 'Pathologic Basis of Disease' 8th Edition.Elsevier. 2011. Page 869.*

Explanation:

Von Meyenberg complexes

- These are small clusters of modestly dilated bile ducts embedded in a fibrous, sometimes hyalinized, stroma located close to or within portal tracts.
- These lesions also known as **'BILE DUCT HAMARTOMAS'**
- These are common incidental finding and without any clinical significance except in the differential diagnosis of metastases to liver

- **Does not contain any pigmented material** .
- They are **not premalignant**

5. Which of the following virus has been found to play a role in the genesis of atherosclerosis?

A. CMV B. HIV
C. EBV D. Coxsackie B

Ans: A. CMV

***Ref:** Robbins and Cotran 'Pathologic Basis of Disease' 8th Edition.Elsevier. 2011. Pg 500*

Explanation:

- **Herpes virus, cytomegalovirus, and Chlamydia pneumoniae** have all been detected in atherosclerotic plaques but not in normal arteries, and seroepidemiologic studies find increased antibody titers to **C. pneumoniae** in patients with more severe atherosclerosis.
- **C. pneumoniae bronchitis** is also associated with **smoking**, a well-established **IHD risk factor**.

6. All the following causes dilated cardiomyopathy *except:*

A. Alcoholism B. Hemochromatosis
C. Fredreich ataxia D. Sarcoidosis

Ans: C. Fredreich ataxia

***Ref:** Robbins and Cotran 'Pathologic Basis of Disease' 8th Edition. Elsevier. 2011. Page 572.*

Explanation:

DILATED CARDIOMYOPATHY (DCM)

- Characterized by ***progressive cardiac dilation and contractile (systolic) dysfunction***, usually with concomitant hypertrophy.
- It is sometimes called **congestive cardiomyopathy**.
- DCM can occur at **any age,** including in **childhood**, but it most commonly occurs between ages **20 and 50 years**.
- It typically presents with **slowly progressing CHF** (e.g., shortness of breath and poor exertional capacity), but patients can slip precipitously from a compensated to a decompensated state.
- The fundamental defect in DCM is **ineffective contraction**.
- Hence in end-stage DCM, the cardiac ejection fraction is typically less than 25%. Secondary mitral regurgitation and abnormal cardiac rhythms are common, and embolism from intracardiac thrombi can occur.
- Fifty percent of patients die within 2 years, and only 25% survive longer than 5 years; death is usually due to progressive cardiac failure or arrhythmia.
- In most cases **cardiac transplantation** is the only definitive treatment *(See the following table)*

Functional Pattern	Left Ventricular Ejection Fraction	Mechanisms of Heart Failure	Causes of Phenotype	Indirect Myocardial Dysfunction (Mimicking Cardiomyopathy)
Dilated cardiomyopathy	<40%	Impairment of contractility (systolic dysfunction)	Genetic Alcohol Peripartum Myocarditis Hemochromatosis chronic anemia; Doxorubicin (Adriamycin) Sarcoidosis Idiopathic	Ischemic heart disease; valvular heart disease; hypertensive heart disease; congenital heart disease
Hypertrophic cardiomyopathy	50% to 80%	Impairment of compliance (diastolic dysfunction)	Genetic; Friedreich ataxia; Storage diseases; Infants of diabetic mother	Hypertensive heart disease; aortic stenosis
Restrictive cardiomyopathy	45% to 90%	Impairment of compliance (diastolic dysfunction)	Amyloidosis; radiation-induced fibrosis; idiopathic	Pericardial constriction

7. A 45-year-old man with cirrhosis due to a1-antitrypsin deficiency receives a liver transplant. He is at increased risk of developing which of the following types of emphysema?

A. Centriacinar B. Paraseptal

C. Panacinar D. Compensatory

Ans: C. Panacinar

Ref: Robbins and Cotran 'Pathologic Basis of Disease' 8th Edition.Elsevier. 2011. Pg 684

Explanation:

Types of Emphysema

1. **Centriacinar (Centrilobular) Emphysema.**
- The central or proximal parts of the acini, formed by respiratory bronchioles, are affected, where as distal alveoli are spared.
- Both emphysematous and normal airspaces exist within the same acinus and lobule.
- The lesions are more common and usually more severe in the upper lobes, particularly in the apical segments.
- The walls of the emphysematous spaces often contain large amounts of black pigment.
- Inflammation around bronchi and bronchioles is common.
- In severe centriacinar emphysema, the distal acinus may also be involved, and differentiation from panacinar emphysema becomes difficult.
- Centriacinar emphysema occurs predominantly in **heavy smokers**, often in association with **chronic bronchitis**.

2. **Panacinar (Panlobular) Emphysema.**
- The acini are uniformly enlarged from the level of the respiratory bronchiole to the terminal blind alveoli.
- The prefix "pan" refers to the entire acinus but not to the entire lung.
- This tends to occur more commonly in the lower zones and in the anterior margins of the lung, and it is usually most severe at the bases.
- This type of emphysema is associated with **α1-antitrypsin (α1-AT) deficiency**.

3. **Distal Acinar (Paraseptal) Emphysema.**
- The proximal portion of the acinus is normal, and the distal part is predominantly involved.
- The emphysema is more striking adjacent to the pleura, along the lobular connective tissue septa, and at the margins of the lobules.
- It occurs adjacent to areas of fibrosis, scarring, or atelectasis and is usually more severe in the upper half of the lungs.
- The characteristic findings are of multiple, continuous, enlarged airspaces from less than 0.5 cm to more than 2.0 cm in diameter, sometimes forming cystlike structures.
- This type of emphysema probably underlies many of the cases of spontaneous pneumothorax in young adults.

4. **Airspace Enlargement with Fibrosis (Irregular Emphysema).**
- The acinus is irregularly involved and almost invariably associated with scarring.
- It may be the most common form of emphysema, because careful search of most lungs at autopsy shows one or more scars from a healed inflammatory process.
- In most instances, these foci of irregular emphysema are asymptomatic and clinically insignificant.

8. **Paroxysmal nocturnal hemoglobinuria occurs due to defective:**

A. CD 55 B. CD 21
C. CD 45 D. CD 34

Ans: A. CD 55

Ref: Robbins and Cotran 'Pathologic Basis of Disease' 8th Edition.Elsevier. 2011. Pg. 652

Explanation:

Paroxysmal nocturnal hemoglobinuria (PNH)

- It results from **acquired mutations** in the phosphatidylinositol glycan complementation group A gene (**PIGA**), an enzyme that is essential for the synthesis of certain cell surface proteins.
- It is the **only hemolytic anemia** caused by an **acquired genetic defect.**
- Proteins are anchored into the lipid bilayer in two ways. Most have a hydrophobic region that spans the cell membrane; these are called **transmembrane proteins**. The others are attached to the cell membrane through a covalent linkage to a specialized phospholipid called **glycosylphosphatidylinositol (GPI).**
- In PNH, these **GPI-linked proteins are deficient** because of somatic mutations that inactivate PIGA.
- PIGA is X-**linked** and subject to **lyonization** (random inactivation of one X chromosome in cells of females).
- PNH is associated with **aplastic anemia**, a marrow failure syndrome that has an autoimmune basis in many individuals.
- PNH blood cells are **deficient in three GPI-linked proteins** that regulate complement activity:

  - ***Decay–accelerating factor, or CD55;***
  - ***Membrane inhibitor of reactive lysis, or CD59; and***
  - ***C8 binding protein.***
- Of these 3 factors, the most important is **CD59**, a potent inhibitor of **C3 convertase** that prevents the spontaneous activation of the alternative complement pathway.
- Red **cells, platelets**, and **granulocytes deficient** in these GPI-linked factors are abnormally susceptible to lysis or injury by complement.
- In red cells this manifests as **intravascular hemolysis**, which is caused by the **C5b-C9 membrane attack complex.**
- The hemolysis is **paroxysmal** and **nocturnal** in **only 25%** of cases
- **Chronic hemolysis** without dramatic hemoglobinuria is more typical.
- The tendency for red cells to lyse at night is explained by a slight decrease in blood pH during sleep, which increases the activity of complement.
- Thrombosis is the leading cause of disease-related death in individuals with PNH.
- About 40% of patients suffer from **venous thrombosis**, often involving the **hepatic, portal, or cerebral veins.**
- Dysfunction of platelets due to the absence of certain GPI-linked proteins contributes to the **prothrombotic state,** as does the **absorption of NO by free hemoglobin**
- About 5% to 10% of patients eventually develop **acute myeloid leukemia** or a **myelodysplastic syndrome**, possibly because hematopoietic stem cells have suffered some type of genetic damage.
- PNH is diagnosed by **flow cytometry**, which provides a sensitive means for detecting red cells that are deficient in GPI-linked proteins such as CD59.

9. Cerebellar hemangioblastoma and retinal tumors are seen in:

A. Von Hippel Lindau syndrome
B. Neurofibromatosis type 1
C. Tuberous sclerosis
D. Neurofibromatosis type 2

Ans: A. Von Hippel Lindau syndrome

Ref: *Chapter 28. CNS, page : 1343: Robbins and Cotran Pathologic Basis of Disease: 8th edition.*

Explanation:

A. The **Von Hippel Lindau gene (VHL)** is tumor suppressor gene located on Chromosome 3p25-p26 and down-regulates expression of vascular endothelial growth factor; hence its dysregulation is associated with **hemangioblastomas** and **retinal tumors.**

B. The **neurofibromatosis type 1 (Chr. 17)** is associated with **optic nerve gliomas, Lisch nodules (pigmented nodules of the iris), café au lait spots (cutaneous hyperpigmented macules).**

C. **Neurofibromatosis type 2 (Chr. 22)** is associated with **8th nerve schwannomas, multiple meningiomas, gliomas and ependymoma of spinal cord**

D. **Tuberous sclerosis complex**:

It is associated with

i. Cortical tubers
ii. Subependymal nodules
iii. Subependymal giant cell astrocytomas
iv. Renal angiomyolipomas
v. Retinal glial hamartomas
vi. Pulmonary lymphangioleiomyomatosis
vii. Cardiac rhabdomyomas
viii. Shagreen patches (cutaneous leathery thickenings)
ix. Ash-leaf patches (hypopigmented areas)
x. Subangual fibromas.

10. Which of the following is a characteristic feature of malignant hypertension?

A. Fibrinoid necrosis
B. Hyalinising and medial hyperplasia
C. Intimal hyperplasia
D. Nephrosclerosis

Ans: A. Fibrinoid necrosis

Ref: *Robbins Pathologic Basis of Disease, 8th edition, Pg:495*

Explanation:

- Fibrinoid necrosis is a characteristic feature of **Malignant hypertension**
- It is also seen in immune vasculitis conditions (HSP), Preeclampsia, Acute Rheumatic fever and Hyperacute graft rejection.

Accelerated* or *Malignant hypertension

- A small percentage, perhaps 5%, of hypertensive persons show a rapidly rising blood pressure that, if untreated, leads to death within a year or two, called *accelerated* or *malignant hypertension.*
- This clinical syndrome is characterized by severe

hypertension (i.e., systolic pressure over 200 mm Hg, diastolic pressure over 120 mm Hg), renal failure, and retinal hemorrhages and exudates, with or without papilledema.

- It may develop in previously normotensive persons but more often is superimposed on pre-existing benign hypertension, either essential or secondary

The characteristic morphological changes in vessels is termed as ***Hyperplastic Arteriolosclerosis***

Hyperplastic Arteriolosclerosis

- This lesion occurs in severe (malignant) hypertension;
- Vessels exhibit "**onion-skin lesions**," characterized by concentric, laminated thickening of the walls and luminal narrowing.
- The laminations consist of smooth muscle cells with thickened, reduplicated basement membranes;
- In malignant hypertension they are accompanied by fibrinoid deposits and vessel wall necrosis **(necrotizing arteriolitis)**, particularly in the kidney.

Benign hypertension

Morphology

The characteristic morphological changes in vessels is termed as **hyaline arteriolosclerosis**

Hyaline Arteriolosclerosis.

- Arterioles show homogeneous, pink hyaline thickening with associated luminal narrowing.
- These changes stem from **plasma protein leakage** across injured **endothelial cells**, and increased smooth muscle cell matrix synthesis in response to chronic hemodynamic stress.
- Although the vessels of elderly persons also frequently show hyaline arteriosclerosis, it is more generalized and severe in individuals with hypertension.
- The same lesions are also a common feature of **diabetic microangiography** (due to hyper-glycembia-induced endothelial cell dysfunction)
- In **nephrosclerosis** due to chronic hypertension, the arteriolar narrowing of hyaline arterio-sclerosis causes diffuse impairment of renal blood supply and causes glomerular scarring.

11. Most common tumor of pineal gland is:

A. Hemangioma
B. Germinomas
C. Teratoma
D. Embryonal Carcinoma

Ans: B. Germinomas

Ref: *Robbin's Pathologic Basis of Disease, 8th ed, Pg: 1163*

Explanation:

PINEAL GLAND

- The rarity of clinically significant lesions (virtually **only tumors**) justifies brevity in the consi-deration of the pineal gland.
- It is a minute, **pinecone-shaped organ** , weigh-ing 100 to 180 mg and lying between the superior colliculi at the base of the brain.
- It is composed of a loose, neuroglial stroma enclosing nests of epithelialappearing pineocytes, cells with photosensory and neuroendocrine functions (hence the designation of the pineal gland as the "**third eye**").
- Silver impregnation stains reveal that these cells have long, slender processes reminiscent of primitive neuronal precursors intermixed with the processes of astrocytic cells.
- The principal secretory product of the pineal gland is melatonin, which is involved in the control of circadian rhythms, including the **sleep–wake cycle**; hence the popular use of melatonin for the treatment of jet lag.
- All tumors involving the pineal are rare
- Most **(50% to 70%)** arise from sequestered **embryonic germ cells**.
- They most commonly take the form of so-called **germinomas**, resembling testicular **seminoma** or **ovarian dysgerminoma**.
- Other lines of germ cell differentiation include embryonal carcinomas, choriocarcinomas, mixtures of germinoma, embryonal carcinoma, and choriocarcinoma, typical teratomas (usually benign).
- Whether to characterize these germ cell neoplasms as pinealomas is still a subject of debate, but most "**pinealophiles**" favor restricting the term pinealoma to neoplasms arising from the pineocytes.

12. c myc on chromosome 8 is seen in:

A. Burkitt's lymphoma
B. Follicular lymphoma
C. Mantle cell lymhoma
D. Body cavity lymphoma

Ans: A. Burkitt's lymphoma

Ref: *Robbins Pathologic Basis of Disease, 8th edition, Pg: 259 & 589*

Explanation:

BURKITT LYMPHOMA

There are three clinical types:

(1) African (endemic) Burkitt lymphoma,

(2) Sporadic (nonendemic) Burkitt lymphoma

(3) Aggressive lymphomas asscioated with HIV.

These 3 types are histologically identical

Morphology

- The tumor exhibits a **high mitotic index** and contains numerous **apoptotic cells**, the nuclear remnants of which are phagocytosed by interspersed benign macrophages.
- These phagocytes have abundant clear cytoplasm, creating a characteristic **"starry sky" pattern**.

Immunophenotype

- These are tumors of mature B cells
- It express surface **IgM, CD19, CD20, CD10, and BCL6**, a phenotype consistent with a germinal center B-cell origin.
- Unlike other tumors of germinal center origin, this **does not express** anti-apoptotic protein **BCL2**.

Molecular Pathogenesis

- *All forms of Burkitt lymphoma are associated with translocations of the **c-MYC** gene on **chromosome 8**.*
- The translocation partner is usually the IgH locus [t(8;14)] but may also be the Ig κ [t(2;8)] or γ [t(8;22)] light-chain loci.
- *All endemic tumors are latently infected with EBV*, which is also present in about 25% of HIV-associated tumors and 15% to 20% of sporadic cases.

Clinical Features

- **Endemic Burkitt lymphoma** often presents as a mass involving the mandible and shows an unusual predilection for involvement of abdominal viscera, particularly the kidneys, ovaries, and adrenal glands.
- **Sporadic Burkitt lymphoma** most often appears as a mass involving the ileocecum and peritoneum.
- Burkitt lymphoma is very aggressive but responds well to intensive chemotherapy.

13. **Klatskin tumor: (Repeat)**

A. Primitive neuroectodermal tumor in chest

B. Cholangiocarcinoma arising from bifurcation of bile duct

C. Lung adenocarcinoma involving apical region

D. Enterochromaffin cell tumor

Ans: B. Cholangiocarcinoma arising from bifurcation of bile duct

Ref: *Benbrahim Z et al. Askin's tumor: a case report and literature review. World J Surg Oncol. 2013; 11: 10.*

Explanation:

- Cholangiocarcinoma arising from bifurcation of bile duct - **Klatsin tumor**
- Lung adenocarcinoma involving apical region - **Pancoast tumor**

Askin tumors - Primitive neuroectodermal tumors (**PNET**) arising from the **chest wall**

Other named Tumors

- **Buschke–Löwenstein tumor-** Giant condyloma acuminatum
- **Ackerman tumor** - Subtype of Verrucous Carcinoma (Carcinoma cuniculatum)
- **Grawitz tumor -** Renal cell carcinoma
- **Krukenberg tumor** - Metastatic secondaries in GIT from an ovarian primary
- **Kuttner's stumor -** Sialadenitis (sialoadenitis) - Inflammation of a salivary gland
- **Potts puffy tumor** - Frontal osteomyelitis with subperiosteal abscess
- **Wilms tumor** - Nephroblastoma affecting children

MICROBIOLOGY

1. **Serum sickness is due to which type of hypersensitivity?**

A. Type I **B.** Type II

C. Type III **D.** Type IV

Ans: C. Type III

Ref: *Ananthnarayan R, Paniker CKJ. Textbook of Microbiology. 8th Edition. Hyderabad: Universities Press; 2009. Pg. 161-168*

Explanation:

HYPERSENSITIVITY

Gell and Coomb classification

- **Type I** - IgE mediated- anaphylaxis and atopy
- **Type II-** cytotoxic or cytolytic
- **Type III-** immune complex mediated
- **Type IV-** T cell mediated

Note: Grave's disease is known as Type V hypersensitivity

Type I hypersensitivity

- **Anaphylaxis**-acute, systemic, potentially fatal form
- **Atopy-** chronic, localized, non fatal, familial form (Coca,1923)
- Type I HS is mediated by IgE antibodies
- Eg of subatances associated with Type I HS:
  - Proteins-foreign serum & vaccines
  - Food-nuts, eggs, milk,seafood
  - Plant pollen
  - Drugs-penicillin, local anesthetics
  - Insect products- venom (bees, wasps, ants) dust mites
  - Mold spores
  - Animal hair and dander

Type II hypersensitivity

Reactions involve combination of IgG or IgM antibodies to cell fixed antigens
Examples of type II reactions

- **Cell surface antigens**
  RBC- transfusion reactions, erythroblastosis fetalis, A.I.H.A
  WBC- neutropenia
  PLATELETS- thrombocytopenia
- **Tissue antigens**
  Goodpasture's syndrome
  Pemphigus

Type III hypersensitivity

- Antibodies (usually IgA) directed against soluble antigens
- Examples of type III hypersensitivity
- **Arthus reaction-** localized hemorrhagic necrosis following SC injection of antigen in sensitized rabbits
- **Serum sickness-** systemic form appears 7-12 days after injection of foreign serum
- Infection (microbial antigen)-kidneys-leptospirosis, malaria, Post streptococcal glomerulonephritis
- Autoimmune diseases- (self antigen)- kidney, skin, joints
- Inhaled antigens (molds, plant pollen)-lung (Farmer's lung)

Type IV hypersensitivity

- Also called delayed hypersensitivity because it takes 48-72 hours to develop
- Involves T_{DTH} cells (subset of T_H cells)
- Cannot be passively transferred by serum
- Examples-contact dermatitis, tuberculin test (48-72 hours) and granuloma (21-28 days)

2. Most common site of infection with *Cryptococcus neoformans* is:

A. Lung **B.** Meninges
C. Skin **D.** Bone

Ans: B. Meninges

Ref: *Ananthnarayan R, Paniker CKJ. Textbook of Microbiology. 8th Edition. Hyderabad: Universities Press; 2009. & Jawetz*

Explanation:

- **Cryptococcosis (torulosis)** is a subacute or chronic infection caused by the **yeast** Cryptococcus neoformans.
- Infection is usually acquired by **inhalation** but may sometimes be through the **skin or mucosa.**
- Most infections are **asymptomatic**. From the lungs the fungus migrates to the CNS where they cause **meningitis**
- The major clinical manifestation is chronic menigitis which can **resemble brain tumor**& **brain abscess**
- Patient may complain of **headache, neck stiffness and disorientation**.
- In addition, there may be lesions in skin, lungs and other organs.
- Cryptococcal meningitis is the most serious type of infection and can resemble tuberculous or other chronic types of meningitis. Its onset is insidious and the course slow and progressive. It is often seen in AIDS.
- **Cutaneous** cryptococcosis varies from **small ulcers to large granulomas**.

3. All are true about streptococcal infections *except:*

A. Throat infection more common in age group of 5-15years
B. Skin infection more common in age <3yrs
C. 15-20% colonization of mucosal surfaces
D. Scarlet fever more common <3yrs

Ans: D. Scarlet fever more common <3yrs

Ref: *Ananthnarayan R, Paniker CKJ. Textbook of Microbiology. 8th Edition. Hyderabad: Universities Press; 2009. & Jawetz, Melnick, & Adelberg's. Textbook of Medical Microbiology, 25th Edition. 2010.*

Explanation:

- **Streptococcus pyogenes** causes **pharyngitis** ('strep throat'), skin infections (impetigo, erysipelas, necrotising fasciitis), toxin mediated disease (scarlet fever, toxic shock-like syndrome) and diseases associated with sequelae of infection, such as acute rheumatic fever and acute glomerulonephritis.
- Streptococcal pharyngitis commonly affects **school going children**. It is rare in children less than 3 years.

- Impetigo (pyoderma) is most often seen in **young children (< 3 years)**, living under conditions of poor hygiene
- **Scarlet fever** is an infectious disease which most commonly affects 4-8 year old children. Symptoms include sore throat, fever and a characteristic red rash. Scarlet fever is usually spread by inhalation. There is no vaccine, but the disease is effectively treated with antibiotics. Most of the clinical features are caused by erythrogenic toxin.

4. **Which of the following activates the classical complement pathway?**

A. Immune complex **B.** Lipopolysaccharide
C. Exotoxin **D.** Zymosan

Ans: A. Immune complex

Ref: *Ananthnarayan R, Paniker CKJ. Textbook of Microbiology. 8th Edition. Hyderabad: Universities Press; 2009.*

Explanation:

Complement-pathways

- **Classic pathway** – Acquired immunity (Activated by antigen antibody complex)
- **Alternate complement pathway** – Innate immunity (Activated by various substances like bacterial endotoxins, fungal cell wall components like zymosan)
- **Mannan/Mannose Binding Lectin pathway** (MBL Pathway) – Innate immunity (Activated by the binding of mannose-binding lectin (MBL) to mannose residues on glycoproteins or carbohydrates on the surface of microorganisms including certain *Salmonella, Listeria,* and *Neisseria* strains, as well as *Cryptococcus neoformans* and *Candida albicans.*)

Sources of Complement

Classical pathway

- C1 –epithelium & fibroblasts
- C3, C4, C6 –C9 –Liver
- C1 –C5 –Macrophages (stimulated by phagocytic events)
- C1 esterase –Liver

Alternate pathway

- Factor B, D, H, I, P -Macrophages (stimulated by phagocytic events)

5. **Which leukotriene is the adhesion factor for the neutrophil on the cell surface to attach endothelium?**

A. B4 **B.** C4
C. D4 **D.** E4

Ans: A. B4

Ref: *Ananthanarayan R, Paniker CKJ. Textbook of Microbiology. 8th Edition. Hyderabad: Universities Press; 2009. Pg. 165*

Explanation:

Leukotrienes

- A substance originally demonstrated in lungs, producing slow, sustained contraction of smooth muscles, and therefore termed **slow reacting substance of anaphylaxis (SRS-A)**, has since been identified as a family of **leukotrienes (LTB4, C4, D4, E4).**
- **LTB4** is a potent mediator of **leukocyte movement** both **in vitro and in vivo**. It mediates interaction of neutrophils (PMNs) with vascular endothelial cells.

6. **Oil and Grease are sterilized by:**

A. Hot air oven **B.** Autoclaving
C. Filtration **D.** Irradiation

Ans: A. Hot air oven

Ref: *Ananthanarayan, Paniker CJ. Textbook of microbiology. 8th Edition. London: John Wiley & Sons; 2009. Pg. 30-38.*

Explanation: *(See table on the next page)*

7. **Which of the following is not true of *Streptococcus pneumoniae*?**

A. Bile insoluble
B. Bleaching on chocolate agar
C. Causes meningitis
D. Possesses capsule

Ans: A. Bile insoluble

Ref: *Ananthanarayan, Paniker CJ. Textbook of microbiology. 8th Edition. London: John Wiley & Sons; 2009. Pg. 218-220.*

Explanation:

- ***Streptococcus pneumoniae*** differs from other streptococci in
  - Morphology: Lanceolate shaped Gram positive cocci arranged in pairs
  - **Bile solubility**
  - **Optochin sensitivity**
  - Possession of specific **polysaccharide capsule**

8. **Ig secreted in secondary immune response is:**

A. Ig G **B.** Ig M

Disinfectant/ Sterilisation	Active against	Use
Ethyl alcohol	Bactericidal but not sporicidal	Skin antiseptics
Methyl alcohol	Active against bacteria and fungal spores	Cabinets & incubators
Isopropyl alcohol	Bactericidal but not sporicidal	Disinfection of suture material, clinical thermometers
Formaldehyde	Bactericidal, sporicidal & virucidal	OT fumigation
Glutaraldehyde	Bactericidal, sporicidal & virucidal (less toxic/ irritant)	Bronchoscopes, endoscopes, cystoscopes
Hypochlorite	Bactericidal, sporicidal & virucidal	Blood spill
Chlorhexidine	Bactericidal, moderate sporicidal & virucidal	Treatment of wounds
Ethylene oxide	Bactericidal, sporicidal & virucidal (highly penetrating gas)	Heart lung machines, respirators, dental equipement
Autoclave	All organisms	Dressings, instruments, media, linen
Hot air oven	All organisms	Glassware, Glass syringes, Grease, oil, liquid paraffin, dusting powder

C. Ig A **D.** Ig E

Ans: A. Ig G

Ref: *Ananthanarayan, Paniker CJ. Textbook of microbiology. 8th Edition. London: John Wiley & Sons; 2009. Pg. 139*

Explanation:

Primary immune response is the antibody response to an initial antigenic stimulus, while response to subsequent stimuli with the same antigen is known as secondary immune response.

Differences between primary and secondary immune response

Primary immune response	Secondary immune response
Slow, sluggish and short-lived	Prompt, powerful and prolonged
Long lag phase	Short or negligible lag phase
Low titre of antibodies that does not persist for long	High titre of antibodies that last longer
Antibody formed is predominantly **IgM**	Antibody formed is pre dominantly **IgG**

Remember M->G (<u>M</u>ahatma <u>G</u>andhi)

9. Coxsackie A virus causes all *except:*

A. Aseptic meningitis
B. Herpangina
C. Hand foot and mouth disease
D. Bornholm's disease

Ans: D. Bornholm's disease

Ref: *Ananthnarayan R, Paniker CKJ. Textbook of Microbiology. 8th Edition. Hyderabad: Universities Press; 2009. Pg. 489.*

Explanation:

Diseases caused by group A Coxsackieviruses

- Herpangina (vesicular pharyngitis)
- Hand-foot-and-mouth disease
- Acute hemorrhagic conjunctivitis

Diseases caused by group B coxsackieviruses

- **Pleurodynia (epidemic myalgia)** or ***Bornholm's disease***:
  - It was first described on the Danish island of Bornholm
  - It is a febrile disedse with stitch- like pain in the chest and abdomen, caused by Group B viruses.
  - The disease may occur sporadically or as epidemics
- ***Myocarditis***: Coxsackie B viruses are the most commonly identified causative agents of viral heart disease in humans
- ***Pericarditis***
- Severe generalized disease of infants

10. Motile clostridia is:

A. Clostridium tetanomorphum
B. Clostridium histolyticum
C. Clostridium septicum
D. Clostridium perfringens

Ans: D. Clostridium perfringens

Ref: *Ananthnarayan R, Paniker CKJ. Textbook of Microbiology. 8th Edition. Hyderabad: Universities Press; 2009. Pg. 249*

Explanation:

- Most Clostridia are **motile** with **peritrichate flagella**.
- The motility is slow and has b-een described as 'stately'.
- Only ***Cl perfringens*** and ***Cl tetani*** **Type VI** are **nonmotile**.

FORENSIC MEDICINE

1. Leading questions are permitted only in:

A. Cross examination **B.** Examination in chief
C. Re-examination **D.** Dying Declaration

Ans: A. Cross examination

Ref: *The Essentials of Forensic Medicine and Toxicology by KS Narayan Reddy. 29th edition. 2010. Pg:*

Explanation:

Leading question

- Leading questions are allowed only during **Cross examination**
- Leading questions are **NOT** allowed during **Examination in Chief (Direct examination)** or **Re-examination**
- Leading question is where one can suggests the desired reply indirectly.
  Example: Were you present in JK Hotel on July 21st?
- The opposite of leading question is **Open question**
  Example: Where were you on July 21?

Procedure in Court

A. Examination in Chief (Direct Examination)

- First examination of the witness, by the lawyer/prosecutor/counsel of the side which summoned
- The objective is to elicit all relevant and convincing facts
- Leading questions are not allowed (only exception is if judge is convinced that witness is hostile

B. Cross Examination

- Lawyer of accused/defence side questions the witness
- The objective is to elicit, remove or modify facts and to test the accuracy of the statement
- Leading questions are ALLOWED

C. Re-Direct Examination or Re-examination

- Done by the lawyer/prosecutor/counsel of the side which summoned
- The objective is to amend or clarify statements made in cross examination
- The witness should not say any new statements during this stage. If so, Cross examination can be done by the lawyer of accused

Questions by Judge can be asked at any stage to clear doubts

2. Green colored urine is seen after ingestion of: (Repeat)

A. Copper sulphate **B.** Phenol
C. Organophosphorus **D.** Cyanide

Ans: B. Phenol

Ref: *The Essentials of Forensic Medicine and Toxicology by KS Narayan Reddy. 29th edition. 2010. Pg: 478*

Explanation:

Refer 2011 forensic medicine question explanation

3. Spalding sign is a feature of:

A. Prematurity **B.** Postmaturity
C. Foetal death **D.** Hydrocephalus

Ans: C. Foetal death

Ref: *The Essentials of Forensic Medicine and Toxicology by KS Narayan Reddy. 29th edition. 2010.*

Explanation:

- In intrauterine **maceration**, the **skull vault** bones may partly **overlap each other**. This is called as **Spalding's sign** and is also detectable by **X-Ray examination** before the birth of the dead fetus
- Spalding sign is a radiological sign showing **loss of alignment & overriding** of cranial vault as a consequence of **IUD** & **maceration of foetus**.
- It takes **2 days to 2 weeks** after death to develop.

Maceration

- It is a process of **aseptic autolysis of a fetus dead in utero**.
- It occurs when the **dead fetus** remains in the utero **for 3 to 4 days** surrounded by liquor amnii but with exclusion of air.
- It does not occur if the dead fetus is born **within 24 hours**.
- It is characterized by **softening** and **degeneration of tissues.**
- The process is **aseptic** because the fetus being enclosed in the membranes is in a sterile condition.

4. **Pin point pupils are seen in all *except:***
A. Cocaine overdose
B. Opium poisoning
C. OPC poisoning
D. Pontine haemorrhage

Ans: A. Cocaine overdose

Ref: *The Essentials of Forensic Medicine and Toxicology by KS Narayan Reddy. 29th edition. 2010.*

Explanation:

Miotic pupils are seen in:

- Phenol
- Chloral hydrate
- OPC
- Barbiturate
- Opioid
- Pontine haemorrhage

Mydriasis occasionally occurs during **opioid rebound** and **withdrawal**

5. **Most common organ to be injured in primary blast injuries is:**
A. Liver
B. Spleen
C. Skin
D. Tympanic membrane

Ans: D. Tympanic membrane

Ref: *The Essentials of Forensic Medicine and Toxicology by KS Narayan Reddy. 29th edition. 2010.*

Explanation:

- Primary blasts can be air blast, underwater blast or solid blast.
- The injury is a result of the wave of pressure created during a blast.
- Most common organ involvement:
  – **Air blast** – ***Tympanic membrane, Lung, Middle ear, cochlea, eyes, bowels***
  – **Underwater blast** – ***GIT***, lungs
  – **Solid blast** – ***Skeleton***, GIT, lungs

6. **ABO antigens are not found in:**
A. Semen **B.** Plasma
C. Sweat **D.** CSF

Ans: D. CSF

Ref: *The Essentials of Forensic Medicine and Toxicology by KS Narayan Reddy. 29th edition. 2010*

Explanation:

ABO antigens

- ABO antigens are found in high concentration in saliva, semen, vaginal and gastric secretions.
- They are found in low titres in sweat, tears and urine.
- Totally absent in nerve tissue, epithelium, skin appendages, bone and cartilage.

PSM

1. **All the following are examples of health promotion *except:***
A. Stop smoking
B. Installation of sanitary latrine
C. Chemoprophylaxis
D. Decreased salt intake

Ans: C. Chemoprophylaxis

Ref: *Textbook of Preventive and Social Medicine, K Park, 22nd edition, page no 40-1*

Explanation:

- Health promotion is simply promoting health. i.e. actions done to improve the level of general health and well being, so that disease initiation process is prevented.
- These actions are not specific for any disease of group of diseases.
- E.g. encourage for healthy lifestyle changes, breastfeeding, balanced nutrition, small family norm, improvement of scio-economic status and clean environment) *(See table on the next page)*
- **Chemoprophylaxis** is **Specific Protection measure** (e.g. immunization, Occupational and automobile safety measures)

2. **One of the following helps deliver of baby in the community:**
A. Health worker female **B.** Anganwadi worker
C. Health assistant female **D.** Village health guide

Ans: A. Health worker female

Ref: *Textbook of Preventive and Social Medicine, K Park, 22nd edition page no 849*

Explanation:

Health worker	Department	Level of health care
Health worker female	H&FW	Sub health center
Anganwadi worker	WCD	a
Health assistant female	H&FW	PHC
Village health guide	Do not exist now, instead ASHA are there who are volunteer health activist, under H&FW	Village

3. **Standard Normal deviate is given by the formula:**
A. (x-‘x/sd) **B.** (x-‘x)2/sd

Level of prevention		Interventions	Examples
Primordial	Prevention of risk factors	Health education	School health education
Primary	Prevention of disease	Health promotion	Life style modification, stop smoking, stop alcoholism
		Specific protection	Chemoprophylaxis, condom usage, wearing helmet, seat belt
Secondary	Prevention of spread of disease and complications	Early diagnosis and prompt treatment	Screening for any disease 2 weeks cough with sputum in case of tuberculosis, any fever case treated as malaria.
Tertiary	Limiting the occurred complication and rehabilitation	Disability limitation	MCR slipper in diabetes before complication, appropriate foot care in diabetes and leprosy
		Rehabilitation	Artificial limb after road traffic accidents

C. $(x-\text{'}x)^2/sd$ **D.** (x+'x)/sd

Ans: A. (x-'x/sd)

***Ref**: Textbook of Preventive and Social Medicine, K Park, 22nd edition, page no 792*

Explanation:

- The distance of a value (x) from the mean ('x) of the curve in units of standard deviation is called "**relative deviate or standard normal deviate**. Usually denoted by **Z.**
- This is important to know area under curve.
- Z also follows normal distribution
- This helps to convert any measurements into normal distribution form and to eliminate the effect of units on measurements.
- To eliminate the effect produced by the choice of units of measurement the data can be put in the unit free form or the data can be normalized.
- Eg: An infant's birth weight can be recorded as 2500 gms or 5.5 pounds

4. **Relative risk is assesses all of the following *except:***

A. Strength of association
B. Biological Plausibility
C. Dose response
D. Temporality

Ans: B. Biological Plausibility

***Ref**: text book of preventive and social medicine, K Park, 22nd edition, page no 75, 86*

Explanation:

- **Relative risk** is calculated through **cohort study** and hence **temporal associated** is confirmed.
- **Relative risk** gives directly idea of **strength of association**, higher the RR, higher the strength of association.
- As exposure level increases different value of relative risk can be calculated.
- For biological plausibility, laboratory type of research is required rather than cohort study, and hence RR cannot comment anything on it.

5. **Median incubation period means:**

A. Time for 50% cases to occur
B. Time between primary case and secondary case
C. Time between onset of infection and period of maximum infectivity
D. Median of several incubation period

Ans: A. Time for 50% cases to occur

***Ref**: Text book of preventive and social medicine, K Park, 22nd edition, page no 62*

Explanation:

- It is relevant in common source single exposure epidemic /point source epidemic.
- This is an important part of understanding natural history of the disease.
- This implies **average incubation period**.
- The gap in time between the onset of the primary case and the secondary case is called the "**serial interval**". This helps to measure incubation period.
- Time between onset of infection and period of maximum infectivity is "**generation time**"
- It is roughly equivalent to incubation period.
- It refers to transmissions of infection, whether clinical or subclinical. However, Incubation period is used only for manifest disease.
(See table on the next page)

6. **In census literacy rate is assessed by:**

A. Attended literacy classes for one year
B. Ability to write signature

Incubation period	Between invasion by an infectious agent and appearance of the first sign/ symptoms
Median Incubation period	The time required for 50 percent of the cases to occur following exposure
Latent period	Equal to IP in non-communicable disease
Serial interval	Between onset of primary case and secondary case
Generation time	Interval between the receipt of infection by a host and maximal infectivity
Period of communicability	During which an infectious agent can be communicated

C. Ability to read and write
D. Attended schooling

Ans: C. Ability to read and write

Ref: *Textbook of Preventive and Social Medicine, K Park, 22nd edition, page no 447*

Explanation:

- **Census** is conducted once in **10 years** in India.
- Literacy rate is assessed those **above 7 years age**
- In census it was first used in **1991 census**
- **A person who can read and write with understanding in any language is considered as literate**
- A person who can merely read but cannot write is not considered literate

7. **Significance of difference between two proportions is best studied by:**

A. 't' test **B.** Chi square test
C. ANOVA **D.** Regression coefficient

Ans: B. Chi square test

Ref: *Textbook of Preventive and Social Medicine, K Park,20th edition, page no:755.*

Explanation:

CHI-SQUARE TEST

- Chi-square (x2) Test is the best method for testing the significance of **difference between two proportions.**
- It has the advantage that it can also be used when more than two groups are to be compared.

8. **All are true about normal response curve *except:***

A. Bell shaped
B. Total area of curve=1
C. SD = 0
D. Mean, mode, median coincide

Ans: C. SD=0

Ref: *Textbook of Preventive and Social Medicine, K Park,21st edition feb 2011,page no:788.*

Explantion:

- The standard normal curve : smooth,bell shaped,perfectly symmetrical curve (based on infinitely large number of observations).
- Total area of curve=1
- Mean=0
- SD=1
- Mean, median and mode all coincides.

9. **Minimum level of free chlorine in potable water is: (Repeat)**

A. 1 mg **B.** 0.5 mg
C. 0.2 mg **D.** 0.7 mg

Ans: B. 0.5mg

Ref: *Park 'Textbook of Preventive and Social Medicine', 22nd edition, Pg: 663 & Community medicine with recent advances, Suryakantha, 3rd edition, Pg: 32.*

Explanation:

- The residual chlorine that remains at the end of one hour contact period is called the 'free residual chlorine'.
- The purpose of residual chlorine is to provide margin of safety against contamination during storage and distribution.
- The minimum concentration of free residual chlorine for drinking purpose should be **0.5 mg/ litre or 0.5 parts per million.**
- Free residual chlorine is detected by **ortho toludine test** using **chloroscope / chlorotex apparatus**.

- During a threat of **outbreak of water borne epidemic** we do **superchlorination** when the free residual chlorine is more than **2mg/litre.** Such high levels may irritate throat, nose and eye. Hence this is followed with **dechlorination** by controlled addition of **sodium thiosulphate** or **activated carbon.**

10. Annual blood smear examination rate in malaria survey is an indicator:

A. Disease rate **B.** Infectivity rate
C. Operational efficiency **D.** Carrier state

Ans: C. Operational efficiency

Ref : *Textbook of Preventive and Social Medicine, K Park,20th edition, page no:227.*

Explanation:

Annual blood examination rate (ABER):

- ABER is given by the formula:

ABER = (Number of slides examined for malarial parasite / Population) x 100

- The WHO Expert Committee on Malaria in 1964 recommended that the monthly number of slides examined should amount to at least 1 per cent of the population. In the Modified Plan of Operation, the minimum prescribed is **10 per cent** of the population in a year.

ABER is an index of operational efficiency.

The annual parasite incidence (**API**) depends upon the annual blood collection and examination rates. A sufficient number of blood slides must be systematically obtained and examined for malaria parasite **to work out accurately annual parasite incidence (API).**

11. Chandler's endemic index is used in:

A. Dengue hemorrhagic fever
B. Malaria
C. Hookworm infestation
D. Cholera

Ans: C. Hookworm infestation

Ref: *Textbook of Preventive and Social Medicine, K Park,20th edition, page no. 215*

Explanation:

Chandler's endemic index – Hookworm Infestation

- **Endemic index** – Chandler worked out an index on the basis of average number of hookworm eggs per gram of faeces for the entire community, as below:
- Average number of eggs per gram of stools :
  - **Below 200** - Hook worm infection is not of much significance
  - **200 - 250** - May be regarded as potential danger
  - **250 - 300** - Minor public health problem
  - **Above 300** - Important public health problem
- **Chandler's index** is still used in epidemiological studies of hookworm disease and also to assess the benefit of mass deworming program.

12. PQLI does not include: (Repeat)

A. Infant Mortality rate
B. Gross national Product
C. Litreacy rate
D. Life expectancy at 1 year of age.

Ans: B. Gross national Product

Ref: *Textbook of Preventive and Social Medicine, K Park, 22nd edition, Pg: 16*

Explanation:

Physical Quality of life index (PQLI)	Consolidates three indicators • Infant mortality • Life expectancy at age one • Literacy • Range – 0 to 100

Human developmental index (HDI)	Consolidates three indicators • Life expectancy at birth (Longevity) • Adult literacy rate and mean year of schooling (Knowledge) • Real GDP per capita (Income) **Notes:** 1. Extra indicator as compare to PQLI is income 2. Infant mortality and life expectancy at age one is conceptually clubbed in HDI as life expectancy at birth Range – 0 to 1

13. Culex mosquito transmits:

A. Yellow fever
B. Dengue fever
C. Tularemia
D. Japanese encephalitis

Ans: D. Japanese encephalitis

Ref: *21st edition Park.*

Explanation:

The diseases transmitted by various insects are

- **Anopheles mosquito**
  - Malaria

- Filaria (not in India)

- **Culex mosquito**
  - Bancroftian Filariasis
  - Japanese Encephalitis
  - West Nile fever
  - Viral Arthritis (epidemic / polyarthritis)
- **Aedes mosquito**
  - Yellow fever (not in India)
  - Dengue
  - Dengue Haemorrhagic fever
  - Chikungunya fever
  - Chikungunya haemorrhagic fever
  - Rift Valley fever
  - Filaria (not in India)
- **Mansonoides mosquito**
  - Malayan (Brugian) filariasis
  - Chikungunya fever
- **Housefly**
  - Typhoid and paratyphoid fever
  - Diarrhoea
  - Dysentry
  - Cholera
  - Gastroenteritis
  - Amoebiasis
  - Helminthic infestations
  - Poliomyelitis
  - Conjucntivitis
  - Trachoma
  - Anthrax
  - Yaws
- **Sandfly**
  - Kala-azar
  - Oriental Sore
  - Sandfly fever
  - Oraya Fever
- **Tsetse Fly**
  - Sleeping Sickness
- **Louse**
  - Epidemic Typhus
  - Relapsing Fever
  - Trench Fever
  - Pediculosis
- **Rat Flea**
  - Bubonic Plague
  - Endemic Typhus
  - Chiggerosis
  - Hymenolepis diminuta
- **Black Fly**
  - Onchocerciasis
- **Reduvid Bug**
  - Chagas Disease
- **Hard Tick**
  - Tick Typhus
  - Viral Encephalitis
  - Viral Fevers
  - Viral Hemorrhagic fevers (eg KFD)
  - Tularemia
  - Tick Paralysis
  - Human Babesiosis
- **Soft Tick**
  - Q Fever
  - Relapsing Fever
- **Trombiculid Mite**
  - Scrub Typhus
  - Rickettsial Pox
- **Itch-mite**
  - Scabies
- **Cyclops**
  - Guinea Worm
  - Fish Tape worm
- **Cockroaches**
  - Enteric Pathogens

14. The extra calorie intake required for a lactating mother is:

A. 400 Kcal **B.** 450 Kcal
C. 500 Kcal **D.** 550 Kcal

Ans: D. 550 Kcal

***Ref:** 21st edition Park*

Explanation:

- In first 6 months of lactation, the extra calories required is **550 kcal.**
- In next 6 months **(7-12** months), the extra calories required is **400 kcal**

  (See table on the next page)

15. Kuppuswamy's socio-economic status classification includes all *except:*

A. Income **B.** Occupations
C. Housing **D.** Education

Ans: C. Housing

***Ref:** Textbook of Preventive and Social Medicine, K Park,21st edition, Feb 2011*

Explanation:

- Kuppuswamy - in India prepared a scale based on **education, occupation and income** which are the three major variables contributing to socio-economic status in urban areas. Similar scales have also been prepared by Pareek and Kulshrestha for use in rural and urban areas.
- Modified Kuppuswamy scale - in India prepared a scale based on **education, occupation of head of the family and monthly income of the family** which are the three major variables contributing to socio-economic status in urban areas.

Summary of RDA for Indians

	Energy Kcal/day	Protein g/day	Calcium	Iron	Vit A	Folic acid
Adult Male	2875 3800 for heavy work	60	400	28	600	100
Adult Female	2225 2925 for heavy work	50	400	30	600	100
Pregnancy	+300	+15	1000	40	600	400
Lactation						
0-6 months	+550	+25 (75)	1000	30	950	150
6-12 months	+400	+18				

- **Prasad scale** – based on income. Commonly used in rural areas.
- **Pareek's scale** – based on education, occupation, caste, level of social participation, land holding, farm power, housing, material possession and family type. It is used in rural areas.

16. Net Reproductive Rate of 1 implies a Couple Protection Rate of: (Repeat)

A. 50 **B.** 60
C. 70 **D.** 80

Ans: B. 60

***Ref**: Textbook of Preventive and Social Medicine, K Park,21st edition feb 2011,page no:452.*

Explanation:

*"To achieve the demographic goal of **NRR - 1** the **couple protection rate** should have to be achieved by **60%** far beyond the present level **(46.6%)**"*

Demographic Indicators

- **Birth rate** - Number of live births during the year per 1000 estimated mid-year population
- **General fertility rate (GFR)** - Number of live births in an area during the year per 1000 midyear female population age 15-44 (or49) in the same year
- **Age specific fertility rate (ASFR)**- Number of live births in a particular age group per 1000 midyear female population of the same age group
- **Total fertility rate** - Average number of children a women would have if she were to pass through her reproductive years bearing children at the same rates as the women now in each age group
- **Gross reproductive rate** - Average number of girl children a women would have if she were to pass through her reproductive years bearing children at the same rates as the women now in each age group
- **Net reproductive rate** - Average number of daughters a newborn girl will bear during her lifetime assuming fixed age-specific fertility and mortality rates.

Also Note

- NRR = number of daughters a newborn girl will bear during her lifetime assuming fixed age-specific fertility and mortatlity rates.
- **TFR** = 2.1 is equivalent to two child norm.
- **NRR** = 1 is equivalent to two child norm, as in NRR we only take into account only female children. NRR = 1 means each women is replaced but a women (her female child).
- **If NRR is less than 1**,then reproductive performance of the population is said to be below replacement level.
- **NRR=1** can be achived only atleast 60% of eligible couples are effectively practising family planning. That is Couple Protection Rate of **60%**

ENT

1. What is the symptom of a person with unilateral abductor paralysis?

A. Dyspnoea on exertion
B. Transient hoarseness
C. Husky voice
D. Inspiratory stridor

Ans: B. Transient hoarseness

***Ref:** Diseases of the Ear Nose and Throat by PL Dhingra, 5th edn. 2010, Page 318*

Explanation:

Unilateral abductor paralysis

- It is due to **unilateral recurrent laryngeal nerve injury**
- The vocal cord lies in the **medial** and **paramedian** position
- Generally patients are **asymptomatic** except for **transient hoarseness** and **no treatment** is required
- Causes include

- Neck trauma
- Benign or malignant thyroid disorders
- Thyroid surgery
- Bronchogenic carcinoma
- Secondaries neck
- Carcinoma of cervical oesophagus

Bilateral abductor paralysis

- It is due to **bilateral recurrent laryngeal nerve injury**
- Bilateral vocal cords will lie in **medial** or **paramedian** position
- Patients have **dyspnoea** and **stridor** which may **worsen** during **respiratory tract infections**
- **Voice** is **not affected** and is good

2. **Regarding acute vestibular neuronitis all are true *except:***

A. Tinnitus and vertigo developing over 1-2 weeks
B. High frequency sensorineural hearing loss
C. Spontaneous nystagmus is present
D. Usually follows an upper respiratory tract infection

Ans: B. High frequency sensorineural hearing loss

Ref: *Diseases of the Ear Nose and Throat by PL Dhingra.5th edn .2010.Page 52*

Explanation:

Vestibular Neuronitis

- Usually follows a **upper respiratory infection**
- Due to direct **viral** involvement on **vestibular ganglion**
- Characterised by **sudden onset of severe vertigo** which may last **few days to 2-3 weeks**
- There are **no cochlear symptoms**
- Other causes of peripheral vertigo are
  - Meniere's disease
  - BPPV
  - Labrynthitis
  - Perilymph fistula
  - Trauma to head

3. **Most common complication of tracheostomy is:**

A. Pneumothorax
B. Surgical emphysema
C. Injury to the large vessels
D. Injury to oesophagus

Ans: B. Surgical emphysema

Ref: *Diseases of the Ear Nose and Throat by PL Dhingra.5th edn .2010.page 340 Tracheostomy A multiprofessional handbook by Claudia Russell and Basil Matta page 51*

Explanation:

- Out of the given options, surgical emphysema is the most common

Complications of Tracheostomy

- Incidence of complications ranges from **5 to 40%**
- Most commonly occurring complications are **haemorrhage, tube obstruction** and **tube displacement**
- Death may occur in **0.5 to 1.6%** of cases and is mostly due to **tube displacement**
- Complications are 2 to 5 fold in emergency tracheotomies in comparison to elective ones

Complications can be divided into

- **Immediate** -Seen during surgery like **haemorrhage, apnoea, Pneumothorax, injury** to **oesophagus**
- **Intermediate**- During first few hours or days like **secondary bleeding, infection, tube block** or **displacement**
- **Delayed** – Seen with prolonged use of tube for weeks like **laryngeal** or **tracheal stenosis, trachea-oesophageal fistula**, and **haemorrhage** due to erosion of a major vessel.

4. **Which of the following is not seen in Meniere's disease?**

A. Vertigo
B. Tinnitus
C. Conductive deafness
D. Sensorineural hearing loss

Ans: C. Conductive deafness

Ref: *Diseases of the Ear Nose and Throat by PL Dhingra.5th edn .2010.Page 112*

Explanation:

- Main pathology in Meniere's disease is distension of the endolymphatic system
- The cochlear duct and Saccule are affected more than the utricle and semicircular canals
- Cardinal symptoms are

1. **Vertigo – episodic**
   - Attacks are in clusters and associated with nausea, vomiting , ataxia and nystagmus
   - There are periods of spontaneous remissions lasting weeks , months or even years
2. **Hearing loss – accompanies or precedes vertigo**
   - Improves after attack, with each attack the hearing loss will add up and gradually the hearing will worsen
3. **Tinnitus – low pitched roaring type**
   - Increases during acute attack

4. **Aural fullness - also fluctuating**
   – May accompany or precede an attack

5. **Which of the following ECG finding is associated with congenital deafness?**

   A. Delta wave **B.** Long QT
   C. Short PR interval **D.** T wave inversion

   Ans: B. Long QT

   Ref: *Diseases of the Ear Nose and Throat by PL Dhingra.5th edn .2010Page 129*

   Explanation:

   Congenital Deafness Associated Syndromes

   Jervelland Lange- Nielsons syndrome
   – Autosomal recessive
   – Repeated syncopal attacks
   – Congenital sensorineural hearing loss
   – Prolonged QT in ECG

   Alports syndrome-
   – Autosomal dominant or X linked
   – Delayed onset of sensorineural hearing loss
   – Hereditary progressive glomerulonephritis
   – Corneal dystrophy

   Pendred syndrome
   – Autosomal recessive
   – Congenital SNHL
   – Goitre

   Usher syndrome
   – Autosomal recessive
   – Delayed onset of SNHL
   – Retinitis pigmentosa
   – Night blindness

   Note: Treacher Collin syndrome and **Aperts syndrome** are associated with **conductive hearing loss**

6. **All the following are features of Gradenigo's syndrome *except:***

   A. Flushing of skin over parotid
   B. Retro orbital pain
   C. VI nerve palsy
   D. Persistent ear discharge

   Ans: A. Flushing of skin over parotid

   Ref: *Diseases of the Ear Nose and Throat by PL Dhingra.5th edn .2010.pg 89*

   Explanation:

   Gradenigo's syndrome

   - Intratemporal complication of atticoantral type of **CSOM**
   - Due to **petrositis**
   - Consists of a Triad which is -
     – **Diplopia due to 6th CN palsy**
     – Deep retro orbital pain due to 5th CN
     – Purulent ear discharge
   - Diagnosis can be made by CT scan or MRI scans
   - Treatment; modified radical or radical mastoidectomy along with IV antibiotics
   - Other Intra temporal complications are
     – Mastoiditis
     – Facial nerve palsy
     – Labrynthitis

7. **Barotraumatic otitis media is a result of:**

   A. Rapid descent while in an aircraft
   B. Rapid ascent while in an aircraft
   C. Sudden acceleration while in a bus
   D. Sudden deceleration while in a bus

   Ans: A. Rapid descent while in an aircraft

   Ref: *Diseases of the Ear Nose and Throat by PL Dhingra.5th edn .2010.pg74*

   Explanation:

   Barotraumatic otitis media

   - Seen in rapid descent during flight, deep water diving
   - **Mechanism**: when the difference between the atmospheric pressure and the middle ear pressure is **>90mmHg** then there occurs' **locking'** of the **Eustachian tube.**
     – Locking occurs because **collapse of soft tissue into the Eustachian tube.**
     – The negative middle ear pressure leads to **transudation**, **hemorrhage** and even **ruptures** of tympanic membrane and round window.
   - Patients will complain of **ear fullness, decreased hearing**, **earache** and **tinnitus**
   - O/E tympanic membrane may **retracted**, **congested** or even **ruptured**, **bubbles** may be seen in the middle ear through the tympanic membrane.
   - **Treatment:** Nasal **decongestants** and **anti-histaminics** and in severe cases a **myringotomy** may be required.

8. **Laryngomalacia is characterized by:**

   A. Usually present at about the age of 5 years
   B. Biphasic stridor
   C. Elongated epiglottis with thin aryepiglottic folds on laryngoscopy
   D. Best treatment by epiglottectomy

   Ans: C. Elongated epiglottis with thin aryepiglottic folds on laryngoscopy

   Ref: *Diseases of the Ear Nose and Throat by PL Dhingra.5th edn .2010.pg314*

Explanation:

Laryngomalacia

- Due to **excessive flaccidity** of the **supraglottis** which gets sucked in during inspiration
- **Most common congenital cause** for **stridor**
- Presents **soon after birth** and **disappears by 2 years** of age
- There is **inspiratory stridor** which **worsens on crying** and **decreases on lying supine**
- O/E long elongated **omega shaped epiglottis** with elongated and **floppy aryepiglottic folds** and prominent arytenoids
- Treatment is mostly **conservative** and **reassurance**
- **Severe cases** may require surgery like **epiglottoplasty, supraglottoplasty**

9. **Treatment of peritonsillar abscess is:**

A. Abscess tonsillectomy
B. Conservative treatment
C. Drainage by Hilton's method
D. Abscess drainage and interval tonsillectomy

Ans: D. Abscess drainage and interval tonsillectomy

Ref: *Diseases of the Ear Nose and Throat by PL Dhingra.5th edn .2010.pg279*

Explanation:

Peritonsillar abscess

Also called as *Quinsy*

- Pus collects between the **capsule of the tonsil and the superior constrictor**
- **Mixed infection** of aerobes and anaerobes
- More common in **adults**
- Presents with **fever, odynophagia muffled or hot potato voice**, halitosis, trismus
- O/E **unilateral tonsillar enlargement** with congestion seen, pushing the uvula to the opposite side, enlarged and tender **jugulodigastric nodes.**
- Treatment is **incision and drainage** at the most prominent point or the junction of anterior pillar with the line drawn from the base of uvula
- Can lead to **parapharyngeal abscess**

OPHTHALMOLOGY

1. **Miotics are useful in which type of squint?**

A. Accomodative squint **B.** Paralytic squint
C. Divergant squint **D.** Congenital squint

Ans: A. Accommodative squint

Ref: *J WHITWELL, Proceedings of the Royal Society of Medicine 07/1958; 51(6):455-7.*

Explanation:

Pilocarpine – Miotic

- Used in **convergence excess** type of **accommodative squint**.
- Pilocarpine causes **ciliary muscle spasm** (as in accommodation) so the patient can see near objects without his attempt to accommodate there by eliminating the convergence.
- It is not used nowadays.

Other uses of pilocarpine:

- In Primary angle closure glaucoma (PACG), to **prevent pupillary block** thereby preventing further attacks.
- Prior to laser peripheral iridotomy in PACG.
- In Primary open angle glaucoma (POAG), **to reduce the IOP** by increasing the trabecular aqeous outflow. It blocks the uveoscleral outflow, so it should not be combined with prostaglandin analogues to reduce IOP.

2. **Extra capsular extraction of lens is not possible in:**

A. Hypermature cataract
B. Immature cataract
C. Lens subluxation
D. Developmental cataract

Ans: C. Lens subluxation

Ref: www.ejournalofophthalmology.com/ejo/ejo18.htmlý; *BASAK Essentials of Ophthalmology,5 th edition, pg no 254,260*

Explanation:

ECCE - It involves the excision of the central part of the anterior capsule [anterior capsulotomy] Followed by the expression of the nucleus & placement of the IOL in the remaining capsular bag.

- Capsule with zonules should be intact so the IOL placed will be in pupillary axis.

ICCE – The whole crystalline lens including the capsule is removed.

Subluxated lens:

- Partially displaced lens still remaining in the pupillary region.
- Causes:
  - Familial ectopia lentis
  - Ectopia lentis et papillae
  - Aniridia
  - Marfan's syndrome [superotemporal subluxation]

– Homocystinuria [inferonasal subluxation]
– Weill marchesani syndrome

Management of subluxated lens:

- Zonular dialysis < 90 degrees – Capsular tension ring [CTR] with ECCE
- 90 – 270 degrees – Modified CTR with loops with ECCE
- > 270degrees - ICCE & anterior vitrectomy with ACIOL, iris fixated IOL or sclera fixated IOL

Capsular tension ring: Fine PMMA made ring which is placed within the capsular bag to give support to the zonules thereby preventing the decenteration of the IOL.

3. **KF ring in Wilson's disease is seen at the level of:**
   A. Descemet's membrane **B.** Epithelium
   C. Endothelium **D.** Stroma

Ans: A. Descemet's membrane

Ref: *BASAK Essentials of Ophthalmology, 5 th edition, pg no 163*

Explanation: *(See the following table)*

- In **KF ring**, the **copper deposits** are seen in the **vertical meridian (6 &12o'clock position)** in the **early stages**.
- It is seen in all Wilson's patients **if CNS** is involved
- With penicillamine therapy , it **disappears**.
- Other manifestations of Wilson's disease are **sunflower cataract & defective accommodation**.

4. **Treatment of congenital dacryocystitis is:**
   A. Dacryocystectomy
   B. Hydrostatic massage
   C. Probing and syringing with antibiotics
   D. Dacryocystorhinostomy

Ans: B. Hydrostatic massage

Ref: *BASAK essentials of ophthalmology, 5 th edition,pg no 387;parson's diseases of the eye 22nd edition pg no.464*

Explanation:

Congenital nasolacrimal duct obstruction/ congenital dacrycyctitis:

- Due to incomplete canalization of the duct , most often the **valve of Hasner.**
- Usually presents at the **3rd week of life** with watering & discharge.

Differential diagnosis:

- Conjuctivitis [ophthalmia neonatorum] – Bilateral, improves with antibiotics.
- Congenital Glaucoma- cornea – hazy, megalocornea, Buphthalmos

Management:

AGE	TREATMENT
<1 year	Lacrimal sac massage **[Creigler's massage]**
10 – 12 months	Probing
1-4 years	Probing, balloon catheterization, silicone tube intubation
>4 years	Dacryocystorhinostomy

Dacryocystorhinostomy:

- A communication is established between the lacrimal sac & the middle meatus of the nose.

Dacryocystectomy:

- Removal of the lacrimal sac.the main aim is to remove the reservoir of the infection .but watering continue throughout the life.
- **Indications**:
  – In extremes of age
  – Fibrotic sac
  – Tumors in the sac
  – TB of the sac
  – Corneal ulcer with chronic dacryocystitis (CDC)
  – Mature cataract with CDC
  – Atrophic rhinitis

5. **Cattle truck appearance on fundus examination is a feature of: (Repeat)**
   A. CRVO
   B. Incomplete CRAO
   C. Incomplete CRVO
   D. Hypertensive retinopathy

Ans: B. Incomplete CRAO

Type of pigment	Disorders	Corneal location
Iron	Kerataconus [**Fleischer's ring]**	Epithelium
	Old opacity **[Hudson Stahli's line]**	Epithelium
	Pterygium [**stocker's line]**	Epithelium
	Filtering bleb **[Ferry's line]**	Epithelium
	Siderosis	Mainly stroma
	Blood staining of cornea	Mainly stroma
Copper	Wilson's disease, chalcosis **[KF ring]**	Descemet's membrane
Melanin	Pigment dispersion syndrome[**Krukenberg spindle]**	Endothelium

Ref: Kanski 7th edition;Clinical Ophthalmology; pg no 563-564

Explanation:

Refer 2011 Opthalmology question explanation

6. **Whorled keratopathy is seen with the use of:**
   A. Digoxin **B.** Amiodarone
   C. Ethambutol **D.** Steroids

Ans: B. Amiodarone

Ref: kanski 7th edition Clinical Ophthalmology page no 862 – 863

Explanation:

Vortex Keratopathy/ Corneaverticillata

- Characterized by **whorl like corneal epithelial deposits**
- In chronological order it starts as **bilateral brown opacities** in the **inferior cornea → whorl like pattern**
- DRUGS –
- **Antimalarials – chloroquine & hydrxychloroquine**
  - No relationship with dosage or duration
  - Reversible on cessation of therapy
  - Other ocular manifestations – **Cataract, bull's eye retinopathy**
- **AMIODARONE – anti arrhythmic drug**
  - Deposits are more in high dose usage & longer duration usage; but slowly reversible with cessation of amiodarone
  - Other ocular manifestations – **Anterior subcapsular lens deposits, Optic neuropathy**

7. **Herbert's pit is seen in:**
   A. Vernal conjunctivitis
   B. Atopic conjunctivitis
   C. Gonococcal conjunctivitis
   D. Chlamydial conjunctivitis

Ans: D. Chlamydial conjunctivitis

Ref: Parson's Diseases of the Eye;21st edition; pg no – 172-175

Explanation:

TRACHOMA:

- Caused by **Chalmydia trachomatis A,B,Ba,C**
- Spread by **3Fs – Fingers, Fomites, Flies**
- Forms epithelial inclusion bodies – **Halberstader Prowazek Inclusion Bodies**
- **Conjunctiva** – upper tarsal follicle which heals to form minute **stellate scars**
- **Arlt's Line** – fibrous band in the tarsal plate
- Limbal follicles – **Herbert Follicles – Herbert Pits**
- Cornea – **Pannus** – lymphocytic infiltration with **vascularisation of cornea**

WHO CLASSIFICATION:[FISTO]

STAGES	FEATURES	TREATMENT
Follicles	≥5 follicles, >0.5mm in upper tarsus	Needs treatment No scarring
Intense	>50% palpebral blood vessels not seen	Uregent treatment Complications +
Scarring	Tarsal conj scarring with white fibrous bands	Inactive
Trichiasis	Atleast one trichiatic lash	Corrective surgery
Opacities	K opacity covering pupillary region	

SAFE STRATEGY:

S – Surgery for trichiasis & entropion
A – Antibiotics
F – Frequent face wash
E – Environmental sanitation

8. **Lagopathalmos is seen in:**
   A. Leprosy **B.** Syphilis
   C. Peripheral neuritis **D.** HZV infection

Ans: A. Leprosy

Ref: Parson's Diseases of the Eye;21st edition, pg no – 176; Basak Diseases of the Eye 5th edition, pg no 117.

Explanation:

Lagophthalmos

- Inadequate closure of the eyelids, resulting in exposure of the eye.
- **Etiology** – nocturnal lagohthalmos
  - Facial nerve palsy – Bell's palsy, leprosy, sarcoid, CSOM, Post mastoidectomy
  - Proptosis & thyroid exophthalmos
  - Comatose patient
  - Cicatrial deformity of the upper lid
- **Clinical features** : Exposure keratitis
- **Neuroparalytic Keratitis** – Exposure keratitis due to facial nerve palsy.
- **Neurotrophic Keratitis** – Keratitis due to corneal anaesthesia – Trigeminal nerve palsy.

9. **Topical steroids is used in:**
   A. Interstitial keratitis
   B. Bacterial keratitis
   C. Fungal kertaitis
   D. Herpetic dendritic keratitis

Ans: A. Interstitial keratitis

Ref: Basak Essentials of ophthalmology 5th edition, pg no 185; kanski 7th edition clinical ophthalmology, pg no 572

Explanation:

Interstitial keratitis:

Inflammation of the corneal stroma without primary involvement of the epithelium or endothelium.

- **Causes:**
  - Congenital syphilis
  - Tuberculosis
  - Cogan's syndrome
- Treatment : **Topical steroids**
- In **Bacterial, fungal & herpetic dendritic keratitis, steroids are contraindicated.**
- In **herpetic disciform keratitis & iridocyclitis, topical steroids are given.**

10. **After injury, when does sympathetic ophthalmitis develop?**

A. Immediately　**B.** After 1-2 weeks
C. After 4-8 weeks　**D.** After 1-2 years

Ans: 4-8 weeks

Ref: *Kanski 7th edition; Clinical Ophthalmolog; page no 465-467*

Explanation:

Sympathetic ophthalmitis

- Bilateral granulomatous panuveitis after penetrating trauma with prolapsed of uvea
- **Injured eye – exciting eye; Normal fellow-sympathizing eye**
- **Causes**:
  - Penetrating injury
  - Intraocular surgeries
  - Cyclophotocoagulation
  - Cyclocryotherapy
- **Site of injury**: Involving CB , iris & lens capsule
- **Pathogenesis**: Autoimmunity against uveal pigments [sequestered antigen]
- **Dalen Fuch's Nodules** – Granulomas between Bruch's & RPE
- **Earliest Symptom**: Loss of accommodation
- **Earliest Sign**: Retrolental flare & cells; KP's at the back of cornea
- Enucleation of the injured eye within 10 days only in eyes with a hopeless visual prognosis
- Treatment: Topical & systemic steroids

MEDICINE

1. **Criteria for transudate pleural effusion all *except:***

A. WBC <1000/cmm　**B.** RBC <5000/cmm
C. Protein <3 g/dL　**D.** Glucose <60mg/dL

Ans: D. Glucose <60mg/dL

Ref: *Harrison's Principles of Internal Medicine 18th edition pg 2178, George Mathew prep manual 1st edition*

Explanation:

Light's criteria for **exudative effusion** are presence of any one:

- Ratio of pleural fluid protein to serum protein > **0.5**
- Ration of pleural fluid LDH to serum LDH **>0.6**
- Pleural fluid **LDH > 2/3** of upper limit of normal serum LDH

However, if serum protein – pleural fluid protein gradient is > 3.1g/dL, it is transudative effusion.

Test	Transudate	Exudate
Protein	<3 g/dL	>3g/dL
P/S Protein	<0.5	>0.5
LDH	<200 IU/L	>200IU/L
P/S LDH	<0.6	>0.6
Glucose	>60mg/dL	<60mg/dL
Leucocytes	<1000/cmm	>1000/cmm
RBC	<5000/cmm	Variable
Causes	CCF, CRF, nephrotic syndrome, cirrhosis, hypoproteinemia	Pneumonia, TB, malignancy, Pulmonary infarction, RA, pancreatitis,

2. **Xanthochromia of CSF seen in all *except:***

A. Bloody tap
B. Carotene
C. Increased antibodies
D. Increased proteins

Ans: A. Bloody tap

Ref: *Harrison's Principles of Internal Medicine, 18th ed, pg e46-1*

Explanation:

- **Xanthochromia** is **yellow discoloration** of CSF supernatant.
- Seen in:
  1. SAH
  2. Jaundice
  3. Increased proteins (>1.5-2 g/L)
  4. Froin's syndrome (spinal subarachnoid block, xanthochromia & excess proteins)

Bloody tap Vs SAH

Bloody tap	SAH
CSF clears on centrifugation	Xanthochromic supernatant CSF
Blood clears in subsequent tubes	Uniformly bloody in all the tubes

Causes of high CSF protein:

1. Guillian-Barre syndrome(GBS)
2. Spinal tumors

3. Meningitis
4. Multiple sclerosis
5. Acoustic neuroma

Albumino-cytological dissociation seen in **GBS**

3. Inheritance of familial hypercholesterolemia:

A. AR **B.** AD
C. XR **D.** XD

Ans: B. AD

Ref: Harrison's Principles of Internal Medicine, 18th edition, page 3148

Explanation:

Familial hypercholesterolemia (FH):

- Homozygous FH is AD, one of the common single-gene disorders
- ***Elevated LDL (500-1000mg/dL***), normal TG
- ***Cutaneous xanthomas***
- ***Premature coronary artery disease***
- Early death in children
- Heterozygous FH , 1in 500 population
- LDL 200-400 mg/dl
- CAD in early age
- ***Tendon xanthomas, arcus lipidalis***
- Treated with statins, cholesterol absorption inhibitor/bile acid sequestrant
- LDL apheresis needed rarely
  (See the following table)

4. Gaint 'a'wave is in all *except:* (Repeat)

A. Complete heart block
B. Tricuspid Stenosis
C. Pulmonary hypertension
D. MR

Ans: D. MR

Ref: Braunwald 5th ed, pg 1073

Explanation:

- **'A' wave** in **JVP** is due to **atrial contraction,** followed by 'X' descent due to atrial relaxation
- **Giant 'A'** is due to
  1. Obstruction at tricuspid valve- **TS, right atrial myxoma**
  2. Non-compliant RV- **PS, PHT, RVMI**
  3. Contraction of atria against a closed TV- **Cannon** 'A' in AV dissociation, junctional rhythm
  4. RV outflow obstruction- **HOCM**
- **TR** – High 'V' wave due to rapid atrial filling à 'CV' wave
- **MR** cause prominent 'A' only in presence of **pulmonary artery hypertension**

5. High SAAG *(serum-ascites albumin gradient)* ascites is seen in all *except:*

A. Cirrhosis of liver
B. Congestive heart failure
C. Chronic renal failure
D. Nephrotic syndrome

Ans: D. Nephrotic syndrome

Ref: Harrison's 18th edition

Explanation:

- The **SAAG** is useful for distinguishing **ascites** caused by **portal hypertension** from **nonportal hypertensive ascites.**
- The SAAG reflects the **pressure within the hepatic sinusoids** and correlates with the **hepatic venous pressure gradient.**
- The SAAG is calculated by **subtracting the ascitic albumin** from the **serum albumin** and does **not change with diuresis.**

SAAG ≥ 1.1 g/dL

- This reflects the presence of portal hypertension and indicates that the ascites is from an increased pressure in the hepatic sinusoids.
- According to Starling's law, a high SAAG reflects the oncotic pressure that counter-balances the portal pressure.
- Possible causes include
  – **Cirrhosis**

Autosomal dominant	Autosomal recessive	X- linked dominant	X-linked recessive
Huntington's disease, Neurofibromatosis type 1, Myotonic dystrophy, Tuberous sclerosis, PCKD, Familial polyposis coli, Hereditory spherocytosis, Von Willebrand disease, Marfan's, Osteogenesis imperfecta, achondroplasia, Familial hypercholesterolemia, Acute intermittent porphyria	Hemochromatosis, cystic fibrosis, á-1 antitrypsin deficiency, thalassemia, sickle cell anemia, CAH, Freidrick's ataxia, spinomuscular atrophy, alkaptonuria, Wilson's disease, homocystinuria	Vit-D resistant rickets Fragile X syndrome Alport's, Charcot-marie tooth disease Rett syndrome	Beckers & Duchen's MD, Haemophila A & B, Fabry's disease Lesch Nyhan Hunter's, Menke's Wiskott-Aldrich Color blindness G6PD deficiency
Y – linked inheritance: Hairy pinna			

- **Cardiac ascites**
- **Fluid overload** due to **chronic renal failure**
- **Sinusoidal obstruction syndrome (venoocclusive** disease)
- Massive **liver metastasis**
- **Hepatic vein thrombosis (Budd-Chiari syndrome**).

SAAG <1.1 g/dL

- It indicates that the ascites is not related to portal hypertension as in **tuberculous peritonitis, peritoneal carcinomatosis**, or **pancreatic ascites**.
- In nephrotic syndrome, due to reduced oncotic pressure (serum albumin), SAAG is < 1.1 g/dL.

6. **Which of the following is characteristic of Cushing's disease?**
   A. Incresed ACTH, increased cortisol
   B. Decreased ACTH, increased cortisol
   C. Increased ACTH, decreased cortisol
   D. Decreased ACTH, decreased cortisol

Ans: A. Incresed ACTH, increased cortisol

Ref: Davidson 21st edition, pg 771

Explanation:

Cushing's disease is due to a pituitary adenoma secreting ACTH.

- Pituitary microadenoma in 90%
- **Cushing's syndrome** is caused by excess activation of the GR (Glucocorticoid receptor)

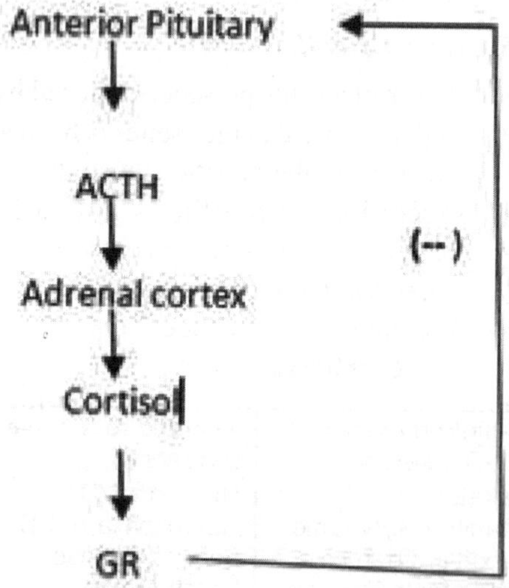

- **Cushing's syndrome** is of two types:

1. **ACTH- dependent Cushing's**
   - Pituitary adenoma secreting ACTH (Cushing's disease)
   - Ectopic ACTH syndrome (Lung carcinoid, small cell ca lung, medullary ca thyroid, pheochromocytoma)
2. **ACTH- independent Cushing's**
   - Iatrogenic (Chronic glucocorticoid therapy),
   - Adrenal adenoma,
   - Adrenal carcinoma

Note:

Pseudo- Cushing's
- Cortisol excess as a part of other illness
- Seen in alcohol excess, chronic depression & primary obesity

7. **Manifestations of vitamin E deficiency includes all *except:***
   A. Hemolysis
   B. Testicular atrophy
   C. Neurological involvement
   D. Thrombocytopenia

Ans: D. Thrombocytopenia

***Ref:** Harrison's Principles of Internal Medicine, 18ed*

Explanation:

Vitamin E

- It includes all stereoisomers of ***tocopherols*** and ***tocotrienols.***
- Vitamin E acts as a ***chain-breaking antioxidant*** and is an efficient ***pyroxyl*** radical scavenger that protects low-density lipoproteins (***LDLs)*** and polyunsaturated fats in membranes from oxidation.
- A network of other antioxidants (e.g., vitamin C, glutathione) and enzymes maintains vitamin E in a reduced state.
- Vitamin E also ***inhibits prostaglandin synthesis*** and the activities of ***protein kinase C*** and ***phospholipase A2.***

Absorption and Metabolism

- After absorption, vitamin E is taken up from ***chylomicrons*** by the liver, and a hepatic -tocopherol transport protein mediates intracellular vitamin E transport and incorporation into very low density lipoprotein ***(VLDL).***
- The transport protein has particular affinity for the RRR isomeric form of -tocopherol; thus, this natural isomer has the most biologic activity.

Requirement

- The RDA for vitamin E is **15 mg/d (34.9 mol or 22.5 IU**) for all adults.
- Dietary deficiency of vitamin E does not exist.
- Vitamin E deficiency is seen along with certain diseases
  - Prolonged malabsorptive diseases

- *Celiac disease*
- Small-intestinal resection
- *Cystic fibrosis*
- Prolonged cholestasis
- *Abetalipoproteinemia*
- Familial isolated vitamin E deficiency (Defect in the tocopherol transport protein)

Clinical Features

- ***Areflexia***
- ***Hemolytic anemia***
- Axonal degeneration of the large myelinated axons
- Posterior column and spinocerebellar symptoms
- ***Peripheral neuropathy***
- ***Ataxic gait***
- Decreased vibration and position sensations.
- ***Ophthalmoplegia***
- ***Skeletal myopathy***
- ***Pigmented retinopathy***
- The laboratory diagnosis of vitamin E deficiency is made on the basis of **low blood levels of Tocopherol (<5 g/mL, or <0.8 mg of tocopherol per gram of total lipids)**.

Treatment: Vitamin E Deficiency

- Symptomatic vitamin E deficiency - **800–1200 mg** of -tocopherol per day.
- Patients with abetalipoproteinemia need high doses- **5000–7000 mg/d**.
- Children - **400 mg/d** orally

Toxicity

- High doses of vitamin E (**>800 mg/D.**
- Nausea, flatulence, and diarrhea
- Reduced platelet aggregation
- Interfere with vitamin K metabolism
- ***Contraindicated*** in patients taking **warfarin** and antiplatelet agents (such as **aspirin** or **clopidogrel**).

8. **Hypocalcemia is associated with:**
   A. Metabolic acidosis
   B. QT prolongation
   C. Hypomagnesemia
   D. Myocardial irritability

Ans: B. QT prolongation

Ref: *Harrison's Principles of Internal Medicine, 18ed*

Explanation:

Clinical Manifestations of Hypocalcemia

- Patients with hypocalcemia may be **asymptomatic** if the decreases in serum calcium are relatively mild and chronic.
- Moderate to severe hypocalcemia is associated with **paresthesias**, usually of the **fingers, toes,** and **circumoral** regions due to **increased neuromuscular irritability.**
- **Chvostek's sign** (twitching of the circumoral muscles in response to gentle tapping of the facial nerve just anterior to the ear) may be elicited.
- **Carpal spasm** may be induced by inflation of a blood pressure cuff to 20 mmHg above the patient's systolic blood pressure for 3 min (**Trousseau's sign**).
- Severe hypocalcemia can induce **seizures, carpopedal** spasm, **bronchospasm, laryngospasm**, and **prolongation of the QT interval**.

Clinical Manifestations of Hypercalcemia

Mild hypercalcemia (up to 11–11.5 mg/dL)

- It is usually asymptomatic
- Recognized only on routine calcium measurements.
- Vague **neuropsychiatric** symptoms, like trouble concentrating, personality changes, or depression
- Assc with **peptic ulcer disease** or **nephrolithiasis**, and increased **fracture risk** .

More severe hypercalcemia (>12–13 mg/dL)

- **CNS** symptoms: Lethargy, stupor, or coma
- **Gastrointestinal** symptoms (nausea, anorexia, constipation, or pancreatitis).
- Decreased **renal concentrating ability**, causing **polyuria** and **polydipsia**.
- **Bone pain** or pathologic **fractures** (in long-standing hyperparathyroidism).
- ECG changes: **Bradycardia, AV block**, and **Short QT interval**

9. **All are true regarding Crohn's disease *except:***
   A. Infertility
   B. Risk of Ca
   C. Medical treatment includes antibiotics, probiotics and TNF alpha blockers
   D. ANCA-positive

Ans: D. ANCA-positive

Ref: *Harrison's Principles of Internal Medicine, 18th edition, pg 2486*

Explanation:

Crohn's disease

- **Most common site-Terminal Ileum** with **rectal sparing, skip areas +**

- It is **transmural**, hence more of **fistula formation**
- More of **systemic symptoms, pain, abdominal mass**
- **Toxic megacolon→ Perforation**
- **Intraabdominal abscess, fallopian tube scarring à infertility**
- **Intestinal obstruction, massive hemorrhage, malabsorption, severe perianal disease**
- **Cobblestoning on endoscope**
- Responds to antibiotics, recurs after surgery
- **ASCA-positive**
- Treatment – **Antibiotics, corticosteroids, sulfasalazine, mercaptopurine, azathioprine, methatrexate, cyclosporine, tacrolimus**
- **Anti-TNF: Infliximab, adalimumab, certolizumab pegol**
- **Anti-integrin**: **Natalizumab**
- **Risk of Ca increases** with **duration & severity** of the disease

10. **All are true about ARDS *except:***

A. Hypercapnia
B. Pulmonary infiltrates
C. Hypoxemia
D. Dyspnea

Ans: A. Hypercapnia

Ref: *CMDT 2013 pg 322, 333, Harrison's Principles of Internal Medicine, 18th edition, pg 2205*

Explanation:

ARDS (Acute Respiratory Distress Syndrome):

- Acute onset respiratory failure
- Bilateral radiological pulmonary infiltrates
- **PCWP < 18mmHg**
- **PaO2/FiO2 < 200** { ALI- Acute lung injuy: Pa/o2/FiO2 < 300}
- Exudative, proliferative & fibrotic phase
- **Causes**- Sepsis, aspiration, shock, lung contusion, near drowning, toxi c fume inhalation
- **Treatment**- Mechanical ventilation with low tidal volume (6ml/kg) and PEEP(10) to keep PaO2 > 55, SpO2 > 88 used along with treating primary condition.

11. **All of the following about grave's disease is true *except:***

A. Cardiac failure is common
B. The Hypertrophy and Hyperplasia of thyroid gland is due to TSH R Ab
C. Remissions and exacerbations are not infrequent
D. It is highly vascular with audible bruit
E. Uniformly enlarged thyroid gland

Ans: B. The Hypertrophy and Hyperplasia of thyroid gland is due to TSH R Ab

Ref: *CMDT 2013, pg 1110*

Explanation:

Grave's Disease

- Grave's disease is an **autoimmune hyperfunctioning** of the **thyroid gland**
- Caused by stimulation of thyroid receptors by **TSHrAb(TSH receptor antibodies)/ TSI(Thyroid-stimulating Immunoglobulin)**
- Increases with high iodine intake & smoking (especially ophthalmopathy)
- Overt **cardiac failure** occurs in only 6-19% , increases with age
- **Sinus tachycardia, (lone) atria fibrillation, thyrotoxic (TT)cardiomyopathy** are other cardiac manifestations.
- Uniformly enlarged gland with **diffuse uptake in radioisotope Tc99 scan** is classical
- FT3 & FT4 are high, TSH is undetectable
- **TSHrAb is positive in 65%**
- **Treatment** : **Propranolol** for **tachycardia**, tremors, anxiety , sweating; thyroid storm; thyroitoxi hypokalemic periodic paralysis
- **Thiourea drugs**: Carbimazole→methimazole, propylthiouracil (PTU)
- For young with mild TT.
- **Methimazole** – Can cause **alopecia, loss of taste**
- In fetus causes
- **Agranulocytosis** seen in 0.3%
- **PTU** is safe in pregnancy
- **Iopanoic acid or sodium iodide** inhibit peripheral T4→T3; in thyroid storm
- **Radioactive iodine (I^{131}):** Contraindicated in pregnant women, no evidence of increased risk of cancer later in life.
- Worsening of ophthalmopathy post radiation & esp in smokers, reduced with steroid cover.
- **Thyroidectomy- Hartley-Dunhill surgey** for pregnant women with uncontrolled thyrotoxicosis or who desire to conceive.

12. **Spirometry finding in Restrictive lung disease profile:**

A. Increased FEV1/FVC Decreased compliance
B. Increased FEV1/FVC Increased compliance
C. Decreased FEV1/FVC Increased compliance
D. Decreased FEV1/FVC Decreased compliance

Ans: A. Increased FEV1/FVC Decreased compliance

Ref: *Davidson 21st ed, pg 651*

Explanation:

SPIROMETRY	COPD	RLD
FEV1	LOW ++	LOW+
VC	LOW+	LOW ++
FEV1/VC	LOW	NORMAL / HIGH
RV	HIGH	LOW
FRC	HIGH	LOW

- TLC: Volume of air in the lungs following maximal inspiration (N= 5-6L)
- FVC: Maximum amount of air exhaled following maximal inspiration (N= 4.8L)
- VT: Volume of air entering & leaving lungs during normal respiration (N+ 500ml)
- RV: Volume of air remaining in the lungs after maximal expiratory effort (1.2L)
- FRC: Volume of air within the lungs at the end of normal respiration (2.5-3L)
- FEV: Volume of air exhaled in a given time during a forced vital capacity effort
  - **Restricitive lung disease:** FVC is reduced because of reduction in intra-thoracic air volume. Eg: ILD, neuromuscular disorders, mechanical factors compressing the lungs like obesity, kyphoscoliosis, pneumothorax. TLC & RV are reduced in all except in neuromuscular disorders
  - **Airway obstruction** show **reduced FEV1/ FVC**. FEV1 is used for follow up of asthma & COPD and in evaluation of bronchodilator response.

13. All are features of obstructive sleep apnea *except:*

A. RVF **B.** LVF

C. Hypoxia **D.** Hypercarbia

Ans: B. LVF

***Ref:** CMDT 2013, pg 318-319, Harrison's 18th ed*

Explanation:

Obstructive sleep apnea / hypopnea syndrome (OSAHS) is a sleep related breathing disorder characterized by:

- Anatomically **narrowed upper airways**
- **Apneic or hypopneic spells** in sleep
- Loud **snoring** during sleep
- Daytime **somnolence, headaches**
- **Weight gain**
- MC in middle age, males, **obese, smoker, hypothyroid, acromegaly**
- Systemic & **pulmonary hypertension, polycythemia**
- **Cor- pulmonale**- which consists of hypoxia, hypercania & RVF
- **Dysrhythmias**
- Diagnosed by **polysomnography**- apneic episodes of 60 seconds
- Must be differentiated from
  - Narcolepsy-seen in children, associated with cataplexy
  - Idiopathic hypersomnolence
- Drugs & depression
- Treatment
- **Indications**
- **Epworth's score > 11, troublesome sleepiness at work/driving, > 15 apnea/hypopnea per hour of sleep**
- Measures: **Weight loss, avoid alcohol**
- **CPAP** (continuous positive airway pressure) & MRS (mandibular repositioning splint)
- Most widely used and effective in RCTs
- **Surgery**:
  1. Uvulopalatopharyngoplasty
  2. Nasal septoplasty
  3. Tracheostomy
  4. Bariatric surgery for obesity
  5. Tonsillectomy (children)
  6. Correct retrognathia in young
- **Atrial pacing** for nocturnal bradycardia
- **Modafinil**: for excess sleep, marginal efficacy only.

14. A 40-year-old man presented with repeated episodes of bronchospasm and hemoptysis. Chest X-ray revealed perihilar bronchiectasis. The most likely diagnosis is:

A. Sarcoidosis

B. Idiopathic pulmonary fibrosis

C. Extrinsic allergic alveolitis

D. Bronchopulmonary aspergillosis

Ans: D. Bronchopulmonary aspergillosis

***Ref:** Harrisons Textbook of Internal Medicine, 17th ed 197 chapter*

Explanation:

- **Perihilar** or **central bronchiectasis** is characteristic of **ABPA**

Allergic Bronchopulmonary Aspergillosis(ABPA)

- Aspergillus may cause a broad spectrum of disease in the human host, ranging from hypersensitivity reactions to direct angioinvasion.
- Aspergillus primarily affects the lungs, causing 4 main syndromes, including:
  1. Allergic Bronchopulmonary Aspergillosis (ABPA),
  2. Chronic Necrotizing Aspergillus Pneumonia or Chronic Necrotizing Pulmonary Aspergillosis

3. Aspergilloma
4. Invasive aspergillosis

- **Allergic bronchopulmonary aspergillosis (ABPA)** is caused by a **hypersensitivity** reaction to the **fungus** and most commonly occurs in those with **asthma and cystic fibrosis** .
- In almost all cases, ABPA represents a **hypersensitivity reaction to A. fumigatus.**
- ABPA occurs in ~1% of patients with asthma and in up to 15% of adults with cystic fibrosis.
- Episodes of bronchial obstruction with mucous plugs leading to coughing fits, "pneumonia," consolidation, and breathlessness are typical.
- Many patients report coughing up thick sputum casts, usually brown or clear.
- **Eosinophilia** commonly develops before systemic glucocorticoids are given.
- The cardinal diagnostic tests include:
  - An elevated serum level of total IgE (usually >1000 IU/mL),
  - A positive skin-prick test to A. fumigatus extract, or
  - Detection of Aspergillus-specific IgE and IgG (precipitating) antibodies.
- **Central bronchiectasis** is characteristic, but patients may present before it becomes apparent.

Diagnostic Criteria For ABPA (Patterson Criteria)

1. Asthma
2. Immediate cutaneous reaction to Aspergillus fumigatus
3. Total serum Ig E > 1000 ng / ml
4. Elevated serum specific Aspergillus IgE, IgG
5. Serum precipitins to Aspergillus antigen
6. Peripheral blood eosinophilia
7. Transient or fixed pulmonary infiltrates
8. Proximal bronchiectasis

Treatment: **Itraconazole** is drug of choice along with glucocorticoids and treatment of asthma. **Voriconazole** may also be given.

15. All the following causes increase in DLCO *except:*

A. Polycythemia
B. Left to right shunt
C. Pulmonary hemorrhage
D. Emphysema

Ans: D. Emphysema

Ref: *Harrison's textbook of internal medicine, 18th ed*

Explanation:

- **Diffusion capacity of lungs (DLCO) or 'transfer factor'** is a measure of gas transfer across the alveolar capillary membrane.
- The transfer of oxygen from the alveoli to form HbO2 can be explained in two steps
  1. Oxygen transfer across the AC membrane and
  2. The chemical combination of oxygen with haemoglobin (Hb).
- The test for lung diffusion capacity of lungs (also known as *transfer factor*) is a measure of the sum of these two functions.
- Diffusion capacity is measured using a surrogate gas i.e. carbon monoxide (CO) and is termed *D*LCO (diffusion capacity of lungs for CO).

Causes of decreased DLCO:

- Reduced respiratory effort
- Respiratory muscle weakness
- Thoracic deformity preventing full inflation
- Interstitial lung disease
- Lung resection
- Emphysema
- Pulmonary oedema
- Pulmonary vasculitis
- Pulmonary hypertension

Causes of increased DLCO:

- Polycythaemia
- Left-to-right shunt
- Pulmonary haemorrhage

16. All the following drugs are used in the treatment of Multidrug resistant tuberculosis *except:*

A. Kanamycin **B.** Ofloxacin
C. Ethionamide **D.** Thiacetazone

Ans: D. Thiacetazone

Ref: *RNTCP*

Explanation:

- Though Thiacetazone has some anti-tubercular activity, it is currently not recommended in the treatement of MDR- Tb.

Multidrug Resistant Tuberculosis

- An MDR-TB suspect who is sputum culture positive and whose TB is due to *Mycobacterium tuberculosis* that are resistant *in-vitro* to isoniazid and rifampicin with or without other anti-tubercular drugs based on DST results from an RNTCP accredited Culture & DST Laboratory.
- MDR-TB, patients who are found to be resistant to rifampicin but sensitive to isoniazid, will also be treated under Category IV treatment. (MDR REGIMEN)

GROUP	DRUGS
Group 1: First-line oral anti-TB agents	Isoniazid (H); Rifampicin (R); Ethambutol (E); Pyrazinamide (Z)
Group 2: Injectable anti-TB agents	Streptomycin (S); Kanamycin (Km); Amikacin (Am); Capreomycin (Cm); Viomycin (Vm).
Group 3: Fluoroquinolones	Ciprofloxacin (Cfx); Ofloxacin (Ofx); Levofloxacin (Lvx); Moxifloxacin (Mfx); Gatifloxacin (Gfx)
Group 4: Oral second-line anti-TB agents	Ethionamide (Eto); Prothionamide (Pto); Cycloserine (Cs); Terizadone (Trd); *para*-aminosalicylic acid (PAS)
Group 5: Agents with unclear efficacy (not recommended by WHO for routine use in MDR-TB patients)	Clofazimine (Cfz); Linezolid (Lzd); Amoxicillin/Clavulanate (Amx/Clv); thioacetazone (Thz); imipenem/cilastatin (Ipm/Cln); high-dose isoniazid (high-dose H); Clarithromycin (Clr)

Category IV regimen

- RNTCP will be using a **Standardised Treatment Regimen** (Cat IV) for the treatment of MDR-TB cases (and those with rifampicin resistance) under the programme.
- Cat IV regimen comprises of 6 drugs- kanamycin, ofloxacin (levofloxacin)†, ethionamide, pyrazinamide, ethambutol and cycloserine during 6-9 months of the Intensive Phase and 4 drugs- ofloxacin (levofloxacin), ethionamide, ethambutol and cycloserine during the 18 months of the Continuation Phase.
- *p*-aminosalicylic acid (PAS) is included in the regimen as a substitute drug if any bactericidal drug (K, Ofl, Z and Eto) or 2 bacteriostatic (E and Cs) drugs are not tolerated.

RNTCP CATEGORY IV REGIMEN: 6 (9) Km Ofx (Lvx) Eto Cs Z E / 18 Ofx (Lvx)Eto Cs E

17. **All the following are present on the ipsilateral side in Lateral medullary syndrome *except:***

A. Diplopia
B. Impaired pain sensation in the body
C. Horner syndrome
D. Facial pain

Ans: B. Impaired pain sensation in the body

Ref: *Harrison's Textbook of Internal Medicine- 18th ed*

Explanation:

- Impaired pain sensation in the body is seen in the contralateral side

Lateral medullary syndrome (WALLENBERG SYNDROME)

Due to occlusion of vertebral artery branches to lateral medulla.

- Post inferior cerebellar a
- Superior cerebellar a
- Middle cerebellar a
- Inferior lateral medullary a

Clinical features

On the side of lesion:

- Pain numbness & impaired sensation over half the face → Due to involvement of descending V nerve nucleus
- **HORNER syndrome** → Due to involvement of descending symphathetic chain
- **Ataxia**
- Nystagmus, diplopia, vertigo, nausea & vomiting → Due to involvement of vestibular nucleus
- Dysphagia, hoarseness, palatal paralysis, vocalcord paralysis → Due to involvement of 9 &10th nerves
- Loss of taste → Due to involvement of nucleus tractus solitarius
- Numbness of arm → cuneate & gracilis nuclei

On opposite site of lesion

- Impaired pain & thermal sense over half of the body → Due to involvement of spino thalamic tract involvement

18. **Which is not a characteristic feature of pseudo tumour cerebri?**

A. Headache
B. Dilated ventricles
C. Increasing opening pressure during LP
D. Papilledema

Ans: B. Dilated ventricles

Ref: *Harrison's Textbook of Internal Medicine- 18th ed*

Explanation:

Pseudo tumour cerebri:

- Headache
- Normal CSF
- Normal or small ventricular size
- CT & MRI are normal
- No focal neurological deficits
- Transient visual obscurations & papilloedema

Causes:

Metabolic causes

1. Hypervitaminosis A
2. Vit A deficiency
3. Steroid therapy
4. Steroid withdrawal
5. Tetracucline
6. Nalidixic acid
7. Irom deficeincy
8. Hyper parathyroidism
9. Adrenal insufficiency
10. Chromic O_2 retention
11. Amiodarone

Infections causes

1. Poliomyelithis
2. Guillian barre syndrome
3. Otitis media

19. All are following are affected in the middle cerebral artery involvement *except:*

A. Hemiplegia **B.** Hemianaesthesia
C. Broca aphasia **D.** Amnesia

Ans: D. Amnesia

Ref: *Harrison's textbook of internal medicine, 18th ed*

Explanation: *(See the following table)*

20. All the following tumors are seen in MEN 1 syndrome *except:*

Artery involved	Areas involved	Symptoms
1. Middle cerebral artery - Cortical branches - Penetrating branches	Supply lateral surface of cerebrum 1. Sensory motor cortex → 2. Motor & sensory speech cent → 3. Optic radiation → Putamen, globus pallidus, genu → Posterior limb of internal capsule	C/L hemiplegia & hemi anesthesia Wernike & broca aphasia (when dominant lobe involved) Homomymous hemi anopia sensory motor hemiplegic syndrome
2. Anterior cerebral artery - Cortical branches - Penetrating branches (HEUBNER'S ARTERY)	Supply medial & superior surface of frontal & parietal lobe. Anterior limb of internal capsule → Part of need of caudate nucleus →	Sensory 7 motor paralys of C/L LL mental changes Bowel bladder incontinence Gait disturbance Ataxic tremor of C/L limbs (frontal ataxia) Apraxia Ideomotor dypraxia
3. Posterior cerebral artery (calcarine cortex)	Primary visual area → Cerebral Ipedumcle → Medical temporal lobe → Thalamus →	C/L homonymons hemoanopia Visual object agnosia Peduncular hemiplagia Amnesia Thalamic syndrome (varying degree of sensory loss & spontaneous lowering pain)
4. Vertebro basilar artery	**BRAINSTEM** a. Midbrain → b. Pons → c. Medulla →	**Weber's syndrome** - I/L 3rd nervepalsy + C/L hemi plagia **Claude's syndrome** - crossed cerebellar abaxia **Millard gubler's syndrome** I/L 7th nerve palsy c C/L hemiplagia Palatal paralysis: I/L post column sensations last ; C/L pain & temp lost

A. Pituitary adenomas
B. Parathyroid tumors
C. Insulinoma
D. Medullary Ca of thyroid

Ans: **D.** Medullary Ca of thyroid

Ref: *Harrison's Textbook of Internal Medicine-18th ed*

Explanation:

MULTIPLE ENDOCRINE NEOPLASIA

MEN I Wermer's	MEN II	
1. Para thyroid tumours 2. Pituitary adenomas 3. Islet cell hyperplasia 4. ZE syndrome, Insulinoma, Glucagenoma, Pancreatic cholera. **Other manifestations:** Fore gut carcinoid, Pheochromocytoma, Lipomas, Angiofibromas.	Medullary CA of thyroid & Pheochromocytoma	
	II A Sipple syndrome	**II B**
	• Hyper parathyroidism • Parathyroid adenoma • Cutaneous lichen amyloidosis • Hirschsprung disease • FMTC (familial medullary thyroid Case)	• Marfinoid habitus • Mucosal neuromes • GIT neuromas

21. All the following causes micronodular cirrhosis *except:*
A. Laennec's cirrhosis
B. Primary biliary cirrhosis
C. Indian childhood cirrhosis
D. Wilson's disease

Ans: **D.** Wilson's disease

Ref: *Harrison's Textbook of Internal Medicine, 18th ed*

Explanation:

Micronodular cirrhosis

- Laennec's cirrhosis
- Jejunoileal bypass
- Primary & secondary biliary cirrhosis
- Indian childhood cirrhosis
- Hemochromatosis

Macro nodular cirrhosis

- Hepatitis B & C
- Wilson's disease
- Alpha 1 antitrypsin deficiency
- Tyrosinemia
- Post necrotic

Both

- Hemochromatosis
- Alcoholic liver disease

22. Photosensitivity is seen in:
A. SLE B. Kawasaki disease
C. Rheumatoid arthritis D. Polyarteritis nodosa

Ans: A. SLE

Ref: *Harrison's Principles of Internal Medicine, 18ed.*

Explanation:

Conditions associated with Photosensitivity

Type	Disease
Genetic	Erythropoietic porphyria Erythropoietic protoporphyria Porphyria cutanea tarda-familial Variegate porphyria Hepatoerythropoietic porphyria **Albinism** **Xeroderma pigmentosum** Rothmund-Thomson syndrome **Bloom syndrome** Cockayne's disease Kindler syndrome **Phenylketonuria**
Metabolic	**Porphyria cutanea tarda**-sporadic **Hartnup disease** Kwashiorkor **Pellagra** **Carcinoid syndrome**
Immediate Delayed	Solar urticaria Drug photoallergy Persistent light reaction/chronic actinic dermatitis
Neoplastic and degenerative	Photoaging **Actinic keratosis** **Melanoma** and nonmelanoma skin cancer
Idiopathic	Polymorphous light eruption Hydroa aestivale Actinic prurigo
Photoaggravated	**Lupus erythematosus** Systemic Subacutecutaneous Discoid **Dermatomyositis** **Herpes simplex** **Lichen planus** actinicus Acnevulgaris (aestivale)

Other Miscellaneous conditions assc with photosensitivity

- Sjögren's syndrome
- Psoriasis
- Atopic eczema
- Erythema multiforme
- Seborrhoeic dermatitis
- Autoimmune bullous diseases
- Mycosis fungoides
- Smith–Lemli–Opitz syndrome
- Sinear Usher syndrome
- Rosacea
- Darier's disease
- Kindler-Weary syndrome

23. Kerley B lines are seen in: (Repeat)

A. Pulmonary edema **B.** Pulonary embolism
C. Pleural effusion **D.** HOCM

Ans: A. Pulmonary edema

Ref: *Harrison's Principles of Internal Medicine, 18ed. & Arun Babu T et al. Pulmonary edema, Recent Advances in Pediatrics, Spl Vol-24, Edited by Suraj Gupte.*

Explanation:

Cardiogenic Pulmonary Edema

Chest radiography

- Cardiomegaly
- Kerley-B lines – Thickening of interlobar septa
- Basilar edema
- Absence of air bronchograms
- Presence of pleural effusion (particularly bilateral)

Echocardiogram

Echocardiography is useful to evaluate left ventricular function, valvular function and pericardial disease.

Pulmonary capillary wedge pressure (PCWP)

PCWP can be measured with a pulmonary arterial catheter. This method helps in differentiating CPE from NCPE. In CPE, PCWP is elevated and large V waves and rapid Y descent may be seen.

Non-Cardiogenic Pulmonary edema (ARDS)

Chest radiography

- Hemodynamic — Peribronchial and Perivascular cuffing, diffuse streakiness- indicated interlobular fluid and distended lymphatics,
- Septal lines - Kerley A & B,
- Butterfly sign - Perihilar opacity (Vascular pedicle > 70 mm),
- Upper zone involvement is an early finding (Vascular re distribution),
- Diffuse patchy opacity - late finding, cardiomegaly.

Types of Kerley Lines

Kerley A lines

- These are longer (at least 2cm and up to 6cm) unbranching lines coursing diagonally from the hila out to the periphery of the lungs.
- They are caused by distension of anastomotic channels between peripheral and central lymphatics of the lungs.
- Kerley A lines are never seen without Kerley B or C lines also present.

Kerley B lines

- These are short parallel lines at the lung periphery.
- These lines represent **interlobular septa**, which are usually **less than 1 cm** in length and parallel to one another at **right angles to the pleura**.
- They are located **peripherally in contact with the pleura** near the lung bases
- These seen in **Congestive Heart Failure** (CHF) and **Interstitial Lung Diseases** (ILD).

Kerley C lines

- These are the **least commonly** seen of the Kerley lines.
- They are **short, fine lines** throughout the lungs, with a **reticular** appearance.
- They represent **thickening of anastomotic lymphatics**

SURGERY

1. Fine needle aspiration cytology is used as a diagnostic modality in all the following thyroid malignancies *except:*

A. Papillary Ca **B.** Follicular Ca
C. Anaplastic Ca **D.** Medullary Ca

Ans: B. Follicular Ca

Ref: *Bailey & Love's Short Practice of Surgery, 25th Edition 792 Sabiston Textbook of Surgery, 19th Edition 909*

Explanation:

- The distinction between a follicular carcinoma and an adenoma can only be made by histological examination
- Invasion of the capsule or of pericapsular blood vessels is necessary to diagnose Carcinoma which can be demonstrated only by histopathology.
- Intraoperative frozen section is not useful

FOLLICULAR CANCER

- Second most common thyroid malignancy (most common-Papillary)

Cinical Features

- 40-60 years
- Female:Male =3:1
- Most commonly presents as asymptomatic thyroid nodule
- Can be associated with Multinodular Goitre in 10%

Diagnosis: Only on Histopathological examination

Management

Based on size of the lesion

•**<2cm** – Hemithyroidectomy followed by Histopathological examination.

If HPE shows

Adenoma – No further treatment

Carcinoma – proceed with Total Thyroidectomy

• **>2cm**- Total thyroidectomy

Thyroid Operations

All thyroid operations can be assembled from three basic elements:

- Total lobectomy
- Isthmusectomy
- Subtotal lobectomy

Total thyroidectomy = 2×total lobectomy + isthmusectomy

Subtotal thyroidectomy = 2×subtotal lobectomy + isthmusectomy

Near-total thryroidectomy = total lobectomy + isthmusectomy + subtotal Lobectomy

Lobectomy = total lobectomy + isthmusectomy

2. **Which of the following is an absorbable suture material?**

A. Polyglycolide **B.** Silk

C. Polypropylene **D.** Cotton

Ans: A. Polyglycolide

Ref: *Bailey & Love's Short Practice of Surgery, 25th Edition 237-8*

Explanation:

Absorbable Suture materials

1. Catgut(plain/chromic)
2. Polyglactin
3. Polyglyconate
4. Polyglycolic acid
5. Polyglycaprone
6. Polydioxanone(PDS)

Non Absorbable Suture materials

1. Silk
2. Linen(cotton)
3. Nylon
4. Surgical steel
5. Polyester
6. Polybutester
7. Polypropelene

3. **Most common artery responsible for hemorrhage in peptic ulcer is:**

A. Gastro epiploic artery

B. Left gastric artery

C. Gastro duodenal artery

D. Superior mesenteric artery

Ans: C. Gastro duodenal artery

Ref : *Sabiston Textbook of Surgery, 19th Edition - 1164*

Explanation:

Peptic ulcer disease (PUD)

- **Most common** cause of **upper GI hemorrhage**
- Approximately 10% to 15% of patients with PUD develop bleeding
- Bleeding is the most common indication for operation and the most common cause for death in PUD.
- **Duodenal ulcers** are **common** then gastric ulcers
- **Source of bleeding** from **Duodenal ulcer** – **Gastroduodenal artery**
- **Source of bleeding** from **Gastric ulcer** - **Left Gastric artery**

Management

- Resuscitation
- Intravenous Proton Pump Inhibitors are started in all patients.
- Upper Gastro Intestinal Endoscopy (UGIE) should be done within 24 hours
- Anti H.Pylori treatment if the patient tests positive for H.Pylori
- Further management is based on findings at UGIE using Forrest classification

Endoscopic Therapy

- For cases of active bleeding as well as those with a visible vessel (Forrest I to IIa).
- In case of an adherent clot (Forrest IIb), the clot is removed and the underlying lesion evaluated.

- Ulcers with a clean base or black spot don't require intervention.
- **Endoscopic options**
  1. Epinephrine injection
  2. Heater probes,
  3. Monopolar or bipolar electrocoagulation,
  4. Laser or argon plasma coagulation (APC)
  5. Hemoclips
- Usually a combination therapy involving injection and coagulation is employed

Indications for Surgery

- Hemodynamic instability despite vigorous resuscitation (>6u transfusion)
- Failure of endoscopic techniques to arrest hemorrhage
- Recurrent hemorrhage after initial stabilization (with up to two attempts at obtaining endoscopic hemostasis)
- Shock associated with recurrent hemorrhage
- Continued slow bleeding with a transfusion requirement >3u/day

Relative Indications

- Rare blood type or difficult crossmatch
- Refusal of transfusion
- Shock on presentation
- Advanced age
- Severe comorbid disease
- Bleeding chronic gastric ulcer for which malignancy is suspected

Forrest Classification

Grade	Description	Rebleeding risk
Ia	Active, pulsatile bleeding	High
Ib	Active, nonpulsatile bleeding	High
IIa	Nonbleeding visible vessel	High
IIb	Adherent clot	Intermediate
IIc	Ulcer with black spot	Low
IIIi	Clean, nonbleeding ulcer bed	Low

4. **Burns grading – Grade 2 indicates involvement of:**
   A. Epidermis
   B. Dermis
   C. Subcutaneous tissue
   D. Deep fascia

Ans: B. Dermis

Ref: *Sabiston Textbook of Surgery, 19th Edition, Pg: 522.*

Explanation:

Depths of burn injury

- **First degree**—injury localized to the ***epidermis***
- **Superficial second degree**—injury to the epidermis and ***superficial dermis***
- **Deep second degree**—injury through the epidermis and ***deep into the dermis***
- **Third degree**—full-thickness injury through the epidermis and ***dermis into subcutaneous fat***
- **Fourth degree**—injury through the skin and subcutaneous fat into ***underlying muscle or bone***

Rule of nines

- Each **upper** limb **9%** Total body surface area (TBSA),
- Each **lower** limb **18%** TBSA
- The **torso 18%** TBSA each side(anterior and posterior)
- The head and neck **9%** TBSA
- Genitalia **1%** TBSA

Parkland's Formula

Total percentage body surface area × weight (kg) × 4 = volume (ml)

- **Half** this volume is given in the **first 8 hours**
- **Second half** is given in the **next 16 hours**

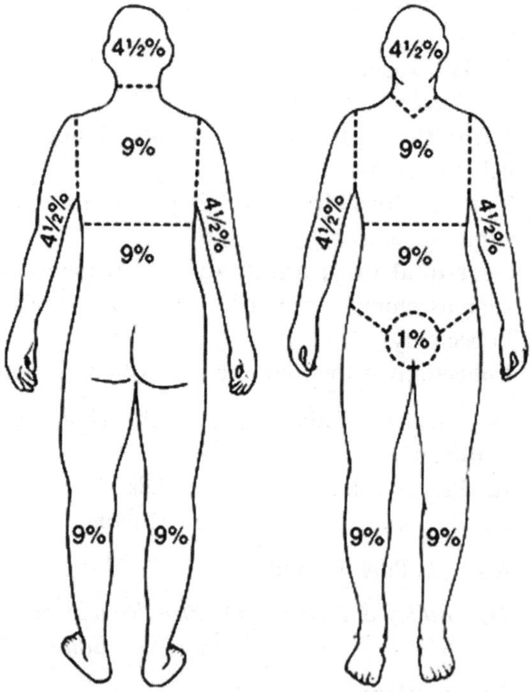

Figure: Rule of Nines in Adults

5. **Treatment of leukoplakia consist of: (Repeat)**
   A. Topical chemotherapy
   B. Excision biopsy of ALL lesions
   C. Ill fitted dencture reposition
   D. Local Radiotherapy

Ans: C. Ill fitted dencture reposition

Ref: *Robbins Pathologic basis of Disease, 8th edition. & Bailey and Love's Short Practice of Surgery 25th Edition*

Explanation:

Leucoplakia

- WHO Defn: 'any white parch or plaque that cannot be characterised clinically or pathologically as any other disease'.
- Multifactorial
- Male to female ratio is 2:1
- ***Tobacco*** smoking and chewing is the single most risk factor

Causes

- The exact underlying cause of leukoplakia is largely unknown & likely to be multifactorial
- **Tobacco -** MC etiologic factor (80%).
- **Alcohol (Not very clear)**
- **Sanguinaria (Bloodroot) -** It is herbal extract which is included in some toothpastes and mouth washes.
- **Ultraviolet radiation**
- **Micro-organisms**
- **Candida**
  - HPV 16 and 18
  - **Epithelial atrophy**
  - Iron deficiency
  - Vitamin deficiencies
  - Oral submucous fibrosis
  - Syphilis
  - Sideropenic dysphagia
- **Tumor suppressor genes** - p53 mutation
- **Trauma**
  - Frictional or irritational trauma leading to keratosis. Eg: Nicotine stomatitis
  - Mechanical trauma- sharp edge on a denture; broken tooth

Clinical features

- Can be small circumscribed white plaque or extensive lesion involving wide areas of the oral mucosa.
- The surface may be smooth or it may be wrinkled, and many lesions are traversed by cracks or fissures.
- The colour of the lesion may be white, yellowish or grey, nodular or speckled on an erythematous base.
- Many lesions are soft whereas other thicker lesions feel crusty. Induration suggests malignant change and is an indication for immediate biopsy. It is important to recognise that it is the speckled or nodular leucoplakias which are the most likely to undergo malignant change.

Potential for malignant change

- Increases with the age of the lesion & Age of patient
- 2.4 per cent at 10 years 4 per cent at 20 years.
- It also showed that as the age of the patient increased so did the risk of malignant transformation: for patients younger than 50 years it was I per cent whereas for those between 70 and 89 years it was 7.5 per cent during a 5-year observation period.

Management

- Tobacco consumption to stop immediately.
- It has been shown that if the patient stops smoking entirely for 1 year the leucoplakia will disappear in 60 per cent of the cases.
- Whenever ***severe epithelial dysplasia or carcinoma in situ is*** present, surgical excision or carbon dioxide laser excision of the lesions is mandatory.
- Small lesions may be excised, the margins of the adjacent mucosa undermined and the defect closed by advancing the margins.
- For larger defects the area should be left to epithelialise spontaneously or alternatively the area can be skin grafted.
- On the tongue the graft is quilted on to the raw area, whereas on the cheek, floor of mouth or palate the graft can be retained in place by suturing a suitable pack overlying it.
- When only ***mild to moderate epithelial dysplasia*** is present the patient should be ***followed up at 4-monthly intervals*** and the lesions recorded in the notes either photographically or diagrammatically.

Premalignant Oral conditions

Definite Premaligant conditions

- Leucoplakia
- Erythroplakia
- Chronic hyperplastic candidiasis.

Not Premalignant, but assc with higher than normal incidence of cancer

- Oral submucous fibrosis
- Syphilitic glossitis
- Sideropenic dysphagia

Not Premalignant Doubtful assc with malignancy

- Oral lichen planus

- Discoid lupus erythematosus
- Dyskeratosis congenita.
- Please note that **Leukoplakia** is diferrent from **Oral Hairy leukoplakia**

Oral Hairy leukoplakia

- Hairy leukoplakia is a distinctive oral lesion that is usually seen in immunocompromised patients.
- Approximately 80% of patients with hairy leukoplakia are infected with the human immunodeficiency virus **(HIV)**
- 20% of lesions are seen in patients who are immunocompromised for other reasons, such as cancer therapy or transplant immuno-suppression.
- Hairy leukoplakia takes the form of white, confluent patches of fluffy (**"hairy"**), hyper-keratotic thickenings, almost always situated on the lateral border of the tongue.
- Unlike thrush, the lesion cannot be scraped off. The distinctive microscopic appearance consists of hyperparakeratosis and acanthosis with "balloon cells" in the upper spinous layer.
- There is **no dysplasia** (It is **not premalignant**)
- Sometimes there is koilocytosis of the superficial, nucleated epidermal cells, suggesting human papillomavirus (HPV) infection, and HPV transcripts have occasionally been found within the cells.
- **EBV** is present in most cells and is **now accepted** as the cause of the condition.
- Sometimes there is superimposed candidal infection on the surface of the lesions, adding to the "hairiness".
- In HIV-positive individuals, with hairy leukoplakia, symptoms of AIDS follow in 2 to 3 years.

6. Testis does not descend beyond ———. (Repeat)

A. 2 months **B.** 4 months
C. 6 months **D.** 8 months

Ref: Bailey & Love's *Short Practice of Surgery 25th Edition Principles Of Paediatric Surgery pg 76*

Ans: B. 4 months

Explanation:

Undescended testis

- This occurs when the **testis** is **arrested** along its normal pathway of descent.
- At birth, about **4%** of **full-term boys** have **unilateral** or **bilateral** undescended testes (**cryptorchidism**), but by **3 months of age this figure is 1.5%** and it changes little thereafter.
- The incidence is **higher** in **preterm** infants because the testis descends through the inguinal canal during the third trimester of pregnancy.
- An **ectopic testis** lies outside its normal line of descent, most often in the **perineum** or **femoral triangle**.
- An undescended testis may be palpable in the groin or at the neck of the scrotum or it may be impalpable if absent or located in the abdomen or inguinal canal.

Useful investigations include:

- **Laparoscopy** – the optimum method of visualising the anatomy
- **Ultrasound scan** – this has a limited role in detecting an inguinal testis in an obese boy;
- **Hormonal** – in cases of bilateral impalpable testes, the presence of testicular tissue can be conûrmed by recording a rise in serum testosterone in response to intramuscular injections of human chorionic gonadotrophin; these boys require specialist endocrine review.
  - **Orchidopexy** is usually undertaken as a day-case procedure. The testis is mobilised through an inguinal incision, preserving the vas deferens and testicular vessels.
  - The associated patent processus vaginalis is ligated and divided and the testis is placed in a subdartos scrotal pouch.
  - **Orchidectomy** is often advised for the unilateral intra-abdominal testis, which cannot be corrected by orchidopexy because of the future risk of malignancy.

The benefits of orchidopexy include:

- **Fertility:** To optimise spermatogenesis the testis needs to be in the scrotum below body temperature at a young age.
  Orchidopexy during the **second year of life** is **currently recommended** by paediatric surgeons. Fertility after orchidopexy for a unilateral undescended testis is near normal. Men with a history of bilateral intra-abdominal testes are usually sterile.
- **Malignancy:** Undescended testes are histo-logically abnormal and at an increased risk of malignancy. The greatest risk is for bilateral intra-abdominal testes. Early orchidopexy for a unilateral undescended testis may reduce the risk but this is not proven.
- **Cosmetic and psychological:** In an older boy a prosthetic testis can be inserted to replace an absent one

7. **Majority of bladder cancers are:**
A. Adenocarcinoma
B. Adenosquamous carcinoma
C. Squamous carcinoma
D. Transitional cell carcinoma

Ans: D. Transitional cell carcinoma

Ref: *Bailey & Love's Short Practice of Surgery, 25th Edition 1334*

Explanation:

Types of Bladder Cancer

- Transitional Carcinoma – 90%
- Squomous cell carcinoma -5 (Associated with bilharzias)
- Adenocarcinoma -1-2% (Arises either from the urachal remnant or from areas of glandular metaplasia)

Note

– Most common type of **Prostrate cancer** – **Adenocarcinoma**
– Most common type of **Renal cell Carcinoma** – **Adenocarcinoma**

8. **Mondor's disease is:**
A. Migratory thrombophlebitis seen in pancreatic Ca
B. Thromboangitis obliterans
C. Thrombosis of deep veins of the leg
D. Thrombophlebitis of superficial veins of breast

Ans: D. Thrombophlebitis of superficial veins of breast

Ref: *Bailey & Love's Short Practice of Surgery, 25th Edition, 833-4*

Explanation:

Mondor's disease

- **Thrombophlebitis of the superficial veins** of the **breast** and **anterior chest wall**
- Can also involve arm

Cause

Idiopathic

Clinical features

- Thrombosed subcutaneous vessel , usually attached to the skin - pathognomonic feature.
- When the skin over the breast is stretched by raising the arm, a narrow, shallow subcutaneous groove alongside the cord becomes apparent.

Differential Diagnoses

- Lymphatic permeation from occult carcinoma

Management

- Conservative
- Restriction of arm movements is advised.
- **Resolves** within few months ***without any complication***
- Association with breast carcinoma is *Coincidental*

9. **Most common cancer arising from a burns scar is:**
A. Adeno carcinoma
B. Fibrosarcoma
C. Squamous carcinoma
D. Adeno squamous carcinoma

Ans: C. Squamous carcinoma

Ref: *Bailey & Love's Short Practice of Surgery, 25th Edition 611*

Explanation:

Squamous carcinoma of Skin

- Second most common form of skin cancer
- Twice more common in men

Risk factors

- UV rays exposure
- Chronic inflammation
  - Chronic sinus tracts
  - Pre-existing scars
  - Osteomyelitis
  - Burns
  - Vaccination points
- Immunosuppression (organ-transplant recipients)
- Chemical carcinogens (arsenicals, tar)
- **HPV5 and HPV16** infection
- Tobacco use

Clinical features

- Lesions vary from smooth nodular to verrucous, papillomatous and ulcerating lesions.
- All variants will eventually ulcerate as they grow.
- The ulcers have a characteristically *everted edge*

Diagnosis - By biopsy

Management

Surgical excision

Lesion < 2 cm – Excision with 4mm margin
Lesion > 2 cm- Excision with 1cm margin

10. **Cork screw esophagus in barium swallow is seen in:**
A. Achalasia cardia
B. Esophageal cancer

C. Diffuse esophageal spasm
D. Diverticulum

Ans: C. Diffuse esophageal spasm

Ref: *Sabiston Textbook of Surgery, 19th Edition 1028*

Explanation:

Diffuse Esophageal spasm

- Hypermotility disorder
- Repetitive, simultaneous, and of high amplitude esophageal contractions
- Motor abnormality of the esophageal body that is more in the lower two thirds.
- Muscular hypertrophy and degeneration of the branches of the vagus observed.

Clinical features

- Chest pain and dysphagia
- Squeezing pressure in the chest that may radiate to the jaw, arms, and upper back mimicking angina
- Symptoms are more during times of emotional stress.
- Regurgitation of esophageal contents and saliva common.

Diagnosis

By esophagraphy and manometric studies

Barium swallow - **Corkscrew esophagus** or **pseudodiverticulosis** due to the presence of tertiary contraction

Manometry

- Simultaneous multipeaked contractions of high amplitude (>120 mm Hg) or long duration (>2.5 seconds)
- Due to spontaneous contractions and intermittent normal peristalsis, standard manometry may
- Not be enough to identify DES.
- An ambulatory manometry has sensitivity of 90% and a specificity of 100% and is preferred.

Management

Pharmacologic or endoscopic treatment preferred
All patients require psychiatric evaluation

Pharmacotherapy

- **Nitrates**,
- **Calcium channel blockers**
- Anticholinergics
- Relative efficacy of each of the drugs not clear

Endoscopic management

- **Bougie dilation** of the esophagus up to 50 or 60 Fr provides relief for severe dysphagia and is 70% to 80% effective.
- **Botulinum toxin** injections have also been tried

Surgery

Indications

- Patients with incapacitating chest pain or dysphagia who have failed medical and endoscopic therapy
- Presence of a pulsion diverticulum of the thoracic esophagus.

Procedure

- A long **esophagomyotomy** is performed through a left thoracotomy or a left video-assisted technique.
- **Dor fundoplication** – to prevent healing of the myotomy site and provide reflux protection

Note:

- Barium Swallow appearance of **Carcinoma esophagus** – **Rat tail appearance**
- Barium Swallow appearance of **Achalasia** - **Bird's Beak appearance** due to dilated esophagus with a distal narrowing
- Gold standard for diagnosing **Achalasia** – **Esophageal manometry**.

11. **Von Hippel Lindau Syndrome is associated with which type of renal neoplasm?**

A. Renal clear cell carcinoma
B. Angiomyolipoma
C. Papillary renal cell carcinoma
D. Renal medullary carcinoma

Ans: A. Renal clear cell carcinoma

Ref: *Campbell Walsh Urology, 10th edition. 2011. Page 1426*

Explanation: *(See table on the next page)*

Site of origin:

- Proximal tubule – Conventional (clear cell) RCC and papillary RCC
- Distal tubule – Oncocytomas
- Collecting duct – Chromophobic and collecting duct RCC
- Calyceal epithelium near renal papillae - Renal medullary carcinoma

Conventional (clear cell) RCC:

- *70-80% of RCCs*
- Worse prognosis
- Aggressive

Renal tumor	Syndrome	Chromosome	Gene	Other features
Conventional/ clear cell RCC	Von Hippel Lindau	3p25-26	VHL gene	Clear cell RCC Hemangioblastomas of the central nervous system Retinal angiomas Pheochromocytoma
Papillary RCC type 1	Hereditary papillary RCC	7q31	c-MET proto-oncogene	Type 1 PRCC
Papillary RCC type 2	Familial Leiomyomatosis and RCC	1q42	Fumarate hydratase	Type 2 PRCC Cutaneous and uterine leiomyomas
Chromophobe RCC	Birt-Hogg-Dubé	17p12q11	BHD1 gene	Chromophobe RCC Oncocytoma Transitional (hybrid oncocytic) tumors Occasional clear cell RCC Cutaneous fibrofolliculomas Lung cysts Spontaneous pneumothorax
Oncocytoma		1p-Loss of Y, 14q Rearrangements of 11q13		Spoke-wheelpattern on angiography Stellate scar on cross-sectional imaging Abundance of mitochondria
Angiomyolipoma	Wunderlich Tuberous Sclerosis (TSc)	TSc – 9 and 16	TSc1 TSc 2	Massive retroperitoneal haemorrhage(10%) Positive for HMB45 Fat (plain CT: $\leq$-20 HU within a renal lesion) - diagnostic hallmark

- Hypervascular
- 3p deletion, VHL gene mutation, Loss of 8p, 9p, 14q and Gain of 5q
- *Respond to immunotherapy*

Chromophilic (papillary) RCC:

- 10-15% of RCCs
- Hypovascular
- ***Seen in End-Stage Renal Disease (ESRD) and Acquired Renal Cystic Disease (ARCD)***
- ***Multicentricity is an important feature (40%)***
- Trisomy 7,17, Loss of Y chromosome
- Type 1: Basophilic
- Type 2: Eosinophilic - aggressive

Chromophobic RCC:

- 3-5% of RCCs
- Prognosis better than conventional RCC
- Hypovascular
- *Mircovesicles on electron microscopy – defining feature*
- *Plant cell appearance*
- *Perinuclear halo*
- *Positive for Hale's colloidal iron* (indicates presence of mucopolysaccharide) – unique to RCC
- *Positive for cytokeratin; Negative for vimentin*
- Loss of 1,6,8,11,18,21,Y; VHL mutations and chromosome 3 abnormalities

Collecting duct (Bellini duct) RCC:

- 1% of RCCs
- Poor prognosis
- Infiltrative
- Affinity for *Ulexeuropaceous*lectin

Renal medullary carcinoma:

- *Exclusively associated with sickle cell trait*
- Infiltrative
- Relatively hypoxic environment plays a role in tumorigenesis

Oncocytoma:

- Histology and mean size (4-6 cm) similar to Chromophobe RCC
- ***Increased uptake on Technetium Sestamibi scan – unique***
- ***Numerous large mitochondria***
- ***Central scar***
- Low grade

Angiomyolipoma (AML):

- Mature adipose tissue, smooth muscle and thick walled vessels seen
- ***HMB 45 positive***

- ***Hyperechoic on ultrasonogram***
- Seen in tuberous sclerosis: 30 years, F:M – 2:1; multicentric
- 5-6th decade; F>>M (if not associated with TS)
- ***Fat on CT (≤ -20HU) diagnostic of AML and excludes RCC***
- ***Pregnancy increases risk of haemorrhage from AML***

12. **One of the following is a contraindication for surgical intervention in varicose veins?**
    A. Symptoms refractory to conservative therapy
    B. Bleeding from a varix
    C. Venous stasis ulcer
    D. Deep venous thrombosis

Ans: D. Deep venous thrombosis

Ref: *Sabiston Text Book of Surgery, 19th edition. 2012. Page 1811*

Explanation:

Deep venous thrombosis (DVT) should be ruled out before intervention in varicose veins.

Indications for intervention in varicose veins:

- Cosmesis
- Symptoms refractory to conservative therapy
- Bleeding from a varix
- Superficial thrombophlebitis
- Lipodermatosclerosis
- Venous stasis ulcer

Indications for IVC filter:

- Recurrent thromboembolism despite adequate anticoagulation
- Chronic pulmonary embolism and resultant pulmonary hypertension
- Deep venous thrombosis in a patient with contraindications to anticoagulation
- Propagating iliofemoral venous thrombus in anticoagulation
- Complications of anticoagulation

Indications for retrievable IVC filter:

- Prophylactic placement in a high-risk trauma patient
- Short-term contraindication to anticoagulation
- Protection during venous thrombolytic therapy
- Extensive ilio-caval thrombosis

Anticoagulation for DVT:

- Treatment of DVT utilises heparin to maintain the aPTT at 60 to 80 seconds, followed by warfarin to obtain an international normalized ratio (INR) of 2.5to 3.0. If unfractionated heparin is used, use a nomogram-based dosing therapy
- Recurrent venous thromboembolism increases if time to therapeutic anticoagulation is prolonged. Hence it is important to reach therapeutic levels within 24 hours
- An initial bolus of 80 U/kg or 5000 units IV bolus is administered
- Maintenance 18 U/kg/hr
- The rate is dependent on a target PTT corresponding to anti-factorXa level of 0.3 to 0.7 unit/mL.
- PTT is to be checked 6 hours after change in heparin dosing
- Warfarin is started on the same day.
- There is no recommended duration of anticoagulant therapy
- Minimum treatment time: 3 months in most cases (Recurrence rate is the same with 3 versus 6 months of warfarin)
- Known hypercoagulable state or venous thrombosis: Lifetime anticoagulation if not contraindicated
- The accepted INR range is 2.0 to 3.0

13. **Most common esophageal motility disorder is:**
    A. Nut cracker esophagus
    B. Esophageal web
    C. Diffuse esophageal spasm
    D. Achalasia cardia

Ans: D. Achalasia cardia

Ref: *Robbins Pathologic basis of disease, 8th ed.*

Explanation:

ACHALASIA CARDIA

- Increased tone of the lower esophageal sphincter (LES), as a result of **impaired smooth muscle relaxation**, is an important cause of **esophageal obstruction.**
- Release of nitric oxide and vasoactive intestinal polypeptide from inhibitory neurons, along with interruption of normal cholinergic signaling, allows the LES to relax during swallowing.
- Achalasia is characterized by the **triad** of:
  - **Incomplete LES relaxation**
  - **Increased LES tone**
  - **Aperistalsis of the esophagus**
- Primary achalasia is caused by failure of distal esophageal inhibitory neurons and is, by definition, idiopathic.
- Degenerative changes in neural innervation, either intrinsic to the esophagus or within the

extraesophageal vagus nerve or the dorsal motor nucleus of the vagus, may also occur.

- Secondary achalasia may arise in **Chagas disease**, in which **Trypanosoma cruzi** infection causes destruction of the myenteric plexus, failure of peristalsis, and esophageal dilatation. **Duodenal**, **colonic**, and **ureteric myenteric plexi** can also be affected in Chagas disease.
- **Achalasia-like disease** may be caused by
  - Diabetic autonomic neuropathy
  - Infiltrative disorders such as malignancy
  - Amyloidosis
  - Sarcoidosis
  - Lesions of dorsal motor nuclei
  - Polio
  - Surgical ablation.
- X-ray: **Absence of Gastric fundus shadow**
- Barium Swallow findings
  - **Bird's beak or rat tail appearance**
  - **Dilatation of proximal esophagus**
  - **Air fluid level** in esophagus
- Treatment options for **primary** and **secondary achalasia** include **laparoscopic myotomy** and **pneumatic balloon dilatation.**
- Heller's Pyloromyotomy
- Pneumatic dilatation
- **Botulinum neurotoxin (Botox) injection**, to **inhibit LES cholinergic neurons**, can also be effective.
- **Calicum channel blockers and nitrates.**

14. Dahlman's procedure is done for management of:

A. Diffuse esophageal spasm
B. Zenker's diverticulum
C. Gastro esophageal reflux
D. Ca esophagus

Ans: B. Zenker's diverticulum

***Ref:** Sabiston Textbook of Surgery, 19th Edition 1023-4*

Explanation:

Pharyngoesophageal (Zenker's) Diverticulum

- **Protrusion of mucosa** and **submucosa posteriorly** above the **cricopharyngeal sphincter** through the natural weak point (**the dehiscence of Killian**) between the oblique and horizontal (cricopharyngeus) fibres of the inferior pharyngeal constrictor.
  - Most common esophageal diverticulum
  - Also known as cricopharyngeal achalasia
  - Usually presents in the seventh decade of life
  - Due to loss of tissue elasticity and muscle tone with age

Clinical Features

- Often initially asymptomatic.
- Sticking sensation in the throat.
- A nagging cough, excessive salivation, and intermittent dysphagia often are signs of progressive disease.
- As the sac increases in size, regurgitation of foul-smelling, undigested material occurs .
- Halitosis, voice changes, retrosternal pain, and respiratory infections - common in older adults.
- The most serious complication - aspiration pneumonia or lung abscess

Diagnosis

- Investigation of choice - **Barium esophagraphy**
- At the level of the cricothyroid cartilage, the diverticulum can be seen filled with barium resting posteriorly alongside the esophagus.
- Lateral views are must because this is usually a posterior structure.
- Neither esophageal manometry nor endoscopy is needed for diagnosis.

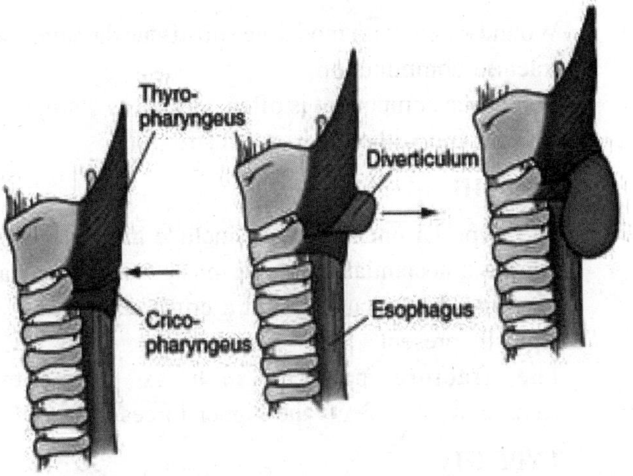

Management

- **Surgical or endoscopic repair of a Zenker's diverticulum** is the gold standard of treatment.
- Traditionally, an open repair through the left neck was advocated.
- Endoscopic exclusion has gained popularity
- Depends on the size of the diverticulum
  - **Small diverticulum (<2 cm),** a myotomy of the proximal and distal thyropharyngeus and cricopharyngeus alone is done.
  - **5 cm** - Diverticulectomy is the treatment of choice In frail patients who may be subject to a higher rate of cervical esophageal leak, a diverticulopexy, without resection, is performed

– **Between 2 and 5 cm- Endoscopic Dohlman procedure**. Endoscopic division of the common wall between the esophagus and diverticulum using a laser or stapler.

ORTHOPEDICS

1. **A segmental compound fracture of tibia with 1 cm skin wound occuring in a farm is classified as:**

A. Type I **B.** Type II
C. Type IIIA **D.** Type IIIB

Ans: C. Type IIIA

***Ref**: Rockwood and Green's Fractures in Adults, 7th Edition*

Explanation:

Compound fractures are classified under the **Gustilo Anderson Classification of Open Fractures**

TYPE I

Low-energy clean wound<1 cm with minimal soft tissue injury and comminution

TYPE II

Wound >1 cm with moderate soft-tissue damage and fracture comminution.
Soft tissue component is often defined as disruption <10 cm and without periosteal stripping

TYPE III

The Type III open fractures include higher energy injuries. Substantial soft tissue injury, with periosteal stripping, has occurred, and a crush component is typically present.
The fracture pattern, such as segmental comminution, reflects the higher forces imparted.

TYPE IIIa

Fracture wound >10 cm with crushed tissue and contamination but usually with adequate soft tissue coverage

TYPE IIIb

Fracture wound >10 cm with crushed tissue and contamination having inadequate soft tissue cover associated with periosteal stripping and often requiring transfer of vascularized tissue for soft tissue coverage

TYPE IIIc

Open fractures associated with a major vascular injury that requires repair for limb salvage

Notes:

- Type I fractures are those with minimal soft tissue injury.
- Skin lacerations are less than or equal to one cm, and are clean, without evidence of deep muscle crushing or foreign debris contamination.
- Additionally, the underlying fracture pattern must be consistent with a low energy injury.
- Examples include spiral diaphyseal fractures or rotational periarticular injuries.
- **Higher energy fracture patterns, such as segmental or bending wedge fractures, should be considered as higher grade open fractures.**
- **Injury being a farm injury is suggestive of contamination. Hence this case would go into Type IIIA.**
- In the event of segmental comminution being present, it would be classified as Type IIIB since segmental comminution is suggestive of more extensive soft tissue and periosteal injury irrespective of the size of the wound.

2. **Minimum intradiscal pressure in vertebral column is seen when a person is:**

A. Standing **B.** Sitting
C. Lying flat **D.** Lying on one side

***Ref**: Katsuhiko Sato, MD, DMSc et al, In Vivo Intradiscal pressure measurement in healthy individuals and in patients with on going back problems, SPINE Volume 24, Number 23, p 2468 –2474*

Ans: C. Lying flat

Explanation:

- In vivo intra discal pressure measurements have shown that the intra discal pressure was highest in the **upright sitting** posture compared to **upright standing**.
- This in turn was **higher** than the **lateral lying down** position.
- The **lowest pressures** were recorded in the **supine and prone positions**.

3. **What is the position of lower limb in anterior dislocation of hip?**

A. Flexion adduction and internal rotation
B. Flexion adduction and external rotation
C. Flexion abduction and internal rotation
D. Flexion abduction and external rotation

Ans: D. In anterior dislocation the leg lies externally rotated, abducted and slightly flexed

***Ref**: Apley's System of Orthopaedics and Fractures 9th edition, p 846.*

Explanation:

- It is not short, because the attachment of rectus femoris prevents the head from displacing upwards.
- Occasionally the leg is abducted almost to a right angle.
- **Anterior dislocation** is **rare** compared with posterior.
- Dislocation of one or even both hips may occur when a weight falls onto the back of a miner or building labourer who is working with his legs wide apart, knees straight and back bent forwards.
- The femoral head will then lie **superiorly** (type I - pubic) or **inferiorly** (type II - obturator).
- Nine out of ten hip dislocations are **posterior**.
- The affected limb will be **shortened** and **internally rotated** in posterior dislocation
- In an **anterior dislocation** the limb will **not be lengthened** , but will be **externally rotated, abducted and slightly flexed**

4. **Which of the following is not a complication of Colle's fracture?**

A. Sudek's osteodystrophy **B.** Non Union
C. Shoulder stiffness **D.** Malunion

Ans: B. Non Union

***Ref**: Apley's System of Orthopaedics and Fractures 9th edition, p 774*

Explanation:

- **Malunion** is common, either because reduction was not complete or because displacement within the plaster was overlooked. The appearance is **ugly**, and **weakness** and **loss of rotation** may persist.
- **Stiffness of the shoulder**, **elbow** and **fingers** from neglect is a common complication. **Stiffness of the wrist** may follow prolonged splintage.
- **Reflex sympathetic dystrophy** or **Sudek's osteodystrophy** is probably quite common, but fortunately it seldom progresses to the full-blown picture of **Sudeck's atrophy**. There may be **swelling** and **tenderness** of the **finger joints,** a warning not to neglect the daily exercises. In about 5 per cent of cases, by the time the plaster is removed the hand is stiff and painful and there are signs of vasomotor instability.
- **Non union** is rare in Colles fracture, though theoretically possible. The distal radius being cancellous is more prone for malunion. The ulnar styloid process often joins by fibrous tissue only and remains painful and tender for several months.

5. **Nerve commonly involved in fracture distal shaft of the humerus is:**

A. Radial
B. Medial
C. Ulnar
D. Circumflex brachial nerve

Ans: A. Radial

***Ref:** Shao YC, Harwood P, Grotz MR, Limb D, Giannoudis PV. Radial nerve palsy associated with fractures of the shaft of the humerus: a systematic review. Bone Joint Surg Br. 2005 Dec;87(12):1647-52. & Wheeless' Textbook of Orthopaedics.*

Explanation:

*" Fractures of the middle and middle-distal parts of the shaft had a significantly higher association with **radial nerve palsy**"*

Palsy Associated with Distal Third fracture of Humerus

- ***Radial nerve*** may be injured by fractures is at junction of mid and distal thirds of humeral shaft, esp if there is lateral displacement of distal fragment
- The radial nerve emerges from spiral groove at this location & is tethered as it pierces the intermuscular septum
- Nerve cannot yield to lateral displacement of distal fragment and therefore may be subject to neuropraxia

6. **In fracture shaft of femur, which nail is commonly used for ORIF?**

A. Kuntscher nail **B.** Austin Moore pin
C. K- wire **D.** Smith-Peterson nail

Ans: A. Kuntscher nail

***Ref**: "Wheeless' Textbook of Orthopaedics - Intramedullary Nailing of Femoral Shaft Fractures". Duke Orthopaedics. & Watson-Jones Fractures and Joint Injuries, 7th edition*

Explanation:

- **Küntscher nail** is an internal fixation device used to maintain the position of the fracture fragments during healing.
- The nail is rigid, having an open slot along its length and has a cloverleaf shape in cross-section.
- It was used in the fixation of diaphyseal fractures in long bones like femur and humerus.

- It has been more or less supplanted by the locked intramedullary nails which are the standard today.
- **Austin Moore pins** are fixation pins used to fix fractures of the neck of femur.
- It is a smooth pin which has two nuts at its end to prevent migration into the joint.
- **K-wires or Kirschner wires** are sterilized, sharpened, smooth stainless steel pins. Introduced in 1909 by Martin Kirschner, the wires are now widely used in orthopaedics and other types of medical and veterinary surgery.
- They come in different sizes and are used to hold bone fragments together (pin fixation) or to provide an anchor for skeletal traction.
- The pins are often driven into the bone through the skin (percutaneous pin fixation) using a power or hand drill.
- **Smith-Petersen Nail** is a triflanged nail for internal fixation of a fracture of the neck of the femur or in trochanteric fracture in combination with a plate.
- It is rarely used at present.

7. **Soap - bubble appearance is seen in:**
   A. Giant cell tumour
   B. Ewing's sarcoma
   C. Adamantinoma
   D. Osteosarcoma

Ans: A. Giant cell tumour

Ref: *Apley's System of orthopaedics and fractures, 9th edition, Tumours*

Explanation:

Giant Cell Tumour

- The X-rays show a radiolucent area situated eccentrically at the end of a long bone and bounded by the subchondral bone plate.
- The endosteal margin may be quite obvious, but in aggressive lesions it is ill-defined.
- The centre sometimes has a **soap-bubble appearance** due to ridging of the surrounding bone.
- The cortex is thin and sometimes ballooned; aggressive lesions extend into the soft tissue.
- The appearance of a 'cystic' lesion in mature bone, extending right up to the subchondral plate, is so characteristic that the diagnosis is seldom in doubt.

Ewing's Sarcoma

- The X-rays usually show an **area of bone destruction** which, unlike that in osteosarcoma, is predominantly in the **mid-diaphysis**.
- New bone formation may extend along the shaft and sometimes it appears as fusiform layers of bone around the lesion – the so-called **'onion - peel'** effect.
- Often the tumour extends into the surrounding soft tissues, with **radiating streaks of ossification** and **reactive periosteal bone at** the proximal and distal margins.
- These features (the **'sunray' appearance and Codman's triangles**) are usually associated with **osteosarcoma**, but they are just as **common in Ewing's sarcoma**.

Adamantinoma

- It has a predilection for the **anterior cortex of the tibia**.
- The X-ray shows a typical **bubble-like defect** in the anterior tibial cortex; sometimes there is thickening of the surrounding bone.

Osteosarcoma

- The X-ray appearances are variable
- Hazy **osteolytic areas** may alternate with unusually dense **osteoblastic areas**.
- The **endosteal margin** is **poorly defined**.
- Often the cortex is breached and the tumour extends into the adjacent tissues; when this happens, streaks of new bone appear, radiating outwards from the cortex – the so-called '**sunburst**' effect.
- Where the tumour emerges from the cortex, reactive new bone forms at the angles of periosteal elevation (**Codman's triangle**).
- While both the **sunburst appearance** and **Codman's triangle** are typical of osteosarcoma, they may occasionally be seen in other rapidly growing tumours.

8. **Trendlenberg's sign is positive in injury to:**
   A. Gluteus maximus
   B. Gluteus medius
   C. Quadriceps femoris
   D. Quadratuslumborum

Ans: B. Gluteus medius

Ref: *Presswood L, Cronin J, Keogh J, Whatman C (2008). Gluteus Medius: Applied Anatomy, Dysfunction, Assessment, and Progressive Strengthening. Strength and Conditioning Journal, 30 (5), 41-53*

Explantion:

- Trendelenburg's sign is found in people with weak or paralyzed abductor muscles of the hip, namely **gluteus medius and minimus**.

- It is named after the German surgeon Friedrich Trendelenburg.
- The Gluteus mediusis far more valuable as a pelvis and lower extremity dynamic stabilizer than it is a pure hip abductor.
- This is apparent when looking at the mechanism of a Trendelenburg Gait
- The role of the gluteus medius during activities such as walking and running is to dynamically stabilize the pelvis in a neutral position during single leg stance.
- Weakness of the right gluteus medius will cause the left hip to drop when standing on the right limb.

9. **Baker's cyst is a swelling which occurs in: (Repeat)**

A. Popliteal fossa **B.** Cubital fossa
C. Lateral malleolus **D.** Medial malleolus

Ans: A. Popliteal fossa

Ref: *Apley's System of Orthopaedics and Fractures. 9th Edition*

Explantion:

- A **Baker's cyst** is produced by bulging of the posterior capsule of the knee and synovial herniation which produce a swelling in the popliteal fossa.
- The lump, which is usually seen in **older people**, is in the **midline of the limb** and at or below the level of the joint.
- It fluctuates but is **not tender**. It becomes **less prominent on knee flexion** as opposed to semimembranosus bursa.
- It is more likely to be caused by **rheumatoid or osteoarthritis**.

10. **Finkelstein's test is done for diagnosis of:**

A. De quervain's tenosynovitis
B. Trigger finger
C. Carpel tunnel syndrome
D. Compartment syndrome

Ans: A. De quervain's tenosynovitis

Ref: *Apley's System of Orthopaedics and Fractures. 9th Edition*

Explantion:

DE QUERVAIN'S DISEASE

- This condition, first described in 1895, is caused by reactive thickening of the sheath around the extensor pollicis brevis and abductor pollicis longus tendons within the first extensor compartment.
- It may be initiatedby overuse but it also occurs spontaneously, particularly in middle-aged women, and sometimes during pregnancy.
- The pathognomonic sign is elicited by **Finkelstein's test.**
- The examiner places the patient's thumb across the palm in full flexion and then, holding the patient's hand firmly, turns the wrist sharply into adduction.
- In a positive test this is acutely painful; repeating the movement with the thumb left free is relatively painless.
- Resisted thumb extension (**hitch-hiker's sign**) is also painful.

11. **French osteotomy is done for correction of:**

A. Osteoarthritis of hip **B.** CTEV
C. Cubitus varus **D.** CDH

Ans: C. Cubitus varus

Explantion:

- **French osteotomy** is a **supra condylar valgus corrective osteotomy** used to correct post-traumatic cubitus varus resulting from a **mal-union of a supracondylar fracture** of the **humerus** in **children**.

12. **Carpal tunnel syndrome is due to compression of: (Repeat)**

A. Median nerve
B. Anterior interosseus nerve
C. Radial nerve
D. Ulnar nerve

Ans: A. Median nerve

Ref: *Wheeless' Textbook of Orthopaedics & Apley's System of Orthopaedics and Fractures, 8th ed.*

Explanation:

Carpal Tunnel Syndrome

- ***Median nerve*** compression syndrome at the wrist;
- ***Most common*** form of ***nerve entrapment***
- Pathophysiology: Nerve compression may result in
  - Ischemia,
  - Focal demyelination
  - Decrease in axonal caliber
  - Axonal loss
- Presence of pain in the wrist and/or fingers and presence of paresthesias in fingers
- Night pain may be especially predictive
- **MRI:** Indicated when atypical CTS due to tumor or anomalous muscle is suspected

- Non Operative Treatment: Carpal tunnel injection/ Median nerve block
- Surgical Treatment: Goals of surgery:
  - Eliminate compression by the tenosynovium;
  - Tenosynovectomy is performed if tissue is bulky, displaces flexor tendons
  - Restore the gliding capacity of the nerve
  - Remove constriction by external epineurium, & liberate fascicles from internal
- Release
  - Surgical Treatment Options:
  - Open surgical release
  - Endoscopic carpal tunnel release

OBS AND GYNAE

1. **Human placenta is:**
   A. Hemochorial
   B. Endothen - esdothelima
   C. Chorio - endothelial
   D. Non-Discoidal

   Ans: A. Hemochorial

   Ref: *DC Dutta's Textbook of Obstetrics, 7th edn, pg 28*

   Explanation:

   Human placenta

   - Starts developing at 6 weeks and completed by 12 weeks
   - Human placenta is **discoid, haemochorial, deciduate**
   - Development of placenta
     - **Fetal part – chorion frondosum**
     - **Maternal part – deciduas basalis**
   - Cleavage of placenta following delivery occurs through deciduas spongiosum
   - Normal weight – 500 gms
   - Functional unit of placenta – **chorionic villi**
   - Umbilical artery has 2 arteries and one vein
   - **Nitabuch's membrane** is **absent** in **placenta accreta**
   - Blood flow in feto placental unit at term 500 ml/ min
   - Oxygen saturation in
     - Umbilical vein –70-80 %
     - Umbilical artery – 50 -60 %
   - Intervillous space is filled with maternal blood
   - Volume of blood in mature placenta – 500 ml

2. **Genital prolapse in a female can be due to all *except:***
   A. Ascites
   B. Complete perineal tear
   C. Chronic cough
   D. Obesity

   Ans: B. Complete perineal tear

   Ref: *DC Dutta's textbook of gynaecology 6th edition, pg 413*

   Explanation:

   COMPLETE PERINEAL TEAR

   - SYMPTOMS
     - Inability to hold flatus and faeces
     - Soreness over perianal region due to constant irritation by stool
     - **Inspite of deficit of perineum, women with CPT do not develop prolapsed. This is because of overactivity of levator ani muscles**

   Aetiology of pelvic organ prolapse

   - Trauma of vaginal delivery to ligaments, endopelvic fascia, levators and perineal body
   - Congenital weakness of supporting structures
   - Postmenopausal atrophy
   - Increased intraabdominal pressure
     - Chronic cough
     - Constipation
     - Ascitis
     - Mass abdomen
   - Heavy work – weight lifting
   - Obesity

3. **Evidence of ovulation has occurred is all *except:***
   A. 10 mm graffian follicles on USG
   B. Progesterone > 5ng/ml
   C. Corpus luteum
   D. Biphasic increase in temperature

   Ans: A. 10 mm graffian follicles on USG

   Ref: *DC Dutta's textbook of obstetrics, 7th edn, pg 224*

   Explanation:

   Diagnosis of ovulation

   - **Indirect methods**
   - ***Menstrual history***
     - Regular menstrual cycle
     - Mittelschmerz
     - Premenstrual syndrome/primary dysmeno-rrhoea
   - ***Basal body temperature***
     - **Biphasic pattern of temperature (0.5 deg. C) in ovulatory cycles**
     - Rise in temperature following ovulation is due to progesterone
   - ***Cervical mucous method***

- Proliferative phase – mucous thin , copious, stretchable (**Spinbarkiet test**)
- Disappearance of fern pattern of mucous beyond 22nd day of cycle suggests ovulation

- ***Vaginal cytology***
  - Maturation index shifts to left in 2nd half of the cycle due to progesterone effect
- ***Hormonal estimation***
  - Serum progesterone ↑
  - Serum LH – LH surge at time of ovulation
    - **Ovulation occurs 34 -36 hrs following LH surge**
    - Coincides about 10-12 hrs following LH peak
    - Urinary LH –kits available
    - Ovulation usually occurs within 14-26 hrs of detection of urinary LH surge
  - Serum estradiol
    - **Peaks 24 hrs prior to LH surge**
    - Coincides 24 -36 hrs prior to ovulation
    - IVF – serum LH and Estradiol measured
- ***Endometrial biopsy***
  - Biopsy done on 21st -23rd day of cycle - secretory endometrium
  - **Subnuclear vacuolation – earliest evidence**
    - Appears 36 -48 hrs following ovulation
- ***USG***
  - Serial TVS during midcycle
  - Precisely measures Graafian follicle
  - Just prior to ovulation measures **18-20 mm**
  - Following ovulation features of recent ovulation in USG
    - Collapsed follicle
    - Fluid in POD
- **Direct method**
  - ***Laparoscopy***
    - Laparoscopic visualisation of recent corpus luteum
    - Detection of ovum in aspirated peritoneal fluid

4. All are sonological markers for downs syndrome *except:*

A. Nuchal transluscency B. Short femur
C. Echogenic bowel D. Hydronephrosis

Ans: D. Hydronephrosis

Ref: *Dutta's Text Book of Obstetrics, 7th edition. pg 106, Williams obstetrics, 23rd edition.*

Explanation:

USG markers of Down's syndrome fetus (soft tissue markers)

- Nuchal fold thickening
- Mild renal pelvis dilatation
- Echogenic intracardiac focus
- Echogenic bowel
- Short femur
- Short humerus

Antenatal Screening for Down's syndrome

- First trimester screening for down's syndrome includes **NT (nuchal translucency)**, **PAPP-A, hCG**
- ***Nuchal translucency > 3.5 mm*** is significant.
- It is done at **11-14** weeks
- Detection rate- **79-87%**
- Triple test and quadruple tests are done in second trimester at **15-20** weeks
- **Triple** test: **hCG, AFP, unconjugated estriol**.
- **Quadruple** test: **triple test + inhibin**
- **Integrated** test: **first trimester** screening + **quadruple** test
- **MSAFP↓, UE3↓, HCG↑, Inhibin A↑** in down's syndrome.

5. The most common breech presentation in a nulliparous woman is:

A. Frank breech B. Complete breech
C. Footling D. Incomplete breech

Ans: A. Frank breech

Ref: *DC Dutta's textbook of obstetrics, 7th edn, pg 374*

Explanation:

Breech

- MC malpresentation
- MC cause – prematurity

Etiology

- **Prematurity**
- Maternal factors - multi
- Fetal factors - anomalies (hydrocephalus)
- Uterine factors - bicornuate, septate, arcuate uterus
- Pelvic factors - contracted pelvis
- Placental factors - placenta praevia, cornuo fundal attachment
- Cord factors - short cord
- Liquor factors - polyhydramnios, oligohydramnios

- **Types of breech**
  - **Complete breech**
    - More common in multi with lax abdominal wall
  - **Incomplete breech**
    - Frank breech (extended breech) – MC in primi

- Footling breech/knee presentation
- **Cord prolapse** **Incidence**
  - Frank breech – 0.5%
  - Flexed breech – 5 %
  - Footling breech – 15%
- **Complicated breech** – breech associated with other obstetric complications like p LSCS, placenta praevia, contracted pelvis etc.
- **Complicated breech delivery** – difficulties encountered during a vaginal breech delivery lke extended arm etc
- **Recurrent breech presentation** – can occur in uterine anomalies like bicornuate or septate uterus
- Denominator – sacrum
- Engaging diameter
  - Buttocks – bitrochanteric (10 cms)
  - Shoulder – bisacromial (12 cms)
  - Head – suboccipito frontal (10 cms)

6. **Shoulder dystocia occurs in delivery of fetus with:**

A. Anencephaly **B.** Hydrocephalus
C. Fetal ascites **D.** Breech

Ans: A. Anencephaly

Ref: *DC Dutta's textbook of obstetrics, 7th edn, pg 406*

Explanation:

SHOULDER DYSTOCIA

- Incidence 0.2 to 1 %
- Anterior or posterior shoulder impacts on maternal symphysis or sacral promontery
- **Predisposing factors**
  - Fetal macrosomia
  - Obesity
  - Diabetes
  - Midpelvic instrumental delivery
  - Postmaturity
  - Multiparity
  - **Anencephaly**
  - Fetal ascites
- **Maternal complications**
  - Postpartum hemorrhage
  - Cervical tears
  - Vaginal tears
  - Perineal tears
  - Operative delivery
- **Fetal Complications**
  - Fetal—asphyxia
  - Brachial plexus injury
  - Klumpke's palsy
  - Fracture humerus
  - Clavicle fracture
  - Sternomastoid hematoma
- **Diagnosis**
  - Definite recoil of head against the perineum[**turtle neck sign**]
  - Inadequate spontaneous restitution
  - Fetal face becomes plethoric
- **Management:**
  1. **Mc Roberts manoever** — Flexing maternal thighs on abdomen straightens sacrum
  2. Suprapubic pressure reduces bisacromial diameter
  3. **Wood's manoever** — Under general anesthesia posterior shoulder rotated anteriorly
  4. **Cleidotomy** — Cutting clavicle in anencephaly or dead fetus
  5. **Zavanelli manoever** — Pushing fetus inside and doing caesarean section or symphysiotomy

7. **Magnesium sulfate as an uterine relaxant is contraindicated in following *except:***

A. Premature rupture of membrane
B. Intrauterine infection
C. Myasthenia gravis
D. Renal failure

Ans: A. Prematre rupture of membrane

Ref: *Practical guide to high risk pregnancy & delivery: Fernando Arias 3rd ed. Pg. 224*

Explanation:

- **Magnesium sulphate** acts by **blocking transmission in the neuromuscular junction.** Hence it is contraindicated in **myasthenia gravis**.
- It is excreted through **kidneys**. Hence, it should be cautiously used in **renal failure** patients.
- **Tocolysis** as such is **contraindicated** in **chorioamnionitis/ intrauterine infection.**
- Hence options b, c & d are ruled out.
- Tocolysis can be given in **preterm PROM** after ruling out chorioamnionitis.
- **Complications of magnesium sulphate therapy**:
  - Muscular weakness
  - Pulmonary edema
  - Respiratory depression
  - Neurotoxicity
  - Neonatal depression
  - Neonatal hyppotonia
  - Neonatal hypocalcemia
  - Intraventricular hemorrhage
- **Drugs that can be used for tocolysis**
  - Nifedipine
  - Magnesium sulphate

- Beta adrenergic drugs like isoxsuprine, ritodrine, terbutaline
- Indomethacine
- Nitroglycerine
- Diazoxide

• Safest tocolytic with least side effects: **Nifedipine.**

8. A pregnant woman with mitral stenosis is most likely to develop cardiac failure in which period?

A. 16wks **B.** 24wks
C. 20wks **D.** 28wks

Ans: D. 28 weeks

Ref: *DC Dutta's Textbook of obstetrics, 7th edn, Pg 276*

Explanation:

• **A heart disease patient is at risk of heart failure during the following periods:**
  - 9 – 11 weeks
  - 28 – 30 weeks
  - During labor
  - Immediately after delivery
  - Post partum 5 days

• **Indications for MTP in heart disease:**
  - Pulmonary hypertension/ eisenmenger's syndrome
  - Marfan syndrome with aortic involvement
  - Aortic coarctation with valvular involvement
  - NYHA III & IV mitral stenosis is a relative indication.

9. Incidence of scar rupture in a pregnant lady with previous LSCS is:

A. 0.2 **B.** 0.5
C. 0.7 **D.** 0.9

Ans: B. 0.5

Ref: *Williams obstetrics, 23rd edition & www.caesarean.org.uk/articles/VBACMM.html*

Explanation:

Incidence of Scar Rupture

The most commonly quoted scar rupture for LSCS, especially by those opposed to and afraid of VBAC is **0.5%, or 1 in 200** chance. (*Ref: Murray, Enkin and Chalmers, 1994*)

Estimated risk of scar rupture:

Type of incision	Incidence of scar rupture
Low transverse	0.2 – 1.5%
Low vertical	1 – 7%
T shaped	4 – 7%
Classical	4 – 7%

10. True statement regarding transverse lie:

A. Cord prolapse is common
B. 3rd degree perineal tear is common
C. Deep transverse arrest can occur
D. More common in primi

Ans: A. Cord prolapse is common

Ref: *DC Dutta's Textbook of obstetrics, 7th edn, DC Dutta's Textbook of gynaecology 6th edition*

Explanation:

• **Cord prolapse** is common in **transverse lie.** Hence, option A is correct.

• Now, if you analyse the other options,
  - **3rd degree perineal tear** can occur only if **vaginal delivery** occurs. But there is no question of vaginal delivery in transverse lie.
  - **Deep transverse arrest** means the **fetal head** is **arrested deep in the pelvic cavity,** sagittal suture is placed in the transverse bispinous diameter and there is no progress in the descent of head even after 1 hr following full dilatation. This condition is a complication of occipitoposterior position.
  - **Transverse lie** is more common in **multiparae,** when compared to **primiparae.**

• **Complications of transverse lie:**
  - PROM
  - Cord prolapse
  - Hand prolapse
  - Neglected shoulder presentation
  - Obstructed labour
  - Dehydration
  - Ketoacidosis
  - Sepsis
  - Rupture uterus

11. Variable deceleration indicates:

A. Head compression **B.** Cord compression
C. Fetal hypoxaemia **D.** Maternal sedation

Ans: B. Cord compression

Ref: *DC Dutta's Textbook of obstetrics, 7th edn, Pg*

Explanation:

• **Variable deceleration** occurs in **Cord compression.**
• **Late deceleration** occurs in **Fetal hypoxemia.**
• **Early deceleration** occurs in **Head compression**

12. Regarding monozygotic twins, which of the following is not true?

A. USG is more useful in the first half of pregnancy
B. Sex discordance can occur rarely

C. Always monochorionic
D. More common following ovulation induction

Ans: C. Always monochorionic

Ref: *DC Dutta's Textbook of obstetrics, 7th edn, Pg 201*

Explanation:

- **Monozygotic twins** are always **identical in sex.**
- Monozygotic twins can be:
  - Diamniotic dichorionic
  - Diamniotic monochorionic
  - Monoamniotic monochorionic
  - Conjoint twins
- Most common cause for **multiple pregnancy – ovulation induction**
- Ultrasound in the first half of pregnancy is best to check for **amnionicity** and **chorionicity.**

13. The placenta is formed from:
A. Decidua basalis
B. Decidua vera
C. Chorion levae
D. Decidua capsularis

Ans: A. Decidua basalis

Ref: *DC Dutta's Textbook of obstetrics, 7th edn, Pg 30*

Explanation:

- **Fetal** contribution for placental formation – **Chorion frondosum**
- **Maternal** contribution – **Decidua basalis**

14. All cause endometrial carcinoma *except:* (Repeat)
A. Fibromyoma
B. HRT
C. OCPs
D. Corpus Cancer Syndrome

Ans: C. OCPs

Ref: *Shaw's textbook of gynecology 15th edition Pg.416*

Explanation:

PREDISPOSING FACTORS FOR ENDOMET RIAL CARCINOMA:

- Hormone replacement therapy after monopause
- Chronic non ovulatory cycles in DUB
- Familial predisposition—familial lynch II syndrome
- Tamoxifen given for breast cancer
- Corpus cancer syndrome—obesity, diabetes and hypertension — 30%
- PCOD
- Fibroid—3%
- Feminising ovarian tumor
  - **OCPs** have **a protective effect** and reduces the risk by **40-50%** and also adding progestogens for 12 days each cycle to oestrogen in HRT reduces its risk to 2%

15. Cervix to body ratio in a postpubertal adolescent girl is: (Repeat)
A. 1:1
B. 2:1
C. 1:2
D. 3:1

Ans: C. 1:2

Ref: *Shaw's Textbook of Gynaecology 15th Edition Pg: 8*

Explanation:

Relationship between the length of cervix and the body of uterus:

- Before puberty - **2:1**
- After puberty - **1:2**
- During reproductive period - **1:3**

16. The level of hCG is maximum during which day of pregnancy:
A. 50-60
B. 60-70
C. 70-80
D. 80-90

Ans: B. 60-70

Ref: *DC Dutta's Textbook of obstetrics, 7th edn*

Explanation:

- **Level of HCG** is highest at **60 -70 days** of pregnancy.
- **HCG** is produced by syncitiotrophoblasts.
- It is responsible for the **rescue and maintenance of corpus luteum** in **the first 6 weeks** of pregnancy.
- **High levels of HCG seen** in:
  - Multiple pregnancy
  - Hydatidiform mole
  - Choriocarcinoma
  - Down's syndrome
- **Low levels seen in:**
  - Ectopic pregnancy
  - Abortion

17. Which is the most common complication during vaginal delivery in diabetic women?
A. Uterine inertia
B. Shoulder dystocia
C. Obstructed labour
D. Post partum haemorrhage

Ans: B. Shoulder dystocia

Ref: Current diagnosis & treatment – Obstetrics and Gynaecology 10th edition pg 316.

Explanation:

- Shoulder dystocia is the most common complication encountered in diabetic women during vaginal delivery, especially when the baby is macrosomic.
- Uterine inertia and PPH can occur if hydramnios is present.

Maternal complications of DM

- Abortion
- Preterm labour
- Pre eclampsia
- Polyhydramnios

Fetal complications of DM

- Hydramnios
- Big baby
- Shoulder dystocia
- Fetal macrosomia
- Sacral agenesis
- Anencephaly and microcephaly
- VSD

Neonatal complications

- Hypoglycemia
- ARDS
- Hyperbilirubinemia
- Polycythemia
- Hypocalcemia

18. Most common cause of spontaneous abortion in first trimester: (Repeat)

A. Chromosomal anomalies
B. Uterine anomalies
C. Antiphospholipid antibody syndrome
D. Hypothyroidism

Ans: A. Chromosomal anomalies

Ref: *Dutta textbook of obstetrics 7th ed pg 160*

Explanation:

COMMON CAUSES OF MISCARRIAGE

First Trimester

- Genetic factors [50%]
- Endocrine [LPD, Thyroid abnormalities, Diabetes]
- Immunological disorders [Autoimmune, Alloimmune]
- Infection
- Unexplained

Second Trimester

- Anatomic
  - Cervical incompetence
  - Bicornuate uterus
  - Septate uterus
  - Uterine synechiae
  - Uterine fibroid
- Maternal medical illness
- Unexplained

PEDIATRICS

1. A 15-month-old child is able to do all the following *except:*

A. Crawl upstairs
B. Make a tower of 5 cubes
C. Name familiar objects
D. Point to familiar things

Ans: B. Make a tower of 5 cubes

Ref: *Nelson's Textbook of Pediatrics. 19th Edition, Page:*

Explanation:

This question is framed from the Nelson table.

(See table on the next page)

2. All the following are true regarding the management of asymptomatic close contacts of whooping cough *except:*

A. Azithromycin is the drug of choice
B. Drug therapy not required in an adequately immunized child
C. Isolation is not required
D. Booster dose is given for under-immunized children

Ans: B. Drug therapy not required in an adequately immunized child

Ref: *Nelson Textbook of Pediatrics, 19th edition. Pg 947*

Explanation:

Management of Household Contacts in Whooping cough

- A **macrolide agent** should be given **promptly** to all household contacts and other close contacts, such as those in daycare, regardless of age, history of immunization, or symptoms.
- Tab. **Azithromycin** is the **drug of choice**. **Erythromycin** can also be used.

EMERGING PATTERNS OF BEHAVIOR FROM 1 TO 5 YR OF AGE

	15 MONTHS
Motor:	Walks alone; crawls up stairs
Adaptive:	Makes tower of **3** cubes; makes a line with crayon; inserts raisin in bottle
Language:	Jargon; follows simple commands; may name a familiar object (e.g., ball); responds to his/her name
Social:	Indicates some desires or needs by pointing; hugs parents
	18 MONTHS
Motor:	Runs stiffly; sits on small chair; walks up stairs with one hand held; explores drawers and wastebaskets
Adaptive:	Makes tower of 4 cubes; imitates scribbling; imitates vertical stroke; dumps raisin from bottle
Language:	10 words (average); names pictures; identifies one or more parts of body
Social:	Feeds self; seeks help when in trouble; may complain when wet or soiled; kisses parent with pucker
	24 MONTHS
Motor:	Runs well, walks up and down stairs, one step at a time; opens doors; climbs on furniture; jumps
Adaptive:	Makes tower of **7** cubes (6 at 21 mo); scribbles in circular pattern; imitates horizontal stroke; folds paper once imitatively
Language:	Puts 3 words together (subject, verb, object)
Social:	Handles spoon well; often tells about immediate experiences; helps to undress; listens to stories when shown pictures
	30 MONTHS
Motor:	Goes up stairs alternating feet
Adaptive:	Makes tower of 9 cubes; makes vertical and horizontal strokes, but generally will not join them to make cross; imitates circular stroke, forming closed figure
Language:	Refers to self by pronoun "I"; knows full name
Social:	Helps put things away; pretends in play
	36 MONTHS
Motor:	Rides tricycle; stands momentarily on one foot
Adaptive:	Makes tower of 10 cubes; imitates construction of "bridge" of 3 cubes; copies circle; imitates cross
Language:	Knows age and sex; counts 3 objects correctly; repeats 3 numbers or a sentence of 6 syllables; most of speech intelligible to strangers
Social:	Plays simple games (in "parallel" with other children); helps in dressing (unbuttons clothing and puts on shoes); washes hands
	48 MONTHS
Motor:	Hops on one foot; throws ball overhand; uses scissors to cut out pictures; climbs well
Adaptive:	Copies bridge from model; imitates construction of "gate" of 5 cubes; copies cross and square; draws man with 2 to 4 parts besides head; identifies longer of 2 lines
Language:	Counts 4 pennies accurately; tells story
Social:	Plays with several children, with beginning of social interaction and role-playing; goes to toilet alone
	60 MONTHS
Motor:	Skips
Adaptive:	Draws triangle from copy; names heavier of 2 weights
Language:	Names 4 colors; repeats sentence of 10 syllables; counts 10 pennies correctly
Social:	Dresses and undresses; asks questions about meaning of words; engages in domestic role-playing

- Visitation and movement of coughing family members in the hospital must be assiduously controlled until erythromycin has been taken for 5 days.
- **Close contacts <7 yr of age** who have received **fewer than 4 doses** of pertussis-containing vaccines should have vaccination initiated or continued to complete the recommended series.
- **Children <7 yr of age** who received a **3rd dose > 6 mo before exposure** or **a 4th dose ≥ 3 yr before exposure** should receive a **booster dose**.
- **Individuals ≥ 9 yr** should be given a **Tdap** (adolescent/adult formulation of tetanus and diphtheria toxoids and acellular pertussis) booster if they have not previously received Tdap and >2 yr have passed since receipt of a diphtheria-containing vaccine.

Age Group	PRIMARY AGENTS		ALTERNATE AGENT	
	Azithromycin	Erythromycin	Clarithromycin	TMP-SMZ
<1 mo	Recommended agent. 10 mg/kg/day in a single dose for 5 days (only limited safety data available)	Not preferred. Erythromycin is associated with infantile hypertrophic pyloric stenosis. Use if azithromycin is unavailable; 40–50 mg/kg/day in 4 divided doses for 14 days.	Not recommended (safety data unavailable)	Contraindicated for infants aged <2 mo (risk for kernicterus)
1–5 mo	10 mg/kg/day in a single dose for 5 days	40–50 mg/kg/day in 4 divided doses for 14 days.	15 mg/kg/day in 2 divided doses for 7 days	Contraindicated at age <2 mo For infants aged =2 mo. TMP 8 mg/kg/day, SMZ 40 mg/kg/day in 2 divided doses for 14 days
Infants (aged ≥6 mo) and children	10 mg/kg in a single dose on day 1 then 5 mg/kg/day (maximum 500 mg) on days 2–5	40–50 mg/kg/day (maximum 2 g/day) in 4 divided doses for 14 days.	15 mg/kg/day in 2 divided doses (maximum 1 g/day) for 7 days	TMP 8 mg/kg/day, SMZ 40 mg/kg/day in 2 divided doses for 14 days
Adults	500 mg in a single dose on day 1 then 250 mg/day on days 2–5	2 g/day in 4 divided doses for 14 days.	1 g/day in 2 divided doses for 7 days	TMP 320 mg/day, SMZ 1,600 mg/day in 2 divided doses for 14 days

3. **All are true regarding osmotic diarrhoea *except:***
   - A. Due to highly osmotic substances in lumen
   - B. Fasting may improve symptoms
   - C. Stool reducing substances are present
   - D. Can be mediated by bacterial toxins

Ans: D. Can be mediated by bacterial toxins

Ref: *Nelson Textbook of Pediatrics, 19th edition.*

Explanation:

Osmotic Diarrhea

- It is caused by the presence of **nonabsorbable solutes** in the gastrointestinal tract.
- The classic example of osmotic diarrhea is **lactose intolerance** due to **lactose enzyme** deficiency in which **lactose** is not absorbed in the small intestine and reaches the colon intact.
- The colonic bacteria **ferment the nonabsorbed lactose** to **short-chain organic acids**, generating an **osmotic load** and causing **water to be secreted** into the lumen.
- Other examples include ingestion of excessive amounts of **carbonated fluids** that exceed the transport capacity, especially in toddlers, and ingestion of magnesium hydroxide and sorbitol, neither of which are absorbed, resulting in an osmotic load.
- **Lactulose**, a synthetic therapeutic disaccharide composed of galactose and fructose, is not digested in the small intestine and is fermented by the colonic bacteria to form organic acids, resulting in osmotic diarrhea.
- Osmotic diarrhea **stops with fasting, has a low pH,** and is **positive for reducing substances.**
- The sum of sodium plus potassium multiplied by two in the stools will be less than the measured stool osmolarity, a finding suggesting the presence of other osmols in the stool.

Causes of Osmotic Diarrhea

Malabsorption of Water-Soluble Nutrients

- Glucose-galactose malabsorption
- Disaccharidase deficiencies (lactase and sucrase-isomaltase)

Excessive Intake of Carbonated Fluids

Excessive Intake of Nonabsorbable Solutes

- Sorbitol
- Lactulose
- Magnesium hydroxide

Osmotic Vs Secretory Diarrhea

	OSMOTIC	SECRETORY
Volume of stool	<200 mL/24 hr	>200 mL/24 hr
Response to fasting	Diarrhea stops	Diarrhea continues
Stool Na^+	<70 mEq/L	>70 mEq/L
Reducing substances	Positive	Negative
Stool pH	<5	>6

4. All are true regarding subacute combined immunodeficiency *except:*

A. Due to deficiency of adenosine deaminase
B. Toxicity of leucocytes due to accumulation of cAMP
C. Both cellular and humoral immunity affected
D. Bone marrow transplantation is the treatment

Ans: B. Toxicity of leucocytes due to accumulation of cAMP

Ref: *Nelson's Textbook of Pediatrics. 19th Edition, Page:*

Explanation:

*"Marked accumulations of **adenosine, 22 -deoxyadenosine**, and **22 -O-methyladenosine** lead directly or indirectly to T-cell apoptosis, which causes the immunodeficiency" (Ref: Nelson)*

Severe Combined Immunodeficiency (SCID)

- Both cellular and humoral immunity affected
- **MC type** is X-linked SCID (X-SCD) due to mutation in Common Cytokine Receptor γ Chain (γC)
- Second most common form of SCID is absence of the enzyme ***adenosine deaminase (ADA)*** (15% patients)
- All patients with SCID have very ***small thymuses*** (<1 g)
- Thymus **fail to descend** from the neck, contain **no thymocytes**, and **lack corticomedullary distinction or Hassall corpuscles.**
- The thymic epithelium appears **histologically normal.**
- Both the **follicular and paracortical areas** of the **spleen** are depleted of **lymphocytes.**
- **Lymph nodes, tonsils, adenoids,** and **Peyer patches are absent** or extremely underdeveloped

Clinical Manifestations

- Affected infants present within the **1st few months** of life with
  - **Recurrent or persistent diarrhea**
  - **Pneumonia**
  - **Otitis media**
  - **Sepsis**
  - **Cutaneous infections**
  - **Growth failure**
- Persistent infections with opportunistic organisms including lead tö death
  - Candida albicans
  - Pneumocystis jiroveci
  - Parainfluenza 3 virus
  - Adenovirus
  - Respiratory syncytial virus
  - Rotavirus vaccine virus
  - Cytomegalovirus (CMV)
  - Epstein-Barr virus (EBV)
  - Varicella-zoster virus
  - Measles virus
  - MMR-V vaccine virus
  - Bacillus Calmette-Guerin (BCG)
- Affected infants also lack the ability to reject foreign tissue and are therefore at risk for severe or fatal **graft versus host disease (GVHD)** from T lymphocytes in nonirradiated blood products or in allogeneic stem cell transplants or less severe GVHD from maternal immunocompetent T cells that crossed the placenta while the infant was in utero.
- These infants also have an **absence of lymphocyte proliferative responses** to **mitogens, antigens,** and **allogeneic** cells in vitro.
- Patients with **adenosine deaminase (ADA) deficiency** have the lowest absolute lymphocyte counts, usually **<500/mm3**.
- **Serum immunoglobulin** concentrations are **low or absent**
- **No antibodies** are **formed** after **immunizations**.
- **T cells** are extremely **low** or **absent**

Treatment

- SCID is a true pediatric emergency.
- Unless immunologic reconstitution is achieved through **stem cell transplantation**, death usually occurs during the 1st yr of life and almost invariably before 2 yr of age.

5. How many permanent teeth will be present in an 8-year-old child?

A. 20 **B.** 24
C. 12 **D.** 16

Ans: C. 12

Ref: *OP Ghai, Textbook of Pediatrics; 7th edition, page : 4*

Explanation:

Permanent teeth erupt in the following order:

First molar → 6-7 years
Central and lateral incisors → 6-8 years

Canine and premolars → 9-12 years
Second molar → 12 years
Third molar → 18 years or later

- So at the age of 8 years first molar, central and lateral incisors would have erupted in each quadrant.
- Hence totally 12 permanat teeth will be present at the age of 8 years.

6. **Breast milk is rich in ____ when compared to cow's milk: (Repeat)**
   A. Lactose **B.** Protein
   C. Fat **D.** Vitamin K

Ans : A. Lactose

Ref: *Care of The Newborn by Meharban Singh 7th Edition, Page No.163 Preventive and social medicine by K.Park, 18th edition, page no.398*

Explanation:

Difference between human and cow's milk (composition per 100 ml)

Constituent	Breast milk	Cow's milk
PROTEIN	1.1g	3.3g
-Casein	0.4g	2.8g
-Soluble protein	0.7g	0.5g
LIPID	3.5g	3.5g
CARBOHYDRATES	7.0g	5.0g
-Lactose	6.5g	4.5g
Calcium	34mg	122mg
Phosphorous	15mg	90mg
Iron	0.29-0.45 mg	0.01-0.38 mg
Folic acid	0.14-0.36μg	0.01-0.06μg
Vitamin B12	0.0008-0.45μg	0.07-1.15μg
Vitamin A	0.5-10 IU	70-220 IU
VitaminC	1.2-10 mg	1.2-1.5 mg
Vitamin D	0.5-10 IU	0.5-4.5 IU
Vitamin K	1.5μg	6μg
ENERGY	67 kcl	65 kcal

7. **Most common complication of mumps in children:**
   A. Orchitis **B.** Aseptic meningits
   C. Myocarditis **D.** Pancreatitis

Ans: B. Aseptic meningitis

Ref: *Nelson's Textbook of Pediatrics. 19th Edition, Page:*

Explanation:

"The most common complications of mumps are ***meningitis, with or without encephalitis****, and* ***gonadal involvement****."*

Common complications

- Aseptic meningitis
- Encephalitis
- Orchitis
- Myocarditis
- Arthritis

Uncommon complications include

- Conjunctivitis
- Optic neuritis
- Pneumonia
- Nephritis
- Pancreatitis
- Thrombocytopenia.
- Thyroiditis

Complications of Mumps

Maternal infection with mumps during the 1st trimester of pregnancy results in increased fetal wastage.

Meningitis and Meningoencephalitis

- Mumps virus is neurotropic and is thought to enter the CNS via the choroid plexus and
- Infect the choroidal epithelium and ependymal cells
- Symptomatic CNS involvement occurs in 10-30% of infected individuals
- CSF pleocytosis has been found in 40-60% of patients with mumps parotitis.
- The meningoencephalitis ***may occur before, along with, or following the parotitis.***
- It most commonly manifests ***5 days after the parotitis.***
- Clinical findings vary with age. Infants and young children have fever, malaise, and lethargy, whereas older children, adolescents, and adults complain of headache and demonstrate meningeal signs.
- CSF in mumps meningitis has a **white blood cell pleocytosis** of 200-600/mm^3 with a predominance of lymphocytes.
- The **CSF glucose** content is **normal** in most patients, but a moderate hypoglycorrhachia (glucose content 20-40 mg/dL) may be seen in 10-20% of patients.
- The CSF **protein** content is **normal or mildly elevated.**
- Less common CNS complications of mumps include transverse myelitis, aqueductal stenosis, and facial palsy.
- Sensorineural hearing loss is rare but has been estimated to occur in 0.5-5.0/100,000 cases of mumps.

Orchitis and Oophoritis

- In adolescent and adult males, **orchitis** is **2nd only to parotitis** as a common finding in mumps.

- Involvement in **prepubescent boys** is **extremely rare**
- **After puberty**, **orchitis** occurs in **30-40%** of males.
- It begins within days following onset of parotitis
- Moderate to high fever, chills, and exquisite pain and swelling of the testes.
- In ≤ **30%** of cases the orchitis is **bilateral**.
- **Atrophy** of the **testes** may occur
- **Sterility is rare** even with bilateral involvement.
- **Oophoritis is uncommon** in postpubertal females but may cause severe pain and may be confused with appendicitis when located on the right side.
- **Mumps Myocarditis** has been linked to later development of **endocardial fibroelastosis.**

SKIN

1. Scabies in children differs from that in adults in that it affects:

A. Webspace **B.** Face

C. Genitalia **D.** Axilla

Ans: B. Face

Ref: *Nelson Textbook of Pediatrics, 19th ed.*

Explanation:

SCABIES

- Scabies is a contagious disease caused by a mite
- Family: Sarcoptidae
- Class : Arachnida
- 2 Main types : Human scabies and animal scabies
- Causative organism: ***sarcoptes scabiei var hominis***

Morphology

- Creamy white, ovoid body
- Size : 0.4×0.2 (female) , 0.2 × 0.15mm (male)
- Time from hatching to adult : 14 -17 days

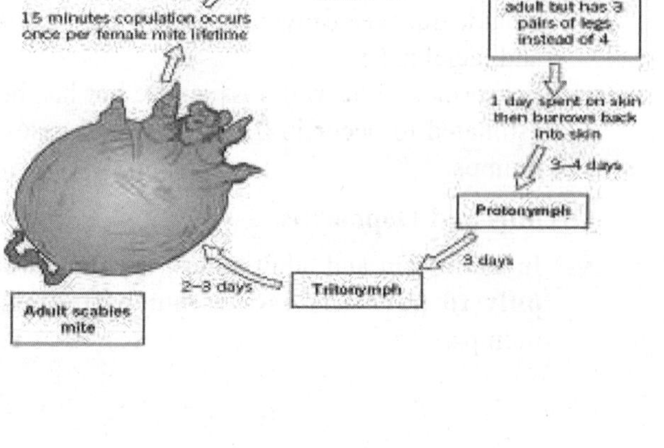

- Average rate of egg laying: **2-3/ day**, (40-50 eggs/ lifetime)
- Average number of female mites
- In adult : **12**
- In infant: **20**
- Lifespan of adult female mite **: 4 – 6 weeks**
- ***Incubation period***
- 1ST episode → **4 weeks**
- Subsequent episode → **2 weeks**
- ***How is scabies transmitted?***
- Scabies is passed from an infected person to another via **prolonged skin contact**, **sexually** and **nonsexually** (ten minutes or more, often through hand holding)
- Infected persons who have **no itching** can pass the mite on to others
- A person can be infected for up to **2 to 6 weeks** before the rash or itching occurs
- Scabies is not transmitted via clothing or bedding

Clinical Features

- Nocturnal itching
- Pathognomic lesions are burrows – slightly raised, brownish, tortuous lesions
- Burrows can be difficult to identify but absence of burrows does not exclude scabies
- Usual sites are wrist, borders of hands, sides of fingers, finger web spaces, instep of feet & genitalia.
- Papular rash.
- The rash is an allergic reaction of the body to the mite, its waste products, and its eggs.
- Sites of rash may not correspond to sites of burrows.
- **Classical sites (Circle of hebra)**
- Axilla, Elbows, Wrist, Hands, Crotch, — all forms a circle
- **Other variants**
- **Nodular scabies**- scrotum, axilla, groins, penis
- **Bullous scabies**
- **Crusted scabies (Norwegian)**
- Neurologic disorders, immunocompromised patients
- widespread erthema, hyperkeratosis, crusting without burrows
- Innumerable mites
- Scabies in clean
- Scabies incognito
- Scabies in infants and children:
- Face, scalp,palms and soles
- Papules, vesicles, nodules in atypical distribution
- Scabies in elderly:
- Atypical,back is commonly involved

- Scabies in hiv/aids:
- Crusted & atypical varieties seen

Complications

- Secondary infections: staphylococcus aureus, streptocooci.
- Eczematization
- Glomerulonephritis
- Urticaria

Diagnosis

- History wise
- H/o nocturnal itching
- Family history of itching
- Typical lesions and their localization
- Diagnostic methods
- Direct examination
- Scrapping & examination ↓ mineral oil
- Probing of burrow with toothpick
- India ink
- Dermoscopy
- PCR
- **Antiscabicidal agents**

  Topical agents

  - Permthrin 5% cream.
  - Lindone (gamma benzene hexachloride) 1% lotion or cream.
  - Benzyl benzoate 10% and 25% lotion or emulsion
  - Malathion 0.5% lotion.
  - Manosulfiram 25% lotion.
  - Crotamition 10% cream.
  - Precipitated sulphur 2%-10% ointment.
  - Esdepallethrine 0.63% aerosol.
  - Ivermection 0.8% lotion.

  Oral drug

  - Ivermection.
- Symptomatic relief of itching
- sedative H1 antihistaminics
- Treatment of secondary infections and eczematization
- Prior to antiscabietic treatment, this should be treated appropriately

Scabies in infants

- Sulphur 2%–10% in petrolatum
- Permethrin 5% cream is approved for use only in infants older than 2 months.
- Ivermectin and lindane are contraindicated
- in infants
- Permethrin 5% cream is the most effective and safe modality
- Benzyl benzoate can be diluted to 12.5% emulsion and used topically.

Scabies in pregnant and lactating women

- 6% sulphur precipitate is recommended.
- Ivermectin, permethrin, and lindane are contraindicated

Crusted scabies

- **Ivermectin** is the drug of choice but multiple doses plus topical agents may be required.
- The hyperkeratosis is treated with a keratolytic agent (5%–10% salicylic acid in petrolatum).
- Nails are cut short and brushed with a scabicidal agent.
- A cure is obtained after a mean treatment of three weeks.

Nodular scabies

- Antiscabitics followed by intralesional steroids

2. **A smear from a genital lesion shows Donovan bodies. The diagnosis is: (Repeat)**

A. Lymphogranuloma venerium
B. Chancroid
C. Granuloma inguinale
D. Syphilis

Ans: C. Granuloma inguinale

Ref: *Thappa DM. Essentials in Dermatology. 1st ed.*

Explanation:

Repeat 2013 dermatology question explanation.

3. **In urticaria pigmentosa, the cell most commonly seen in skin on microscopy is:**

A. Mast cell **B.** Langerhan's cell
C. Plasma cells **D.** Lymphocytes

Ans: A. Mast cell

Ref: *Rook's Dermatology, 8th ed.*

Explanation:

Urticaria pigmentosa

- It is the most common type of **cutaneous mastocytosis**
- Occurs due to the accumulation of mast cells in the skin
- Caused by a point mutation at amino acid 816 of the proto-oncogene **c-kit**
- The skin lesions are Itchy Small, Yellow Tan To Reddish Brown Macules scattered all over the body
- Mild **Trauma** such as **scratching** or **rubbing** the lesions may cause **urtication** and **erythema** around macules **(Darier's sign)**
- Symptoms exacerbated by temperature, spicy foods, alcohol and drugs

- **Diagnosis**: HPE shows **mast cell infiltration** of the **dermis**
- **Treatment**: Avoidance of **precipitating factors** and **antihistaminics**
- **Nifedipine**, a calcium channel blocker may reduce mast cell degranulation
- Another mast cell stabilizer **Gastrocrom**, a form of **cromoglicic acid** has also been used to reduce mast cell degranulation.

4. **Koebner's phenomenon is seen in all the following *except:***

   A. Lichen planus **B.** Psoriasis
   C. Warts **D.** Pityriasis rosea

   Ans: D. Pityriasis rosea

   Ref: *Principles of diagnosis in dermatology. In: Thappa DM, editor. Essentials in Dermatology, 2nd edn., NewDelhi: Jaypee brothers medical publishers (P) Ltd 2009;16-30*

   Explanation:

- **Koebner or isomorphic phenomenon**: Occurrence of morphologically identical lesion in traumatized uninvolved skin resulting in linear alignment of lesions
- Named after Heinrich Koebner
- Types:
  - **Koebner phenomenon**
    - Psoriasis
    - Vitiligo
    - Eczema
    - Dermatitis herpetiformis
    - Bullous pemphigoid
  - **Pseudokoebner phenomenon**
    - Warts
    - Molluscum contagiosum (pseudo because of direct inoculation by the organisms)
  - **Reverse Koebner phenomenon**
    - Area of psoriasis clears following injury
    - Granuloma annulare lesions clear following biopsy
  - **Remote reverse Koebner phenomenon**
    - Spontaneous repigmentation of vitiligo at sites distant from sites of skin grafting

5. **Air-borne contact dermatitis can be diagnosed by:**

   A. Skin biopsy
   B. Patch test
   C. Prick test
   D. Estimation of serum IgE levels

   Ans: B. Patch test

   Ref: *Eczema. In: Thappa DM, editor. Essentials in Dermatology, 2nd edn., NewDelhi: Jaypee brothers medical publishers (P) Ltd 2009;99-113. & Atopic dermatitis, Eczema and non infectious immunodeficiency disorders. In: James WD, Berger TG, Elston DM, editors. Andrew's diseases of the skin: Clinical Dermatology, 11th edn., China: Saunders Elsevier 2011; 62-87.*

   Explanation:

- **Patch test** – Application of allergens suspected to be the cause of allergic contact dermatitis to intact uninflamed skin in non irritating concentration
- Diagnostic of **allergic contact dermatitis** (airborne contact dermatitis is a type of allergic contact dermatitis wherein the allergens are airborne like pollen, cement, etc)
- Patch test – **Delayed hypersensitivity** (type IV hypersensitivity)
- Reading done **two days** later
- **Prick test**
  - **Type** I hypersensitivity reaction, used to detect allergy to a host of allergens like food, dust, insects, drugs, etc
  - Done in **atopic dermatitis, chronic urticaria, allergic rhinoconjunctivitis, bronchial asthma**
  - Reading done in **15 minutes**
- Serum IgE levels are nonspecifically elevated in allergic conditions characteristically high levels are seen in **atopic dermatitis** and very high levels in **hyper IgE syndrome**
- Skin biopsy reveals nonspecific features of **spongiosis** seen in all cases of dermatitis and not specific for airborne contact dermatitis.

6. **How many bacilli should be there in the tissue for slit skin smear to be positive for Hansen's disease?(Repeat)**

   A. 10 baccili / gram of tissue
   B. 10^2 baccili / gram of tissue
   C. 10^3 baccili / gram of tissue
   D. 10^4 baccili / gram of tissue

   Ref: *Rook's Textbook of dermatology*

   Ans: D. 10^4 baccili / gram of tissue

   Explanation:

- **At least 10^4 bacilli** should be present **per gram tissue** for **1+ bacteriological index** in slit skin smear.
- Maximum number of bacilli in a highly bacillated lepromatous leprosy patient is $\mathbf{10^{12}}$.
- Average density of bacilli in lepromatous leprosy **is 2.5 billion per 1 cm^3 tissue.**

7. **Fishnet appearance in immunoflorescence is seen in: (Repeat)**

A. Pemphigus vulgaris
B. Bullous pemphigoid
C. Dermatitis herpetiformis
D. Darier disease

Ans: A. Pemphigus vulgaris

Ref: *Vesiculobullous disorders. In: Thappa DM, editor. Essentials in Dermatology, 2ndedn.,NewDelhi:Jaypee brothers medical publishers (P) Ltd 2009;114-26*

Explanation:

- Pemphigus is an autoimmune blistering disorder characterized by ***autoantibody formation*** against the intercellular cementing substance called ***desmogleins***
- The mechanism of cell separation is called ***acantholysis***- loss of intercellular substance causing separation of the epidermal keratinocytes which become roundedà result in intraepidermal blister
- These large rounded keratinocytes with large nucleus, perinuclear halo and peripheral condensation of cytoplasm are called the ***acantholytic cells*** – seen in Tzanck smear
- **Types of pemphigus:**
  - Pemphigus vulgaris (variant-pemphigus vegetans)- most common type
  - Pemphigus foliaceus (variant-pemphigus erythematosus; endemic pemphigus or fogoselvagem)
  - Paraneoplastic pemphigus
  - Drug induced pemphigus
  - IgA pemphigus
  - Neonatal pemphigus
- **Clinical features:**
  - Fluid filled bullae→rupture→painful erosions with no tendency to spontaneous healing
  - Painful mucosal erosions- oral (most common; almost in all cases in pemphigus vulgaris); genital mucosa, pharynx, larynx,conjunctiva, urethra
  - ***Bulla spread sign/Asboe Hansen sign-positive***
  - ***Nikosky sign***- peeling of skin leaving behind erosions when tangential pressure applied over areas of normal looking skin or over bony prominences (other conditions-staphylococcal scalded skin syndrome, toxic epidermal necrolysis)
- **Diagnosis:** Tzanck smear- acantholytic cells; histopathology; direct and indirect immunofloresence
- **Treatment:** ***systemic steroids*** are mainstay of treatment
- Adjuvants- cyclophosphamide, azathioprine, methotrexate, mycophenolate mofetil, dapsone, plasmapheresis, iv immunoglobulins; biological agent- Rituximab (anti CD20)

(See table on the next page)

ANESTHESIOLOGY

1. The following anaesthetic drug causes pain on intravenous administration:

A. Midazolam **B.** Propofol
C. Ketamine **D.** Thiopentone sodium

Ans: B. Propofol

Ref: *Miller text book of Anaesthesia. 6th edition.*

Explanation

- **Following measures can prevent the pain on Propofol injection**
- Select a **Big vein**
- Inject Propofol in a **continuous running drip**
- Mixing Propofol with **lignocaine 1%** decreases pain on injection or prior injection of lignicaine 1% decreases pain on injection
- Special Preparations containing **1% Propofol in 16% polyoxyethylated castor oil** decreases the pain
- Prior injection with **fentanyl** decreases pain to some extent

2. Malignant hyperthermia is caused by:

A. Succinyl Choline **B.** N2O
C. Atropine **D.** Dantolene

Ans: A. Succinyl Choline

Ref: *Miller textbook of Anaesthesia. 6th edition*

Explanation:

Malignant Hyperthermia

It is a clinical syndrome observed during GA associated with rapidly increasing temperature of >1degree/5 min

Etiology

It is due to the abnormality of Ryanodine receptor which is a calcium releasing channel of sarcoplasmic reticulum.

The abnormality leads to excessive accumulation of calcium which causes sustained contraction of the muscle

Risk Factors

- Duchenne Muscular Dystrophy
- Arthrogryposis multiplex congenital

Characteristics of Various Pemphigus Disorders (High Yield table)

Features	Pemphigus vulgaris	Pemphigus foliaceus	Bullous pemphigoid	Dermatitis herpetiformis
Antigen	Desmoglein 3	Desmoglein 1	BP 180, BP 230	Unknown
Level of split	Intraepidermal - suprabasal	Intraepidermal- subcorneal	Subepidermal	Subepidermal
Mechanism of blister	Acantholysis	Acantholysis	Basement membrane zone disruption	Basement membrane zone disruption
Age	40-60 years	40-50 years	>60 years	20-55 years
Symptoms	Pain	Pain (less severe)	Pruritus	Intensely pruritic
Type of blister	Flaccid bullae on normal or erythematous skin	Transient blisters	Tense bullae on normal or erythematous or urticated skin	Grouped erythematous papules and papulovesicles; vesicles excoriated
Nature of erosion	Painful erosions with no tendency to spontaneous healing	Crusted moist scaly erosions	Erosions heal spontaneously	-
Distribution	Scalp, face, trunk, axilla, groins, pressure sites	Seborrheic distribution	Flexural aspect of limbs, lower abdomen, groin, axilla	Extensor aspect of limbs (elbows, knees), buttock, nasal cleft, shoulder, upper back, face, scalp
Bulla spread sign	+	Transient vesicles	+/-	Vesicles not seen as excoriated
Nikolsky sign	+	+	-	-
Mucosal involvement	Almost in all patients; may be presenting or the only feature (80-90%)	Uncommon	Rare; never presenting feature; desquamative gingivitis (40%)	Common but asymptomatic
Tzanck smear	Acantholytic cells	Acantholytic cells	Eosinophils	Neutrophils
HPE	Suprabasal cleft with row of tomb stone appearance	Subcorneal split	Subepidermal blister with eosinophils	Neutrophilic microabscess at tips of dermal papillae
DIF	Intercellular **IgG** deposists throughout the *epidermis* in fish net pattern	Intercellular **IgG** deposists in upper *epidermis*	Linear **IgG** and **C3** deposists in *basement membrane zone*	Granular **IgA** deposists in *dermal papilla*
IIF	Antibody titres correlate with disease severity	Antibody titres correlate with disease severity	Antibody titres do not correlate with disease severity	Negative or anti basement membrane zone or dermal autoantibodies. Antithyroid or antigliadin antibodies present
Associations	Thymoma, myasthenia gravis, lymphoma, bronchogenic carcinoma	-	Gastric carcinoma, diabetes, rheumatoid arthritis, psoriasis	Gluten sensitive enteropathy
Main stay of treatment	Steroids+adjuvants	Steroids+adjuvants	Steroids+adjuvants	Dapsone Gluten free diet

- Osteogenesis imperfect
- Congenital strabismus
- Central core diseases
- History of Neuroleptic malignant syndrome
- Masseter spasm with succinyl choline

Causative Agents

Muscle Relaxants: Succinyl choline – **MC drug**

Inhalational agents

- Halothane – **MC agent**
- Isoflurane
- Desflurane
- Enflurane
- Sevoflurane
- Methoxyflurane

Local Anesthetic: Lignocaine

Other drugs:

- Tricyclic antidepressants
- MAO inhibitors
- Phenothiazines

Clinical features

- Hyperthermia
- Hypoxia
- Cyanosis
- Hyperkalemia
- Muscle rigidity
- Tachycardia
- Hypertension
- Cardiac Arrhythmias
- Renal Failure
- DIC
- Pulmonary edema
- Cerebral edema
- Death

Investigations

- Severe Metabolic acidosis (pH < 7)
- Increased end tidal CO2
- Increased CPK levels
- Increased Myoglobin

Treatment

- Stop all anesthetics immediately
- Hyperventilation with 100% O2
- Control Temperature by ice cooling and ice cold saline
- Correct acidosis with Sodium bicarbonate
- Correct electrolyte imbalance – Hyperkalemia
- Maintain urine output

Specific therapy

DANTROLENE – 2mg/kg every 5 minutes to a maximum of 10 mg /kg

3. Fixed performance device:

A. Venturi mask
B. Nasal cannula
C. Simple mask
D. Non rebreathing mask

Ans: A. Venturi mask

Ref: *Ajay Yadav, Short Textbook of Anesthesia, 1st edition, pg 37.*

Explanation:

Oxygen Delivery Systems

- Oxygen is given thru fixed and variable performance devices.
- ***Fixed performance*** devices deliver a flow of oxygen equal to or in excess of peak inspiratory flow
- ***Variable performance*** devices use the deadspace of the nasopharynx or face masks as a reservoir of oxygen. They cannot deliver high inspired concentrations of oxygen.
- The oxygen delivery systems are classified into High flow delivery & low flow delivery systems

High flow delivery systems

- These work on ***Venturi Principle*** which states that if a gas is passed through a narrow orifice at high pressure it creates shearing forces around the orifice which entrain room air in specific ratio.
- The inspiratory gas flow should be 3 – 4 times the minute volume
- These high flow system include venture mask which delivers accurate inspired oxygen (FiO2) (Error is only 1-2%)

VENTURI MASK:

- These are 'Fixed performance' oxygen delivery devices, delivering accurate oxygen concentration.
- 'Fixed performance' because the performance is not affected by changes in patient's tidal volume and respiratory rate.
- The venture mask are available in different colours

Colour	Flow rate of O2 (Litre per min)	Delivered O2 (FiO2)
Blue	02	24%
White	04	28%
Orange	06	31%
Yellow	08	35%
Red	10	40%
Green	15	60%

- The maximum oxygen that can be delivered by venture mask is 60%

Low flow oxygen delivery systems

- These include
  - Nasal cannula
  - Simple mask (Mary Carterall mask)
  - Oxygen tents
  - Non rebreathing mask
  - Rebreathing mask
  - Polymask
- The advantage is that these are very cheap and can be used in wards, preoperative and postoperative rooms and these are better tolerated by patients as compared to high flow systems.
- The disadvantage is that the delivered oxygen (FiO2) accuracy cannot be predicted (Compared to venturi mask which delivers accurate concentration)
- These **low flow systems** are **'variable performance' devices**, since their performance is affected by changes in patient's tidal volume and respiratory rate.

Oxygen Mask: Very commonly used in wards. Also known as Mary carterall mask

Oxygen flow rate/min	Delivered oxygen (FiO2)
5-6 litres	40%
6-7 litres	50%
7-8 litres	60%

- So maximum concentration of oxygen that can be delivered by oxygen mask is **60%**
- Increasing rate **beyond 8 litres** will not increase the FiO2 to more than **60%**
- Attaching reservoir bag can increase FiO2 to **80%**

Nasal Cannula: The tip of nasal cannula should lie in nasopharynx

Flow rate (litre/min)	FiO2
1	24%
2	28%
3	32%
4	36%
5	40%
6	44%

- So, Maximum oxygen which can be delivered by nasal cannula is **44%**

Non rebreathing masks: Can deliver upto **80%** of oxygen

Rebreathing mask: When tightly fit, they can provide 100% oxygen

RADIOLOGY

1. Rat tail tapering of lower esophagus in barium swallow is seen in:

A. Diffuse esophageal spasm
B. Achalasia cardia
C. Ca esophagus
D. Gastroesophageal reflux

Ans: C. Ca esophagus

Ref: Multiple sources

Explanation:

X-Ray Findings - Abdomen (Contrast)

A. Barium

- **Bird's Beak deformity** of lower oesophagus - **Achalsia cardia** (Barium Swallow)
- **Rat tail tapering** of lower oesophagus - **Carcinoma oesophagus** (Barium Swallow)
- **Cork screw oesophagus - Diffuse oesophageal spasm** (Barium Swallow)
- Commonest radiological appearance of **gastric carcinoma** (in barium meal follow through) is - **filling defect in antrum / body of stomach**
- **Trifoliate duodenum - Chronic duodenal ulcer with scarring** (Barium Meal)
- **Hour Glass stomach - Peptic ulcer**
- **Cup & Spill / Cascade stomach - Volvulus** of stomach
- Constriction of transverse duodenum - superior mesenteric artery syndrome
- **Bull's eye lesion** (in barium meal) - **Leiomyosarcoma**
- **Single-bubble appearance - Pyloric stenosis**
- **Double-bubble sign - Duodenal atresia,** duodenal stenosis, annular pancreas
- **Triple-bubble sign - Jejunal atresia**
- **Coffee bean sign - Strangulation** of incompletely obstructed loop of small intestine
- **String of Beads - Small bowel obstruction**
- **Coiled spring appearance-Intussusception**
- **Pincer-shaped ending** in barium enema - **Intussusception**
- **Bird of Prey sign - Sigmoid volvulus**

– **Moulage sign** (flocculation of barium, with mucosal thickening) - seen in - **malabsorption** syndrome
– **String sign of Kantor - Crohn's** disease
– **Pipe-stem appearance (Loss of Haustrations)- Ulcerative Colitis** (Barium Enema)
– **Saw-tooth appearance** and / or diverticula - Diverticular disease / **Diverticulosis** (Barium Enema)
– **Scalloping of edge** of **sigmoid** colon on barium enema - **Ulcerative colitis**
– **Napkin ring sign - Annular carcinoma** of **colon**
– **Porcelain gall bladder - Carcinoma** of **gall bladder**
– **Pad sign** - Carcinoma **pancreas** (Barium Meal)

B. ERCP (Endoscopic retrograde cholangiopancreatography)
– **Scrambled-egg appearance** - Carcinoma of **pancreas**
– **Chain of Lakes appearance - Chronic pancreatitis**
– **Double duct sign - Carcinoma** of **pancreas**

C. PTC (Percutaneous transhepatic cholangiography)
– **Meniscus sign - Choledocholithiasis**

2. Rigler's sign in plain abdominal X-ray is seen in:

A. Perforated peptic ulcer
B. Ascites
C. Intussusception
D. Portal vein obstruction

Ans: A. Perforated peptic ulcer

***Ref:** Multiple sources*

Explanation:

- Rigler sign in seen in pneumoperitoneum , like in perforated viscus.

X-Ray Findings - Abdomen (Plain)

- **Football sign / Cupola Sign / Rigler's Sign - Pneumo-peritoneum**
- **Gasless abdomen - acute pancreatitis**
- Appearance of **jejunum** - characterised by **valvulae conniventes**
- Appearance of **ileum - characterless**
- Appearance of **large intestine - Haustrations**
- **Stippled Calcification** - Type of calcification in Plain X-ray abdomen in **Neuroblastoma**
- **Curvilinear Calcification** - Type of calcification in Plain X-ray abdomen in **Wilm's tumor**
- Calcification in region of **pancreas - chronic pancreatitis**
- **Solitary splenic calcification > 1cm** - most commonly seen in - **Splenic artery aneurysm**
- **Calcification** in the wall of **urinary bladder** and **ureter - Schistosomiasis**

3. Drooping water lilly sign seen in:

A. Spleen tumor
B. Liver tumour
C. Supra renal mass
D. Superior pole renal mass

Ans: D. Superior pole renal mass

***Ref:** Callahan MJ. The drooping lily sign. Radiology. 2001 Apr;219(1):226-8.*

Explanation:

Drooping lily sign

- It is a **urographic sign** in some patients with a **duplicated collecting system.**
- It refers to the inferolateral displacement of the opacified lower pole moiety due to an obstructed (and unopacified) upper pole moeity.
- The enlarged, obstructed upper pole of kidney is the pathology
- Causes are **HYDRONEPHROSIS OF THE UPPER POLE COLLECTING SYSTEM** due to **obstructing ectopic ureterocele** or **ectopic insertion of the upper pole ureter**
- Usually due to a nonopacified, hydronephrotic upper pole collecting system
- The appearance of the lower pole collecting system is reminiscent of a lily flower that is wilting or drooping

Important X-Ray Findings - Abdomen (Plain)

- ***Football sign/Cupola Sign/Rigler's Sign*** - pneumo-peritoneum
- ***Gasless abdomen*** - acute pancreatitis
- ***Appearance of jejunum*** - characterised by valvulae conniventes
- ***Appearance of ileum*** - characterless
- ***Normal Appearance of large intestine*** - Haustrations
- ***Stippled Calcification*** - Type of calcification in Plain Xray abdomen in Neuroblastoma
- ***Curvilinear Calcification*** - in Plain X-ray abdomen in Wilm's tumor

- ***Calcification in region of pancreas*** - chronic pancreatitis
- ***Solitary splenic calcification > 1cm*** - - Splenic artery aneurysm
- ***Calcification in the wall of urinary bladder and ureter*** - Schistosomiasis

4. **Cold lesion on bone scan suggest:**
   A. Osteomyelitis
   B. Lytic lesion
   C. Metastasis
   D. Sequestrum

   Ans: C. Metastasis

   Ref: *Internet Source: http://radiology.med.miami.edu/documents/2009Bone_Scan_All.pdf*

   Explanation:

Interpretation of Bone scans

Regional Hyperactivity may be due to:

a. Normal bone growth and remodeling
b. Increased Blood Flow (trauma, heterotopic ossification)
c. Reactive osteoblastic activity (active infections, tumors)
d. Reparative bone process (healing fractures, tumors, infections)
e. Hyper-metabolic activity (metabolic disorders)

They induce an increase in blood flow and osteoblastic activity,which enhance Ca / Phosphate local accretion into the hydroxyapatite matrix

Cold Spots may be caused by:

a. ***Malignant Tumors***
   – Lung (2-4%)
   – Breast (5%)
   – Renal (10%)
   – Neuroblastomas (bone marrow mets)
   – Thyroid (most cases)
   – Multiple Myeloma (most cases)
b. ***Bone Abscesses (they are surrounded by activity)***
c. ***Bone ischemia (AVN, sickle cell, etc.)***
d. ***Hemangiomas (normal or decreased activity)***

5. **Cobra head appearance is seen in:**
   A. Ureterocele
   B. Wilm's Tumor
   C. Horse shoe kidney
   D. Vesicoureteral reflux

   Ans: A. Ureterocele

   Ref: *Harrison's online. 18th ed*

   Explanation:

Some Important Features in Contrast Radiographs

- **Spider leg** appearance —— **Polycystic** kidney
- **Cobra head** appearance — **Ureterocele**
- **Flower vase** appearance of ureters — **Horse shoe** kidney
- **Sandy** patches — **Schistosomiasis** of bladder
- **Soap bubble** appearance — **Hydronephrosis**
- **Apple core** lesion on barium — **Ca colon**
- **Claw appearance** on barium enema — **Intussusception**
- **Saw tooth** appearance —— **Diverticula** of colon
- **Birds beak** appearance of esophagus on barium meal — **Achalasia**
- **Cork screw** appearance of esophagus on barium meal — **Diffuse esophageal spasm**
- ***String sign of kantor***—— **Crohn's** dissease
- **Thumb printing** sign — **Ischemic colitis**
- **EGG SHELL CALCIFICATION** —— **Silicosis, Sarcoidosis, Scleroderma, Histoplasmosis, Amyloidosis, lymphoma** following radiotherapy

6. **String sign of Kantor is seen in:**
   A. Crohn's disease **B.** Ulcerative colitis
   C. Ca Colon **D.** Typhoid colitis

   Ans: A. Crohn's disease

   Ref: *http://www.learningradiology.com*

   Explanation:

String Sign of Kantor

- Seen in **Crohn's disease**
- Finding seen on contrast studies using primarily **barium**
- It is caused by **severe spasm secondary to irritability of the loop** producing the appearance of a **frayed cotton string**
- At first, **edema** and **spasm narrow the loop** but the narrowing is at least **partially distensible**
- Eventually the wall of the ileum may become **fibrotic** and the **lumen fixed** in diameter

Imaging Findings

- Persistently **narrowed** but potentially distensible **terminal ileum**
- First sign of Crohn's ileitis is usually **shallow aphthous ulcers**
- **Short, linear ulcers** along the **mesenteric border** may also be seen with Crohn's ileitis
- Induration of the surrounding fat may cause the loop to be separated from the other small bowel loops (**Proud loop**)

PSYCHIATRY

1. **Which of the following is not seen in a case of borderline personality disorder?**
   A. Identity crisis
   B. Dissociative events
   C. Risk taking behaviour
   D. Strong interpersonal relationships

Ans: D. Strong interpersonal relationships

***Ref**: Synopsis of psychiatry, Kaplan & Sadock, 10th edition*

Explanation:

Borderline personality disorder

- It is a type of personality disorder.
- It is typically seen in females, especially in young adults.
- The basic problem in borderline personality disorder [BPD] is **'poor self-image'** resulting in abnormal way of perceiving, experiencing, thinking, feeling and behaving in this group.
- The sense of poor self is reflected by frequent **identity crisis** and **chronic inner emptiness**.
- They have higher level of sensitivity over real/perceived (the latter is more) rejection, failure.
- **Emotional dyscontrol** is common as evidenced by anger outbursts.
- They find **difficulty in focussing** and are more **prone to develop dissociation**.
- These people form as well as **break relationships quickly** and **over trivial reasons**.
- Their actions are **impulsive** in nature and **carry no planning**.
- They are more **prone to hurt themselves** (self-injurious behaviour in the form of frequent wrist slashing, tablet poisoning etc.,) and others (**temper tantrums**)
- Mood stabilizers like **Valproate** have been found useful (the **ONLY personality disorder** where **pharmacotherapy found effective so far**).
- **Dialectic behaviour therapy (DBT)** is the psychotherapeutic method found useful.

2. **Reversible dementia is a feature of:**
   A. Alzheimer's disease
   B. Pick's disease
   C. Multiinfarct dementia
   D. Hypothyroidism

Ans: D. Hypothyroidism

***Ref**: Harrison's Textbook of Internal Medicine*

Explanation

Dementia

- It is a syndrome characterized by
  – Memory disturbances (typically acquisition & recent memory are impaired)
  – Agnosia (inability to recognise like one's name)
  – Aphasia (inability to talk properly)
  – Apraxia (inability to do which were done with ease before)
  – Executive dysfunction (unable to perform the previously performed/learned activities)
- Dementia is basically due to degeneration of neurons of brain.
- Depending upon the site, it may be cortical (Alzheimer's disease) or subcortical (Parkinson's disease) or mixed (Vascular/Multi-infarct dementia).
- While the degeneration is progressive, sometimes if the cause is removed or treated, the dementia resolves.
- Hence, depending upon the "reversibility", there are

1. **Irreversible dementias** (Alzheimer's disease, Multi-infarct dementia)
2. **Reversible** [FEDUP]
   – *Failure of other organs* (CCF, COPD→Respiratory failure, Renal failure, etc.)
   – *Endocrine* (hypothyroidism, hypoparathyroidism, hypoadrenalism, diabetes)
   – *Drugs* (chemotherapy)
   – *Under/Over minerals & vitamins* (defieciency states esp. Vitamin B1,2,6,12) (Toxicity due to chronic exposure / ingestion of to aluminium, arsenic, lead)
   – *Psychiatric conditions* (depression, schizophrenia)

3. **Which of the following is a classical symptom of depression?**
   A. Altered sleep pattern
   B. Weight loss
   C. Guilt
   D. Decreased appetite

Ans: C. Guilt

***Ref**: Synopsis of psychiatry, Kaplan & Sadock, 10th edition*

Explanation

Depression

- It is a common psychiatric syndrome characterized by persistent & pervasive sad mood.
- Because of such sad mood, the person might feel guilty, which in turn gives rise to thoughts like **worthlessness, hopelessness & helplessness (Cognitive triad of Beck)**, which in turn put him/her at risk of ending life (ie., suicide).
- The other symptoms mentioned in the question do occur in any psychiatric disorder.
- So, the best answer would be "Guilt" which is pathognomonic of depression.

4. Which of the following is a first rank symptom in Schizophrenia?

A. Delusions
B. Thought insertion
C. Perceptional hallucinations
D. Word salad

Ans: B. Thought insertion

Ref: Synopsis of psychiatry, Kaplan & Sadock, 10th edition

Explanation

- Schneider described a set of symptoms which were characteristic (but not pathognomonic) of schizophrenia.
- They are grouped as follows
- **Auditory hallucinations** of following characteristics
  - Voices heard arguing/discussing or giving instructions/commanding (2nd person)
  - Voices heard commenting on one's actions (running commentary, usually describing the patient in the 3rd person)
  - Thought echo (thoughts being heard aloud in one's mind)
  - Thought insertion (thoughts are ascribed to other people who are intruding into the patient's mind)
  - Thought withdrawal (feeling that one's thoughts are being sucked by means like chips)
  - Thought broadcasting (also called thought diffusion- where one's thoughts are known to others by means of internet/mobile etc)
- **Somatic passivity experiences** (delusions of control / of being controlled i.e, he/she is nothing but a doll & his/her speech/activities are controlled by external agents/alien forces)
- **Delusional perception** (Sudden delusional idea after a normal perception e.g., suddenly believing that one is the king after seeing a horse!)

5. Which of the following is not seen in Korsakoff's syndrome? (Repeat)

A. Clear consciousness
B. Inability to learn new things
C. Hallucinations
D. Confabulation

Ans: C. Hallucinations

Ref: Synopsis of psychiatry, Kaplan & Sadock, 10th edition

Explanation

Wernicke's encephalopathy

- It is a condition which is **acute in onset** (cf. Korsakoff psychosis is **insidious**)
- It is characterized by the triad:
  1. **Confusion** (delirium tremens)
  2. **Ataxia** (in-coordination of movements)
  3. **Nystagmus** (due to **opthalmoplegia** and / or vestibular dysfunction). [CAN- the Mnemonic]
- Chronic alcohol intake depletes **thiamine** (Vitamin B1) by various mechanisms.
- During acute intoxication, such deficiency results in degeneration of paraventricular regions of brain (**mammillary bodies, thalamus** and **hypothalamus**).
- The treatment is **'THIAMINE'** IV **250-500mg/** day as slow infusion for first five days, followed by oral route (100mg tds) for at least 15days.
- It is **reversible** if treated early.
- Otherwise, the condition progresses into "**Korsakoff's psychosis**", which is characterized by **amnesia** (both **anterograde & retrograde**) [declarative memory deficit], **confabulation** (to fill up the gaps in memory), **apathy & lack of insight**.
- Less than 20% only respond to thiamine and often need as long as two years to show moderate improvement.

Other neuropsychiatric disorders due to alcohol are:

- Cerebellar degeneration,
- Central Pontine Myelinosis &
- Corpus callosum demyelination (Marchiafava-Bignami disease).

Riboflavin deficiency

- Mucositis (Chelitis, Stomatitis, Glossitis)

- Dermatitis (Seborrheic)
- Normochromic, normocytic anemia.

Folate deficiency - Depression.

Vitamin B12

- Depression & Psychosis (both folate and Vit.B12 cause mental disorders either directly or by increasing homocysteine levels in brain).

6. **The type of treatment which can be used for mental retardation is:**

A. Psychoanalysis
B. Family therapy
C. Transaction analysis
D. Rapid emotive treatment and response

Ans: B. Family therapy

Ref: Synopsis of psychiatry, Kaplan & Sadock, 10th edition

Explanation

Mental retardation [MR] is a syndrome characterized by

- Low IQ (Intelligence Quotient) compared to others of one's age, sex, socio-economic & educational background
- Poor adaptation (due to developmental delay)

The causes of MR are diverse

- Prenatal (illnesses of parents, chromosomal anomalies)
- Perinatal (difficult labor)
- Postnatal (meningitis)
  - Most cases of MR are not curable, hence rehabilitation is the key.
  - In rehabilitation, family therapy is the first one, where the parents / care-givers are taught about the illness, its prognosis, complications, methods to deal with behavioural problems and methods of training.

Grades of MR are based on IQ level (normal is 90-110)

- Profound (<20)
- Severe (20-35)
- Moderate (35-50)
- Mild (50-70)
- Borderline intelligence (70-90)
  - The other options mentioned in the question need good level of cognitive development (in other words, maturity), hence not at all applicable to patients with MR.
  - For patients with MR, behaviour therapy (based on techniques like reinforcement) is useful. Drugs in MR are two types -1. Treating primary / co-morbid disorders (like epilepsy), 2. Treating psychiatric problems (anti-psychotics).

7. **Déjà vu phenomenon means:**

A. Feeling that familiar things look unfamiliar
B. Feeling that unfamiliar things look familiar
C. Unable to recall the familiar name
D. Feeling detached from one's own body

Ans: B. Feeling that unfamiliar things look familiar

Ref: Synopsis of psychiatry, Kaplan & Sadock, 10th edition

Explanation

- Altered state of consciousness, sense of self and surroundings is a frequent symptom in psychiatry.
- They occur in following situations
  - Organic conditions like epilepsy
  - Substance related like cannabis intoxication
  - Psychiatric disorders like schizophrenia, dissociative disorder
  - Isolated phenomena
- **Déjà vu** is when a person has strong feeling that an event or experience currently being experienced has been experienced in the past, whether it has actually happened or not (mostly the latter).
- **Jamais vu** is the opposite of déjà vu, where a person feels it strange in familiar situation.
- **Presque vu** is when a person is temporarily unable to recall a word or name but with effort, he/she could do it.
- **Depersonalization** is a subjective experience of unreality in one's sense of self.
- **Derealisation** is experiencing 'unreality' of the outside world.

8. **Good prognostic factor in schizophrenia:**

A. Insidious onset
B. Positive symptoms
C. Disorganized subtype
D. Absence of depression

Ans: B. Positive symptoms

Ref: *A Short Textbook of Psychiatry by Niraj Ahuja, 7th edition. 2011. Jaypee. Page 62*

Explanation: *(See table on the next page)*

Prognostic Factors in Schizophrenia

Sl no	Good prognostic factors	Poor prognostic factors
1	Acute or abrupt onset	Insidious onset
2	Onset > 35 years (Late Onset)	Onset < 20 years (Early Onset)
3	Presence of precipitating stressor	
4	Good premorbid adjustment	Poor premorbid adjustment
5	Catatonic Subtype	Disorganised, simple, undifferentiated, chronic catatonic subtypes
6	Short duration (< 6 months)	Chronic course (> 2 years)
7	Presence of Depression	Absence of Depression
8	Predominance of Positive symptoms	Predominance of Negative symptoms
9	Family history of mood disorder	Family history of Schizophrenia
10	First episode	Past history of Schizophrenia
11	Pyknic (Fat) Physic	Asthenic (Thin) physique
12	Female sex	Male sex
13	Good social support	Poor social support or unmarried
14	Presence of confusion, perplexity, or disorientation in the acute phase	Flat or blunted affect
15	Proper treatment, good treatment, concordance	Absence of proper treatment
16	Good response to treatment	Poor response to treatment
17	Outpatient treatment	Long term hospitalization
18	Normal cranial CT scan	Evidence of ventricular enlargement on CT scan

9. **Tactile hallucinations are seen in all *except:***
   A. Delirium tremens
   B. Amphetamine abuse
   C. Opiod withdrawal
   D. Frontal lobe tumor

Ans: D. Frontal lobe tumor

Ref: *A Short Textbook of Psychiatry by Niraj Ahuja, 7th edition. 2011. Jaypee. Pages 31, 38, 43, 48*

Explanation:

DELIRIUM TREMENS (DT)

- It is the most severe alcohol withdrawal syndrome
- Occurs within 2 - 4 days of complete abstinence from heavy alcohol drinking in about 5% of patients
- Clinical course is short and recovery occuring within 3 - 7 days
- This is an organic brain syndrome (Delirium) with features of:
  - Clouding of consciousness with disorientation in time and place
  - Poor attention span and distractability
  - Visual, auditory hallucinations and illusions, which are often vivid and very frightening
  - Tactile hallucinations of insects crawling over the body
  - Marked autonomic disturbance with tachycardia, fever, hypotension, sweating and pupillary dilatation
  - Psychomotor agitation and ataxia
  - Insomnia, with reversal of sleep-wake pattern
  - Dehydration with electrolyte imbalance
- Death can occur in 5 - 10% of patients due to cardiovascular collapse, infection, hyperthermia or self-inflicted injury.

Amphetamine Abuse

- Amphetamine refers to a phenyl-iso-propylamine or methyl-phenethylamine.
- It is a powerful CNS stimulant with peripheral sympathetomimetic effects.
- It acts primarily on norepinephrine release in brain along with an action on the release on dopamine and serotonin.
- Street name - Ecstasy or XTC

Signs of Symptoms

- Acute intoxication causes Paranoid hallucinatory syndrome which closely mimics paranoid schizophrenia.
- Diagnosis can be confirmed by elevated urinary amphetamine levels.
- Chronic intoxication leads to severe and compulsive craving for the drug
- A high degree of tolerance can develop requiring subsequent high doses
- Tactile hallucinations in clear consciousness can occur

OPIOID WITHDRAWAL

- The onset of withdrawal symptoms typically occurs within 12 - 24 hours, peaks within 24 - 72 hours and subsides within 7 - 10 days
- The characteristic symptoms include
  - Lacrimation
  - Rhinorrhoea
  - Pupillary dilatation
  - Sweating
  - Diarrhoea
  - Yawning
  - Tachycardia
  - Mild Hypertension
  - Insomnia
  - Raised body temperature
  - Muscle cramps
  - Generalised myalgia
  - Severe anxiety
  - Piloerection
  - Nausea and vomiting
  - Anorexia
  - Tactile hallucinations

The withdrawal symptoms are managed by

- Substitution of drugs like Methadone
- Clonidine
- Naltrexone with clonidine
- Other drugs like - LAAM (levo-alpha-acetyl-methadol), propoxyphene, diphenoxylate, buprenorphine and lofexidine

FRONTAL LOBE SYNDROME

Frontal involved causes two types of syndromes

A. Orbito frontal syndrome (Pseudo-psychopathic)
- Disinhibition
- Jocularity
- Impulsivity
- Impaired sight
- Impaired judgement

B. Frontal convexity type (Pseudo-depressive)
- Apathy
- Lack of initiative
- Retardation
- Perseveration

Hallucinations are not seen in Frontal lobe involvement.

JIPMER–2006

ANATOMY

1. **All are branches of mandibular nerve *except:***
   A. Auriculotemporal **B.** Zygomatic
   C. Inferior alveolar nerve **D.** Lingual

Ans: B. Zygomatic

Ref: Gray's Anatomy, 40th edition, pg. 535

Explanation:

Mandibular Nerve

- It is the **largest** of the three branches of **trigeminal** division
- It is the nerve of **first brachial arch**
- It is a **mixed nerve** consist of large sensory and small motor root
- Its sensory root arise from trigeminal ganglion and motor root arise directly from the pons
- From middle cranial fossa both the root emerge through the foramen ovale
- Immediately below the foramen both the root unite to form trunk of mandibular nerve in the infratemporal fossa
- The trunk intervenes between tensor veli palate medial and lateral pterygoid laterally
- It divides into anterior and posterior division
- **Branches**
  - ***From the trunk***
    1. Nervous spinosus
    2. Nerve to medial pterygoid
  - ***From the anterior division (3 motor 1 sensory)***
    1. Masseteric nerve
    2. Deep temporal nerve
    3. Nerve to lateral pterygoid
    4. Buccal nerve-sensory nerve
  - ***From the posterior division (3 sensory 1 motor)***
    1. Auriculotemoral nerve
    2. Inferior alveolar nerve
    3. Lingual nerve
    4. Nerve to mylohyoid-motor nerve (also supplies anterior belly of digastric

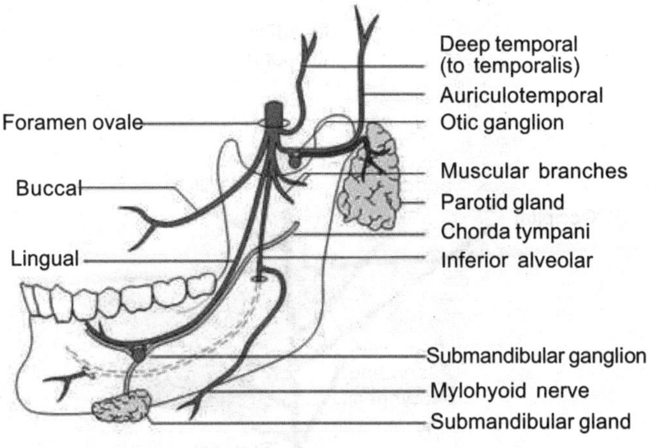

Note: Mandibular nerve block can be given in trigeminal neuralgia

2. **Not a branch of external carotid artery:**
   A. Superior thyroid artery
   B. Lingual artery
   C. Ascending pharyngeal artery
   D. Ophthalmic artery

Ans: D. Ophthalmic

Ref: Gray's Anatomy, 40th edition, pg. 399

Explanation:

- **Common carotid artery** lies within the carotid sheath of deep cervical fascia, together with the **internal jugular vein** and **vagus nerve.**
- At the level of the upper border of the thyroid cartilage (C4), the common carotid artery bifurcates into external and internal carotid arteries.
- The **external carotid artery** gives off:
  - Superior thyroid
  - Lingual
  - Posterior auricular artery
  - Facial
  - Occipital
  - Ascending pharyngeal—only medial branch
  - Terminal branches, maxillary and superficial temporal arteries.

Mneumonic–**S**ister **L**ouis **P**owdered **F**ace **O**ften **A**ttract **M**edical **S**tudents **(SLPFOAMS)**.

- External carotid artery branches anastomose with branches of the internal carotid arteries on the scalp, forehead and face, and in the orbit, nasopharynx and nasal cavity, and with branches of the subclavian artery in the pharynx, larynx and thyroid glands.

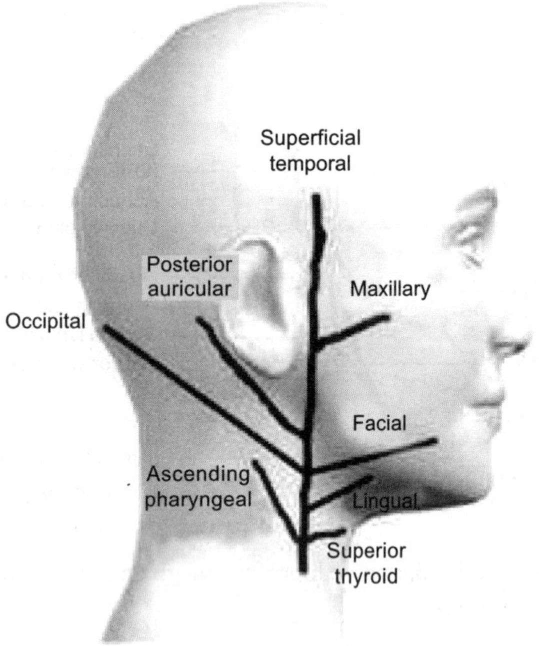

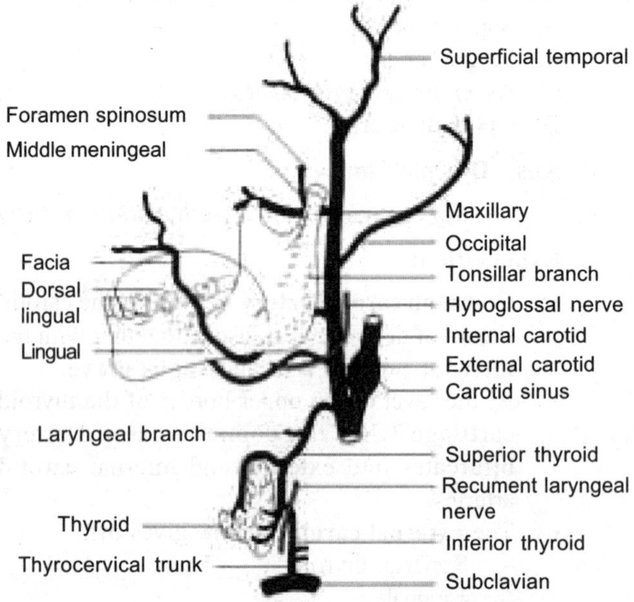

3. **Nasolacrimal duct opens into: (Repeat)**
   A. Inferior meatus **B.** Superior meatus
   C. Middle meatus **D.** Sphenoethmoidal recess

Ans: A. Inferior meatus

Ref: *Gray's Anatomy, 40th edition, pg. 550*

Explanation:

- Lateral wall of the nose has **3 concha 3 meatus**
- The **inferior concha** is an **independent bone.**
- The space under cover of the inferior concha is known as the **inferior meatus**– ***largest meatus***
- During postnatal development, the ostium of the nasolacrimal duct moves upwards and is increasingly hidden under the over-arching inferior concha.
- The **middle and superior concha** are parts of **ethmoidal labyrinth**
- The space undercover the middle concha and superior concha is called middle meatus and superior meatus respectively
- The area intervening between the **superior concha** and **nasal roof** is called as **supreme meatus**

	Contents
Supreme meatus	Opening of spenoidal sinus
Superior meatus	Posterior ethmoidal sinus
Middle meatus	Bulla ethmoidalis
	Hiatus semilunaris
	Openings of maxillary and ethmoidal sinus
Inferior meatus	Naso lacrimal duct

4. **Lymphatic follicles are not seen in**
   A. Thymus **B.** Tonsil
   C. Lymph node **D.** Spleen

Ans: A. Thymus

Ref: *Juinquera Textbook of histology*

Explanation:

- Histology of thymus varies with the age
- It is a **lobulated** lymphoid organ
- It has **outer cortex** with densely packed **lymphocytes without lymphoid follicles**
- It has **inner medulla** contains **more epithelial reticular cells** and **Hassal's corpuscle**

5. **Following is not a derivative of first arch: (Repeat)**
   A. Stapes **B.** Malleus
   C. Maxilla **D.** Mandible

Ans: A. Stapes

Ref: *Gray's Anatomy, 40th edition, pg. 596*

Explanation: *(See table on the next page)*

6. **The parasympathetic supply to otic ganglion comes from: (Repeat)**
   A. 7th cranial nerve **B.** 8th cranial nerve
   C. 9th cranial nerve **D.** 3rd cranial nerve

Ans: C. 9th cranial nerve

Ref: *Gray's Anatomy, 40th edition, pg. 495*

Explanation:

Pharyngeal Arches and Their Derivatives

Arch number	Arch name	Embryonic cartilage	Cartilage derivative	Muscle	Nerve	Artery
1	**Mandibular**	Quadrate Meckel's	• Incus • Malleus • Anterior ligament of malleus • Spine of sphenoid • Sphenomandibular ligament • Genial tubercle of mandible	• Tensor tympani • Muscles of mastication • Mylohyoid • Anterior belly of digastric • Tensor veli palatini	**Trigeminal (V)** **Mandibular division**	• First aortic arch artery [transitory]
2	**Hyoid**	Reichert's	• Stapes • Styloid process of temporal bone • Stylohyoid ligament • Lesser horn and upper part of body of hyoid bone	• Stapedius • Stylohyoid • Facial muscles, including • Buccinator • Platysma • Posterior belly of digastric	**Facial** (VII)	• Stapedial artery [transitory]
3	Third		• Greater horn and lower part of body of hyoid	• Stylopharyngeus	**Glossopharyngeal** (IX)	• Common carotid artery, first part of internal carotid artery
4	Fourth		• Thyroid cartilage • Corniculate cartilage • Cunieform cartilage	• Pharyngeal and extrinsic laryngeal muscles, levator veli palatini	**Vagus** (X) **Pharyngeal** branch	• Proximal part of subclavian artery on the right side • Arch of aorta between origins of left common carotid and left subclavian arteries
6	Sixth		• Arytenoid cartilages	• Intrinsic laryngeal muscles	**Vagus** (X) recurrent **laryngeal** branch	• Part between the pulmonary trunk and dorsal aorta • Becomes **ductus arteriosus on left,** disappears on right

- This is a small, oval, flat reddish-grey ganglion situated just below the foramen ovale.
- It is a peripheral parasympathetic ganglion related topographically to the mandibular nerve, but connected functionally with the glossopharyngeal nerve. *(See the following figure)*

Inferior salivatory nuclei
↓ Through tympanic branch
Glossopharyngeal nerve (9th CN)
↓
Tympanic plexus
↓
Lesser petrosal nerve
↓
Otic ganglion
↓
Auriculotemporal nerve
↓
Parotid gland

7. Common carotid artery is derived from:

A. Third arch B. Second arch
C. Fourth arch D. Sixth arch

Ans: A. Third arch

Ref: *Gray's Anatomy, 40th edition, pg. 399*

Explanation:

Refer explanation above question

8. Lens is derived from: (Repeat)

A. Surface ectoderm **B.** Neuroectoderm
C. Mesoderm **D.** Endoderm

Ans: A. Surface ectoderm

Ref: *Gray's Anatomy, 40th edition, pg. 700*

Explanation:

Embryology of Eye

- The developing eye appears in the **22 days** embryo as a pair of shallow grooves on the sides of the forebrain
- Optic vesicle forms as a out pocketings of the forebrain which comes in contact with the **surface ectoderm**
- The optic vesicle begins to invaginate to form **optic cup**
- The cells of surface ectoderm initially in contact with the optic vesicle begin to elongate and form the lens placode which develops into lens **vesicle**
- The lens develops from the lens vesicle
- The posterior cells become filled with a very high concentration of proteins (**crystallins**) which **render them transparent**; they also become densely packed within the lens as **primary lens fibres**.
- Cells at the equatorial region of the lens elongate and contribute secondary lens fibres to the body of the lens in a process which continues into adult life
- The polarity and growth of the lens appear to depend on the differential distribution of soluble factors which promote either cell division or lens fibre differentiation and are present in the anterior chamber and vitreous humour respectively.
- Congenital cataracts can be associated with mutations in genes that encode structural lens proteins, particularly **crystallin proteins**.
(See the following table)

9. Red nucleus is present in:

A. Upper pons **B.** Lower pons
C. Midbrain **D.** Medulla

Ans: C. Midbrain

Ref: *Gray's Anatomy, 40th edition, pg. 280*

Explanation:

Red Nucleus

- The red nucleus is a pink, ovoid mass, approximately 5 mm in diameter and lying **dorsomedial** to the **substantia nigra**
- The tint appears only in fresh material and is caused by a **ferric iron pigment** in its **multipolar** neurons.
- Small multipolar neurones occur in all parts of the nucleus.
- The magnocellular element is considered phylogenetically old, which accords with the parvocellular predominance in primates.
- Rostrally, the red nucleus is poorly demarcated, and it blends into the reticular formation and caudal pole of the interstitial nucleus.
- It is traversed and surrounded by fascicles of nerve fibres, including many from the **oculomotor** nucleus.

10. Type of neuron present in the autonomic ganglion:

A. Unipolar **B.** Bipolar
C. Multipolar **D.** Apolar

Ans: C. Multipolar

Ref: *Gray's Anatomy, 40th edition, pg. 225*

Explanation:

- Autonomic ganglia appear as bulbous dilatations in autonomic nerves.
- Some are located within certain organs, especially in the **walls of the digestive tract**, where they constitute the **intramural ganglia.**
- These ganglia are devoid of connective tissue capsules, and their cells are supported by the stroma of the organ in which they are found.

Embryogenic Origin of Eye structures

Surface ectoderm	Neural ectoderm	Mesoderm	Neural crest
• Conjunctival epithelium	• Iris epithelium	• ***Extraocular muscle***	• Corneal endothelium
• Corneal epithelium	• Ciliary epithelium	• Corneal stroma	• Trabecular meshwork endothelium
• ***Crystalline lens***	• ***Sphincter pupillae***	• ***Sclera***	• ***Ciliary muscle***
• Tarsal glands	• ***Dilator pupillae***	• Iris stroma	• Part of vitreous
• Lacrimal glands	• Part of vitreous	• ***Choroid***	• Uveal melanocytes
	• Part of retina	• Vessels	• Meningeal sheaths of optic nerve
	• Part of RPE	• Part of vitreous	• Ciliary ganglion
	• Part of optic nerve		

- Autonomic ganglia usually have ***multipolar*** neurons
- As with craniospinal ganglia, autonomic ganglia have **neuronal perikaryons** with **fine Nissl bodies**
- A layer of ***satellite cells*** frequently envelops the neurons of autonomic ganglia.
- In intramural ganglia, only a few satellite cells are seen around each neuron.

11. One of the following is not derived from the endoderm:

A. Kidney
B. Urinary bladder
C. Liver
D. Pancreas

Ans: A. Kidney

***Ref:** Langmann Embryology, 11th edition*

Explanation: *(See the following table)*

12. Waldeyer's fascia is between:

A. Rectum and urinary bladder
B. Rectum and sacrum
C. Bladder and uterus
D. Pubis and bladder

Ans: B. Rectum and sacrum

***Ref:** Gray's Anatomy, 40th edition, pg.1139*

Explanation: *(See the following figure)*

- **Fascia of Waldeyer** is between **rectum and sacrum**
- The **upper third of the rectum** is covered by peritoneum on its **anterior** and **lateral** aspects.
- It is related **anteriorly** to the sigmoid colon or loops of ileum if these lie in the pelvis, otherwise

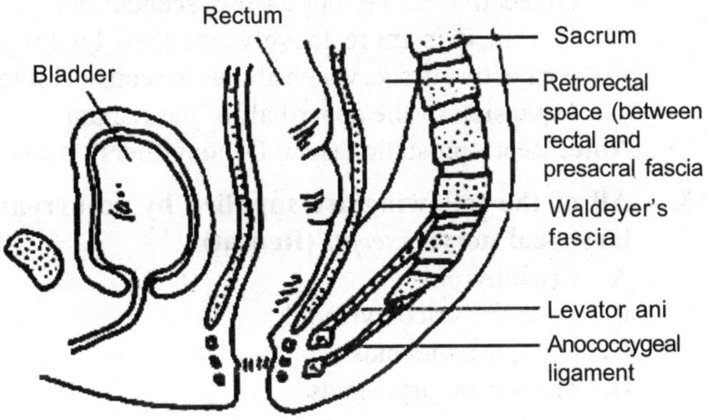

it is related to the urinary bladder in males, or the cervix and body of the uterus in females.

- The **middle third of the rectum** is covered by peritoneum only on its **anterior** aspect.
- The peritoneum is reflected superiorly onto the urinary bladder in males to form the rectovesical pouch, or onto the posterior vaginal wall in females to form the recto-uterine pouch (**Pouch of Douglas**).
- The level of this reflection is higher in males; the rectovesical pouch is approximately 7.5 cm (about the length of the index finger) from the anorectal junction.
- In females the recto-uterine pouch is approximately 5.5 cm from the anorectal junction.
- In the male neonate, peritoneum extends on to the front of the rectum as far as the lower limit of the prostate.
- Superiorly the peritoneum is firmly attached to the muscle layer of the sigmoid colon by fibrous

Ectoderm	Mesoderm	Endoderm
• Central nervous system • Peripheral nervous system • Sensory epithelia of the eye, ear, and nose • Epidermis and its appendages (hair and nails) • Mammary glands • Pituitary gland • Subcutaneous glands • Enamel of teeth • **Neural crest cells**, derived from neuroectoderm, give rise to the cells of the spinal, cranial (cranial nerves V, VII, IX and X) and autonomic ganglia • Ensheathing cells of the peripheral nervous system • Pigment cells of the dermis • Muscle • Connective tissues • Bone of pharyngeal arch origin • Suprarenal medulla • Meninges (coverings) of the brain and spinal cord.	• Connective tissue • Cartilage • Bone • Striated muscles • Smooth muscles • Heart • Blood • Lymphatic vessels • Kidneys • Ovaries • Testes • Genital ducts • Serous membranes lining the body cavities (pericardial, pleural and peritoneal) • Spleen • Cortex of suprarenal glands.	• Epithelial lining of the gastrointestinal and respiratory tracts • Parenchyma of the tonsils • Thyroid and parathyroid glands • Thymus • Liver • Pancreas • Epithelial lining of the urinary bladder and most of the urethra • Epithelial lining of the tympanic cavity • Tympanic antrum • Pharyngotympanic (auditory) tube.

connective tissue, but as it descends onto the rectum it is more loosely attached by fatty connective tissue, which allows for considerable expansion of the upper half of the rectum

Note: Recto-prostatic fascia, Denonvilliers' fascia

13. **All of the following are supplied by recurrent laryngeal nerve *except:* (Repeat)**
A. Cricothyroid
B. Posterior cricoarytenoid
C. Oblique arytenoids
D. Transverse arytenoids

Ans: A. Cricothyroid

Ref: *Gray's Anatomy, 40th edition, pg. 700*

Explanation:

Nerve Supply of Larynx

Motor

- All intrinsic muscles of the laryngx are supplied by **recurrent laryngeal nerve** except for **cricothyroid** which is supplied by **external laryngeal nerve**

Sensory

- **Upto** the level of **vocal fold** is supplied by **internal laryngeal nerve**
- **Below** the level of **vocal cord** is supplied by **recurrent laryngeal nerve**

14. **All the following glands are supplied by facial nerve *except:***
A. Parotid **B.** Submandibular
C. Lacrimal **D.** Nasal

Ans: A. Parotid

Ref: *Gray's Anatomy, 40th edition, pg.700*

Explanation:

- Preganglionic nerves travel in the **lesser petrosal branch** of the **glossopharyngeal** nerve and synapse in the **otic ganglion.**
- Postganglionic secretomotor fibres reach the gland via the **auriculotemporal nerve.**

Gustatory sweating (Frey's syndrome or auriculotemporal syndrome)

- Gustatory sweating (auriculotemporal syndrome) commonly occurs following **parotid surgery** or other surgery or trauma that results in opening of the parotid capsule.
- It is thought to reflect **aberrant innervation of sweat glands** on the face by **regrowing parasympathetic secretomotor axons** that would previously have innervated the parotid gland.
- Frey's syndrome is characterized by **sweating, warmth and redness of the face** as a result of **salivary stimulation by the smell or taste of food.**
- The management of Frey's syndrome is difficult.
- **Denervation by tympanic neurectomy** or **auriculotemporal nerve avulsion** have been advocated, but are often not curative.
- The symptoms can be managed by the **subcutaneous infiltration of purified botulinum toxin** into the affected area, and use of antiperspirant.

15. **Omphalocoele is associated with:**
A. Spina bifida
B. Cardiac defects
C. Chromosomal abnormalities
D. Malignancies

Ans: B. Cardiac defects

Ref: *Langmann Embryology, 11th edition*

Explanation:

Omphalocele

- Omphalocele represents **ventral body wall defect** but it does not arise from failure in body wall closure. Instead due to the midgut loop fails to return to the abdominal cavity.
- It is associated with **cardiac** abnormalities and neural tube defect
- Chromosomal abnormalities present in **15%** of cases
- Increase in **alpha feto protein**

Exomphalos

- It is a ventral wall defect with midline herniation of the intra-abdominal contents into the base of the umbilical cord.
- Herniated viscera are covered by the peritoneum internally and amnion externally.

Meckel's Diverticulum

- **Failure of obliteration** of the **vitello-intestinal duct** connecting the **midgut to the yolk sac** results in Meckel's diverticulum.
- This may present as a short segment of vitelline duct attached to the original ventral side of the ileum.
- It may remain attached to the umbilicus as a **fistula**; or it may remain as a ligamentous attachment to the umbilicus.

Gastroschisis

- Gastroschisis is a **para-umbilical defect** of the **anterior abdominal** wall associated with evisceration of the abdominal organs.

- The organs are not enclosed in membranes, thus gastroschisis can be detected by prenatal ultrasonography and differentiated from exomphalos.
- Gastroschisis is thought to result from **periumbilical ischaemia** caused by vascular compromise of either the umbilical vein or arteries.
- The incidence of this condition appears to be increasing, especially in babies born to young women less than 20 years old.
- High incidence of associated **congenital anomalies**

Congenital Volvulus

- Congenital volvulus arises if the **midgut** loop does not rotate appropriately.
- **Left-sided colon** occurs if the midgut loop has not rotated at all; mixed rotation results in the caecum lying inferior to the pylorus; failure of attachment of the peritoneum appropriately may result in the small intestine being attached at only two points on the posterior abdominal wall.
- All of these arrangements lead to a risk of volvulus, which may result in necrosis of the gut.

16. Epoophoron is a remnant of:(Repeat)

A. Wolffian duct **B.** Paramesonephric duct
C. Wolffian body **D.** Allantoic duct

Ans: C. Wolffian body

Ref: *Gray's Anatomy, 40th edition, pg.1305*

Explanation: *(See the following table)*

17. Stylopharyngeus is supplied by:

A. Glossopharyngeal nerve
B. Oculomotor nerve
C. Accessory nerve
D. Abducent nerve

Ans: A. Glossopharyngeal nerve

Ref: *Gray's Anatomy, 40th edition, pg.564*

Explanation:

Note:

- All muscles of **pharynx** are supplied by **cranial accessory nerve** through **vagus** except **stylophayngeus** which is supplied by **glossopharyngeal nerve**
- All muscles of **palate** are supplied by **cranial accessory nerve** except **tensor palate** which is supplied by **mandibular nerve**
- All the muscles of **facial expression** are supplied by **facial nerve** except **levator palpebrae superioris**
- All muscles of **tongue** are supplied by **hypoglossal** except **palatoglossus** which is supplied by **cranial accessory nerve**
- All muscles of **larynx** are supplied by **recurrent**

Gonad	Testis	Ovary
Gubernacular cord	Gubernaculum testis	Ovarian and round ligaments
Mesonephros (Wolffian body)	Appendix of epididymis (?)	Appendices vesiculosae (?)
	Efferent ductules	Epoöphoron
	Lobules of epididymis	
	Paradidymis	Paroöphoron
	Aberrant ductules	
Mesonephric duct (Wolffian duct)	Duct of epididymis	Duct of epoöphoron (Gartner's duct)
	Vas deferens	
	Ejaculatory duct	
	Part of bladder and prostatic urethra	Part of bladder and urethra
Paramesonephric (Müllerian) duct	Appendix of testis	Uterine tube
		Uterus
	Prostatic utricle	Vagina (?)
Allantoic duct	Urachus	Urachus
Cloaca:		
Dorsal part	Rectum and upper part of anal canal	Rectum and upper part of anal canal
Ventral part	Most of bladder	Most of bladder and urethra
	Part of prostatic urethra	
Urogenital sinus	Prostatic urethra distal to utricle	
	Bulbo-urethral glands	Greater vestibular glands
	Rest of urethra to glans	Vestibule
Genital folds	Ventral penis	Labia minora
Genital tubercle	Penis	Clitoris
	Urethra in glans	

laryngeal nerve except **cricothyroid** which is supplied by **external laryngeal nerve**

18. Upper 1st molar is supplied by:

A. Superior alveolar nerve
B. Inferior alveolar nerve
C. Mental nerve
D. Lingual nerve

Ans: A. Superior alveolar nerve

Ref: *Gray's Anatomy, 40th edition, pg.500*

Explanation:

Branches of Maxillary Nerve

In the Cranium

- Middle meningeal nerve in the meninges.

From the Pterygopalatine Fossa

- Infraorbital nerve through infraorbital canal.
- Zygomatic nerve (zygomaticotemporal nerve, zygomaticofacial nerve) through inferior orbital fissure
- Nasal branches (nasopalatine) through sphenopalatine foramen
- Superior alveolar nerves (Posterior superior alveolar nerve, Middle superior alveolar nerve, Anterior superior alveolar nerve)
- Palatine nerves (Greater palatine nerve, Lesser palatine nerve), including the Nasopalatine nerve
- Pharyngeal nerve

In the Infraorbital Canal

- Anterior superior alveolar nerve
- Infraorbital nerve

On the Face

- Inferior palpebral nerve
- Superior labial nerve

Superior Alveolar Nerves

Anterior superior alveolar nerve innervates

- All anterior teeth
- Premolars
- Mesiobuccal root of the first maxillary molar

Posterior superior alveolar nerve innervates

- Second and third maxillary molars
- Two of the three roots of the maxillary first molar (all but the mesiobuccal root)

Middle superior alveolar nerve innervates

- Sinus mucosa
- Roots of the maxillary premolars
- Mesiobuccal root of the first maxillary molar
- It is not always present in majority of cases. In such cases, posterior superior alveolar nerve innervates the premolars and molars.

19. Posterior cord of brachial plexus contains all *except:*

A. Long thoracic nerve of Bell
B. Axillary
C. Radial
D. Upper subscapular

Ans: A. Long thoracic nerve of Bell

Ref: *Gray's Anatomy, 40th edition, pg.820*

Explanation:

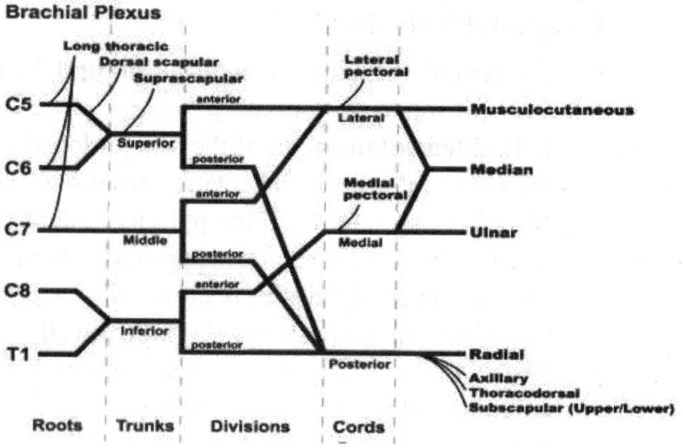

Lateral cord	Lateral pectoral	C5, 6, 7
	Musculocutaneous	C5, 6, 7
	Lateral root of median	C(5), 6, 7
Medial cord (M4U)	Medial pectoral	C8, T1
	Medial cutaneous of forearm	C8, T1
	Medial cutaneous of arm	C8, T1
	Ulnar	C(7), 8, T1
	Medial root of median	C8, T1
Posterior cord (ULTAR)	Upper subscapular	C5, 6
	Thoracodorsal	C6, 7,8
	Lower subscapular	C5, 6
	Axillary	C5, 6
	Radial	C5,6,7,8, (T1)
Root	Dorsal scapular nerve	C5
	Long thoracic nerve of bell	C5,6,7
Trunk	Nerve to subclavius	C5,6
	Suprascapular nerve	C5,6

20. Oblique popliteal ligament attaches to:

A. Semimembranosus **B.** Semitendinosus
C. Sartorius **D.** Adductor magnus

Ans: A. Semimembranosus

Ref: *Gray's Anatomy, 40th edition, pg.1393*

Explanation:

Oblique Popliteal Ligament

- It is an expansion of **semimembranosus tendon** which blends with the **posterior capsule**

- It is pierced by **middle genicular nerve and** vessels which also supply the **cruciate ligament and synovial membrane**
- Terminal part of posterior division of ***obturator nerve*** also pierces the oblique popliteal ligament
- It is attached to **intercondylar line** and **lateral femoral condyle:**

21. **Prostate is supplied by:**
A. Sympathetic + Parasympathetic
B. Parasympathetic
C. Sympathetic
D. None

Ans: A. Sympathetic + Parasympathetic

Ref: *Gray's Anatomy, 40th edition, pg.1245*

Explanation:

- The **superior hypogastric plexus** conveys the **sympathetic nerves** from the pre-ganglionic fibres are derived from **L1 and L2**
- The **parasympathetic fires** are derived from the **pelvic splanchnic nerves** which convey pre-ganglionic fibres from **S2, S3 & S4**. They are **secretomotor** to the glands.
- The **somatic pudendal nerve** supplies the **external urethral sphincter**
- Nerves containing **neuropeptide Y** and **vasointestinal polypeptide (VIP)** are localized in the **subepithelial connective tissue**, in the **smooth muscle layers** of the gland, and in the walls of its blood vessels.

PHYSIOLOGY

1. **Pneumotaxic centre is situated in:**
A. Medulla
B. Pons
C. Midbrain
D. Reticular activating system

Ans: B. Pons

Ref: *Guyton & Hall, Respiratory Center, In: Textbook of Medical Physiology,12th ed., Philadelphia, Saunders, Elsevier, 2012, p 506.*

Explanation:

Pneumotaxic Center

- Located dorsally in the **nucleus parabrachialis** of the **upper pons**
- Transmits signals to the **inspiratory area**
- Control the **"switch-off"** point of the inspiratory ramp (control the duration of the filling phase of the lung cycle).
- When the signal is strong, inspiration lasts for 0.5 second, when the pneumotaxic signal is weak, inspiration continues for 5 or more seconds.
- Secondary effect: Increases the rate of breathing (limitation of inspiration also shortens expiration; i.e. strong signal can increase upto 30 to 40 breaths/minute; weak pneumotaxic signal may reduce the rate to only 3 to 5 breaths per minute).

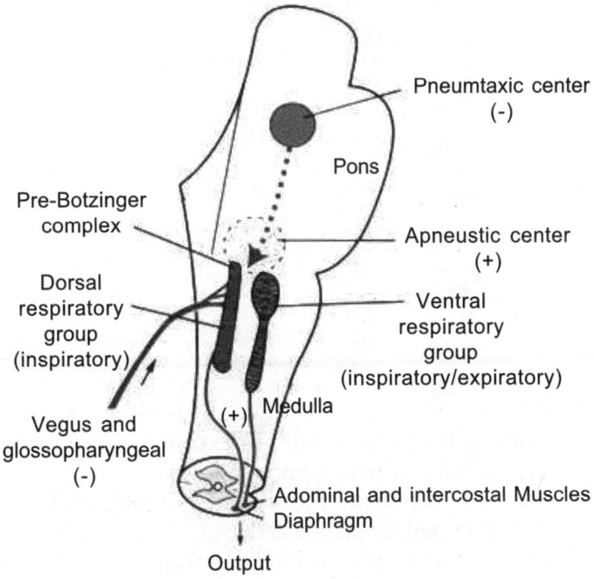

2. **Intrinsic factor is secreted by:**
A. Parietal cells **B.** Chief cells
C. Mucus cells **D.** G cells

Ans: A. Parietal cells

Ref: *Guyton & Hall, Gastric Secretion, In: Textbook of Medical Physiology, 12th ed, Philadelphia, Saunders, Elsevier 2012, p 777*

Explanation:

- **Stomach mucosa** has 2 types of tubular glands
  1. **Oxyntic glands (Gastric glands)-** secrete **hydrochloric acid, pepsinogen, intrinsic factor** and **mucus.**
  2. **Pyloric glands** - **mucus** for protection of the pyloric mucosa from the stomach acid; also secrete the hormone **gastrin.**

  Stomach oxyntic gland is composed of three types of cells:
  1. **Mucous neck cells** - secrete mainly **mucus**
  2. **Peptic (or chief) cells** - secrete large quantities of **pepsinogen**
  3. **Parietal (or oxyntic) cells** - secrete **hydrochloric** acid and **intrinsic factor**

  (See figure on the next page)

Structure of Gastric Glands and Cell Types

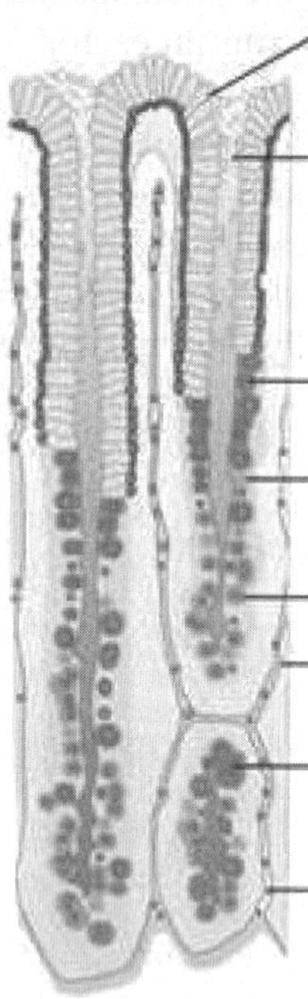

3. **All are true about inhibin *except:***
   A. It is a steroidal compound
   B. FSH stimulates the secretion of inhibin B
   C. Secreted by sertoli cells
   D. Inhibin B inhibits FSH secretion

   Ans: A. It is a steroidal compound

Ref: *Pal GK, Male Reproductice System In: Textbook of Medical Physiology, 2nd ed, Ahuja Publishing House 2011; 54: 450*

Explanation:

Inhibin

Source

- Sertoli cells (testes)
- Granulosa cells (ovaries)

Types

- Inhibin A
- Inhibin B

Structure

- It is made up of α and β subunits; they are polypeptides
- Activin is made up of only β subunits (no α subunit)
- Inhibin A - α, β**A**; Inhibin B - α, β**B**

Functions

- **FSH stimulates the secretion of inhibin** from the granulosa cells. Inhibin B coincides with change is FSH concentration
- In turn, **inhibin B suppresses FSH.**
- Inhibin A coincides with pattern of progesterone.
- It regulates spermatogenesis in males

4. **Melatonin is secreted by:**
   A. Mammillary body **B.** Pineal gland
   C. Posterior pituitary **D.** Hypothalamus

   Ans: B. Pineal gland

Ref: *Pal GK, Pineal gland, In: Textbook of Medical Physiology, 2nd ed, Ahuja Publishing House, 2011; 51: 418-19*

Explanation:

Pineal Gland Secretes

- Melatonin
- Arginine vasotocin
- Arginine vasopressin
- Oxytocin
- Proopiomelanocortin

Synthesis of Melatonin

Tryptophan

↓

5 Hydroxy tryptophan

↓

Serotonin (5 Hydroxy Tryptamine)

↓

N-Acetyl serotonin (N-Acetyl % Hydroxytryptamine)

↓

Melatonin (N-Acetyl 5 Methoxytryptamine)

Functions

- **Diurnal change** in melatonin coordinates **endocrinal responses** of the body
- **Inhibits gonadal** functions
- Influences **melanophores** and skin color in lower animals.
- Mechanism
  - ML1A,1B receptors - By increasing cAMP
  - ML2 receptor - By increasing IP_3, DAG

5. **Substance causing mesangial relaxation:**
   A. Histamine **B.** cAMP
   C. ADH **D.** Angiotensin II

   Ans: B. cAMP

Ref: *Pal GK, Glomerular Filtration, In: Textbook of Medical Physiology, 2nd ed, Ahuja Publishing House 2011; 61: 513*

Explanation:

Mesangial Cell Contraction is by

- Angiotensin II
- Norepinephrine
- Endothelin
- ADH
- PDGF
- PAF
- Histamine
- Thromboxane A2
- PGF_2
- Leukotriene

Mesangial Cell Relaxation is by

- Dopamine
- ANP
- cAMP
- PGE_2
- Nitric oxide
- Bradykinin

6. **De-afferentation of muscle explains:**
   A. Influence of vestibulo spinal tract on alpha fibers
   B. Influence of vestibulo spinal tract on gamma fibers
   C. Influence of reticulo spinal tract on alpha fibers
   D. Influence of reticulo spinal tract on gamma fibers

   Ans: D. Influence of reticulo spinal tract on gamma fibers

Ref: *Pal GK, Regulation of Posture and Movement, In: Textbook of Medical Physiology, 2nd ed, Ahuja Publishing House 2011; 114: 859.*

Explanation:

- ***Dorsal rhizotomy*** causes **de-afferentation (Ia fibers).**
- De-afferentation abolishes input from muscle spindle to spinal cord.
- Experimentally, even after de-afferentation, influence of vestibulo spinal tract on alpha fibers is not affected. But, gamma motor neuron (controlled by reticulo spinal tract) mediated response in extra fusal fibers (muscle contraction at rest, i.e., muscle tone) is lost
- Hence, **Vestibulo spinal tract** mainly influences **alpha motor neuron.**
- **Reticulo spinal tract** mainly influences **gamma fibers**

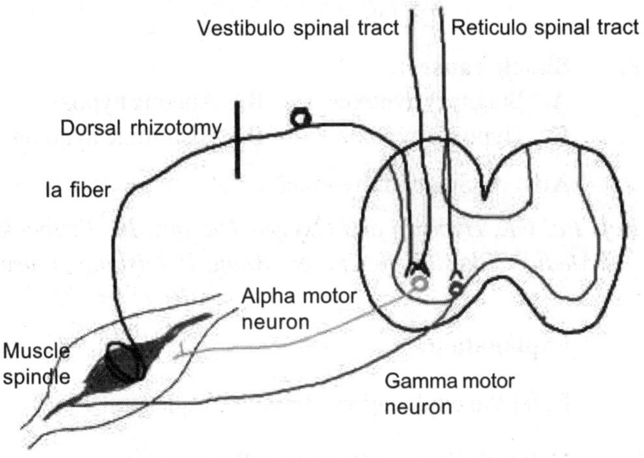

7. **Carbon monoxide poisoning causes which type of hypoxia?**
   A. Anemic hypoxia **B.** Hypoxic hypoxia
   C. Stagnant hypoxia **D.** Histotoxic hypoxia

   Ans: A. Anemic hypoxia

Ref: *Pal GK, Hypoxia and Oxygen Therapy, In: Textbook of Medical Physiology, 2nd ed, Ahuja Publishing House 2011; 94: 754-55*

Explanation:

Hypoxia

- Hypoxia is O_2 deficiency at the tissue level.
- Types
  - **Hypoxic hypoxia** - **PO_2** of the arterial blood is reduced. Eg:
    - High altitude (low PO_2 in inspired air)
    - Hypoventilation (airway obstruction, respiratory muscle paralysis)
  - **Anemic hypoxia** - arterial **PO_2 is normal** but the amount of hemoglobin available to carry O_2 is reduced. Eg:
    - Anemia
    - Carbon monoxide poisoning – CO has more affinity (for Hb) than O_2; release of CO from CO-Hb is slow; hence O_2 cannot bind with Hb
    - Altered Hb - Methemoglobin
  - **Stagnant or ischemic hypoxia** - blood flow to a tissue is so low that adequate O_2 is not delivered to it despite a normal PO_2 and hemoglobin concentration Eg:
    - Heart failure, shock, vascular obstruction
  - **Histotoxic hypoxia** - amount of O_2 delivered to a tissue is adequate, but because of the action of a toxic agent, the tissue cells cannot make use of the O_2 supplied to them Eg:
    - Cyanide poisoning

◦ Diphtheria

8. **Shock causes:**
   A. Stagnant hypoxia **B.** Anemic hypoxia
   C. Hypoxic hypoxia **D.** Histotoxic hypoxia

   Ans: A. Stagnant hypoxia

Ref: *Pal GK, Hypoxia and Oxygen Therapy, In: Textbook of Medical Physiology, 2nd ed, Ahuja Publishing House 2011; 94: 754-55*

Explanation:

Refer the explanation of previous question

9. **Calmodulin acts through all *except:***
   A. MLCK
   B. Calcium-calmodulin kinase
   C. Phosphorylase kinase
   D. Phosphodiesterse

   Ans: D. Phosphodiesterase

Ref: *Pal GK, Mechanism of Hormone Action, In: Textbook of Medical Physiology, 2nd ed, Ahuja Publishing House 2011; 42: 318*

Explanation:

Calmodulin

- Has 148 amino acid
- Has four sites for calcium
- When it binds with calcium, it changes its shape and initiates multiple effects (activation or inhibition of protein kinases).
  – Eg: activates **myosin light chain kinase** (phosphorylation increases the ATPase activity) cause smooth muscle contraction.

(See the following figure)

- Calmodulin also acts through phosphorylase kinase, calcium-calmodulin kinase I, II & III
- Phosphodiesterse degrades cAMP to 5'AMP

10. **Function of thyroid hormones:**
    A. Inhibits beta myosin heavy chain
    B. Increases cholesterol
    C. Inhibits ovulation
    D. Increases diastolic blood pressure

    Ans: A. Inhibits beta myosin heavy chain

Ref: *Pal GK, The Thyroid Gland, In: Textbook of Medical Physiology, 2nd ed, Ahuja Publishing House 2011; 46: 352-55*

Explanation:

Physiological Actions of Thyroid Hormone

- **Basal metabolism**

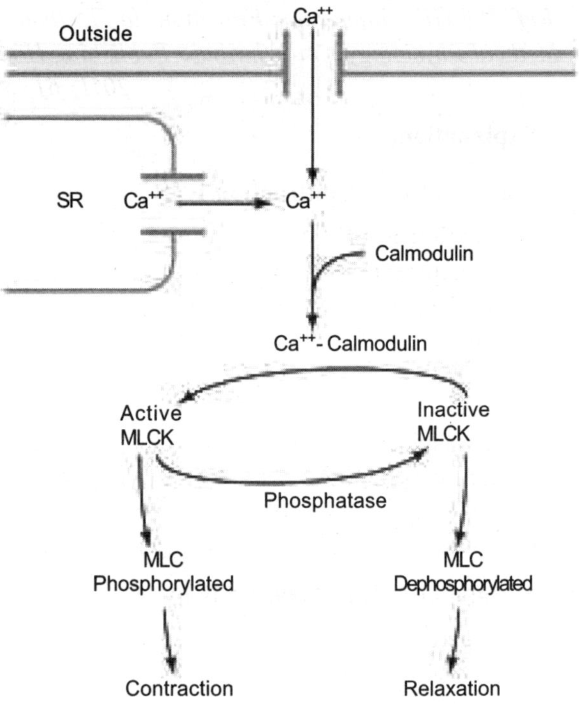

  – ↑ rate of oxygen consumption
  – ↑ Na^+ K^+ ATPase activity
  – Thermogenic action
- **On nervous system**
  – Proliferation of axons, branching of dendrites
  – Development of synapse
  – Formation of neurotransmitter
  – ↑ receptors
  – Myelination
- **On growth and development**
  – Promoting gene expression for GH
  – Linear growth of bone
  – ↑ osteoid action, bone remodeling
  – Teeth eruption and development
- **On CVS**
  – ↑ ***Heart rate*** - ↑number of β receptors on SA node; ↑ sensitivity of β receptor for catecholamine
  – ↑ ***Myocardial contractility***
    ◦ By inducing expression of myosin heavy chain (↑ α MHC activity; suppress β MHC activity)
    ◦ ↑ Ca ATPase activity
  – ***Blood pressure***
    ◦ ↑ HR, stroke volume - ↑ systolic BP
    ◦ Thermogenic cutaneous vasodilation - ↓peripheral resistance - ↓ diastolic BP
- **On metabolism**
  – ***Carbohydrate***
    ◦ ↑ glucose absorption
    ◦ ↑ hepatic gluconeogenesis
    ◦ ↑ glycogenolysis

- *Fat*
  - ↑ lipolysis, stimulate cholesterol synthesis – also ↑oxidation and bile excretion – net reduction in plasma cholesterol, total lipid
- *Protein*
  - Proteolysis and turnover

- **Synergize net effect of catecholamines**
- **On respiratory system**
  - ↑ oxygen utilization
  - Stimulate erythropoiesis
- **On GIT**
  - Enhance the motility
  - ↑ appetite, food intake
- **Skeletal muscle**
  - ↑ expression of MHC genes
- **On reproductive system**
  - Female – follicular maturation, ovulation
  - Male – spermatogenesis
- **On kidney**
  - ↑ renal blood flow, GFR

11. Touch and pressure sensation are carried by: (Repeat)

A. Alpha fibers **B.** Beta fibers
C. Gamma fibers **D.** Delta fibers

Ans: B. Beta fibers

Ref: *Pal GK, Nerve, In: Textbook of Medical Physiology, 2nd ed, Ahuja Publishing House 2011; 18: 164*

Explanation:

Classification of Nerve Fibers

Type of fiber	Physiological role	Diameter (μm)	Conduction velocity (m/s)
A			
α	Proprioception; somatic motor	12–20	70–120
β	Touch Pressure	5–12	30–70
γ	Motor to muscle spindles	3–6	15–30
δ	Pain Cold Touch	2–5	12–30
B	Preganglionic autonomic	<3	3–15
C			
Dorsal root	Pain, temperature, some mechanoreception	0.4–1.2	0.5–2
Sympathetic	Postganglionic sympathetic	0.3–1.3	0.7–2.3

12. Major adrenocortical hormone in blood is:

A. Cortisol **B.** Corticosterone
C. Aldosterone **D.** Deoxy corticosterone

Ans: A. Cortisol

Ref: *Guyton & Hall, Synthesis and Secretion of Adrenocortical Hormones, In: Textbook of Medical Physiology, 12th ed, Philadelphia, Saunders, Elsevier 2012, p 924*

Explanation: *(See table on the next page)*

13. Sleep spindle and K complexes are seen in: (Repeat)

A. REM **B.** NREM Stage II
C. NREM Stage III **D.** NREM Stage IV

Ans: B. NREM Stage II

Ref: *Pal GK, Reticular Formation, EEG and Sleep, In: Textbook of Medical Physiology, 2nd ed, Ahuja Publishing House, 2011; 119: 895-96*

Explanation:

Sleep

- It is defined behaviorally by four criteria
  - Reduced motor activity
  - Decreased response to stimulation
  - Stereotypic postures (in humans, for example, lying down with eyes closed)
  - Relatively easy reversibility (distinguishing it from coma, hibernation and estivation)
- EEG pattern repeats in every **90 minutes**
- Non-REM phase
  - 4 stages
- REM phase
  - Late part of night
  - 25% of total sleep period

Non-REM Sleep (Slow Wave Sleep)

- Stage 1
  - Beta to alpha rhythm
- Stage 2
  - Amplitude increases
- **Sleep spindle** (12-14 Hz; 50 μV; for about 2 seconds) and **K complexes** (high amplitude)
- Stage 3
  - High amplitude; low frequency
- Stage 4
  - Delta rhythm
- **Autonomic and visceral changes**
  - ↓ heart rate and BP
  - ↓ body temperature
  - Slow regular respiration
  - ↓ GI activity
  - ↓ muscle tone
  - No rapid eye movement

Adrenal Steroid Hormones in Adults

Steroids	Average plasma concentration (free and bound, μg/100 ml)	Average amount secreted (mg/24 hr)	Glucocorticoid activity	Mineralocorticoid activity
Adrenal Steroids				
Cortisol	12	15	1.0	1.0
Corticosterone	0.4	3	0.3	15.0
Aldosterone	0.006	0.15	0.3	3000
Deoxycorticosterone	0.006	0.2	0.2	100
Dehydroepiandrosterone	175	20	-	-

Paradoxical sleep (REM Sleep)

- Features
  - Rapid eye movements
  - EEG
    - High frequency; low voltage rhythm
    - PGO spikes (**Ponto-Geniculo-Occipital**)
  - Difficult to arouse; likely to wakeup spontaneously
  - **Dream is remembered**
  - ↑ sympathetic system (↑ HR, BP, Respiration)
  - **Penile erection**
  - Decreased muscle tone (except extraoccular and middle ear)

14. To cause hemorrhagic shock, least volume of blood loss should be:

A. 30% **B.** 40%
C. 20% **D.** 50%

Ans: C. 20%

Ref: *Klingensmith ME, Chen LE, Glasgow SC, Goers TA, Melby SJ, Reticular Formation, EEG and sleep, In: Washington Manual of Surgery, 5th Edn, Lippincott Williams & Wilkins 2008; 7: 145*

Explanation: *(See the following table)*

15. All are true about Gap junction *except:*

A. Permits amino acids upto 1000 Da mol wt.
B. Opening of gap junction does not depend on trans membrane voltage
C. Halothane closes gap junction reversibly
D. Gap junction is made up of connexon is made up of six identical connexins

Ans: B. Opening of gap junction does not depend on trans membrane voltage

Ref:

1. *Pal GK, Functional Organization of Cell, In: Textbook of Medical Physiology, 2nd ed. Ahuja Publishing House, 2011; 3: 19*
2. *Pollard TD, Earnshaw EC, Intercellular Junctions, In: Cell Biology, 2nd ed. 31: 573-79*

Explanation:

Gap Junctions - Nexus

- Made up of ***connexons*** – trans-membrane protein
- Each connexon is made up of six identical connexins (protein)
- Allow upto 1 KDa molecules
  Eg:
  - Ions (Electrical synapse)
  - 2nd messengers
  - Peptides
- Opening depends on
  - Trans mb volt
  - H^+, Ca^{++} ion
  - Protein kinase
- Eg. Skin, GIT, Heart, Skeletal muscle, Glial cell
- **Oleamide**, a fatty acid amide produced by the brain, blocks gap junctional communication and induces sleep
- Organic alcohols (**heptanol and octanol**) and general anesthetics (**halothane**) can also close gap junction channels reversibly; also nonspecific

Signs and Symptoms for Different Classes of Shock

	Class I	Class II	Class III	Class IV
Blood loss (mL)	Upto 750	750–1,500	1,500–2,000	>2,000
Blood loss (% blood volume)	Upto 15%	15%–30%	30%–40%	>40%
Pulse rate	<100	>100	>120	>140
Blood pressure (mm Hg)	Normal	Normal	Decreased	Decreased
Pulse pressure (mm Hg)	Normal or increased	Decreased	Decreased	Decreased
Urinary output (mL/hr)	>30	20–30	5–15	Negligible
CNS/Mental Status	Slightly anxious	Mildly anxious	Anxious and confused	Confused and lethargic

Mutations in Connexin Subunit (Human)

- **Cx-26β2** - Dominant and recessive mutations with deafness; skin disease
- **Cx-30β6** - Recessive deafness; skin disease
- **Cx-31β3** - Recessive deafness; skin disease
- **Cx-32β1** - X-linked point mutations, defective myelin, peripheral nerve degeneration; deafness
- **Cx-43α1** - Deafness
- **Cx-50α8** - **Cataracts** in lens of the eye

16. **Intestinal motility is enhanced by all *except:***
    A. CCK **B.** Motilin
    C. Secretin **D.** Gastrin

Ans: C. Secretin

Ref: *Pal GK, Gastro Intestinal Hormones, In: Textbook of Medical Physiology, 2nd ed, Ahuja Publishing House 2011; 26: 895-96*

Explanation:

Functions - Gastrin

- Stimulation of **gastric acid** and **pepsin** secretion
- ↑ Growth of **gastric mucosa** (Trophic action)
- ↑ **Gastric motility**
- ↑ **LES tone** - Prevents reflux esophagitis
- ↑ **Insulin** secretion, stimulate **exocrine pancreas**
- Stimulates **histamine** secretion from ECL

Functions - CCK

- **Contraction of gallbladder** - releasing bile
- Secretion of **pancreatic juice** also trophic effect
- **Enhance intestinal motility**
- Augments contraction of pyloric sphincter to prevent reflux of duodenal contents into stomach
- Acts as **GUT FACTOR** stimulating glucagon secretion
- Role in anorexia, anxiety and analgesia

Functions of Secretin

- **Neutralizes acidity of chyme** by secreting more alkaline & more voluminous pancreatic juice
- Secretes **Bicarbonate from liver, pancreas and duodenal Brunners Glands**
- Promote normal growth and maintenance of pancreas
- Enhances action of cholecystokinin
- **Reduces gastric secretion and motility**
- Counteracts blood glucose level spikes by triggering increased release of insulin after oral load of glucose

Motilin

- Secreted by the **enterochromaffin cells & Mo cells** in the stomach and large intestine
- Motilin 7 and erythromycin act through G-protein coupled receptors in the duodenal entric neurons
- Motilin determines the length of the inter-digestive period as it **increases the motility** of the gut

17. **Fick's principle is used to calculate:**
    A. Cardiac output **B.** Pulse pressure
    C. Cardiac axis **D.** LVET

Ans: A. Cardiac output

Ref: *Pal GK, Cardiac Output. In: Textbook of Medical Physiology, 2nd ed, Ahuja Publishing House 2011; 74: 608*

Explanation:

- In Fick's method, the following variables are measured:
  - **Oxygen consumption** in ml of pure gaseous oxygen per minute
  - **Oxygen concentration** of blood taken from the **pulmonary artery**
  - **Oxygen concentration** of blood from a cannula in a **peripheral artery**

$$\text{Cardiac Output} = \frac{\text{Oxygen consumption}}{\text{Arteriovenous oxygen difference}} \times 100$$

- **Fick's principle** can also be used in **renal physiology** to calculate **renal blood flow.**
- Pulse pressure is the difference between systolic and diastolic pressure
- Cardiac axis is measured using ECG
- Left ventricular ejection time is estimated with carotid pulse tracing

BIOCHEMISTRY

1. **Tay-Sach's disease is due to the deficieny of:**
   A. Hexoaminidase A **B.** Sphingomyelinase
   C. β-glucocerebrosidase **D.** Galactocerebrosidase

Ans: A. Hexoaminidase A

Ref: *Harper's Illustrated Biochemistry, 28th edition*

Explanation:

Lipid Storage Disorders

- Defects in lysosomal enzymes concerned with the degradation of complex lipids
- These lipids accumulate in lysosomes→ lysis→ tissue destruction
- Since brain and nervous tissue have ↑concentration of sphingolipids, symptoms usually severe
- Depends also on extent of enzyme deficiency

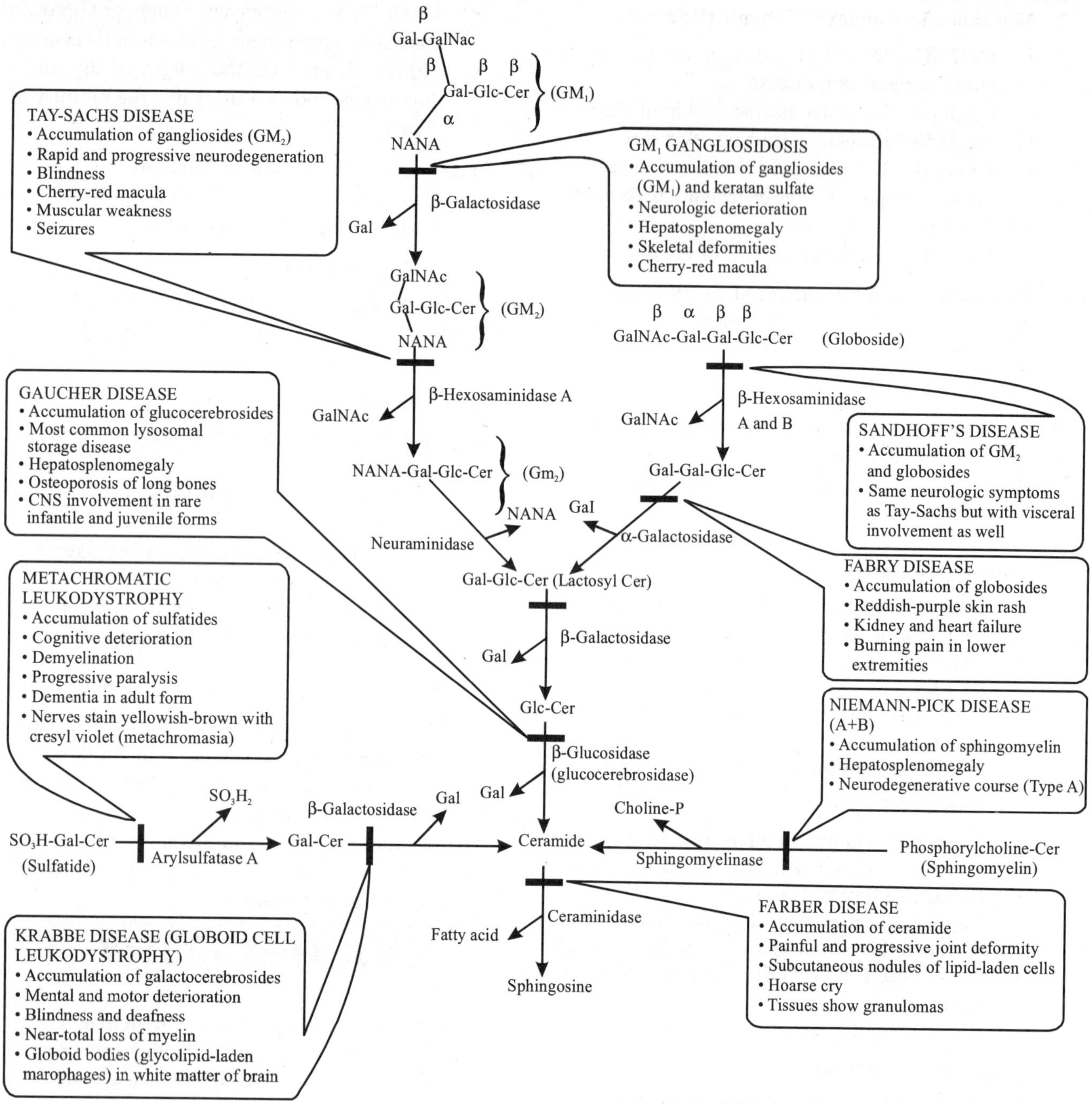

2. **Cirrhosis does not occur with:**

A. Calcium **B.** Copper
C. Alcohol **D.** Iron

Ans: A. Calcium

Ref: *Harper's Illustrated Biochemistry, 28th edition*

Explanation:

- **Iron overload,** hemochromatosis - Disorder of iron storage, excessive intestinal absorption and deposition of excessive iron which can cause a triad of:
  - Pigmentation of skin
  - Damage to the pancreas causing diabetes mellitus
  - Cirrhosis of liver (**Bronze Diabetes**)

Alcohol consumption results in fatty liver, alcoholic hepatitis and cirrhosis of liver in the last stage.

Wilson's Disease:

- Failure to synthesize ceruloplasmin
- Impairment in binding of Cu; Excretion defect
- Free Cu in plasma
- Hepatolenticular degeneration
- Abnormal Cu deposition in liver and lenticular

nucleus of brain-hepatic and brain necrosis, eyes – **kayser fleischer ring**

- ↓ Cu and ceruloplasmin in plasma
- ↑ Cu excretion in urine

3. **Following amino acid form an integral part of collagen synthesis:**

A. Lysine **B.** Leucine
C. Arginine **D.** Glutamic acid

Ans: A. Lysine

Ref: *Harper's Illustrated Biochemistry, 28th edition*

Explanation:

Collagen

- Collagen is a fibrous protein
- Most abundant structural protein
- Accounts for **25%** of the total body proteins
- Found in skin, joints, skeleton, tendons, cartilage, cornea and blood vessels
- Unusual right-handed **triple helix**
- 3 polypeptide chains, an unusual amino acid composition
- **33% glycine, 10% proline, 10% hydroxy-proline (Hyp)**
- The sequence **Gly-X-Y-Gly-X-Y** is **repetitive**
- Hydroxylated amino acid (pro, lys) characteristic of collagen
- Synthesized **post-translationally**, a step requiring **vitamin C.**
- Vitamin C deficiency symptoms explained by disturbances in collagen biosynthesis.
- Collagen molecules tend to associate with one another to form larger, more complex cylindrical fibrils (diameter 20-500 nm)
- At either end, the individual collagen molecules are **cross-linked via** modified **lysine residues.**
- This gives tensile strength to collagen
- Extent of cross-linking increases with age

4. **Erythrocyte glutathione reductase deficiency is seen in deficiency of:**

A. Riboflavin **B.** Folic acid
C. Vitamin C **D.** Vitamin E

Ans: A. Riboflavin

Ref: *Glatzle D, Korner WF, Christeller S, Wiss O. Method for the detection of a biochemical riboflavin deficiency. Stimulation of NADPH2-dependent glutathione reductase from human erythrocytes by FAD in vitro. Investigations on the vitamin B2 status in healthy people and geriatric patients. Int.J Vitam Res 1970;40:166-183*

Explanation:

- **Glutathione**, in reduced form (**GSH**), **maintains cell membrane integrity** against oxidative stress by acting as a substrate for the reduction of peroxides to less damaging alcohols by **glutathione peroxidase.**
- Glutathione reductase facilitates this process by catalysing the conversion of oxidized glutathione (GSSG) to GSH, thereby maintaining an adequate level of intracellular GSH.
- Optimal glutathione reductase activity depends on adequate availability of **flavin adenine dinucleotide** (FAD), a coenzyme derived from **riboflavin (vitamin B-2).**
- Thus **glutathione reductase activity** is **suboptimal** in individuals with **riboflavin deficiency**.
- Riboflavin (vitamin B-2) is a water soluble B vitamin that serves as a **precursor of FAD** and **flavin** mononucleotide.
- These two compounds are important coenzymes in a variety of electron transfer reactions during energy producing, biosynthetic, detoxifying and electron scavenging processes.

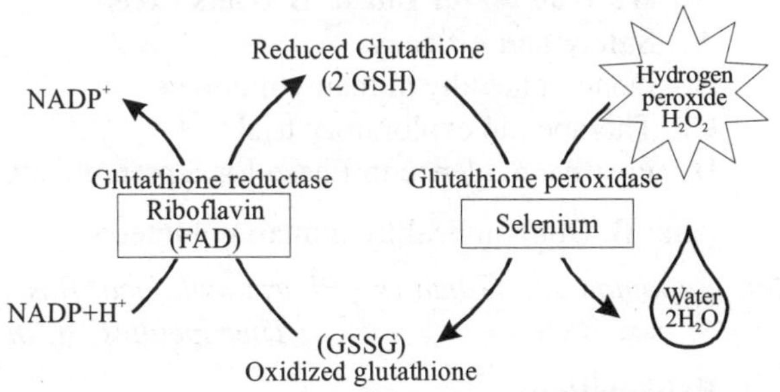

5. **Putrescene – a polyamine is formed by decarboxylation of:**

A. Arginine **B.** Ornithine
C. Citrulline **D.** Adenine

Ans: B. Ornithine

Ref: *Harper's Illustrated Biochemistry, 28th edition*

Explanation:

- **Polyamines** include **putrescine, spermidine, spermine.**
- **Ornithine** is a major **precursor** for synthesis of polyamines.

Conversion of ornithine to putrescine is catalyzed by **Ornithine Decarboxylase.**

(*See* figure on the next page)

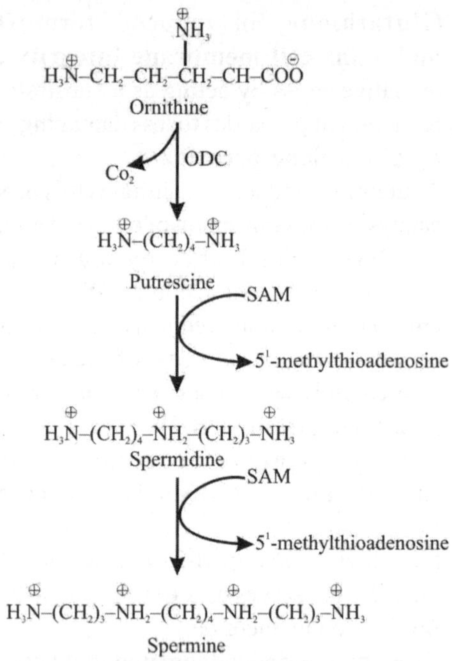

PHARMACOLOGY

1. **All are true about Phase II trials *except:***
   A. Safety and efficacy
   B. Done in healthy human volunteers
   C. Therapeutic exploratory trial
   D. Positive evidence in Phase I is a prerequisite

   Ans: B. Done in healthy human volunteers

***Ref:** Goodman and Gilman's "Pharmacological Basis of Therapeutics" 12th ed*

Explanation:

- Phase II trial is done on **Patients** (Phase I done on healthy human volunteers)
- It is done for assessing the **safety and efficacy**
- If Phase I trial indicates any serious adverse effects, Phase II cannot be done

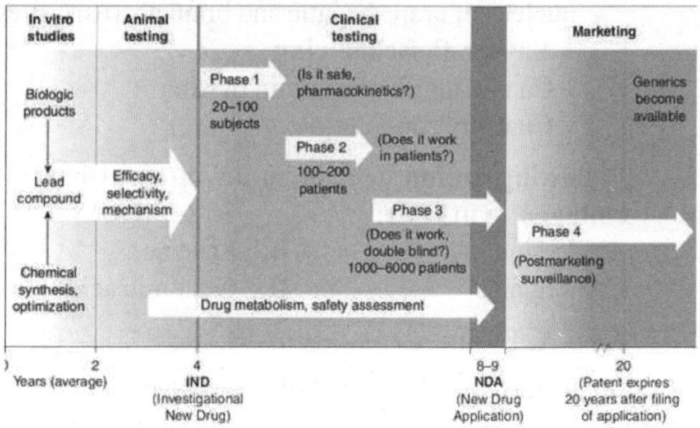

- Positive evidence and absence of serious adverse effects from Phase I are prerequisite for proceeding with Phase II trial. *(See the following table and figure)*

2. **All are true about Nefopam *except:***
   A. Non opioid
   B. Decreases PG synthesis
   C. Causes seizures
   D. Prevents shivering

   Ans: B. Decreases PG synthesis

***Ref:** Essentials of Medical Pharmacology by K.D.Tripathi, 6th ed & Internet Source*

Explanation:

Nefopam

- It is a centrally-acting but **non-opioid analgesic** drug of the **benzoxazocine** chemical class
- It is widely used for the relief **pain** as an alternative to opioid analgesic drugs.
- The mechanism of action of nefopam is not well understood, although inhibition of **serotonin**, **dopamine** and **noradrenaline** reuptake is thought to be involved in its analgesic effects and there may be other modes of action such as through **histamine H3 receptors** and **glutamate**

PHASE I **First in Human**	**PHASE II** **First in Patient** **(therapeutic exploratory)**	**PHASE III** **Multi-Site Trial** **(therapeutic confirmatory)**	**PHASE IV** **(Post-marketing surveillance)**
10-100 participants	50-500 participants	A few hundred to a few thousand participants	Many thousands of participants
Usually healthy volunteers; occasionally patients with advanced or rare disease	Patients	Patients	Patients in treatment with approved drug
Open label	Randomized and controlled (can be placebo-controlled); may be blinded	Randomized and controlled (can be placebo-controlled) or uncontrolled; may be blinded	Open label
Safety and tolerability	Efficacy and dose ranging	Confirm efficacy in larger population	Adverse events, compliance, drug-drug interactions
Months to 1 year **Success rate: 50%**	1-2 years Success rate: 30%	3-5 years Success rate: 25-50%	No fixed duration —

- Recently, nefopam has been found to act as a **voltage-gated sodium channel blocker**, and this may in part or fully mediate its **anti-nociceptive** effects
- Nefopam has additional action in the **prevention of shivering**.
- Nefopam at a dose of **30–120 mg** is significantly **more effective** than **aspirin** as an analgesic although with a greater incidence of side effects such as **sweating, dizziness, nausea and rarely seizures and even death,** especially at higher doses.
- **Less potent** than **morphine** but produce **fewer side effects**
- Does not **produce respiratory depression** and has much less abuse potential
- Also used to treat **severe hiccups**

3. **Bromocriptine inhibits: (Repeat)**

A. Prolactin	**B.** Vasopressin
C. Imipramine	**D.** Levodopa

Ans A. Prolactin

Ref: *Essentials of Medical Pharmacology by K.D.Tripathi, 6th ed p.235*

Explanation:

- **Prolactin** is under predominant inhibitory control of hypothalamus through PRIH which is dopamine that acts on pituitary lactotrope D2 receptor.
- **Dopamine agonists - ↓Plasma Prolactin levels**
- **Dopamine antagonists - ↑Plasma Prolactin levels**
- **Dopaminergic agonists**
  - Dopamine
  - Bromocriptine
  - Cabergoline
- **Dopaminergic antagonists**
  - Chlorpromazine
  - Haloperidol
  - Metoclopramide
  - Dopamine depleters (Reserpine, Methyldopa)

4. **All of the following are useful against MRSA *except:***

A. Vancomycin	**B.** Linezolid
C. Retapamulin	**D.** Streptogramin

Ans: C. Retapamulin

Ref: *Basic & Clinical Pharmacology Katzung, 12th ed. p.1063. Essentials of Medical Pharmacology by K.D.Tripathi 6th ed*

Explanation:

Retapamulin

- It is a semi-synthetic **pleromutilin** derivative effective in the treatment of uncomplicated superficial skin infection caused by **group A β-hemolytic streptococci and S aureus, excluding MRSA.**
- Topical retapamulin 1% ointment is indicated for use in adult and pediatric patients, above 9 months, for the treatment of **impetigo**.
- Recommended treatment regimen is twice-daily application for 5 days.

Quinupristin/Dalfopristin

- Belongs to **streptogramins** is a combination of two semisynthetic pristinamycin antibiotics
- Combination exerts synergistic **inhibition** of bacterial **Protein synthesis**.
- It is active against
  - Most gram-positive cocci including MRSA, some VRSA and some VRE
  - Neisseria, Legionella and Chlamydia pneumoniae.
- The combination is bactericidal against streptococci and staphylococci but bacteriostatic against E. faecium.

Linezolid

- Belongs to the class **'Oxazolidinones'** which is available for the treatment of resistant gram-positive coccal (aerobic and anaerobic) and bacillary infections.
- It is active against
  - MRSA, VRSA & VRE
  - Penicillin-resistant Strep. pyogenes, Strep. viridans and Strep. pneumoniae,
  - Tuberculosis
  - Corynebacterium
  - Listeria
  - Clostridia
  - Bact. fragilis.
- It is primarily bacteriostatic
- Gram negative bacteria are not affected

5. **Heparin induced thrombocytopenia is reversed by:**

A. Warfarin	**B.** Enoxaparin
C. Danaparoid	**D.** Ardeparin

Ans: C. Danaparoid

Ref: *Goodman and Gilman's "Pharmacological basis of therapeutics" 12th ed p.859 & Essentials of Medical Pharmacology by K.D.Tripathi 6th ed pg.600*

Explanation:

- **Danaparoid** is a heparinoid preparation containing mainly **heparin sulfate**, obtained from **pig gut mucosa**
- Used in heparin induced thrombocytopenia (HIT)

Heparin-Induced Thrombocytopenia

- Heparin-induced thrombocytopenia (platelet count <150,000/mL or a 50% decrease from the pretreatment value) occurs in about **0.5%** of medical patients **5-10 days** after initiation of therapy with heparin.
- The incidence of heparin-induced thrombocytopenia and thrombosis is **higher** in **surgical patients and in women than men** (2:1)
- The development of **IgG antibodies** against **complexes of heparin** with '**Platelet factor 4**' appears to cause reactions in HIT.
- These complexes activate platelets by binding to **FcγIIa** receptors, which results in platelet aggregation, release of more platelet factor 4, and thrombin generation.
- The antibodies also may trigger **vascular injury** by binding to platelet factor 4 attached to endogenous heparin sulfate on the endothelium.
- **Heparin**, **LMWH** and **fondaparinux** should be **discontinued immediately**
- The diagnosis of heparin-induced thrombocytopenia can be confirmed by a **heparin-dependent platelet activation assay** or an **assay for antibodies** that react with **heparin/platelet factor 4** complexes
- Because thrombotic complications may occur after cessation of therapy, an alternative anticoagulant such as **lepirudin, argatroban, or fondaparinux** should be administered to patients with heparin-induced thrombocytopenia

> – **Idraparinux**, a hypermethylated version of fondaparinux, underwent phase III clinical testing. This drug has a $t_{1/2}$ of 80 hours and is given subcutaneously on a **once-weekly** basis.
> – To overcome the lack of an antidote, a biotin moiety was added to idraparinux to generate **idrabiotaparinux**, which can be neutralized with intravenous **avidin**.

6. **NMDA antagonist used in Alzheimer's disease is:**

A. Memantine	**B.** Rivastigmine
C. Donepezil	**D.** Galantamine

Ans: A. Memantine

Ref: *Goodman and Gilman's "Pharmacological Basis of Therapeutics" 12th ed p.622*

Explanation:

Memantine

- It is used either as an adjunct or an alternative to **cholinesterase inhibitors** in **Alzheimer's disease**, and is also commonly used to treat other neurodegenerative dementias.
- Memantine is a **noncompetitive antagonist** of the **NMDA-type glutamate receptor**.
- It interacts with the **Mg^{2+} binding site** of the channel to prevent excessive activation while sparing normal function.
- Adverse effects of memantine include **headache** or **dizziness**, but are usually mild and reversible.
- The drug is excreted by the **kidneys** and **dosage** should be **reduced** in patients with severe **renal impairment.**

7. **Which one of the following is not an NMDA receptor?**

A. Kappa	**B.** Kainate
C. AMPA	**D.** Glutamate

Ans: A. Kappa

Ref: *Basic & Clinical Pharmacology, Katzung 12th ed. p.367*

Explanation:

- Kappa is an opioid receptor whereas the others are NMDA receptors.
  Below is a table summarizing different receptors and their transducer mechanisms.
  (See table on the next page)

8. **Which drug is used to suppress lactation? (Repeat)**

A. Bromocriptine	**B.** Metoclopramide
C. Domperidone	**D.** Prolactin

Ans: A. Bromocriptine

Ref: *Basic & Clinical Pharmacology, Katzung 12th ed.*

Explanation:

- Dopamine agonists suppress prolactin release very effectively in patients with hyperprolactinemia.
- **Bromocriptine and cabergoline** are ergot derivatives with a high affinity for dopamine D_2 receptors. Quinagolide, a drug approved in Europe, is a non ergot agent with similarly high D_2 receptor affinity.
- **ADR***:* Dopamine agonists can cause nausea, headache, light-headedness, orthostatic hypotension and fatigue. Psychiatric manifestations occasionally occur, even at lower doses, and may take months to resolve.
- **Erythromelalgia** occurs rarely. High dosages of ergot-derived preparations can cause cold-induced peripheral digital vasospasm. Pulmonary infiltrates have occurred with chronic high-dosage therapy.
- **Cabergoline** appears to cause nausea less often than bromocriptine.

	Receptor subtypes	Agonist	Antagonist	Mechanism
Glutamate	N-Methyl D-aspartate (NMDA)	NMDA	2-amino-5-phosphonovalerate Dizocilpine	Excitatory
	AMPA	AMPA	CNQX	Excitatory
	Kainate	Kainic acid Domoic acid		
	Metabotriopic	ACPD Quisqualate	MCPG	Inhibitory (Presynaptic)
GABA	GABA -A	Muscimol	Bicuculline Picrotoxin	Inhibitory
	GABA -B	Baclofen	2-hydroxy Saclofen	Inhibitory
Dopamine	D1		Phenothiazines	Inhibitory
	D2	Bromocriptine	Phenothiazine Butyrophenones	Inhibitory
Acetylcholine	Muscarinic M1	Muscarine	Pirenzepine Atropine	Exciatatory
	Muscarinic M2	Muscarine Bethanechol	Atropine Methoctramine	Inhibitory
	Nicotinic	Nicotine	Dihydro beta erythroidine Alpha-bungarotoxin	Exciatatory

9. Rate of elimination of drug is:

A. Clearance **B.** T1/2

C. Biotransformation **D.** Bioavailability

Ans: A. Clearance

Ref: *Basic & Clinical Pharmacology, Katzung 12th ed. P.38*

Explanation:

- **Clearance** of a drug is the factor that predicts the rate of elimination in relation to the drug concentration

Clearance = rate of elimination/plasma concentration

- **Biotransformation**: It is a chemical modification (or modifications) made by human body on a chemical compound.
- Drug biotransformations have 2 classical reactions: Phase I and Phase II.

(See the following figure)

- **Bioavailability**: It is the fraction of administered drug that reaches the systemic circulation. Bioavailability is expressed as the fraction of administered drug that gains access to the systemic circulation in a chemically unchanged form.

10. Ondansetron is not useful for:

A. Chemotherapy-induced nausea and vomiting

B. Postoperative and postradiation emesis

C. Reduce craving in alcoholism

D. Chemotherapy induced hyperuricemia

Ans: D. Chemotherapy induced hyperuricemia

Ref: *Basic & Clinical Pharmacology, Katzung 12th ed. P.397. 1099*

Explanation:

- 5-HT 3-receptor antagonists are the primary agents for the prevention of acute **chemotherapy-induced nausea and emesis.**
- 5-HT 3-receptor antagonists are used to prevent or treat **postoperative nausea and vomiting**. Because of adverse effects and increased restrictions on the use of other antiemetic agents, 5-HT 3-receptor antagonists are increasingly used for this indication.
- Most 5HT3 antagonist cause **QT interval prolongation** (Maximum effect with **Dolosetron)**
  - Drugs that have shown efficacy in maintaining abstinence and reducing craving in chronic alcoholism:
    - **Ondansetron**, a serotonin 5-HT 3-receptor antagonist
    - **Topiramate**, a drug used for partial and generalized tonic-clonic seizures
    - **Baclofen**, a GABA B receptor antagonist

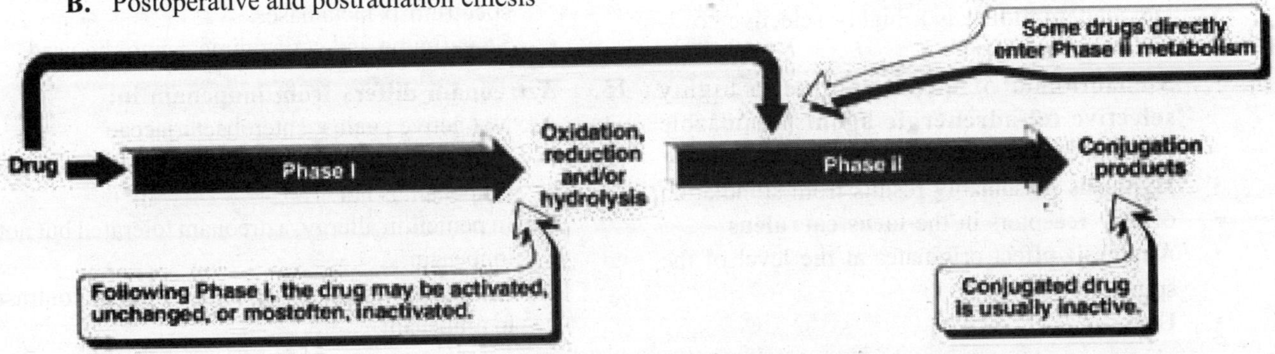

11. Longest acting triptan:

A. Rizatriptan **B.** Zolmitriptan
C. Naratriptan **D.** Frovatriptan

Ans: D. Frovatriptan

Ref: *Basic & Clinical Pharmacology, Katzung 12th ed. P.286*

Explanation:

From the table given below, the longest acting triptan is frovatriptan with half life of 27 hours.

Triptan drugs	**Routes**	**Onset of action (hours)**	**Half life (hours)**
Almotriptan	Oral	2.6	3.3
Eleitriptan	Oral	2	4
Frovatriptan	Oral	3	27
Naratriptan	Oral	2	5.5
Rizatriptan	Oral	1-2.5	2
Sumatriptan	Oral, Nasal, Subcut Rectal	1.5	2
Zolmitriptan	Oral, Nasal	1.5-3	2.8

12. Least sedative anti-histaminic is:

A. Cetrizine **B.** Hydroxyzine
C. Chlorpheniramine **D.** Carbinoxamine

Ans: A. Cetrizine

Ref: *Basic & Clinical Pharmacology, Katzung 12th ed. P.279*

Explanation:

- All except cetrizine are first generation anti-histaminics
- The classical side effect of first generation anti-histaminics is **sedation**.

13. Dexmedetomidine is a new drug used in:

A. General anaesthesia **B.** Treatment of VRSA
C. Hypertension **D.** Multiple sclerosis

Ans: A. General anaesthesia

Ref: *Basic & Clinical Pharmacology, Katzung 12th ed. P.445*

Explanation:

- **Dexmedetomidine** is a highly selective α 2-adrenergic agonist
- S-enantiomer of medetomidine, a highly **selective α2-adrenergic agonist** imidazole derivative that is used in veterinary medicine.
- **Hypnosis** presumably results from stimulation of α2 receptors in the **locus caeruleus**
- **Analgesic** effect originates at the level of the spinal cord
- **Uses**
  - **Dexmedetomidine** is principally used for the **short-term sedation** of intubated and ventilated patients in an ICU setting.
  - In the operating room, dexmedetomidine may be used as an adjunct to general anesthesia or to provide sedation, eg, during awake fiberoptic tracheal intubation or regional anesthesia.
  - It is also tried in postoperative shivering

14. Drug of choice for treating extended spectrum beta lactamase (ESBL) organism is:

A. Aztreonam **B.** Imipenem
C. Cefipime **D.** Ceftazidime

Ans: B. Imipinem

Ref: *Basic & Clinical Pharmacology, Katzung 12th ed. P.800-802*

Explanation:

- **Aztreonam** is a **monobactum** and has structural similarities to **ceftazidime**; hence, its **gram-negative spectrum** is **similar** to that of the third-generation **cephalosporins**.
- It is stable to many β lactamases with the notable exceptions being AmpC β lactamases and **extended-spectrum β lactamases**.
- A **carbapenem** is indicated for infections caused by susceptible organisms that are resistant to other available drugs, eg, P **aeruginosa**, and for treatment of mixed aerobic and anaerobic infections.
- **Carbapenems** are highly active in the treatment of **enterobacter** infections because they are resistant to destruction by the β lactamase
- Carbapenems are also the treatment of choice for infections caused by extended-spectrum β -lactamase (ESBL) producing gram-negative bacteria.
- **Cefepime** a fourth-generation cephalosporin is more resistant to hydrolysis by chromosomal β lactamases (eg, those produced by Enterobacter). However, like the third-generation cephalosporins, it is **hydrolyzed** by extended-spectrum β lactamases.
- So cefipime and ceftazidime cannot be used.

15. Aztreonam differs from imipenam in:

A. Not active against enterobacteriaceae
B. Aztreonam is effective against ESBL whereas imipenam is not
C. In penicillin allergy, aztreonam tolerated but not imipenam
D. Aztreonam does not penetrate CSF in contrast to imipenam

Ans. C. In penicillin allergy aztreonam tolerated but not imipenam

Ref: *Basic & Clinical Pharmacology, Katzung 12th ed. P.800-802*

Explanation:

- **Penicillin-allergic patients** tolerate **aztreonam** without reaction.
- In patients with a history of penicillin anaphylaxis, aztreonam may be used to treat serious infections such as pneumonia, meningitis, and sepsis caused by susceptible gram-negative pathogens.
- Patients allergic to penicillins may be allergic to carbapenems (imipenam) as well.
- Option **A:** Both are active against enterobacteriaceae
- Option **B**: Imipenam is effective against extended spectrum beta lactamase.
- Option **D:** Both drugs penetrate the cerebrospinal fluid.

16. True statement regarding salicylate poisoning is:

A. Resp alkalosis followed by metabolic acidosis
B. Poisoning causes coupling of oxidative phosphorylation
C. Acidifying the urine promotes salicylate excretion
D. Hemodialysis is not possible

Ans. A. Resp alkalosis followed by metabolic acidosis

Ref: *Basic & Clinical Pharmacology, Katzung 12th ed. P.1035-1036*

Explanation:

Salicylate Poisoning

- Acute ingestion of more than **200 mg/kg** is likely to produce intoxication.
- **The first sign of salicylate toxicity** is often **hyperventilation** and **respiratory alkalosis** due to medullary stimulation.
- **Metabolic acidosis follows**, and an **increased anion gap** results from **accumulation of lactate** as well as **excretion of bicarbonate** by the kidney to **compensate for respiratory alkalosis.**
- Poisoning causes **uncoupling of oxidative phosphorylation** and disruption of normal cellular metabolism.
- For moderate intoxications, **intravenous sodium bicarbonate** is given to **alkalinize the urine** and promote **salicylate excretion** by **trapping** the **salicylate** in its ionized, polar form.
- For severe poisoning (eg, patients with severe acidosis, coma and serum **salicylate level > 100 mg/dL**), **emergency hemodialysis** is performed to remove the salicylate more quickly.

PATHOLOGY

1. Anti-mitochondrial antibodies are seen in:

A. Primary biliary cirrhosis
B. Autoimmune hepatitis
C. Sclerosing cholangitis
D. Secondary biliary cirrhosis

Ans: A. Primary biliary cirrhosis

Ref: *Robbins Pathologic Basis of Disease, 8th edition*

Explanation:

- The presence of serum anti-mitochondrial antibodies (AMA) is a highly specific indication of **primary biliary cirrhosis (PBC).**
- Detectable serum AMA with a titer **over 1:40** is significant
- PBC is a progressive inflammatory liver disease characterized by autoimmune-mediated destruction of intrahepatic bile ducts.
- It primarily occurs among women aged **40-60** years.
- Probable diagnosis of PBC is based on meeting 2 of the following 3 criteria:
  – Positive serum anti-mitochondrial antibody (**AMA**) result (titers >1:40)
  – **Cholestatic pattern** of liver enzymes for more than **6 months**
  – **Histopathologic** evidence of **Asymmetric destruction** of **intrahepatic bile ducts**

Serum AMA targets non-organ-specific mitochondrial antigens numerically classified as **M1-M9.**

(See table on the next page)

2. Lymphocyte predominance subtype of Hodgkin's disease is characterized by:

A. CD 15 **B.** CD 30
C. CD 20 **D.** EBV

Ans: C. CD 20

Ref: *Robbins Pathologic Basis of Disease, 8th edition*

Explanation:

Lymphocyte Predominance Type

- This uncommon "**nonclassical**" variant of HL accounts for about **5%** of cases.
- Involved nodes are effaced by a nodular infiltrate of small lymphocytes admixed with variable numbers of macrophages.
- "Classical" Reed-Sternberg cells are usually difficult to find. Instead, this tumor contains so-called **L&H (lymphocytic and histiocytic)**

Distinguishing Features of the Major Intrahepatic Bile Duct Disorders

	Secondary Biliary Cirrhosis	Primary Biliary Cirrhosis	Primary Sclerosing Cholangitis
Etiology	Extrahepatic bile duct obstruction: biliary atresia, gallstones, stricture, carcinoma of pancreatic head	Possibly autoimmune	Unknown, possibly autoimmune; 50% to 70% associated with IBD
Sex predilection	None	Female to male, 6 : 1	Female to male, 1 : 2
Symptoms and signs	Pruritus, jaundice, malaise, dark urine, light stools, hepatosplenomegaly	Same as secondary biliary cirrhosis; insidious onset	Same as secondary biliary cirrhosis; insidious onset
Laboratory findings	Conjugated hyperbilirubinemia, increased serum alkaline phosphatase, bile acids, cholesterol	Same as secondary biliary cirrhosis, serum IgM autoantibodies (especially M2 form of anti-mitochondrial antibody)	Same as secondary biliary cirrhosis, plus elevated serum IgM, >hypergammaglobulinemia
Important pathologic findings before cirrhosis develops	Prominent bile stasis in bile ducts, bile ductular proliferation with surrounding neutrophils, portal tract edema	Dense lymphocytic infiltrate in portal tracts with granulomatous destruction of bile ducts	• Periductal portal tracts fibrosis, • Segmental stenosis of extrahepatic and intrahepatic bile ducts

variants, which have a multilobed nucleus resembling a **popcorn kernel ("popcorn cell")**.

- Eosinophils and plasma cells are usually scant or absent.
- **L&H variants express B-cell markers typical of germinal-center B cells**
- CD 20 and BCL -6 positive and negative for CD 15 and CD 30
- They are usually EBV negative

(See the following table)

3. **Wire loop lesion seen in lupus nephritis is due to:**
   A. Capillary wall thickening
   B. Basement membrane thickening
   C. Subepithelial deposits
   D. Sclerosis of mesangium

Ans: A. Capillary wall thickening

Ref: *Robbins Pathologic Basis of Disease, 8th edition*

Explanation:

*"Prominent **subendothelial deposits** create a **homogeneous thickening of the capillary wall**, which are seen by light microscopy as a "**wire-loop**" lesion. Such wire loops are often found in both focal and diffuse proliferative (**class III or IV) lupus nephritis**, which reflects active disease"* *(Ref: Robbins)*

Lupus Nephritis

- Lupus nephritis results from the deposition of circulating immune complexes, which activate the complement cascade leading to **complement-**

Subtypes of Hodgkin Lymphoma

Subtype	Morphology and Immunophenotype	Typical Clinical Features
Nodular sclerosis	• Frequent lacunar cells and occasional RS cells • Background infiltrate composed of T lymphocytes, eosinophils, macrophages and plasma cells • Fibrous bands dividing cellular areas into nodules • RS cells ***CD15+, CD30+; usually EBV-***	• Most common subtype • Usually stage I or II disease • Frequent mediastinal involvement • No sex predilection • Most patients young adults
Mixed cellularity	• Frequent mononuclear and diagnostic RS cells • Background infiltrate rich in T lymphocytes, eosinophils, macrophages, plasma cells • RS cells ***CD15+, CD30+; 70% EBV+***	• 50% stage III or IV disease • Males • Females • Biphasic incidence, peaking in young adults and again in adults older than 55
Lymphocyte rich	• Frequent mononuclear and diagnostic RS cells • Background infiltrate rich in T lymphocytes • RS cells ***CD15+, CD30+; 40% EBV+***	• Uncommon • Males • Females • Seen in older adults
Lymphocyte depletion	• Reticular variant: Frequent diagnostic RS cells and variants and a paucity of background reactive cells • RS cells ***CD15+, CD30+; most EBV+***	• Uncommon • Presents with advanced disease • Common in older males & in HIV
Lymphocyte predominance	• Frequent L&H (popcorn cell) variants in a background of follicular dendritic cells and reactive B cells • RS cells ***CD20+, CD15-, C30-; EBV-***	• Uncommon • Young males with cervical, axillary lymphadenopathy or mediastinal LN

mediated damage, leukocyte infiltration, activation of **procoagulant factors**, and release of various **cytokines**.

- The presence of antiphospholipid antibodies trigger a **thrombotic microangiopathy**.
- The most common clinical sign of renal disease is **proteinuria**, but **hematuria, hypertension,** varying degrees of **renal failure**, and active **urine sediment** with **red blood cell casts** can also be present.
- **Anti-dsDNA antibodies** that fix complement correlate best with the presence of renal disease.
- **Hypocomplementemia** is common in patients with acute lupus nephritis **(70–90%)**.
- **Class I** nephritis describes **normal glomerular histology** by any technique or normal light microscopy with minimal mesangial deposits on immunofluorescent or electron microscopy.
- **Class II** designates mesangial immune complexes with **mesangial proliferation**. Both class I and II lesions are typically associated with minimal renal manifestation and normal renal function.
- **Class III** describes **focal lesions** with proliferation or scarring, often involving only a segment of the glomerulus.
- **Class IV** - global, diffuse proliferative lesions. **Most common type: Worst Renal prognosis**.
- The **class V** lesion describes **subepithelial immune deposits** producing a **membranous** pattern

Classification for Lupus Nephritis

Class I	Minimal mesangial	Normal histology with mesangial deposits
Class II	Mesangial proliferation	Mesangial hypercellularity with expansion of the mesangial matrix
Class III	Focal nephritis	Focal endocapillary ± extracapillary proliferation with focal subendothelial immune deposits and mild mesangial expansion
Class IV	Diffuse nephritis	Diffuse endocapillary ± extracapillary proliferation with diffuse subendothelial immune deposits and mesangial alterations
Class V	Membranous nephritis	Thickened basement membranes with diffuse subepithelial immune deposits; may occur with class III or IV lesions and is sometimes called mixed membranous and proliferative nephritis
Class VI	Sclerotic nephritis	Global sclerosis of nearly all glomerular capillaries

4. Most common site for peripheral aneurysm is:

A. Popliteal **B.** Profunda femoral
C. Femoral **D.** External iliac

Ans: A. Popliteal

Ref: *Robbins Pathologic Basis of Disease, 8th edition & Harrison online Chapter 249.*

Explanation:

"Popliteal artery aneurysms are the most common peripheral artery aneurysms".

Popliteal Artery Aneurysm

- **Popliteal artery** aneurysms are the **most common** peripheral artery aneurysms.
- Approximately **50%** are **bilateral**.
- Associated with aneurysms of other arteries, especially the **aorta**.
- The most common clinical presentation is **limb ischemia** secondary to **thrombosis** or **embolism**.
- **Rupture** occurs less frequently.
- Other complications include **compression** of the adjacent **popliteal vein or peroneal nerve**.
- Popliteal artery aneurysm can be detected by **palpation** and confirmed by **duplex ultrasonography**.
- **Repair** is **indicated** for **symptomatic** aneurysms or when the diameter exceeds **2–3 cm**, owing to the risk of thrombosis, embolism or rupture

5. Which of the following is a multilineage stimulator?

A. IL 1 **B.** IL 2
C. IL 3 **D.** Stem cell factor

Ans: C. IL 3

Ref: *Robbins Pathologic Basis of Disease, 8th edition*

Explanation: *(See figure on the next page)*

6. To assess prognosis and effect of treatment in a case of AML, which of the following is used?

A. Cytogenetics **B.** Flow cytometry
C. FAB classification **D.** Leukocyte count

Ans: A. Cytogenetics

Ref: *Robbins Pathologic Basis of Disease, 8th edition & Harrisons, 18th edition.*

Explanation:

"Chromosome findings at diagnosis are currently the most important independent prognostic factor." ***(Ref: Harrison)*** *"For patients in complete remission, immunophenotyping to detect minute populations of blasts, reverse transcriptase*

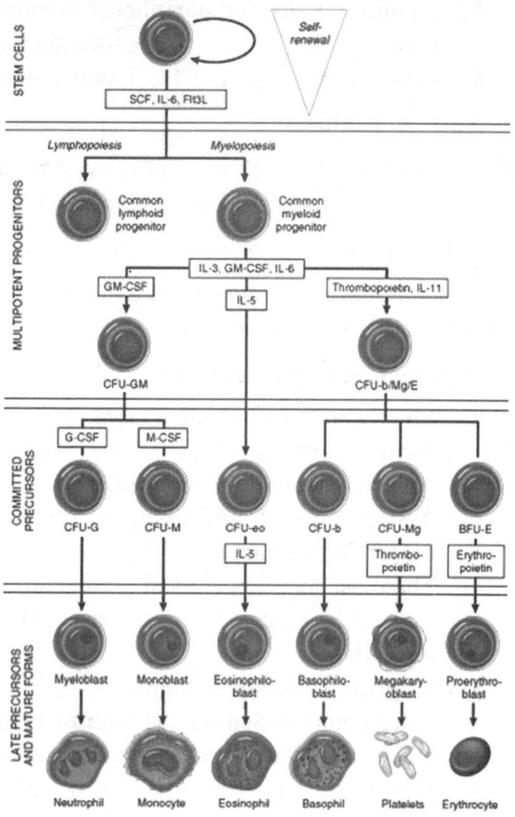

*polymerase chain reaction (RT-PCR) to detect AML-associated molecular abnormalities, and either metaphase **cytogenetics** or **interphase cytogenetics** by fluorescence in situ hybridization (FISH) to detect AML-associated **cytogenetic aberrations** are currently being investigated to assess whether residual disease that has clinical significance is present **following treatment**."* *(Ref: Harrison)*

Prognostic Factors in AML

Good prognostic factors

- t(15;17)
- t(8;21)
- inv(16)
- No cytogenetic abnormality

Poor prognostic factors

- Complex karyotype
- t(6;9)
- inv(3), or
- Deletion 7
- Hyperleukocytosis (>100,000/L)

7. **The term 'sequence' in genetics means:**
   A. Order of nucleotides within DNA
   B. Order of aminoacids in tRNA
   C. ?
   D. ?

   Ans: A. Order of nucleotides within DNA

Ref: Robbins Pathologic Basis of Disease, 8th edition, Pg. 471 & Internet Sources

Explanation:

What is Sequence?

- A nucleic acid sequence is a succession of letters that indicate the order of nucleotides within a **DNA (using GACT) or RNA (GACU)** molecule.
- By convention, sequences are usually presented from the **5' end to the 3' end**.
- Because nucleic acids are **normally linear (unbranched) polymers**, specifying the sequence is equivalent to defining the covalent structure of the entire molecule.
- For this reason, the nucleic acid sequence is also termed the **primary structure**.

8. **Stellate granuloma is seen in:**
   A. Cat's scratch disease
   B. Syphilis
   C. Lymphogranuloma venereum
   D. Actinomycosis

   Ans: A. Cat's scratch disease

Ref: Robbins Pathologic Basis of Disease, 8th edition

Explanation:

- **Cat-scratch disease** Gram-negative bacillus
- Rounded or **stellate granuloma** containing central granular debris and recognizable neutrophils are characteristic lesions in Cat-scratch disease
- Giant cells uncommon

Note: 'Stellate abscess' is seen in **lymphogranuloma venereum**

9. **Mannose 5 Phosphate pathway is required in entry to:**
   A. Lysosome **B.** Mitochondria
   C. Golgi apparatus **D.** Nucleus

   Ans: A. Lysosome

Ref: Robbins Pathologic Basis of Disease, 8th edition

Explanation:

Lysosomal Storage Diseases

- Lysosomes are key components of the **"intracellular digestive tract"**.
- They contain a **battery of hydrolytic enzymes**, which have two special properties.
  - First, they function in the **acidic milieu** of the lysosomes.
  - Second, these enzymes constitute a special category of **secretory proteins** that are

destined **not** for the **extracellular fluids** but for **intracellular organelles**. This latter characteristic requires special processing within the **Golgi apparatus**.

- Similar to all other secretory proteins, **lysosomal enzymes (acid hydrolases)** are synthesized in the endoplasmic reticulum and transported to the **Golgi apparatus**.
- Within the Golgi complex they undergo a variety of **post-translational modifications**, of which one is very important.
- This modification involves the attachment of terminal **mannose 6-phosphate** groups to some of the oligosaccharide side chains.
- The phosphorylated mannose residues serve as an "**address label**" that is recognized by specific receptors found on the inner surface of the **Golgi membrane**.
- Lysosomal enzymes bind these receptors and are thereby segregated from the numerous other secretory proteins within the Golgi.
- Small transport vesicles containing the receptor-bound enzymes are pinched off from the Golgi and proceed to fuse with the **lysosomes**.
- Thus, the enzymes are targeted to their intracellular abode, and the vesicles are shuttled back to the Golgi.
- Genetically determined errors in this sorting mechanism may give rise to one form of **lysosomal storage disease.**

Mucolipidoses (MLS)

- **I-cell disease (ML II)** and **pseudo-Hurler polydystrophy:** Deficiency of phosphorylating enzymes essential for the formation of **mannose-6-phosphate** recognition marker.
- Acid hydrolases lacking the recognition marker cannot be targeted to the lysosomes but are secreted extracellularly as **Mucopolysaccharide** and **glycolipid.** *(See the following figure)*

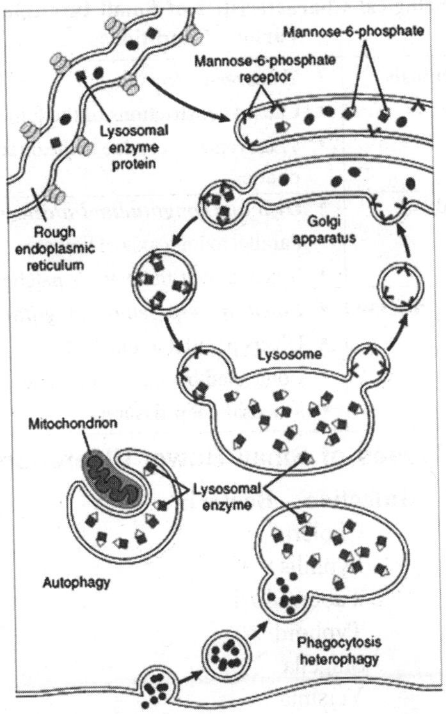

Mannose Receptors

- Mannose receptors and Scavenger receptors are involved in **binding** and **ingesting microbes**.
- The **macrophage mannose receptor** is a **lectin** that binds **terminal mannose** and **fucose** residues of **glycoproteins** and **glycolipids**.
- These sugars are typically part of molecules **found on microbial cell walls**, whereas mammalian glycoproteins and glycolipids contain terminal sialic acid or N-acetylgalactosamine.
- Therefore, the **mannose receptor** recognizes **microbes** and **not host cells.**
- **Macrophage scavenger receptors** bind a variety of **microbes** in addition to **modified LDL** particles.
- Macrophage **integrins**, notably **Mac-1 (CD11b/CD18)**, may also bind **microbes** for **phagocytosis**.
- The efficiency of **phagocytosis** is greatly enhanced when microbes are **opsonized** by specific proteins (**opsonins**) for which the phagocytes express **high-affinity receptors**.
- The major opsonins are **IgG antibodies**, the **C3b** breakdown product of complement, and certain plasma **lectins**, notably **mannan-binding lectin**, all of which are recognized by specific receptors on leukocytes.

10. Small intestinal tuberculous ulcer is characteristically:

A. Transverse ulcer **B.** Longitudinal ulcer
C. Multiple oval ulcers **D.** Serpiginous ulcers

Ans: A. Transverse ulcer

Ref: *Robbins Pathologic Basis of Disease, 8th edition, & Karnam US, Rosen CM, Raskin JB. Small Bowel Ulcers. Curr Treat Options Gastroenterol. 2001 Feb;4(1):15-21.*

Explanation:

*"The gross pathology is characterized by **transverse** ulcers, fibrosis, thickening and stricturing of the bowel wall, enlarged and matted mesenteric lymph nodes, omental thickening, and peritoneal tubercles". (See the table on next page)*

Morphological Characteristics of Small Intestinal Ulcers in Various Conditions

Tuberculosis	• ***Transverse ulcers*** • Causes constrictions of the lumen • Transverse ulcers due to the direction of lymphatics
Typhoid	• ***Oval and longtitudinal ulcers*** • Parallel to long axis of bowel • Situated over the peyer's patches
Crohn's disease	• ***Linear or serpigenous longtitudinal ulcers*** • Ulcers parallel to one another • Connected by short transverse ulcers • Mucosal deep fissures

Causes of Small Bowel Ulceration

- **Infection - Bacteria**
  - Cholera
  - Syphilis
  - Tuberculosis
  - Typhoid
  - Shigella
  - Yersinia
- **Infection - Virus, Parasites & Fungal**
  - CMV
  - Ascariasis
  - Hookworm infestation
  - Strongyloidosis
  - Amoebiasis
  - Aspergillosis
  - Histoplasmosis
- **Neoplasia**
  - Adenoma
  - Leiomyoma
  - Carcinoid
  - Lymphoma
  - Kaposi sarcoma
  - Histiocytosis
  - Mets
- **Congenital**
  - Intestinal atresia
  - Meckel's diverticulum
  - Ectopic gastric mucosa
- **Vascular**
  - Thromboembolism
  - SLE
  - Polyarteritis nodosa
  - Mesenteric insufficiency
  - Behcet's syndrome
- **Iatrogenic/Drug Induced**
  - NSAIDS
  - Digoxin
  - Steroids
  - Radiation
  - Immunosuppression
- **Toxic**
  - Arsenic
  - Acute jejunitis - Beta toxin producing Clostridium perfringens
- **Inflammatory**
  - Celiac disease
  - Crohn's disease
  - Diverticulitis
- **Idiopathic**
  - Idiopathic chronic ulcerative enteritis
- **Misc**
  - Uremia
  - Amyloidosis
  - Zollinger Ellison syndrome

11. One of the following is not a characteristic of apoptosis:

A. Cell shrinkage
B. Chromatin condensation
C. Bleb formation
D. Karyolysis and karyorhexxis

Ans: D. Karyolysis and karyorhexxis

Ref: *Robbins Pathologic Basis of Disease, 8th ed, Pg:3*

Explanation:

Apoptosis

- **Apoptosis** is a pathway of cell death that is induced by a tightly regulated suicide program in which cells destined to die activate enzymes that degrade the cells' own nuclear DNA and nuclear and cytoplasmic proteins.
- Apoptotic cells break up into fragments, called **apoptotic bodies**, which contain portions of the cytoplasm and nucleus.
- The plasma membrane of the apoptotic cell and bodies remains intact, but its structure is altered in such a way that these become "tasty" targets for phagocytes.
- The dead cell and its fragments are rapidly devoured, before the contents have leaked out, and therefore cell death by this pathway does not elicit an inflammatory reaction in the host.
- Apoptosis is different from necrosis.

Characteristics of Necrosis

- Loss of membrane integrity
- Enzymatic digestion of cells
- Leakage of cellular contents
- Inflammatory reaction

Morphology of Apoptosis

- The following morphologic features, some best seen with the electron microscope, characterize cells undergoing apoptosis.

- **Cell shrinkage**. The cell is smaller in size; the cytoplasm is dense; and the organelles, though relatively normal, are more tightly packed.
- **Chromatin condensation**: This is the most characteristic feature of apoptosis. The chromatin aggregates peripherally, under the nuclear membrane, into dense masses of various shapes and sizes. The nucleus itself may break up, producing two or more fragments.
- **Formation of cytoplasmic blebs and apoptotic bodies**: The apoptotic cell first shows extensive surface blebbing, then undergoes fragmentation into membrane-bound apoptotic bodies composed of cytoplasm and tightly packed organelles, with or without nuclear fragments.
- **Phagocytosis of apoptotic cells or cell bodies, usually by macrophages**: The apoptotic bodies are rapidly ingested by phagocytes and degraded by the phagocyte's lysosomal enzymes.
- **Plasma membranes** are thought to **remain intact** during apoptosis, until the last stages, when they become permeable to normally retained solutes.
- On histologic examination, in tissues stained with hematoxylin and eosin, the apoptotic cell appears as a round or oval mass of intensely eosinophilic cytoplasm with fragments of dense nuclear chromatin.
- Because the cell shrinkage and formation of apoptotic bodies are rapid and the pieces are quickly phagocytosed, considerable apoptosis may occur in tissues before it becomes apparent in histologic sections.
- **Apoptosis—in contrast to necrosis—does not elicit inflammation**, making it more difficult to detect histologically. *(See the following table)*

Features of Necrosis and Apoptosis

Feature	Necrosis	Apoptosis
Cell size	Enlarged (swelling)	Reduced (shrinkage)
Nucleus	Pyknosis → karyorrhexis → karyolysis	Fragmentation into nucleosome-size fragments
Plasma membrane	Disrupted	Intact; altered structure, especially orientation of lipids
Cellular contents	Enzymatic digestion; may leak out of cell	Intact; may be released in apoptotic bodies
Adjacent inflammation	Frequent	No
Physiologic or pathologic role	Invariably pathologic (culmination of irreversible cell injury)	Often physiologic, means of eliminating unwanted cells; may be pathologic after some forms of cell injury, especially DNA damage

MICROBIOLOGY

1. **Warthin Finkeldy cells are found in:**
   A. Measles
   B. Mumps
   C. Molluscum contagiosum
   D. Herpes simplex infection

Ans: A. Measles

Ref: Ananthanarayan, Paniker CJ. Textbook of Microbiology 8th Edition & John Wiley & Sons, 2009

Explanation:

- **Guarneri bodies** - Vaccinia
- **Bollinger bodies** - Fowlpox
- **Molluscum bodies** - Molluscum contagiosum
- **Tzanck cells** - Multinucleated giant cells found in Herpes simplex infection
- **Warthin Finkeldy cells** - Type of multinucleate giant cell found in hyperplastic lymph nodes early in the course of measles
- **Clue cells** are epithelial cells of the vagina with distinctive stippled appearance due to presence of intracellular bacteria

2. **SARS is due to:**
   A. Hantavirus
   B. Orthomyxovirus
   C. Coronavirus
   D. Respiratory syncytial virus

Ans. C. Coronavirus

Ref: Jawetz, Melnick & Adelberg's Textbook of Medical Microbiology, 25th Edition. 2010

Explanation:

Severe Acute Respiratory Syndrome (SARS)

- It is a novel coronavirus which belongs to serogroup 2 and is closely related to human coronavirus OC43.
- The receptor for the SARS virus is **Angiotensin-converting enzyme 2.**
- SARS virus originated in a **non-human host** and acquired the ability to infect humans.
- Chinese **horseshoe bats** are natural reservoirs of SARS-like coronaviruses.
- The outbreak of SARS erupted in southern China in late 2002 and by the time it waned in mid-

2003, had resulted in over 8000 cases in 29 countries, with over 800 deaths (case fatality rate of 9.6%). It spread by close contact with affected individuals.

Clinical Features

- The SARS coronavirus causes severe respiratory disease.
- The incubation period averages about **6 days**.
- Common early symptoms include fever, malaise, chills, headache, dizziness, cough and sore throat, followed a few days later by shortness of breath.
- Many patients have abnormal chest radiographs.
- Some cases progress rapidly to **acute respiratory distress**, requiring ventilator support.
- Death from progressive respiratory failure occurs in nearly **10%** of cases, with the highest death rate among the elderly.

Diagnosis

- Most patients (> 95%) with SARS develop an antibody response to viral antigens detectable by a **fluorescent antibody test or ELISA**.
- SARS virus **RNA** was detectable in plasma by **PCR**, with viremia most readily detectable between **days 4 and 8 of infection.**

3. **Prozone phenomenon is due to: (Repeat)**
   A. Antigen excess
   B. Antibody excess
   C. Excessive immune complex
   D. Acute phase reactants

Ans. B. Antibody excess

Ref: *Ananthanarayan, Paniker CJ. Textbook of Microbiology. 8th Edition. John Wiley & Sons; 2009. Pg. 104*

Explanation:

- Antigen and antibody can combine in various proportions.
  - **State of antibody excess – Prozone**
  - **Optimal ratio – Zone of equivalence**
  - **State of antigen excess – Postzone**

(See the following figure)

- The prozone is very important in **serodiagnosis**
- Sera rich in antibody may sometimes give a false negative precipitation or agglutination result
- E.g. Patients with **Brucellosis** are known to exhibit prozone phenomenon
- The serum should be diluted several times when prozone phenomenon is suspected

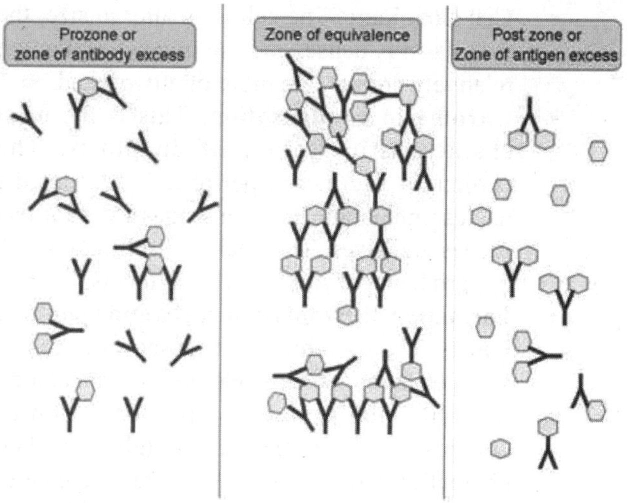

4. **Which of the following is not a coccidian parasite?**
   A. Isospora **B.** Toxoplasma
   C. Blastomyces **D.** Cyclospora

Ans. C. Blastomyces

Ref: *Parija SC. Textbook of Medical Parasitology. 3rd Edition. John Wiley & Sons; 2004*

Explanation:

Coccidian Parasites

- Coccidian parasites are classified as:
  - ***Intestinal coccidian parasites***
    - Cryptosporidium parvum
    - Cyclospora cayetanensis
    - Isospora belli
  - ***Tissue (Non-intestinal) coccidian parasites***
    - Toxoplasma gondii
    - Sarcocystis hominis
- The intestinal coccidian parasites are the causative agents of chronic diarrhea in AIDS patients.
- Of the intestinal coccidian parasites, Cryptosporidium parvum is most refractory to treatment.
- Toxoplasma gondii is a coccidian parasite which is known to be transmitted transplacentally resulting in congenital toxoplasmosis.
- **Blastomyces dermatitidis**
  - It is true fungal pathogen associated with deep mycosis.
  - It is a dimorphic fungus.
  - It causes acute or chronic pyogranulomatous infection of respiratory system disseminating to skin, bones and GU systems.

5. **Which of the following is catalase positive? (Repeat)**
   A. Staph epidermidis **B.** Enterococcus
   C. Streptococcus **D.** Pneumococcus

Ans. A. Staph epidermidis

Ref: *Ananthanarayan, Paniker CJ. Textbook of microbiology. 8th Edition. London: John Wiley & Sons; 2009. Pg. 52, 159*

Explanation:

- **Catalase test:**
  - When a bacterial colony is placed in hydrogen peroxide, if it produces catalase enzyme there will be prompt effervescence.
- **Catalase positive organisms:**
  - Staphylococcus aureus
  - Coagulase negative staphylococci such as S. epidermidis
  - Micrococci
  - Pseudomonas
  - Candida
  - Coliforms
    - Citrobacter, Enterobacter, E.coli, Klebsiella (which are all lactose +)
    - Shigella, Yersinia, Proteus and Salmonella (which are all lactose -)
    - Serratia (a slow lactose fermenter)
- Although **Shigella dysenteriae type 1** is a coliform, it is **catalase negative.**
- **Streptococcus, pneumococcus and enterococcus** are **catalase negative.**
- In patients with **chronic granulomatous disease**, a familial condition with disorder of phagocytosis, recurrent infections due to **catalase positive organisms** are more common as the leucocytes are unable to kill catalase positive bacteria following phagocytosis.

6. **Toxoplasma infection in first trimester causes:**

A. Chorioretinitis	**B.** Cardiac defects
C. Neural tube defects	**D.** Hearing defects

Ans. A. Chorioretinitis

Ref: *Parija SC, Textbook of Medical Parasitology. 3rd Edition. London: John Wiley & Sons; 2004. Pg. 175*

Explanation:

Toxoplasma Gondii

- It is an **obligate intracellular parasite,** residing in **reticulendothelial** cells and nucleated cells of the host.
- Three major morphologic forms are present (All forms are infectious)
  - **Tachyzoites** – Humans and cats
  - **Tissue cyst** – Humans and cats
  - **Oocyst** – Cats only
- **Congenital toxoplasmosis**
  - It occurs when a non-immune pregnant woman becomes infected during pregnancy
  - It is due to transplacental transmission of the **tachyzoites**
  - If the infection occurs during first trimester, it can result in
    - **Abortion or Stillbirth (Most common)**
    - **Congenital toxoplasmosis (17%)**
  - If infection occurs during last trimester, the symptoms are mild and the babies may be asymptomatic at birth.
  - About **65%** of the babies suffer from congenital toxoplasmosis due to infection during last trimester.
  - The classical clinical triads of congenital toxoplasmosis are:
    - **Chorioretinitis**
    - **Cerebral calcifications**
    - **Convulsions.**
  - Microcephaly, hydrocephalus, organomegaly and mental retardation are the less frequent manifestations.

7. **Hyper infective syndrome is seen in:**

A. Enterobius	**B.** Strongyloidosis
C. Ascariasis	**D.** Trichuriasis

Ans. B. Strongyloidosis

Ref: *Parija SC. Textbook of Medical Parasitology. 3rd Edition. London: John Wiley & Sons; 2004. Pg. 297*

Explanation:

Hyperinfection Syndrome

- It is caused by **Strongyloides stercoralis** in patients with **reduced immunity.**
- It occurs due to:
  - Immunosuppressive therapy: Corticosteroids, chemotherapeutic agents, radiation, etc
  - Organ transplantation
  - Underlying illnesses such as hematological malignancy (Leukemia), autoimmune diseases (SLE), AIDS, end stage renal disease and malnutrition
- It is characterized by **massive larval invasion** of the **lung** and **CNS.**
- **Severe diarrhea** and **paralytic ileus** are also common due to large number of larva in the intestine.
- **Eosinophilia** is characteristically **absent**
- **Thiobendazole** is used for treatment . However the response is very poor.

- **Mortality rate** is **very high** despite treatment.
- All patients with strongyloidosis should be treated before administration of immunosuppressive therapy, to prevent this complication.

8. **Which parasite is not found in muscle?**
   A. Trichuris **B.** Toxoplasma
   C. Trichinella **D.** Sarcocystis

Ans. A. Trichuris

Ref: *Parija SC. Textbook of Medical Parasitology. 3rd Edition. London: John Wiley & Sons; 2004*

Explanation:

Trichuris Trichiura

- It is commonly known as **whipworm**
- Larvae hatches in the **small intestine** and develops in **villi** of **small intestine**
- **No tissue migratory phase**, unlike other nematodes such as Ascaris and Hookworm

Toxoplasma

- **Tissue cyst** is the resting form found in various organs of the body including **muscles**
- Seen in chronic stage of infection.
- They contain hundreds of slow growing forms called **bradyzoites.**
- Size - 40 – 50 mm

Trichinella Spiralis

- Trichinellosis is a disease of swine.
- Man is an accidental host.
- Both adult and larval stages are found in the same host.
- The larva deposited in the intestinal mucosa is carried by the circulation and encysted in **striated muscle.**

Muscular Sarcocystosis

- Acquired by ingestion of food contaminated by sporocysts in dog/cat faeces
- Sporocysts exist in the intestine and release sporozoites, which enter the lumen of arteries
- In the vascular endothelium the sporozoites develop into schizonts, which give rise to merozoites
- The **merozoites** invade the **skeletal muscles** and develop into mature sarcocysts

9. **The Entamoeba species that is morphologically identical to E. histolytica is:**
   A. E. coli **B.** E. dispar
   C. E. hartmanni **D.** E. gingivalis

Ans. B. E. dispar

Ref: *Parija SC. Textbook of Medical Parasitology. 3rd Edition. London: John Wiley & Sons; 2004. Pg 26-47*

Explanation:

- Trophozoites and cysts of E. histolytica/ E.dispar/E.moshkovskii are similar in morphology in light microscopy.
- E.dispar/ E.moshkovskii are non-pathogenic Entamoeba spp.

Differences Between Pathogenic and Non-pathogenic Amoeba

Properties	E. histolytica	E. dispar
Agglutinate concanavalin A	+	-
Caecal ulceration in weaning rat	+	-
Phagocytosis of RBC	+	-
Adherence to epithelial cells	+	-
Zymodemes	II, VI, VII, XI, XII, XIII, XIV	I and III

10. **A liquid medium which selective favours the growth of pathogenic bacteria and inhibits the commensal bacteria is known as:**
    A. Enriched medium **B.** Selective medium
    C. Enrichment medium **D.** Differential medium

Ans. C. Enrichment medium

Ref: *Ananthanarayan, Paniker CJ. Textbook of microbiology. 8th Edition. London: John Wiley & Sons; 2009. Pg. 40*

Explanation:

Types of Culture Media with Examples

- **Enriched Media**
  - Basal media which is enriched with blood, serum or egg
  - Eg. Blood agar, Loeffler's serum slope, Lowenstein-Jensen medium
- **Enrichment Media**
  - Liquid medium which selectively favours the growth of certain pathogenic bacteria and inhibits the commensal bacteria
  - Eg. Tetrathionate broth, selenite F broth, Alkaline peptone water
- **Selective Media**
  - Solid medium which selectively favours the growth of certain pathogenic bacteria and inhibits the commensal bacteria
  - Eg. Deoxycholate citrate agar (DCA), Thiosulphate citrate bile salt sucrose agar (TCBS), Wilson-Blair medium
- **Differential Media**
  - A medium that brings out differing characteristics of bacteria and thus helping to distinguish between them
  - Eg. MacConkey's medium

11. Vector for Visceral leishmaniasis in India is

A. Phlebotomus orientalis
B. Phlebotomus major
C. Phlebotomus argentipes
D. Lutzomyia longipalpis

Ans. C. Phlebotomus argentipes

Ref: *Parija SC. Textbook of Medical Parasitology. 3rd Edition. London: John Wiley & Sons; 2004. Pg 90*

Explanation:

Vectors Involved in Various Visceral leishmaniasis

- ***Indian visceral leishmaniasi****s* – Phlebotomus argentipes
- ***Infantile visceral leishmaniasis*** – Phlebotomus major, P. perniciosus, P. longicuspis
- ***Sudanese visceral leishmaniasis*** – Phlebotomus orientalis, P. martini
- ***South American visceral leishmaniasis*** – Lutzomyia longipalpis

Indian Visceral Leishmaniasis

- Caused **Leishmania donovani**
- It is an anthroponotic disease (**Not a zoonotic** disease)
- Affects mainly **young adults**
- Post kala-azar dermal leishmaniasis is common
- **Lymph node** involvement is uncommon

12. Which of the following is not the function of complements?

A. Cell lysis **B.** Antiviral action
C. Promotes phagocytosis **D.** Toxin neutralization

Ans. D. Toxin neutralization

Ref: *Ananthanarayan, Paniker CJ. Textbook of microbiology. 8th Edition. London: John Wiley & Sons; 2009. Pg 120*

Explanation:

Functions of Complement

- It mediates **immunological membrane damage (cytolysis, bacteriolysis)**
- It amplifies the inflammatory response and participates in the pathogenesis of certain hypersensitivity reactions.
- It exhibits **antiviral activity**
- It **promotes phagocytosis** and **immune adherence**.
- It also interacts with the **coagulation**, **fibrinolytic** and **kininogenic** systems of blood.

13. Definitive host for Echinococcus granulosus is:

A. Man **B.** Dog
C. Cattle **D.** Pig

Ans. B. Dog

Ref: *Parija SC. Textbook of Medical Parasitology. 3rd Edition. London: John Wiley & Sons; 2004. Pg 221*

Explanation:

Echinococcus Granulosus

- Causes cystic echinococcosis or **hydatid disease** in man and other herbivorous animals.
- Adult tape worms are found attached to the wall of the intestinal mucosa of dogs and wild canines – **Definitive hosts.**
- Larval stage is found in humans and other herbivorous animals – **Intermediate hosts.**
- Man is an accidental intermediate host.
- Man acquires the infection by ingestion of food contaminated with infected dog faeces or while handling infected dogs.

14. True about mesosomes are all *except:*

A. Site of bacterial respiration
B. They are invagination of plasma membrane
C. They coordinate nuclear division
D. They are more prominent in Gram negative bacteria

Ans. D. They are more prominent in Gram negative bacteria

Ref: *Ananthanarayan, Paniker CJ. Textbook of microbiology. 8th Edition. London: John Wiley & Sons; 2009. Pg 18*

Explanation:

Mesosomes

- Are also known as **chondroids.**
- They are vesicular, convoluted or multilaminated structures formed as **invaginations of the plasma membrane** into the cytoplasm.
- They are more prominent in **Gram-positive** bacteria.
- They are the principal sites of **respiratory enzymes** in bacteria and are analogous to the mitochondria of eukaryotes.
- Mesosomes are often seen in relation to the nuclear body and the site of synthesis of cross-wall septa, suggesting that they coordinate nuclear and cytoplasmic division during binary fission.

15. All are true about plasmid *except:*

A. Cannot replicate
B. Vectors for gene transfer

C. Circular DNA molecules found in bacteria
D. Are also present in yeasts

Ans. A. Cannot replicate

Ref: *Ananthanarayan, Paniker CJ. Textbook of microbiology. 8th Edition. London: John Wiley & Sons; 2009. Pg. 60*

Explanation:

Plasmids

- Plasmids are **circular DNA molecules** present in the cytoplasm of bacteria, capable of autonomous replication (**independent replicons)**
- Plasmid are involved in transmission of drug resistance
- Plasmids have become important **vectors in genetic engineering** because of their ability to transfer genes from one cell to another
- Plasmids may also be seen in **yeasts**, which are eukaryotes.

16. Plasmid DNA–Chromosomal DNA combines to form:

A. Mesosome **B.** Ribosome
C. Transposon **D.** Episome

Ans. D. Episome

Ref: *Ananthanarayan, Paniker CJ. Textbook of microbiology. 8th Edition. London: John Wiley & Sons; 2009. Pg. 60, 67*

Explanation:

- Plasmid DNA may sometimes be integrated with chromosomal DNA are known as **Episome**
- **Transposons**
  - They are structurally and genetically **discrete segments of DNA** that have the ability to move around in a **'cut-and-paste' manner** between **chromosomal and extrachro moso mal DNA** molecules within cells.
  - A transposon is a segment of DNA with one or more genes in the centre, and the two ends carrying **'inverted repeat' sequences** of nucleotides-nucleotide sequences comple mentary to each other but in the reverse order.
  - They are also known as **'jumping genes'**.

17. All mycobacteria produces pigment *except:*

A. M. kansasii **B.** M. simiae
C. M. avium **D.** M. scrofulaceum

Ans. C. M. avium

Ref: *Ananthanarayan, Paniker CJ. Textbook of microbiology. 8th Edition. London: John Wiley & Sons; 2009. Pg 360-1*

Explanation:

Classification of Atypical Mycobacteria (Runyons classification)

Atypical mycobacteria/Non-tuberculous mycobacteria/Mycobacteria Other Than Tubercle bacilli

- **Group I – photochromogens**
  - Produce pigment when exposed to light but not in dark
  - E.g. *M marinum, M simiae, M kansasii*
- **Group II – scotochromogens**
  - Form pigment even in dark
  - E.g. *M scrofulaceum, M gordonae*
- **Group III – non photochromogens**
  - Do not form pigment even on exposure to light
  - E.g. *M avium, M intracellulare, M xenopi, M ulcerans*
- **Group IV – rapid growers**
  - Capable of rapid growth, colonies developing within 7 days
  - E.g. *M fortuitum, M chelonae*

18. Most common cause of traveller's diarrhea is:

A. EHEC **B.** ETEC
C. EPEC **D.** EIEC

Ans. B. ETEC

Ref: *Ananthanarayan, Paniker CJ. Textbook of microbiology. 8th Edition. London: John Wiley & Sons; 2009. Pg 276-7*

Explanation:

There are 5 classes of *E. coli* that cause diarrheal diseases:

- Enterotoxigenic *E. coli* (ETEC)
- Enteroinvasive *E. coli* (EIEC)
- Enterohemorrhagic *E. coli* (EHEC)
- Enteropathogenic *E. coli* (EPEC)
- Enteroaggregative *E. coli* (EAggEC).

ETEC

- Fimbrial adhesins e.g. CFAI, CFAII, K88, K99
- Non invasive
- Produce labile toxine (LT) and/or Stable toxin (ST) toxin
- Watery diarrhea in travelers ***(Traveller's Diarrhea)***
- No inflammation, no fever

EIEC

- Nonfimbrial adhesins, possibly outer membrane protein
- Invasive, penetrate and multiply within epithelial cells
- Does not produce shiga toxin

- Dysentery-like diarrhea (mucous, blood)
- Severe inflammation, fever

EPEC

- Non fimbrial adhesin (intimin)
- Moderately invasive (not as invasive as Shigella or EIEC)
- Does not produce LT or ST; some reports of shiga-like toxin
- Usually **infantile diarrhea**; watery diarrhea similar to ETEC
- Some inflammation, no fever

EAggEC

- Produce ST-like toxin (EAST) and a hemolysin
- **Persistent diarrhea** in young children without inflammation, no fever

EHEC

- Moderately invasive
- Produce shiga toxin
- Pediatric diarrhea
- Copious bloody discharge (hemorrhagic colitis)
- Intense inflammatory response, may be complicated by hemolytic uremia

Shiga Toxin-Producing *Escherichia coli* (STEC)

- A type of enterohemorrhagic *E. coli* (EHEC) bacteria
- Hemolytic uremic syndrome

19. False regarding active immunity is:

A. Induced by infection or immunogens
B. Effective only after lag period
C. No negative phase
D. Booster effect on subsequent dose

Ans. C. No negative phase

Ref: *Ananthanarayan, Paniker CJ. Textbook of microbiology. 8th Edition. London: John Wiley & Sons; 2009. Pg. 87, 139*

Explanation:

Differences Between Active and Passive Immunity

Active immunity	Passive immunity
Actively produced by host's immune system	No active participation of host's immune system
Induced by infection or immunogens	Readymade antibodies are transferred
Long lasting effective protection	Transient, less effective
Immunological memory present	No memory
Effective only after lag period	Immediate immunity
Booster effect on subsequent dose	Subsequent dose less effective
Negative phase may occur	No negative phase
Not applicable in immunodeficient	Applicable in immunodeficient

Negative Phase

- When an antigen is injected into a individual already carrying the specific antibody in circulation, a temporary fall in the level of the circulating antibody occurs due to the combination of the antigen with the antibody. This is negative phase.
- It is followed by an increase in the titre of the antibody exceeding the initial level.
- In active immunity when the antigen is introduced, negative phase may occur, before formation of new antibodies.

FORENSIC MEDICINE

1. All are true about lithium toxicity *except:*

A. Dysarthria is the first sign
B. Increased liver enzymes
C. Activated charcoal is specific treatment
D. Renal failure

Ans: B. Increased liver enzymes

Ref: *A Short Textbook of Psychiatry by Niraj Ahuja, 7th edition. 2011. Jaypee. & Katzung Pharmacology*

Explanation:

Adverse Effects and Complications of Lithium Therapy

A. NEUROLOGIC AND PSYCHIATRIC ADVERSE EFFECTS

- **Tremor** is one of the most common adverse effects of lithium treatment, and it occurs with therapeutic doses.
- **Propranolol** and **atenolol**, which have been reported to be effective in essential tremor, also alleviate **lithium-induced tremor**.
- Other reported neurologic abnormalities include **choreoathetosis, motor hyperactivity**, **ataxia**, **dysarthria** and **aphasia**.
- **Psychiatric disturbances** at toxic concentrations are generally marked by mental confusion and withdrawal.

B. DECREASED THYROID FUNCTION

- Lithium probably decreases thyroid function in most patients exposed to the drug, but the effect is reversible or nonprogressive.

C. NEPHROGENIC DIABETES INSIPIDUS AND OTHER RENAL ADVERSE EFFECTS

- **Polydipsia** and **polyuria** are common but reversible concomitants of lithium treatment, occurring at therapeutic serum concentrations.
- The principal physiologic lesion involved is loss of responsiveness to antidiuretic hormone

(nephrogenic diabetes insipidus). Lithium-induced diabetes insipidus is resistant to vasopressin but responds to amiloride.

D. EDEMA

- **Edema** is a common adverse effect of lithium treatment and may be related to some effect of lithium on sodium retention.

E. CARDIAC ADVERSE EFFECTS

- The **bradycardia-tachycardia** ("sick sinus") syndrome is a definite contraindication to the use of lithium because the ion further depresses the sinus node.
- **T-wave flattening** is often observed on ECG but is of questionable significance.

F. USE DURING PREGNANCY

- Renal clearance of lithium increases during pregnancy and reverts to lower levels immediately after delivery.
- Lithium is transferred to nursing infants through **breast milk,** in which it has a concentration about one-third to one-half that of serum.
- Lithium toxicity in newborns is manifested by lethargy, cyanosis, poor suck and Moro reflexes, and perhaps hepatomegaly.
- An earlier report suggested an increase in the frequency of cardiac anomalies, especially **Ebstein's anomaly**, in lithium babies.

G. MISCELLANEOUS ADVERSE EFFECTS

- **Transient acneiform eruptions.**
- **Folliculitis** is less dramatic and probably occurs more frequently.
- **Leukocytosis** is always present during lithium treatment, probably reflecting a direct effect on leukopoiesis rather than mobilization from the marginal pool.

2. **Which of the following is not characteristic of criminal negligence?**

A. No specific violation of law needs to be proved
B. If found guilty, can be imprisoned
C. Gross negligence leading to death
D. Guilt should be proven beyond doubt in court

Ans: A. No specific violation of law needs to be proved

Ref: *The Essentials of Forensic Medicine and Toxicology by KS Narayan Reddy. 29th edition. 2010. Pg: 34*

Explanation:

Criminal Negligence: When a doctor shows gross absence of skill and care during treatment resulting in death of patient.

Medical Negligence is Considered to be Criminal Negligence if.

A. When a doctor shows gross absence of skill or care during treatment resulting in serious injury to or death of a patient
B. When a doctor performs an illegal act.
C. When an assaulted person dies, the defence may attribute the death to the negligence or undue interference in the treatment of the deceased by the doctor.

Section 304-A IPC Deals with Criminal Negligence

"Whosoever causes the death of any person by doing any rash or negligent act not amounting to culpable homicide shall be punished with imprisonment upto 2 years or with fine or with both."
(See the following table)

3. **Heart blocks are caused by.**

A. Yellow oleander poisoning
B. Organophosphorus poisoning
C. Phenol poisoning
D. Methyl alcohol poisoning

Ans: A. Yellow oleander poisoning

Ref: *The Essentials of Forensic Medicine and Toxicology by KS Narayan Reddy. 29th edition. 2010*

Explanation:

Yellow Oleander (Thevetia Peruviana)

- Seeds contain highly toxic cardiac glycosides including Thevetins A and B and Neriifolin.

Difference between Civil and Criminal Negligence

Trait	Civil Negligence	Criminal Negligence
Offence	No specific or clear violation of law needs to be proved	Must have specifically violated a particular criminal law in question
Negligence	Simple absence of care and skill	Gross negligence, inattention or lack of competency
Conduct of physician	It is compared to a generally accepted simple standard of professional conduct	Not compared to a single test
Consent for act	Good defence; cannot recover damages	Not a defence; can be prosecuted
Trial by	Civil Court	Criminal Court
Evidence	Strong evidence is sufficient	Guilt should be proved beyond doubt
Punishment	Liable to pay damages	Imprisonment

- A wide variety of bradyarrhythmias and tachyarrhythmias occur following ingestion.
- Continuous ECG monitoring for at least 24 h is necessary to detect arrhythmias.
- Longer monitoring is appropriate in patients with severe poisoning.

Supportive Care

- Correction of dehydration with normal saline is necessary, and antiemetics are used to control severe vomiting.

Electrolytes

- **Hypokalemia** worsens toxicity due to digitalis glycosides, and **hyperkalemia** is life-threatening. Both must be corrected.
- Hyperkalemia is due to extracellular shift of potassium rather than an increase in total body potassium and is best treated with **insulin-dextrose infusion.**
- Intravenous calcium increases the **risk of cardiac arrhythmias** and is not recommended in treating **hyperkalemia**.

Gastric Decontamination

- The place of emesis induction and gastric lavage has not been investigated, although they are used in practice.
- Single-dose activated charcoal is probably beneficial
- Activated charcoal is clearly safe.

Arrhythmia Management

- Bradyarrhythmias are commonly managed with atropine, isoprenaline, and temporary cardiac pacing in severe cases.
- Tachyarrhythmias have a poor prognosis and are more difficult to treat.
- Lidocaine is the preferred antiarrhythmic.
- The role of intravenous magnesium is uncertain.
- Digoxin-specific antibody fragments are effective in reverting life-threatening cardiac arrhythmias.
- **Digoxin-specific antibody fragments** remain the **only proven therapy** for yellow oleander poisoning.

Other Therapies

- Activated charcoal
- Atropine
- Isoprenaline
- Antiarrhythmics
- Intravenous magnesium

4. **Methanol poisoning is treated by all *except:***

A. Ethanol **B.** Fomepizole
C. Hemodialysis **D.** Forced alkaline diuresis

Ans: D. Forced alkaline diuresis

Ref: *The Essentials of Forensic Medicine and Toxicology by KS Narayan Reddy. 29th edition. 2010*

Explanation:

Methyl Alchohol (Methanol) Poisoning

- Methanol has a high toxicity in humans.
- The median lethal dose is **100 mL.**
- Methanol is toxic by two mechanisms:
  - Methanol (whether it enters the body by ingestion, inhalation, or absorption through the skin) can be fatal due to its **CNS depressant properties** in the same manner as ethanol poisoning.
  - It is metabolized to **formic acid** (which is present as the formate ion) via formaldehyde in a process initiated by the enzyme alcohol dehydrogenase in the liver.
- Methanol is converted to formaldehyde via alcohol dehydrogenase (ADH) and formaldehyde is converted to formic acid (formate) via aldehyde dehydrogenase (ALDH).
- Formate is toxic because it inhibits mitochondrial cytochrome C oxidase, causing the symptoms of **hypoxia** at the cellular level and **metabolic acidosis**.

Clinical Features

- The initial symptoms of methanol intoxication include central **nervous system depression, headache, dizziness, nausea, lack of coordination and confusion**.
- Sufficiently large doses can cause **unconsciousness** and **death**.
- **Death** due to **respiratory failure.**
- Physical examination may show **tachypnea.**
- Ophthalmologic examination may show **dilated pupils** with **hyperemia** of the **optic disc** and **retinal edema**.

Treatment

- Methanol poisoning can be treated with the antidotes **ethanol or fomepizole.**
- Both drugs act to reduce the action of alcohol dehydrogenase on methanol by means of competitive inhibition, so it is excreted by the kidneys rather than being transformed into toxic metabolites.
- Further treatment may include giving sodium bicarbonate for metabolic acidosis, and

hemodialysis or **hemodiafiltration** can be used to remove methanol and formate from the blood.
- **Folinic acid or folic acid** is also administered to enhance the metabolism of formate.

PSM

1. A case of chicken pox should be isolated for a period of:

A. 6 days B. 10 days
C. 12 days D. 14 days

Ans: A. 6 days

Ref: *Park 22nd edition pg 112*

Explanation:

Disease	**Isolation**
Measles	From onset of catarrhal stage through 3rd day of rash
Chicken pox	Until all lesions crusted about 6 days of rash
H zoster	6 days after onset of rash
Influenza	3 days after onset
Polio	2 weeks for adult, 6 weeks pediatrics
Hepatitis	3 weeks
Pertussis	4 weeks or until paroxysms ceases
Mumps	Until swelling subsides
TB	Until 3 weeks of effective chemotherapy

- Chicken pox and herpes zoster have same period of isolation i.e. till 6 days of rash.
- Pertussis and mumps till the major symptom subsides i.e. paroxysmal cough in pertussis and swelling in mumps.

2. In RNTCP the most effective tool for case finding is:

A. Sputum examination B. Radiology
C. Culture D. Mantoux test

Ans: A. Sputum examination

Ref: *Park 22nd edition*

Explanation:

- The case finding tool in RNTCP is **Sputum examination**.
- In the previous program NTP there was **over reliance on X-ray** as the case finding tool.
- **X-ray** had low specificity and had lot of **difference in opinion** in reporting of the X-ray **(poor inter rater reliability)**, hence the case finding tool in RNTCP is sputum examination.
- In RNTCP, X-ray is used only to diagnose a small proportion of cases such as – sputum negative cases and extra pulmonary tuberculosis such as pleural and pericardial effusion.

3. Most common cause of blindness in India is:

A. Cataract B. Refractive error
C. Glaucoma D. Diabetes

Ans: A. Cataract

Ref: *Park pg 372*

Explanation:

- The national survey on blindness 2006-07.
- Cause for blindiness in India
  - **Cataract** 62.6%
  - **Refractive error** 19.7%
  - **Glaucoma** 5.8%
- Hence the most common cause for blindness in India is cataract.

4. Indalone belong to following type of insecticide:

A. Stomach poison B. Contact poison
C. Repellant D. Block respiration

Ans: C. Repellant

Ref: *Park 22nd edition pg 728*

Explanation:

- Indalone is a repellant. The repellants act by inhibiting the attraction of the insect to the pheromones released by warm blooded organisms.
- **Example of repellants are:**
  - Meta diethyltoluamide
  - Benzyl benzoate
  - Indalone
  - Dimethyl phthalate
  - Ethyl hexanediol

5. 'Confounding bias' in a case control study can be removed by:

A. Double blinding
B. By properly recalling events
C. Matching
D. By selecting representative population

Ans: C. Matching

Ref: *Park 22nd edition*

Explanation:

- Confounder is a variable which is an **independent risk factor** for disease and is **non-causally** associated with the **exposure**.
- That is the variable should be related to the disease and to the risk factor under study like shown in the following figure:

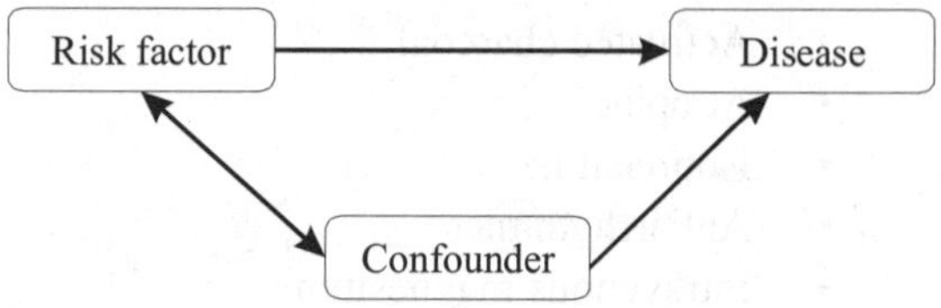

- To remove the effect of confounding at the design-stage, matching is done, i.e., cases and controls are similar with respect to confounding variable.

6. **A village has a total of 100 under five children. The coverage with measles vaccine in this age group is 60%. Following the occurrence of measles case in a child after a visit outside, 12 children developed measles. The secondary attack rate of measles is:**
   A. 12% **B.** 33%
   C. 30% **D.** 15%

   Ans: B. 33%

   Ref: *Park 22nd edition*

   Explanation:
   - Population of under five child = 100
   - Total population susceptible = 39 (total children – unimmunized – index case) = 100-40-1
   - **Secondary attack rate = number of exposed person developing the disease within the range of the incubation period**
   - Numerator = 12
   - Denominator = 39
   - = 12/39 × 100 = 33.3%
   - = 66.7% (67%)

7. **Who is ASHA?**
   A. Worker of a Non-Governmental Organization
   B. Community level voluntary worker for health
   C. Government health worker
   D. Helper of anganwadi

   Ans: B. Community level voluntary worker for heath

   Ref: *Park 22nd edition*

   Explanation:
   - **ASHA (Accredited social health activist)** are involved in health care of community under the National Rural Health Mission.
     - Accredited social health activists (ASHAs) are community health workers instituted by the Government of India's Ministry of Health and Family Welfare (MoHFW) as part of the National Rural Health Mission (NRHM
     - The mission began in 2005; full implementation was targeted for 2012. Once fully implemented, there is to be "an ASHA in every village" in India, a target that translates into 250,000 ASHAs in 10 states.

   Roles and Responsibilities

   ASHAs are local women trained to act as health educators and promoters in their communities. Their tasks include:
   - Motivating women to give birth in hospitals.
   - Bringing children to immunization clinics.
   - Encouraging family planning (e.g., surgical sterilization).
   - Treating basic illness.
   - Injury with first aid.
   - Keeping demographic records.
   - Improving village sanitation.
   - ASHAs are also meant to serve as a key communication mechanism between the healthcare system and rural populations.

   Selection
   - ASHAs must primarily be **female residents of the village** that they have been selected to serve, who are likely to remain in that village for the foreseeable future.
   - **Married, widowed or divorced women are preferred** over women who have yet to marry since Indian cultural norms dictate that upon marriage a woman leaves her village and migrates to that of her husband.
   - ASHAs must have **class eight education or higher**, preferably be between the ages of **25 and 45**, and are selected by and accountable to the gram panchayat (local government).
   - If there is no suitable literate candidate, a semi-literate woman with a formal education lower than eighth standard, may be selected.

   Remuneration
   - Although ASHAs are considered volunteers, they receive outcome-based remuneration and financial compensation for training days.
   - For example, if an ASHA facilitates an **institutional delivery** she receives **Rs. 600** and the mother receives **Rs. 1400**.
   - ASHAs also receive **Rs. 150** for each child **completing an immunization session** and **Rs. 150** for each individual who undergoes family planning.

8. **The limiting amino acid in Bengal gram is:**
   A. Methionine **B.** Lysine
   C. Leucine **D.** Tryptophan

   Ans: A. Methionine

   Ref: *Park 22nd edition pg 564*

   Explanation:
   - **Cereals** lack **lysine** and **pulses** lack **methionine**.
   - These are called the **limiting amino acid**. A food containing both pulses and cereals would be

complete food, as the deficiency of lysine in cereals is supplemented by the lysine in pulses.

- Also **methionine** is compensated by the **cereals.**
- This is called the supplementary action of protein.

9. What is not true about Chi square test?

A. Non-parametric test
B. Continuous variables
C. Proportion
D. Compares more than 2 groups

Ans: B. Continuous variables

Ref: *Park 22nd ed*

Explanation:

Categorical Variable:

- E.g. Gender, blood group, presence or absence of diabetes mellitus.
- The data is summarised as proportions.
- Chi-square is used to test the statistical significance between two proportions. It is a non-parametric test. It can compare more than two proportions also.

Continuous Variable:

- E.g age, blood pressure, haemoglobin.
- If the values follow a normal distribution then they are summarised as mean and standard deviation. Parametric tests such as t test, ANOVA are used to identify statistical significance in them.
- If the distribution of the values is skewed (with extreme low or high value) then they are summarised as median and interquartile range.
- Non-parametric tests such as Wilcoxon, Mann-Whitney test are used to identify statistical significance in them.

10. All of the following are tests for milk pasteurization *except:*

A. Methylene blue **B.** Phosphatase test
C. Standard plate count **D.** Coliform count

Ans: A. Methylene blue

Ref: *Park 22nd edition page 608*

Explanation:

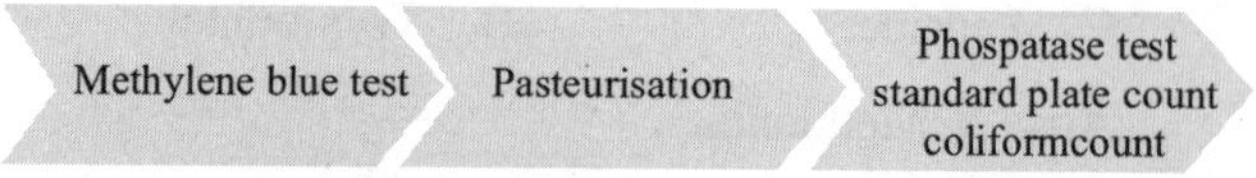

- **Methylene blue** is used to check microorganism in milk.
- This test is done when the milk is accepted for pasteurization.
- The time take for the blue colour imparted by methylene blue to milk to disappear.
- The milk which remains blue to longest is considered to be of best quality.

To **test pasteurized milk** we use three tests:

1. **Phosphatase test** based on the principle that the temperature required for pasteurization destroys the phosphatase in raw milk. Hence if pasteurization is complete no phosphatase will be detected in milk.
2. Standard plate count.
3. Coliform count.

11. All of the following are milk borne diseases *except:*

A. Brucellosis
B. Pasturella
C. Streptococcal infections
D. Viral hepatitis

Ans: B. Pasturella

Ref: *Park 22nd edition pg 607*

Explanation:

MILK BORNE DISESASE

Infections of animal – transmitted to man:

- Tuberculosis
- Brucellosis
- Streptococcal infections
- Staphylococcal enterotoxin poisoning
- Salmonellosis
- Q fever
- Cow pox
- Foot and mouth disease
- Anthrax
- Leptospirosis
- Tick-borne encephalitis

Infections primary to man – transmitted through milk:

I. Diarrhoeal diseases:

- Typhoid/Para-typhoid fevers
- Shigellosis
- Cholera
- E. Coli

II. Non-Diarrhoeal diseases:

- Streptococcal infections
- Staphylococcal food poisoning
- Diphtheria
- Tuberculosis
- Enteroviruses
- Viral hepatitis.

12. Maternal mortality rate the denominator is:

A. 1000 live births **B.** 100 live births
C. 1000 total births **D.** 100 total births

Ans: A. 1000 live births

Ref: *Park 22nd edition*

Explanation:

The denominator **1000 live births** is the best choice. Strictly speaking

Maternal mortality ratio: Number of maternal deaths during a given time period per 100,000 live births during same time period. In many countries reporting and recording of live birth is more complete than that of total births. Hence live birth is taken as the denominator in most indicators. The denominator of 100,000 is taken so as to avoid decimals when in the maternal mortality decreases to a great extent.

Maternal mortality rate: Number of maternal deaths in a given period per 100,000 women of reproductive age during the same time period.

13. **Regarding mid-day meal programme, true statement is:**

A. 1/3 of calories and 1/2 of protein is supplemented
B. 1/2 of calories and 1/3 of protein is supplemented
C. 1/3 of calories and 1/3 of protein is supplemented
D. 1/2 of calories and 1/2 of protein is supplemented

Ans: A. 1/3 of calories and 1/2 of protein is supplemented

Ref: *Park 22nd edition*

Explanation:

Mid-day meal programme

- Aka School lunch programme
- It is in operation since 1961 throughout the country
- The objectives
- To attract more children to schools
- Retaining them
- Increasing literacy rates

Principles

- The meal should be a **supplement** and **not a substitute** to the home diet.
- The meal should supply atleast **one-third of the total energy** requirement and **half of total protein** needs.
- The cost of the meal should be reasonably low.
- The meal should be prepared easily in schools. No complicated process should be involved.
- **Locally available foods** should be used.
- The **menu** should be **frequently changed** to avoid monotony.
- **Every child** in every Government and Government assisted Primary Schools with a prepared mid-day meal with a minimum content **of 300 calories** and **8-12 grams** of protein **each** day of school for a **minimum of 200 days**.

14. **Amount of residual chlorine to be present after contact time should: (Repeat 2013)**

A. 0.5 mg/dl
B. 1 mg/dl
C. 1.5 mg/dl
D. 2 mg/dl

Ans: A. 0.5 mg/dl

Ref: *Park's Textbook of Preventive and Social Medicine,20th edition, page 625*

Explanation:

- The free chlorine should be available in water for at least **one hour** to kill the bacteria and viruses.
- This one hour period is called **contact period.**
- After chlorination or addition a chlorination agent the water should be used only **after one hour contact** period.
- The minimum recommended concentration of **free residual chlorine is 0.5 mg/L for one hour**.
- The free residual chlorine provides a margin of safety against subsequent microbial contamination such as may occur during storage and distribution.
- **Residual chlorine** is assessed by **ortho toludine test**.
- An ideal disinfect of water should have a residual effect.
- Other methods of purification such as usage of ozone, filteration does not have residual effect.
- Horrocks apparatus is used to assess chlorine demand.
- Chlorination is one of the important method of water purification.
- Chlorine kills pathogenic **bacteria**, but it has **no effect on spores, cysts, ova and certain viruses** (e.g., **polio, viral hepatitis**) except in high doses; it oxidizes iron, manganese and hydrogen sulphide; it destroys some taste and odour-producing constituents; it controls algae and slime organisms; and aids coagulation.

15. **The minimum contact period after chlorination:**

A. ½ hour
B. 1 hour
C. 2 hours
D. 3 hours

Ans: B. 1 hour

Ref: *Park's Textbook of Preventive and Social Medicine,20th edition, page 625*

Explanation:

Refer to the above explanation.

ENT

1. **Bony septal perforation is seen:**
   A. Syphilis **B.** Leprosy
   C. TB **D.** Lupus

   Ans: A. Syphilis

   Ref: *Diseases of the Ear, Nose and Throat by PL Dhingra. 5th edn .2010 page 166*

   Explanation:

   Septal Perforation

   - Most common cause is **trauma** which can be due to **surgery** like **SMR**, **cauterization** for **epistaxis, nose picking** etc
   - Perforation in **cartilaginous part**
     – Lupus
     – Tuberculosis
     – Leprosy
   - **Syphilis** causes destruction of **bony septum**
   - **Wegners disease** causes total destruction
   - Also seen in workers exposed to **chromic plating**, **soda ash** manufacturing and those exposed to **arsenic.**
   - Other causes like:
     – **Nasal myiasis**
     – **Rhinolith**
     – **Septal abscess**
     – **Prolonged use of cocaine**
     – **Prolonged use of steroid sprays**
   - Small perforations cause a **whistling sound** on inspiration and expiration whereas large ones will cause crusting and epistaxis
   - Treatment consists of treating the cause, alkaline nasal douches for removing the crusts, local flaps or sialastic buttons for closure.

2. **Modified Young's operation is done for:**
   A. Atrophic rhinitis **B.** Allergic rhinitis
   C. Acute sinusitis **D.** Chronic sinusitis

   Ans: A. Atrophic rhinitis

   Ref: *Diseases of the Ear, Nose and Throat by PL Dhingra. 5th edn. 2010 page 170*

   Explantation:

   Young's Operation

   - It is done as a treatment of **atrophic rhinitis**
   - It involves **closure of the nasal cavity** affected with atrophic rhinitis by creating **mucocutaneous flaps.**
   - These flaps are sutured together in two layers: first the mucosal layer, then the skin layer.
   - The **nasal cavity** is kept **closed for a period of 9 months.**
   - Re-examination is done after 9 months - if the crusts have disappeared, a revision surgery is performed and the nasal cavity is reopened.
   - The theory behind this procedure is that the closed nasal cavity has time to heal.

3. **Subjective interference is present in:**
   A. Pure tone audiometry
   B. Impedance audiometry
   C. Otoacoustic emission
   D. Brainstem evoked potential

   Ans: A. Pure tone audiometry

   Ref: *Dhingra page 27*

   Explanation:

   A. PTA is subjective test.
   B. Impedance audiometry, OAE and BERA are objective tests.

   Otoacoustic Emission (OAE)

   OAE are low intensity sounds produced by the outer hair cells of a normal cochlea.
   Sedation does not affect OAE.
   Types are:
   A. **Spontaneous OAE** – Healthy individuals with hearing loss < 30 dB.
   B. **Evoked OAE** – Elicited by a sound stimulus and are of the following type:
      i. Transient evoked OAE (TEOAE)- evoked by clicks.
      ii. Distortion product OAE (DPOAE) – two tones are simultaneously presented to the cochlea to produce distortion products.

   Uses

   A. Screening test of hearing in neonates
   B. Differentiate between a cochlear and retro-cochlear lesion

   OAE may be absent in:

   A. 50% of normal population
   B. Lesions of the cochlea
   C. Middle ear disorders
   D. Hearing loss > 30 dB

   BERA – Brainstem Evoked Response Audiometry

   - Also called **BAER or BAEP or ABR** (auditory brainstem response)
   - In this electric potentials are generated in response to several click stimuli or tone bursts and picked up from the vertex by surface electrodes

- Tests the integrity of central auditory pathway
- Non invasive test
- Normally **7 waves** are seen in the first 10 milliseconds
- **I, III and V waves** are **most important**
- Absolute latency, inter wave latency and the amplitude of the waves is measured
- Site for generation of waves are
  i. Wave I – distal CN VIII
  ii. Wave II – proximal CN VIII
  iii. Wave III – cochlear nucleus
  iv. Wave IV – superior olivary complex
  v. Wave V – lateral lemniscus
  vi. Wave VI and VII – inferior colliculus

Uses

- Screening for hearing in infants
- Threshold estimation in infants
- To diagnose retro cochlear pathology and brainstem lesions
- Monitor VIII N in surgery of acoustic neuroma

4. Most common presentation of nasopharyngeal carcinoma is: (JIPMER 2011 Repeat)

A. Epistaxis
B. Cervical lymphadenopathy
C. Nasal obstruction
D. Hearing loss

Ans: B. Cervical lymphadenopathy

Ref: *Diseases of the Ear, Nose and Throat by PL Dhingra. 5th edn .2010 page 265*

Explanation:

Nasopharyngeal Carcinoma

- Most commonly seen in the Chinese population
- Bimodal age distribution
- Risk factors are burning of incense sticks, preserved salted fish and decreased intake of vitamin C
- Types of Nasopharyngeal carcinoma
  Type I - squamous cell carcinoma
  Type II - non keratinizing carcinoma
  Type III - undifferentiated carcinoma
- **Presents most commonly as cervical lymph node (60%)**
- Most common region is posterior cervical
- Also presents as hearing loss, nasal block, epistaxis and cranial nerve palsy **(most common VIN)**
- Other cranial nerves which can be involved are II, III, IV, VI, V, IX, X XI, Horner's syndrome
- Diagnosis is with CT scan and MRI scans
- Treatment is with radiotherapy and chemotherapy (cisplatin +/- 5FU)

5. Otalgia referred pain is carried by all *except:*

A. CN VII **B.** CN VIII
C. CN X **D.** C2, C3

Ans: B. CN VIII

Ref: *Diseases of the Ear, Nose and Throat by PL Dhingra.5th edn .2010 page 143*

Explanation:

It is pain in the ear due to lesions in distant regions.

i. Via VN – auriculo temporal nerve
Dental – caries, apical abscess
Oral cavity – benign/malignant ulcers on tongue
Temporomandibular joint disorders
Sphenopalatine neuralgia

ii. Via IX N – Jacobson's nerve (tympanic branch)
Oropharynx – acute tonsillitis, quinsy, ulcer in soft palate, post tonsillectomy
Base of tongue – malignancy, ulcer
Enlarged styloid process

iii. Via X N – Arnold's nerve
Ulcer/malignancy of vallecula, epiglottis, larynx, oesophagus

iv. Via C2 and C3 spinal nerves – cervical spondylosis , cervical injury

6. Rinne's positive means

A. Conductive hearing loss in ipsilateral ear
B. Conductive hearing loss in opposite ear
C. Normal hearing
D. AC < BC

Ans: C. Normal hearing

Ref: *Diseases of the Ear Nose and Throat by PL Dhingra. 5th edn .2010 page 26*

Explanation:

Rinne's Test

- It is a tuning fork test and is used to assess hearing status in a patient
- In Rinne's test air conduction (AC) is compared with bone conduction (BC)
- **Rinne's positive** is **AC>BC** and is seen in **normal hearing** and **SNHL**
- **Rinne's negative** is **AC < BC** and is seen in **conductive hearing loss**

7. After Caldwell Luc operation, the person experience loss of sensation over cheek, this is due to involvement of which nerve?

A. Mandibular nerve **B.** Vagus nerve
C. Maxillary nerve **D.** Facial nerve

Ans: C. Maxillary nerve

Ref: Diseases of the Ear Nose and Throat by PL Dhingra. 5th edn. 2010 page 421

Explanation:

Caldwell Luc Operation

- In this the **maxillary sinus** is entered through the **canine fossa** by a **sublabial** approach
- **Indications** are:
  1. Blow out fracture of orbit
  2. Removal of foreign body in maxillary sinus
  3. Oro antral fistula
  4. Dental cyst
  5. Recurrent antrochoanal polyp
  6. Vidian neurectomy
  7. Approach to pterygopalatine fossa for ligation of maxillary artery
- **Contraindicated in age < 17 years**
- **Complication**s are:
  1. Post op bleeding
  2. Anaesthesia of the cheek due to stretching of the infra orbital nerve (branch of maxillary nerve)
  3. Anaesthesia of teeth
  4. Sublabial fistula
  5. Injury to nasolacrimal duct

OPHTHALMOLOGY

1. **Left homonymous hemianopia is due to lesion in:**

A. Optic chiasma **B.** Left optic radiation
C. Right optic radiation **D.** Right optic tract

Ans: C. Right optic tract

Ref: Kanski's Clinical Ophthalmology 6th edition and Harrison's Online

Explanation:

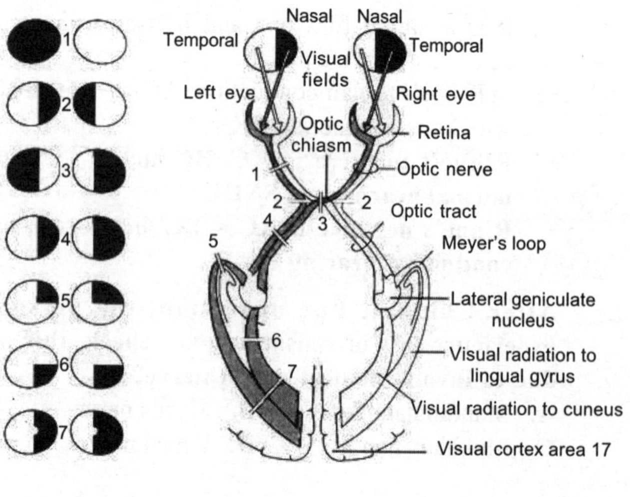

Visual field defect no	Name	Site of lesion
1	Monocular field defects	Optic nerve
2	Binasal hemianopia	Lateral parts of optic chiasma
3	Bitemporal hemianopia	Central part of optic chiasma
4	Homonymous hemoanopia, incongruous, macular involved	Optic tract
5	Superior homonymous quadrantanopia	Temporal lobe
6	Inferior homonymous quadrantanopia	Parietal lobe
7	Homonymous hemianopia, congruous, macular sparing	Occipital cortex

2. **Giant papillary conjunctivitis is caused by**

A. Contact lens **B.** Trichiasis
C. LASIK **D.** LASEK

Ans: A. Contact lens

Ref: Kanski clinical ophthalmology 6th edition; page 218, 234

Explanation:

Conjunctival papillae: Hyperplasic conjunctival epithelium with fibrovascular core and subepithelial infiltration with inflammatory cells.

Three types of papillae:

Micropapillae – mosaic like red dots
Macropapillae - < 1mm in size
Giant papillae - > 1mm in size

Causes of Giant Papillary Conjunctivitis

- Repeated mechanical irritation of the conjunctiva
- Ocular prostheses
- Extruding scleral buckles
- Exposed ocular sutures
- Filtering bleb
- Elevated corneal scars
  - Giant papillary conjunctivitis symptoms and signs, such as **papillary changes in the tarsal conjunctiva**, have been associated with the use of all types of contact lenses (eg, rigid, hydrogel, silicone hydrogel, piggyback, scleral, prosthetic).

Incidence of giant papillary conjunctivitis with various types of contact lenses

- Soft contact lens wearers: **1% to 45%**
- Conventional soft contact lens: **34%**
- Extended wear disposable soft contact lens wearers **-5%**
- Frequent replacement contact lens (every one day to twelve weeks): **21.27%**
- Rigid gas permeable lens wearers: Very low **(1% to 5%).**

3. **Most dangerous complication of trachoma is**
   A. Ptosis B. Pannus
   C. Herbert pits D. Follicles

Ans: B. Pannus, if trichiatic lash is in the option, then that is the answer

Ref: Parson's Diseases of the Eye;21st edition; pg 172-175

Explanation:

TRACHOMA

- Caused by chalmydia trachomatis A, B, Ba, C
- Spread by 3Fs – Fingers, Fomites, Flies
- Forms epithelial inclusion bodies – **Halberstader Prowazek inclusion Bodies**
- **Conjunctiva** – upper tarsal follicle which heals to form minute stellate scars
- **Arlt's Line** – fibrous band in the tarsal plate
- Limbal follicles – **Herbert Follicles – Herbert Pits**
- Cornea – **Pannus** – Lymphocytic infiltration with vascularisation of cornea

WHO Classification of Trachoma

Stages	Features	Treatment
Follicles	≥5 follicles, >0.5 mm in upper tarsus	Needs treatment No scarring
Intense	>50% palpebral blood vessels not seen	Urgent treatment Complications +
Scarring	Tarsal conj scarring with white fibrous bands	Inactive
Trichiasis	Atleast one trichiatic lash	Corrective surgery
Opacities	K opacity covering pupillary region	

4. **Roving movement of eyeball in a 6-year-old child is due to:**
   A. Cerebellar dysfunction
   B. Brainstem dysfunction
   C. Congenital
   D. All the above

Ans: D. All the above

Ref: Parson's Diseases of the Eye 21st edition; pg no. 494; Kanski Clinical Ophthalmology 6th edition pg 830- 833

Explanation:

NYSTAGMUS

- Nystagmus is a repetitive, involuntary, **To & fro** oscillations of the eye.
- Each cycle of movement is initiated by an involuntary defoveating drift which move the eye away from the object of interest, followed by a corrective refixating saccadic movement.

CLASSIFICATION:

Based on Etiology:

Physiological:
- End gaze nystagmus
- Optokinetic nystagmus
- Vestibular nystagmus

Pathological:

Congenital–Infantile, Nystagmus blockage syndrome

Acquired– **A.** Secondary to visual loss,

B. Toxic/metabolic –
- Alcohol
- Lithium
- Barbiturates
- Phenytoin
- Salicylates
- Benzodiazepines
- Wernicke encephalopathy
- Thiamine deficiency

C. Neurological–involving midbrain, cerebellum, brainstem, vestibular apparatus pathology

D. Functional–coal miners nystagmus

Based on Pattern of Manifestation:

- ***Manifest*** – Nystagmus is present when both the eyes are normally open.
- ***Latent*** –No movement is present when both the eyes are open but nystagmus is elicited only when either eye is covered.
- ***Manifest latent*** – Nystagmus is present when both the eyes are open, it increases when either eye is closed.

Based on the Direction of the Nystagmus:

The direction of the fast phase of the nystagmus is the direction of the nystagmus **Horizontal, vertical, rotator**

Based on Pattern of Movement:

- ***Jerky*** – saccadic movement with slow defoveating drift and a fast corrective saccadic movement
- ***Pendular*** – non saccadic in that both the foveating and defoveating movements are slow and equal in velocity

5. **Anterior staphyloma is seen in:**
   A. Sloughing corneal ulcer
   B. Scleritis
   C. Glaucoma
   D. Pathological myopia

Ans: A. Sloughing corneal ulcer

Ref: Parson's Disease of the Eye 21st edition, pg 222–223

Explanation:

Staphyloma

Types	Site	Causes
Anterior	Involving part or the whole of the cornea; lined by iris	Sloughing corneal ulcer
Intercalary	Limbus and 2 mm from the limbus; lined by ciliary body	Perforating injuries Marginal corneal ulcer Anterior scleritis Scleromalacia perforans Post surgical wound site Secondary glaucoma
Equatorial	2-8 mm from the limbus [vortex vein entry]; lined by the choroid	Scleritis, Pathological myopia, Chronic uncontrolled glaucoma
Posterior	Posterior pole; lined by the choroid	Same as equatorial

- Staphyloma is characterized by an **ectasia of the outer coats** [cornea, sclera or both] of the eye with an incarceration of the uveal tissue

Management:

- Treat the cause
- IOP control
- Observation
- Local excision with sclera or corneal patch graft

6. **Treatment of irregular astigmatism**
   A. Spectacles
   B. Contact lens
   C. Intra ocular contact lens
   D. Tattooing

Ans: B. Contact lens

Ref: *Parson's Diseases of the Eye 21st edition pg no: 77, Basak Essentials of Ophthalmology 5th edition pg no.77*

Explanation:

ASTIGMATISM

- The incident parallel rays of light do not come to appoint focus on the retina, due to reacraction varies in different meridian.

Few Definitions:

- **Regular astigmatism** – Principal meridians are perpendicular.
- **With-the-rule astigmatism** – The vertical meridian is steepest (a rugby ball or American football lying on its side).
- **Against-the-rule astigmatism** – The horizontal meridian is steepest (a rugby ball or American football standing on its end).
- **Oblique astigmatism** – The two meridians are perpendicular to each other but not along the principal meridians. The steepest curve lies in between 120 and 150 degrees and 30 and 60 degrees.
- **Irregular astigmatism** – Principal meridians are not perpendicular. The surface is so distorted it **cannot be corrected with spectacles.**
- Children tend to have with-the-rule astigmatism and elderly people tend to have against-the-rule astigmatism.

Causes of irregular astigmatism:

- **Ectasias** – Keratoconus, Pellucid marginal degeneration
- **Post surgical** – Refractive surgeries [radial keratotomy, Lasik, Lasek, PRK], Penetrating keratoplasty
- **Scars** – Salzmann's nodular degeneration, Post trauma
- **Eyelid lesions** – Tumors, Chalazion

MEDICINE

1. **POEMS syndrome is associated with all *except:***
   A. Osteolytic multiple myeloma
   B. Hypertrichosis
   C. Papilledema
   D. Amenorrhea

Ans: A. Osteolytic multiple myeloma

Ref: *Harrison's 18th edn, pg 3080*

Explanation:

POEMS syndrome

- **Polyneuropathy**, ***o*rganomegaly**, ***e*ndocrinopathy**, ***m*ultiple myeloma**, and **skin changes**.
- It is associated with **osteosclerotic myeloma, Waldenstorm's macroglobulinemia, MGUS** but not the classical osteolytic multiple myeloma
- Elevations in **IL-1β, IL-6, TNF-α and VGEF** implicated
- **Polyneuropathy:** Sensory and motor deficits characterised by distal, symmetrical weakness spreading proximally
- Hepatomegaly and lymphadenopathy occur in about two-thirds of patients, and splenomegaly is seen in one-third.

- **Endocrine**:
  - **Amenorrhea** in women
  - **Impotence** and gynecomastia in men
  - Hyperprolactinemia
  - Papilledema
  - Type 2 diabetes mellitus
  - Hypothyroidism
  - Adrenal insufficiency
- **Skin changes:**
  - **Hyperpigmentation**
  - **Hypertrichosis**
  - Skin **thickening**
  - **digital clubbing**
- **Others**
  - Peripheral edema
  - Ascites
  - Pleural effusions
  - Fever
  - Thrombocytosis.
- Not all the components of POEMS syndrome may be present initially.
- Treatment: Like myeloma. **Plasmapheresis does not appear** to be of benefit in POEMS syndrome.

2. **Asthenospermia means:**
   A. Immotile sperms
   B. Absent sperms
   C. Dead sperms
   D. Dysmorphic sperms

Ans: A. Immotile sperms

Ref: *Harrison's 18th edn.*

Explanation:

Azoospermia - Absence of sperm in the ejaculate.
Aspermia - Zero volume ejaculate.
Oligospermia - Low numbers of sperm.
Asthenospermia - Poor sperm motility.
Teratospermia - Abnormal morphology (shape) of sperm.

3. **Bulls eye retinopathy is seen in toxicity of: (Repeat)**
   A. Chloroquine **B.** Mefloquine
   C. Primaquine **D.** Quinine

Ans: A. Chloroquine

Ref: *CMDT, 2013, pg 197*

Explanation:

Adverse Effects of Chloroquine

- **Ocular**- Irreversible retinal damage,
- **CNS**- Seizures, Tinnitus, Nerve deafness
- **GIT**- Anorexia, nausea, vomiting
- **Skin pigmentation**

4. **Martel's sign is seen in**
   A. Rheumatoid arthritis **B.** Gonococcal arthritis
   C. Gout **D.** TB arthritis

Ans: C. Gout

Ref: *Harrison's 18th edn.*

Explanation:

Martel's sign: ***Cystic*** changes, well-defined ***erosions*** with ***sclerotic margins*** (often with overhanging bony edges), and ***soft tissue masses*** are characteristic features of ***advanced chronic tophaceous gout.***

Rheumatoid Arthritis: X-ray Features

- Juxta-articular osteopenia
- Soft tissue swelling
- Symmetrical joint space loss
- Subchondral erosions
- Subluxation and collapse

Gonococcal Arthritis:

- DGI (Disseminated gonococcal infection): Migratory arthritis of wrists, hands, knees, feet and ankle associated with papules over trunk and extensor aspect of the distal extremities.
- Gonococcal septic arthritis: Suppurative, single joint-hip, knee, ankle, wrist.

Tubercular Arthritis:

- 1% of pulmonary and 10% of extrapulmonary cases
- Chronic granulomatous monoarthritis: Hips, knees, ankle
- Poncet's disease – Reactive symmetric polyarthritis
- No mycobacteria in the joints, symtoms resolve with ATT

5. **Drug of choice for low excretors of uric acid in renal failure is:**
   A. Bromobenzene **B.** Allopurinol
   C. Febuxostat **D.** Probenecid

Ans: A. Bromobenzene

Ref: *Harrison's 18th edn, pg 3182*

Explanation:

Treatment of Gout

- **Uricosuric agents** (Increases excretion in under excretors, 24h urine uric acid <600 mg)
- Probenecid and sufinpyrazone is used if renal function is normal
- Bromobenzene can be used in renal failure
- Drugs with **mild uricosuric effects** are: losartan, fenofibrate, amlodipine
- Overproducers and in renal failure – Allopurinol, xanthine oxidase inhibitor

- Needs dose adjustment in CRF, causes toxic epidermal necrolysis
- **Febuxostat**– Specific xanthine oxidase inhibitor, no dose adjustment in CRF
- **Pegloticase**– New urate-lowering biological agent, in patients allergic to/not responding to allopurinol
- Colchicines anti-inflammatory prophylaxis for acute flares of gout, dose is lowered in renal failure
- Acute attack– NSAIDS, colchicines and glucocorticoids, anakinra (IL-1β)
- Low purine diet (Red meat, seafood, offal), good hydration

6. **Immunological mucocutaneous syndrome is similar to infection caused by:**

A. Staph aureus **B.** Pneumococcus
C. Coxsackie **D.** Herpes

Ans: D. Herpes

Ref: *Harrison's 18th edn, pg 390, 1456*

Explanation:

- **Erythema multiforme (EM)** is a condition which produces target like, symmetric skin lesions on knees, elbows, palms and soles which spread centrifugally.
- Caused by **drugs** like **sulfa, penicillin, phenytoin**; infections due to **Herpes simplex virus (HSV)** and **Mycoplasma pneumonia.**
- Associated with fever rash and diffuse mucocutaneous lesions.
- Subdivided into: EM minor due to HSV and EM major due to HSV, Myco pn, drugs.
- EM major has involvement of **mucous membranes.**
- EM can also follow **vaccinations, radiation therapy**, environmental toxins like **oleoresin** in **poison ivy**.

7. **Which lipoprotein levels are indirectly proportional to coronary artery disease?**

A. HDL **B.** LDL
C. Cholesterol **D.** TG

Ans: A. HDL

Ref: *Harrison's 18th edn, pg 1987; Davidson 21st edn, pg 451*

Explanation:

- Increased levels of **atherogenic lipoproteins**, especially **LDL, IDL, lipoprotein (a)** and **chylomicron** contribute to the development of atherosclerosis
- Their increased plasma concentration and reduced diameter favour subendothelial accumulation of these lipoproteins
- After oxidation, they are not cleared normally, trigger an inflammatory response
- They are taken up by macrophages to form foam cells, which have abnormal effect on the endothelium
- **HDL removes cholesterol** from the **tissues** to the **liver**, where it is metabolized and excreted in bile
- HDL also counteracts some components of the inflammatory response, such as expression of vascular adhesion molecules by the endothelium.
- **Low HDL** associated with **high TG predispose** to **atherosclerosis** and **CAD**

7.A **Microcytic anemia is seen in deficiency of:**

A. Vitamin B2 **B.** Vitamin B5
C. Pyridoxine **D.** Folic acid

Ans: C. Pyridoxine

Ref: *Davidson 21st edn, pg 127*

Explanation:

Pyridoxine (Vitamin B6) Deficiency

- It is seen with **INH, Penicillamine**
- Pyridoxine is used in INH induced **peripheral neuropathy, sideroblastic anemia**
- Therapeutic uses
  - **Antiemetic** in **radiation induced nausea**
  - **Nausea in pregnancy**
  - **Carpal tunnel syndrome**
  - **Premenstrual syndrome**
- Chronic high doses can cause **sensory polyneuropathy**

(See table on the next page)

Sideroblastic Anemia

- It results from defective incorporation of iron into heme molecule in the cytoplasm of cells
- **Causes:** Congenital or Acquired
  - Myelodysplastic syndromes
  - Copper
  - B6 deficiencies
  - Zinc overdose
  - Alcohol
  - ATT
- Microcytic hypochromic picture, siderocytes with basophilic iron deposits (**Pappenheimer bodies**)
- Serum **iron** is **high** and **TIBC** is **low, S. Ferritin** is **high**
- **Ringed sideroblasts** are seen in bone marrow with **Prussian blue** staining

Nutrient	Clinical finding	Contributing factors
Thiamine- B1	• Dry and wet beriberi • Wernicke's encephalopathy Korsakoff's psychosis	• Alcoholism • Chronic diuretic use • Hyperemesis
Riboflavin- B2	• Seborrhea • Magenta tongue • Angular stomatitis • Cheilosis	
Niacin- B3	• **Pellagra:** • Diarrhea • Dementia • Dermatitis • Death • Glossitis	• Alcoholism • B2 deficiency • B6 deficiency
Pyridoxine- B6	• Seborrhea • Glossitis • Neuropathy • Depression • Convulsions • Microcytic anemia	• Alcoholism • INH
Folate	• Megaloblastic anemia • Atrophic glossitis • Depression • ↑ homocysteine	• Alcoholism • Sulfasalazine • Pyrimethamine • Triamterene
Vitamin B12	• Megaloblastic (pernicious) anemia subacute combined degeneration of the cord • ↑ homocysteine • ↑ methylmalonic acid	• Gastric atrophy • Terminal ileal disease • Vegans • H2 blockers • Chronic metformin use

8. **Chloride receptor defect is responsible for:**

A. Cystic fibrosis
B. Wilson's disease
C. Alpha-1 antitrypsin deficiency
D. Hemochromatosis

Ans: A. Cystic fibrosis

***Ref:** Harrison's 18th edn, pg 2149*

Explanation:

Cystic Fibrosis

- Autosomal recessive
- Mutation in **CFTR** (cysic fibrosis transmembrane conductance regulator) gene
- Clinical Features
  - **Bronchiectasis**
  - Exocrine pancreatic insufficiency
  - Intestinal dysfunction
  - Abnormal sweat gland function
  - Urogenital dysfunction
- CF airway **epithelia** exhibit **abnormal Cl- secretion and Na+ absorption**
- Predisposes to infections, **Staph. aureus, Pseud.aeruginosa**. Others are **H.influenza, Alcaligenes, Burkholderia, Proteus**, E.coli, **Klebsiella, Aspergillus**
- Lack of CFTR Cl- channel in the apical membrane of pancreas, **failure to secrete $NaHCO_3$ and water, destruction** of the **pancreas**
- In the sweat glands, inability to absorb Cl- from the sweat leads to **high Cl- concentrations** in **sweat** measured after iontophoresis of cholinergic agents
- Spirometry: ↑ RV/TLC, ↓ FVC and ↓ FEV1
- CXR- hyperinflation, brochiectasis, **right upper lobe (Earliest** involved)
- Clubbing, pneumothorax, hemoptysis, corpulmonale
- **GIT:** Meconium ileus, DIOS, protein and fat malabsorption, diabetes later
- **GUT:** Late onset puberty, azoospermia, female infertility
  - **Treatment**
- Gene therapy of CFTR gene
- Clearance of secretions with hypertonic saline, antibiotics
- Recombinant human DNAse to degrade DNA in sputum
- **Pancreatic enzyme replacement**, Vit E and K, Insulin
- **Megalodiatrizoate enema** for acute intestinal obstruction

- **Urodeoxycholic** acid for cholestatic liver disease
- Predisposed to **renal stones** and **osteoporosis**

9. **Erythropoietin is increased in all *except:***

A. CML
B. MDS
C. Essential thrombocytosis
D. Polycythemia vera

Ans: D. Polycythemia vera

Ref: *Harrison's 18th edition, pg 456, 898*

Explanation:

Erythropoeitin is low in polycythemia vera, elevated in secondary causes.

Polycythemia Vera:

- Most common myeloproliferative disorder, clonal disorder of a multipotent hematopoietic progenitor cell in which erythrocytes, granulocytes and platelets accumulate without any recognizable physiological stimulus
- Mutation in the **JAK2 V617F gene** on chromosome **9** (70-95%) is responsible in pathogenesis
- **High hemoglobin/hematocrit**: Male > 17g/dL (Htc > 60%); female > 15g/dL (Htc > 55%)
- **Splenomegaly**, Aquagenic pruritis
- **Hyperviscosity** syndrome
  - Neurological synptoms
  - Hypertension
  - Arterial and venous thrombosis
  - Erythromelalgia due to thrombocytosis
  - Hyperuricemia
- Confirmed with elevated red cell mass, male > 36 mL/kg; female > 32 mL/kg
- **Low erythropoietin** levels
- ↑ WBC, ↑ basophils, thrombocytosis
- Smoker's polycythemia- ↑ carboxyhemoglobin, ↓ oxygen saturation
- **Gaisbock's syndrome**- Spurious erythrocytosis due to reduced plasma volume

Secondary Causes of Polycythemia:

1. **Hypoxia:**
- CO intoxication
- High altitude
- Pulmonary diseases
- R → L shunts
- Sleep apnea
- Hepatopulmonary syndrome

2. **Renal Diseases:**
- Cysts
- Renal artery stenosis

3. **Tumors:**
- Hypernephroma
- Hepatoma
- Cerebellar hemangioblastoma
- Uterine myoma
- Meningioma

4. **Drugs:**
- Androgens
- Recombinant erythropoietin

5. **Familial:**
- Erythropoietin receptor mutation
- VHL mutation (Chuvash syndrome)
- 2,3 BPG mutation

10. **Splenomegaly is a feature of all *except:***

A. Aplastic anemia **B.** CML
C. Thalessemia **D.** Hypersplenism

Ans: A. Aplastic anemia

Ref: *Harrison's 18th edn, pg 467*

Explanation:

Aplastic anemia is pancytopenia with hypocellular bone marrow. It does not produce any organomegaly.

- Causes of massive splenomegaly:
  - CML
  - Myelofibrosis
  - Hairy cell leukemia
  - Chronic malaria
  - Kala azar
  - Extrahepatic portal vein thrombosis
- Other causes:
  - Acute malaria
  - Typhoid
  - Infectious mononucleosis
  - Infective endocarditis
  - Leptospirosis
  - Tuberculosis
  - Viral hepatitis
  - HIV
  - SLE
  - Rheumatoid arthritis
  - HIV
  - Hemolytic anemia

Mechanisms of Splenomegaly:

1. **Hypertrophy/hyperplasia** related to specific splenic function: RES hyperplasia in hereditary spherocytosis, thalassemia; immune hyperplasia as in infectious mononucleosis, SLE
2. **Passive congestion**: As in portal hypertension
3. **Infiltrative diseases**: Lymphomas, Myeloproliferative disorders

11. **All of the following can cause aplastic anaemia *except:***
A. Fanconi's anaemia
B. Wiskott-Aldrich syndrome
C. Dyskeratosis congenital
D. Reticular dysgenesis

Ans: B. Wiskott-Aldrich syndrome

***Ref:** Harrison's 18th ed, pg 887*

Explanation:

Inherited Cytopenias	Acquired Cytopenias
Fanconi's anemia Dyskeratosis congenital Shwachman–Diamond syndrome Reticular dysgenesis Amegakaryocytic thrombocytopenia Familial aplastic anemias Preleukemia (monosomy 7) Nonhematological (Down, Dubowitz, Seckel)	**Aplastic anemia** **Secondary To :** Radiation Drugs and chemicals Viruses: EBV; non A,B,C Hepatitis, Parvovirus B19, HIVImmune diseases–Eosinophilic fasciitis, hyperimmunoglobulinemia, thymoma PNH Pregnancy Idiopathic
Cytopenias: Congenital PRCA (Diamond-Blackfan syndrome) Kostmann's syndrome Schwachman-Diamond syndrome Reticular dysgenesis Amegakaryocytic thrombocytopenia Thrombocytopenia with absent radii	**Cytopenias** PRCA Drugs and toxins Pure white cell aplasia Idiopathic amegakaryocytic thrombocytopenia

Wiskott-Aldrich Syndrome (WAS)

- X-linked recessive, due to WASP gene mutation; immune dysfunction affecting T lymphocyte
- Recurrent bacterial infections, eczema, bleeding
- Predisposes to lymphoma and autoimmune disorders
- Diagnosed by intracellular immunofluroscence analysis of WAS protein (WASP)
- Treatment: Prophylactic antibiotics, IgG supplementation, topical treatment of eczema
- Splenectomy for thrombocytopenia
- Allogenic HSCT is curative

12. **Pancytopenia is seen in all *except:***
A. Wiskott-Aldrich syndrome
B. Fanconi's anaemia
C. Schwartzmann Diamond syndrome
D. Kostmann's syndrome

Ans: A. Wiskott-Aldrich syndrome

***Ref:** Harrison's 18th ed. pg 887*

Explanation:

Refer to the above explanation.

13. **All of the following drugs are indicated in immediate post MI period *except:***
A. CCBs B. Morphine
C. Enalapril D. Aspirin

Ans: A. CCBs

***Ref:** Harrison's 18th edn, pg 2028*

Explanation:

Management of acute MI: Remember **'MONA'**

Morphine:

- Effective analgesic for chest pain, it allays anxiety
- It may reduce cardiac output and BP by reducing sympathetic vasoconstriction
- Can cause diaphoresis, nausea, bradycardia or heart block

Oxygen:

- In case the patient is hypoxic, it helps to limit the infarct size in the first 6-12 hours.

Nitrates:

- Sublingual nitroglycerin abolishes pain
- It decreases myocardial oxygen demand by decreasing the preload and improves the myocardial oxygen supply by dilating the coronaries
- Contraindicated in BP< 90, right ventricular infarction, recent PDE-I intake

Aspirin:

- Effective for all the acute coronary syndromes including STEMI
- Rapid inhibition of COX-1 in platelets and reduction in TXA2 occurs with absorption from buccal mucosa of chewed aspirin tablet
- Causes gastritis, peptic ulcer bleed, peforation, increased risk of bleeding, asthma

– **ACE Inhibitors and ARBs** reduce the mortality rate after STEMI by reducing the ventricular remodeling by reducing the risk of CHF

– **Beta-blockers (BB)**, by IV route are used for control of chest pain in STEMI by diminishing the myocardial oxygen demand and hence ischemia. Oral BB started with in first 24 hours in patients without : signs of heart failure, hypotension <100, risk of cardiogenic shock, HR <60, PR interval > 0.24, 2nd/3rd degree heart block, asthma

– **CCBs** may increase the mortality if used in acute settings

14. **Nocturnal angina and diaphoresis is a predominant symptom in:**

A. Chronic AR B. Chronic MR
C. Acute AR D. Acute MR

Ans: A. Chronic AR

Ref: *Harrison's 18th edn pg 1942*

Explanation:

Chronic AR

- Myocardial ischemia occurs due to elevated myocardial oxygen demand by LV dilatation, hypertrophy, LV systolic tension
- Coronary filling may be compromised as coronary filling occurs during diastole when the arterial pressure and driving force is low'! Decreased supply
- Hence, it causes nocturnal angina associated with severe diaphoresis
- Other symptoms are palpitations, dyspnea, signs of CCF
- Jarring of whole body, **head bobbing, Quinke's** sign, **water hammer** pulse, **Duroziez's** sign, **Traube's** sign, wide pulse pressure
- High pitched EDM at the 3rd left ICS, **Austin Flint murmur** due to diastolic displacement.

Acute AR

- Caused by infective **endocarditis, trauma, aortic dissection**
- LV cannot dilate to maintain stroke volume, rapid rise in LV diastolic pressure → LA and PA wedge pressure
- Rapid pulmonary edema and cardiogenic shock
- Soft S1, not so wide pulse pressure, soft EDM

15. **All of the following causes cirrhosis *except:***

A. Wilson's disease B. Hemochromatosis
C. Paracetamol D. Cystic fibrosis

Ans: D. Cystic fibrosis

Ref: *Harrison's 18th edn, pg 2592*

Explanation:

Causes of Cirrhosis

- Alcoholism
- Chronic viral hepatitis – HBV, HCV
- Cardiac cirrhosis
- Autoimmune hepatitis
- Nonalcoholic steatohepatitis
- Biliary cirrhosis
- Hemochromatosis
- Wilson's disease
- α_1- Antitrypsin deficiency
- Cystic fibrosis
- Cryptogenic cirrhosis

16. **All are seen is tumor lysis syndrome *except:* (Repeat)**

A. Hypercalcemia B. Hypocalcemia
C. Hyperphosphatemia D. Hyperkalemia

Ans: A. Hypercalcemia

Ref: *Harrison's Principles of Internal Medicine, 18th edition, pg 2274*

Explanation:

Refer Medicine 2013 question explanation

Tumor lysis Syndrome (TLS)

- Characteristic biochemical changes in Tumor lysis Syndrome
  - Hyperuricemia
  - Hyperkalemia
  - Hypocalcemia
  - Hyperphosphatemia
  - Acidosis
  - Acute renal failure.

17. **Hypernatremic hypovolemia causes all *except:***

A. Cerebral haemorrhage
B. Cerebral thrombosis
C. Pontine myelinolysis

Ans: B. Cerebral thrombosis

Ref: *Harrison's 18th edn, pg 349*

Explanation:

Causes of Hyponatremia

- Cerebral edema
- Acute hyponatremic encephalothy
- Nausea, headache, vomiting
- Seizure, brainstem herniation, coma, death
- Respiratory failure, ARDS
- Chronic hyponatremia causes subtle gait and cognitive abnormalities
- ODS (**Osmotic demyelination syndrome**), Central Pontine Myelinosis (CPM)
- Seen during rapid correction of hyponatremia
- Due to delayed accumulation of organic osmolytes into the brain cells
- It mainly affects **Pons**, also **cerebellum, thalamus, putamen, cerebral** cortex and **subcortex**
- Presents as **quadriparesis, dysphagia, dysarthria, diplopia, locked-in syndrome, LOC**

- Risk factors – **Alcoholism, Malnutrition, Hypokalemia**

18. Kussmaul sign is seen in all *except:* (Repeat)

A. Severe TS **B.** RVF
C. RV infarct **D.** Constrictive pericarditis

Ans: B. RVF

***Ref:** Harrison's 18th edn, pg 1976*

Explanation:

Kussmaul's Sign

- It is seen in the JVP, which shows a rise/lack of fall during inspiration
- Seen in
  - Chronic constrictive pericarditis
  - Tricuspid stenosis
  - Right ventricular infarction
  - Restrictive cardiomyopathy
  - Massive pulmonary embolism
  - Advanced LV systolic heart failure.

19. All are autosomal recessive *except:* (Repeat)

A. Haemochromatosis **B.** Sickle cell anaemia
C. Friederich ataxia **D.** Huntington's chorea

Ans: D. Huntington's chorea

***Ref:** Harrison's Principles of Internal Medicine, 18th edition, page 3148*

Explanation:

(See the following table)

20. Angina equivalent is a term given to:

A. Breathlessness **B.** Sweating
C. Chest pain **D.** Palpitations

Ans: C. Chest pain

***Ref:** Circulation Journal, Aug 14, 2007*

Explanation:

- An **anginal equivalent** is a symptom other than chest pain, occurring in a patient at high cardiac risk.
- Anginal equivalents are considered to have the same importance as angina pectoris in patients presenting with elevation of cardiac enzymes/ ECG changes which are diagnostic of myocardial ischemia.
- Such symptoms are:
  - Shortness of breath
  - Diaphoresis
  - Extreme fatigue
  - Pain at other sites like neck or jaw pain.

21. Most common Ig seen in multiple myeloma: (Repeat)

A. IgG **B.** IgM
C. IgA **D.** IgE

Ans: A. IgG

***Ref:** Harrison's Principles of Internal Medicine, 18th edition,*

Explanation:

Also refer Medicine 2013 question explanation.

Multiple Myeloma

- Multiple myeloma is a malignant proliferation of plasma cells derived from a single clone.
- ***Characteristics***
  - *Lytic bone lesions*
  - Anemia with high ESR
  - Roulex formation of red cells
  - Renal failure
  - Infections
  - Hypercalcemia
- ***Triad of Multiple myeloma***
  - *Marrow plasmacytosis* >10%
  - Lytic bone lesions
  - Serum and /or urine M component
- Monoclonal plasma cells(κ,λ light chain restricted) in BM or as a tumor (solitary plasmacytoma)
- ***End organ damage***:
  - Lytic bony lesions
  - Anemia

Autosomal dominant	Autosomal recessive	X-linked dominant	X-linked recessive
Huntington's disease, Neurofibromatosis type 1, Myotonic dystrophy, Tuberous sclerosis, PCKD, Familial polyposis coli, Hereditary spherocytosis, Von Willebrand disease, Marfan's, Osteogenesis imperfecta, achondroplasia, Familial hypercholesterolemia, Acute intermittent porphyria	Hemochromatosis, cystic fibrosis, α-1 antitrypsin deficiency, thalassemia, sickle cell anemia, CAH, Freidrick's ataxia, spinomuscular atrophy, alkaptonuria, Wilson's disease, homocystinuria	Vit-D resistant rickets Fragile X syndrome Alport's, Charcot-Marie tooth disease Rett syndrome	Beckers & Duchen's MD, Haemophila A & B, Fabry's disease Lesch Nyhan Hunter's Menke'sWiskott-Aldrich Color blindness G6PD deficiency
Y – linked inheritance: Hairy pinna			

- Hypercalcemia
- Renal failure with paraproteinemia (mostly IgG or IgA)
- S. electrophoresis for M band (β,γ) ; Urine Bence Jones protein for light chains
- Non secretory myeloma– no paraproteins, poor prognosis
- X-rays axial skeleton– skull, spine, long bones, ribs for lytic lesions
- PET or MRI useful for early lesions
- Radionuclide scan not useful
- Must be differentiated from smoldering myeloma and MGUS
- **Treatment:** Thalidomide/lenolidamide+ high dose dexamethasone
- Bortezomib, Autologous hematopoietic SCT
- Localized RT for vertebral collapse
- Bisphosphonates for malignant hypercalcemia (beware of their osteonecrosis jaw!)
- **Prognosis**

Stage	β2 microglobulin	Albumin	Survival
Stage 1	<3.5 mg/L	≥3.5 g/dL	>5 yrs
Stage 2	3.5-5.5 mg/L		
Stage 3	>5.5 mg/L		<2 yrs

22. **All are seen in alkaptonuria *except:***
A. Cardiac disease B. Ochronosis
C. Arthritis D. Seizures

Ans: D. Seizures

Ref: Harrison's 18th edition, pg 3219

Explanation:

Alkaptonuria

- Autosomal recessive
- Due to **deficiency** of **homogentisic acid oxidase**
- **Clinical features**
  - Oochronosis
  - Arthritis
  - Cardiac valve involvement
  - Coronary artery calcification
  - Pigmented heart valves, sclera, joint, skin and renal calculi
  - Urine darkens on standing
- **Nitisinone** used to reduce urinary excretion of homogentisic acid

23. **All are true about systemic sclerosis *except:***
A. Genetic component
B. Calcinosis cutis
C. Pulmonary artery hypertension
D. Anticentromere antibodies

Ans: A. Genetic component

Ref: Harrison's 18th edn, pg 2757

Explanation:

- **ANA** is **positive** in all
- **Scl-70 and anticentromere** abs specific for **scleroderma**
- **Scl-70** mostly seen in **diffuse cutaneous scleroderma**
- **Anticentromere abs** seen more in **limited cutaneous scleroderma** and **Pulm artery hypertension**
- Abs **to β_2GPI** → Ischemia of fingers
- 1.6% prevalent of **family** history
- High risk of other autoimmune disorders like **SLE, RA**

Systemic Sclerosis

(Aka Systemic Scleroderma)

Diffuse

- Most common type in childhood
- Symmetric thickening and hardening of the skin (sclerosis) with fibrous and degenerative changes of viscera

Limited

- Rare in childhood
- Previously known as CREST (calcinosis cutis, Raynaud phenomenon, esophageal dysfunction, sclerodactyly, and telangiectasia) syndrome

Systemic Sclerosis

- The skin manifestations of SSc include.
- Early phase of **edema.**
- **Induration** and **fibrosis** of skin
- **Loss of subcutaneous fat,** sweat glands and hair follicles.
- **Atrophic skin** becomes shiny and waxy in appearance.
- **Flexion contractures** develop at the elbows, hips and knees associated with secondary muscle weakness and atrophy.
- **Small oral stoma** with decreased mouth aperture.
- **Skin ulceration** over pressure points, such as the elbows, may be associated with subcutaneous calcifications.
- Severe **Raynaud phenomenon** causes ulceration of the fingertips with subsequent loss of tissue pulp and tapered fingers (**sclerodactyly**).
- Resorption of the distal tufts of the distal phalanges may occur (**acro-osteolysis**).
- Hyperpigmented postinflammatory changes surrounded by atrophic depigmentation gives a **salt-and-pepper appearance.**

- Pulmonary disease is the most common visceral manifestation of SSc and includes both arterial and interstitial involvement (**alveolitis**).
- Symptoms range from asymptomatic disease to exercise intolerance, dyspnea at rest, and right-sided heart failure.
- **Pulmonary arterial hypertension (PAH)** is a poor prognostic sign.
- Gastrointestinal tract disease is seen in 25% of children with the disease.
- Common manifestations include **esophageal** and **intestinal dysmotility** resulting in **dysphagia**, **reflux**, dyspepsia, **gastroparesis**, bacterial overgrowth, **dilated bowel loops** and **pseudo-obstruction**, dental caries, as well as **malabsorption** and **failure to thrive.**
- Renal arterial disease can cause chronic or severe episodic **hypertension.**
- **Cardiac fibrosis** is associated with arrhythmias, ventricular hypertrophy and decreased cardiac function.
- **Mortality** from juvenile systemic sclerosis is most commonly a result of **cardiopulmonary disease.**

24. Infectious mononucleosis is characterized by all *except:*

A. Atypical lymphocytes
B. Increased B cells
C. Absolute lymphocytosis

Ans: B. Increased B cells

Ref: *Harrison's 18th edn, pg 1467*

Explanation:

Infectious Mononucleosis

- It is caused by EBV
- Fever, cervical nodes , hepatosplenomegaly and rash
- Lymphocytosis with atypical lymphocytes (CD 8+)
- Abnormal LFT
- **CNS complications:**
  - Meningitis
  - Encephalitis
  - Cranial nerve palsies
  - GBS
  - Transverse myelitis
- **Splenic rupture**, upper airway obstruction, bacterial superinfection can occur

25. Urine of a UTI patient has a pH of more than 8, the probable organism is:

A. E coli **B.** Proteus
C. Klebsiella **D.** Candida

Ans: B. Proteus

Ref: *Harrison's 18th edn, pg 1245*

Explanation:

Proteus UTI

- Causes only 1% UTI in healthy women
- Causes 5% of hospital acquired UTI
- 15% of catheter associated UTI
- Produces **urease**, which hydrolyses **urea→ Ammonia→ Alkaline urine**
- Alkaline urine→ precipitation of organic and inorganic compounds→ **Struvite** and **Carbonate-Apatite crystals, Staghorn calculi** and forming **Biofilm on catheter.**

26. Angiokeratoma is seen in: (Repeat)

A. Fabry's disease **B.** Pompe's disease
C. Hurler's disease **D.** Gaucher's disease

Ans: A. Fabry's disease

Ref: *Harrison's 18th edn, pg 2349, 3191*

Explanation:

Fabry's Disease

- X- linked disorder, deficient **lysosomal α-galactosidase A** activity
- Childhood males
- **Painful acroparesthesias**
- **Cutaneous angiokeratoma**
- **Corneal dystrophy**
- **Hypohidrosis**
- The lesions are red-blue in colour, in **bathing – suit distribution,**
- **Angiokeratoma** is also seen in:
  - **Fordyce scrotal angiokeratoma**
  - Arthropod bites
  - Cherry hemangiomas
  - Bacillary angiomatosis (Bartonella hensalae, B.quintana)
- Atypical mycobacteria, sporotrichosis, Nocardia and Leishmaniasis also produce red popular lesions
- Cardiomyopathy, cerebrovascular disease, renal injury (renal failure, FSGS, zebra bodies, Maltese cross) due to small vessel vasculitis
- Treated with **ACE inhibitors** and recombinant **α-galactosidase A,** Renal transplantation

27. Most common source of systemic emboli is:

A. Varicose veins **B.** Mural thrombi
C. Cardiac thrombi **D.** Pulmonary embolism

Ans: B. Mural thrombi

Ref: Kumar & Robbin, Pg 91

Explanation:

Systemic Thromboembolism

- **80%** from **cardiac mural thromboembolism**
- **75%** of it is from **LV infarcts**
- **25%** with **dilated LA**
- Aortic aneurysm, atherosclerotic plaque, valvular vegetations, paradoxical embolism
- Common arterial embolisation sites– **Lower extremities (75%),** CNS (10%), intestines, kidneys and spleen
- **Pulmonary thromboembolism** occurs most commonly from **DVT**

28. Giant 'A' wave is in all *except:* (Repeat)

A. Complete heart block
B. Tricuspid stenosis
C. Pulmonary hypertension
D. MR

Ans: D. MR

Ref: Braunwald 5th ed, pg 1073; The Jugular Venous Pressure and Pulse Contour– Clinical Methods, 3rd ed, HK Walker

Explanation:

Refer Medicine 2013 question explanation.

Normal mean jugular venous pressure is 6-8 cm H_2O

- **'A' wave:** Occurs before carotid upstroke, after the P wave in ECG, caused by atrial contraction filling the RV at the end diastole.
- **'C' wave:** During the carotid upstoke, caused by transmission of carotid impulse through the jugular veins OR by bulging of the tricuspid valve into the RA in early systole.
- **'X' descent:** Movement of the lower portion of RA towards RV in late systole.
- **'V' wave:** Passive RA filling during late systole and early diastole.
- **'Y' descent:** Abrupt termination of downstroke of V wave in early diastole after the tricuspid valve opens and RV passively fills.
- 'A' wave in JVP is due to atrial contraction, followed by 'X' descent due to atrial relaxation
- **Giant 'A' is due to**
  1. Obstruction at tricuspid valve— TS, right atrial myxoma
  2. Non-compliant RV— Pulmonary stenosis, COPD with pulmonary hypertension, restrictive cardiomyopathy, RVMI
  3. Contraction of atria against a closed TV- Cannon 'A' in AV dissociation, junctional rhythm
  4. RV outflow obstruction- HOCM
- **Cannon 'A' waves**: Right atrial contraction occurs against a closed tricuspid valve
  1. Complete heart block
  2. Atrial contraction during a ventricular ectopic
- TR – High 'V' wave due to rapid atrial filling → rapid 'CV' wave
- MR cause prominent 'A' only in presence of pulmonary artery hypertension
- **Absent 'A' waves:** In atrial fibrillation

29. Increased lung compliance is seen in:

A. Emphysema **B.** Bronchial asthma
C. Chronic bronchitis **D.** Bronchiectasis

Ans: A. Emphysema

Ref: Harrison's 18th edn, pg 2087

Explanation:

Lung compliance: is defined as **change in lung volume for every unit change in pressure**

- Compliance (stretchability) = 1/ elasticity (stiffness)
- Greater the compliance = easier for the lungs to expand
- Compliance depends upon = tissue elasticity (25%) + surface tension (75%)
- Surfactant synthesized by alveolar type 2 cells
- Increased collagen= decrease compliance
- Restrictive lung disease (fibrosis) = increases collagen= decreases compliance
- Obstructive lung disease (emphysema) = collagen and elasticity decrease = increases compliance
- Compliance increases with age
- Laplaces law states collapsing pressure is inversely proportional to the radius of the alveoli
- **Emphysema**: ***Increased RV & FRC***
- **Restrictive lung: *Decreased FRC & TLC***

30. Residual volume of lung in an average adult male is: (Repeat)

A. 3.0 L **B.** 0.9 L
C. 1.2 L **D.** 1.9 L

Ans: C. 1.2 L

Ref: Davidson, 21st ed, pg 651

Explanation:

Refer Medicine 2013 question explanation.

- TLC: Volume of air in the lungs following maximal inspiration (N= 5-6L)
- FVC: Maximum amount of air exhaled following maximal inspiration (N= 4.8L)
- VT: Volume of air entering and leaving lungs during normal respiration (N+ 500 ml)
- RV: Volume of air remaining in the lungs after maximal expiratory effort (1.2L)
- FRC: Volume of air within the lungs at the end of normal respiration (2.5-3L)
- FEV: Volume of air exhaled in a given time during a forced vital capacity effort

31. Priapism is seen in all *except:*

A. Sickle cell anaemia
B. Megaloblastic anaemia
C. Scorpion sting
D. Spinal injury

Ans: B. Megaloblastic anaemia

Ref: *Harrison's 18th edition, pg 375, 855*

Explanation:

Priapism

- It refers to **persistent and painful erection**
- **Causes of priapism** are:
  - Spinal/pelvic injury
  - Scorpion /poisonous spider venom
  - Alcohol
  - Marijuana
  - Cocaine
  - PDE-5 inhibitors like sildenafil,tadalafil, vardenafil
  - Prostaglandin E1-alprostadil
  - Warfarin
  - Heparin
  - Hypercoagulable states

32. Artemesinin is best used for:

A. Relapse of malaria
B. Cerebral malaria
C. Chronic malaria
D. Recrudescent malaria

Ans: B. Cerebral malaria

Ref: *CMDT 2013, pg 1492*

Explanation:

- **Treatment of cerebral malaria:**
  - IV **Quinine**: Needs continuous cardiac monitoring; can cause QTc prolongation, hypoglycemia
  - IV **Artesunate** has better efficacy and safer than quinine, 2.4 mg/kg IV BD, then OD
  - **Exchange transfusion** if parasite index is > 10%
  - **Artemisinin (qinghaosu)** acts rapidly against erythrocytic stages of malarial parasites. It is effective against complicated and multidrug resistant malaria. Due to their short half life, recrudescence is high if used alone, hence not useful for prophylaxis also.
- **Chloroquine sensitive falci and vivax:** Chloroquine 1g, 500mg at 6, 24, 48 hrs, followed by Primaquine 15mg for 14 days
- **Chloroquine resistant, uncomplicated falciparum**: Oral quinine, Mefloquine, Doxy, Clindamycin, Oral Artesunate

SURGERY

1. Migratory thrombophlebitis is seen in: (Repeat)

A. Pancreatic adenocarcinoma
B. Promyelocytic leukemia
C. Hodgkin's lymphoma
D. Prostate Ca

Ans: A. Pancreatic adenocarcinoma **D.** Prostate Ca

Ref: *Robbins and Cotran, Pathologic Basis of Disease: 8th edition*

Explanation:

"Migratory thrombophlebitis, known as the Trousseau sign, occurs in about 10% of adenocarcinoma of pancreas patients and is attributable to the elaboration of platelet-aggregating factors and procoagulants from the carcinoma or its necrotic products." *Ref: Robbins*

Migratory Thrombophlebitis (Trousseau Syndrome)

- It is associated with a significant risk of underlying **malignancy**, esp **Pancreas, Lung** and **Prostate.**
- The **veins** of the **neck, chest, abdomen**, and **lower extremities** are involved either sequentially or simultaneously.
- The **hypercoagulable state** associated with cancer is **multifactorial** in origin, and may be induced by **inflammatory cytokines, acute-phase reactants, circulating tissue factor** and **cancer microparticles.**

2. Perinerual spread is seen in:

A. Adenoid cystic carcinoma
B. Pleomorphic adenoma
C. Mucoepidermoid Ca
D. Warthin's tumor

Ans: A. Adenoid cystic carcinoma

Ref: Robbins and Cotran Pathologic Basis of Disease, 8th edition

Explanation:

*"Although slow growing, **adenoid cystic carcinomas** are relentless and unpredictable tumors with a tendency to invade **perineural** spaces" **Ref: Robbins***

Adenoid cystic carcinoma

- It is a relatively uncommon tumor.
- Found in the minor salivary glands in 50% of cases (especially in **Palate**).
- Among the major salivary glands, the **parotid** and **submandibular** glands are the most common locations.

Morphology

- Small, poorly encapsulated, infiltrative, gray-pink lesions.
- Microscopically, small cells having dark, compact nuclei and scant cytoplasm.
- These cells tend to be disposed in **tubular**, **solid**, or **cribriform patterns** reminiscent of **cylindromas** arising in the **adnexa of the skin.**
- The spaces between the tumor cells are filled with a **hyaline material** which represents **excess basement membrane.**
- Has a tendency to invade **perineural spaces** and are **recurrent**.
- **>50%** disseminate widely to distant sites such as **bone, liver** and **brain.**
- 5-year survival rate is about **60% - 70%.**

3. **Circumcision is contraindicated in:**
   A. Phimosis
   B. Ballooning of prepuce
   C. Hypospadias
   D. Ca penis

Ans: C. Hypospadias

Ref: Bailey and Love's Short Practice of Surgery 25th Edition

Explanation:

*"Most of the procedures for hypospadias make use of **prepuceal skin** and so **circumcision should be avoided** until repair is done."*

Contraindications for Circumcision

- In infants with certain genital structure abnormalities
- Misplaced urethral opening (as in hypospadias and epispadias)
- Curvature of the head of the penis (chordee)
- Ambiguous genitalia
- This is because the **foreskin** may be **needed** for **reconstructive surgery**.

Circumcision is also avoided in:

- Premature infants
- Clinically unstable infants
- Undiagnosed bleeding conditions

3. **Vertical banded gastrectomy is done in:**
   A. Gastric ulcer
   B. Obesity
   C. Ca stomach
   D. Gastric outlet obstruction

Ans: B. Obesity

Ref: The Washington Manual of Surgery, 6th edition

Explanation:

Surgical Options for Treating Obesity

Bariatric Surgery

Indications

- Patients with a body mass index of greater than 40, or
- Greater than 35 with associated comorbidities.
- Who have failed intensive efforts using medical means

Benefits of surgery

- Reversal of the disease processes associated with severe obesity.
- **Hypertension** resolves in **50%** and improves in another **25%** of patients.
- NIDDM is reversed in **two-thirds** of cases.
- Incidence of new-onset diabetes is decreased.

Mechanism

- Gastric restriction produces a **small gastric reservoir.**
- Produces **early satiety.**
- Reduces oral intake.
- **Malabsorption** of varying degrees is induced by bypass of selected portions of the proximal small bowel.

Procedures

Vertical Banded Gastroplasty

- Aka "**stomach stapling**" or a **Vertical sleeve gastroplasty**
- Low incidence of metabolic derangement because it **maintains GI tract continuity**.
- An **end-to-end anastomosis (EEA)** stapler is used to create a window in the midbody of the stomach.

- A vertical staple line then is placed from the angle of His to the window to partition the stomach, leaving a small reservoir.
- A mesh band is then positioned through the hole, around the lesser curve, to restrict the size of the passage for the food bolus.
- Complications are rare and include **breakdown of the suture line** and **erosion of the mesh band** into the **gastric wall,** resulting in **perforation**.
- Metabolic complications and **malnutrition** are less frequent than with procedures that include a malabsorptive component.
- Mortality is less than **1%.**
- Weight loss is approximately **45%** of excess body weight at **1 year.**

Roux-en-Y Gastric Bypass (RYGBP)

- Currently the most popular procedure.
- A 30-mL proximal gastric pouch is created either by transection or by using a stapling device.
- A 1-cm diameter anastomosis is then performed between the pouch and a Roux-en-Y limb of small bowel.
- This results in a **small reservoir**, a small passage for pouch emptying, and bypass of the duodenum and proximal jejunum.
- The length of the Roux limb directly correlates with the degree of postoperative weight loss.
- Mortality is **1%,** most commonly secondary to a leak at the gastrojejunostomy, which occurs in 2–4% of patients.
- Late complications include **incisional hernia, stomal stenosis** and **ulcer.**
- Nutritional complications include **folate**, vitamin **B12, iron** and **calcium** deficiency.
- Weight loss is **70% o**f excess weight at **1 year.**
- **Reversal** of **NIDDM** occurs rapidly, often **within 2 weeks.**
- **Dumping syndrome** occurs in most patients, which reinforces dietary behavior modification.

Jejunoileal Bypass

- It is a purely malabsorptive procedure.
- High rate of long-term complications, including diarrhea, **bypass or stasis enteritis** (characterized by abdominal pain and distention), **excessive flatulence, electrolyte abnormalities, cholelithiasis, hepatic dysfunction,** and **nephrolithiasis** secondary to **hyperoxaluria**.
- The long-term mortality rate is **10%.**
- As a result, this **procedure is no longer performed** for obesity.

Laparoscopic Bariatric Surgery

Indications for bariatric surgery are the same as those for traditional open procedures.

Contraindications

- These are relative contraindications
- A body mass of index of greater than 60
- Previous upper abdominal surgery
- Evidence of an excessively large liver
- Presence of a ventral hernia

Procedures in Laparoscopy

- **Gastric stapling** operations rely on the concept of restricting the volume of oral intake.
- The vertical banded gastroplasty, RYGBP, and the adjustable gastric banding are procedures amenable to a laparoscopic approach.
- **RYGBP** appears to be most beneficial in producing long-term weight loss.
- Patients who have undergone RYGBP tend to have **dumping**, which motivates them to avoid high-calorie foods.
- A laparoscopic **adjustable gastric band (AGB),** commonly called a Lap-Band, A Band, or LAGB, is an inflatable silicone device placed around the top portion of the stomach, intended to slow consumption of food.

Complications

Immediate postoperative period (are same as in open gastric bypass)

- Wound infection
- Bleeding
- Deep venous thrombosis
- Pulmonary embolism
- Anastomotic leakage
- Myocardial infarction
- 1–2% mortality.
- Delayed complications are less common than in open surgery and include **anastomotic stricture** and rare **incisional hernias.**

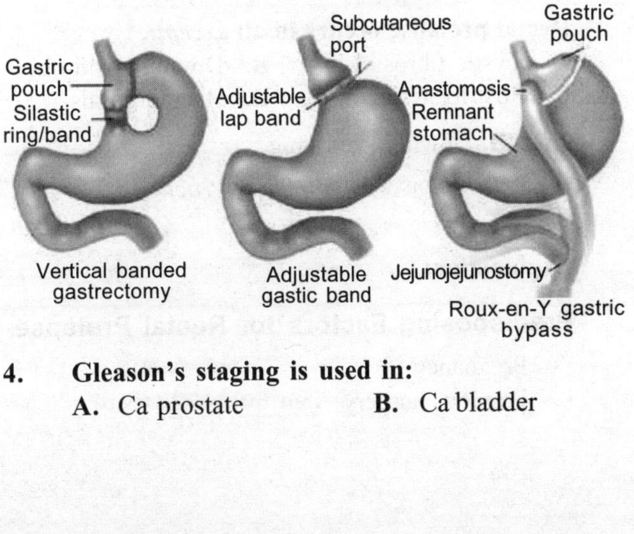

Vertical banded gastrectomy

Adjustable gastic band

Roux-en-Y gastric bypass

4. **Gleason's staging is used in:**
   A. Ca prostate **B.** Ca bladder

C. Ca pancreas **D.** Ca colon

Ans: A. Ca prostate

Ref: Bailey & Love's Short Practice of Surgery, 25th Edition & Internet Sources

Explanation:

The Gleason Grading System

- It is used to help evaluate the prognosis of men with **prostate cancer.**
- It also predicts prognosis and helps guide therapy.
- Scoring based upon its **microscopic appearance** on **histopathology.**
- Cancers with a higher Gleason score are more **aggressive** and have a **worse prognosis.**
- The pathologist assigns a Gleason score based on the sum of two numbers:
  - The **first number** is the **grade of the most common tumor pattern.**
  - The **second number** is the **grade of the second most common pattern.**
- If there are three patterns the first number is the most common and the second is the one with the highest grade.

Gleason Sacle

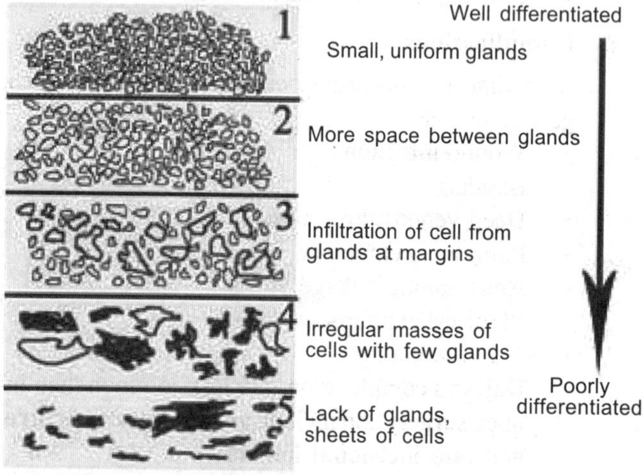

5. **Rectal prolapse occurs in all *except:***

A. Cystic fibrosis **B.** Down's syndrome
C. Post-hysterectomy **D.** Haemorrhoids

Ans: B. Down's syndrome

Ref: Bailey & Love's Short Practice of Surgery, 25th Edition

Explanation:

Predisposing Factors for Rectal Prolapse

- Pregnancy
- Previous surgery
- Pelvic neuropathies
- Neurological disease
- High gastrointestinal helminth loads esp, whipworm
- COPD
- Cystic fibrosis

Rectal Prolapse

A. Partial Prolapse

- The mucous membrane and submucosa of the rectum protrude outside the anus for approximately **1-4 cm.**
- When the prolapsed mucosa is palpated between the finger and thumb, it is evident that it is composed of **no more than a double layer of mucous membrane** (cf. complete prolapse).
- Occurs in children and elderly.

In infants

- Immature sacral curve and reduced resting anal tone which offers diminished support to the mucosal lining of the anal canal (Mann) predisposes to this condition.

In children

- Partial prolapse often commences after an attack of **diarrhoea**, as a result of **severe whooping cough**, or from **loss of weight** and consequent **diminution in the amount of fat in the ischiorectal fossae.**

In adults

- The condition in adults is usually associated with **third-degree haemorrhoids.**
- In the female, a **torn perineum** predisposes to prolapse, and in the male straining from **urethral obstruction.**
- In old age, both partial and complete prolapse are associated with **atony of the sphincter** mechanism.
- Partial prolapse may follow an **operation for fistula-in-ano** where a large portion of muscle has been divided. Here the prolapse is usually **localised** to the **damaged quadrant** and is **seldom progressive.**
- Prolapsed mucous membrane is **pink**; prolapsed internal haemorrhoids are **plum coloured** and more **pedunculated.**

Treatment

- **In infants and young children**
  - **Digital reposition.**
  - **Submucous injections**: Injections of 5 per cent phenol in almond oil are carried out under general anaesthesia.

- Thiersch's operation.

- **In adults**
  - **Submucous injections:** May be successful in early partial prolapse.
  - **Excision of the prolapsed mucosa**.

B. Complete Prolapse

- Aka **procidentia** is less common than the partial prolapse.
- The protrusion consists of **all layers of the rectal wall** and is a descending hernia-en-glissade of the rectum downwards through the levator ani.
- The process starts with the **anterior wall of the rectum** where the supporting tissues are weakest, especially in **women**.
- It is commonly **10-15 cm** in length.
- On palpation, it is thicker than a partial prolapse (due to double thickness of the entire rectal wall).
- Complete prolapse is **uncommon** in **children**, but is more common in the elderly.
- Women are six times more often affected than men.
- In women, prolapse of the rectum is commonly **associated with prolapse of the uterus**, or a past history of a **gynaecological operation**, e.g. **hysterectomy.**
- Assciated with **faecal incontinence** in 50% cases.

Treatment

- Surgery is required and the operation can be performed via the perineal or the abdominal approaches. Whenever possible, an abdominal rectopexy is recommended, but when the patient is elderly and very frail, or is suffering from injury or disease of the spinal cord, or in very early life, a perineal operation is indicated.

Perineal Approach

- **Delorme's operation** (Now the preferred perineal operation).
- **Thiersch's operation.**
- **Postanal repair (Parks).**
- **Perineal rectosigmoidectomy (Altemeier)**

Abdominal Approach

- The principle of all abdominal operations for rectal prolapse is to replace and hold the rectum in its proper position. They are recommended in patients with complete prolapse, who are otherwise in good health.
  - **Wells' operation.**
  - **Ripstein's operation.**
  - **Lahaut's operation.**

6. **Goblet sign is seen in:**

A. Ureteral tumor	**B.** Ureteral calculi
C. TB	**D.** Schistosomiasis

Ans: A. Ureteral tumor

Ref: *Daniels RE 3rd. The Goblet Sign. Radiology. 1999 Mar210(3):737-8*

Explanation:

The Goblet Sign

- It is a cup-shaped collection of contrast material that is seen just distal to an intraluminal filling defect of the ureter.
- It is perhaps best demonstrated at retrograde ureterography.
- It can also be seen during intravenous urography when there is partial or no obstruction of the ureter.
- The Goblet sign is a clue that the ureteral filling defect is a **mass** rather than a calculus.
- The slow expansion of a polypoid intraluminal tumorous mass from a **uroepithelial carcinoma** causes dilatation of the ureter distal as well as proximal to the mass.
- Propulsion of the mass distally during ureteral peristalsis further contributes to the dilatation of the ureter distal to the tumor and thus causes the cup-shaped collection of contrast material.
- On the other hand, the **ureteral lumen just distal** to a **mechanical obstruction** caused by a **calculus** will have a **narrowed appearance** due to wall spasm and edema.
- Dilatation proximal to either a tumor or calculus varies with the degree of obstruction.

7. **Indication for surgery in a case of hydatid cyst are all *except:***

A. Cyst > 5 cm	**B.** Cyst in liver
C. Cyst in lung	**D.** Cyst in brain

Ans: B. Cyst in liver

Ref: *Nelson*

Explanation:

- Cysts in liver alone is not an indication for surgery.

Management of Hydatid Cysts

- For simple, accessible cysts surrounded by tissue, ultrasound- or CT-guided Percutaneous Aspiration, Instillation (hypertonic saline or another scolicidal agent) and Re-aspiration **(PAIR)** is the preferred therapy.
- Spillage with PAIR is uncommon, but prophylactic albendazole therapy is routinely

administered >1 wk prior to PAIR or surgery and continued for 1 mo thereafter.

- **PAIR** is contraindicated in **pregnancy** and for **bile-stained cysts**, which should not be injected with a scolicidal agent because of increased risk for biliary complications.

Indications for Surgery in Hydatid Cyst

- Presence of **large liver cysts** with **multiple daughter cysts**
- **Single** superficially situated **liver cysts** with high risk of rupture
- Infected cysts
- Cysts communicating with the biliary tree
- Exerting pressure on adjacent vital organs
- Cysts in the lung, brain, kidney or bones.

Procedure

- For conventional surgery, **the inner cyst wall** (only laminate and germinal layers are of parasite origin) can be easily peeled from the fibrous layer, although some studies suggest that removal of the whole capsule has a **better outcome**.
- The cavity should then be **topically sterilized** and either closed or **filled** with **omentum**.
- Considerable care must be taken to **avoid spillage of cyst contents**, because cyst fluid contains viable **protoscolices**, each capable of producing **secondary cysts** wherever it lodges.

8. **Most common type of Fistula in ano:**

A. Intersphincteric B. Trans-sphincteric
C. Suprasphincteric D. Extrasphincteric

Ans: A. Intersphincteric

Ref: *Bailey & Love's Short Practice of Surgery, 25th Edition, 1263 and Sabiston Textbook of Surgery, 19th Edition. pg 1394-5*

Explanation:

Park's Classification of Fistula in Ano

Based on the relation of fistulous tract with the external sphincter.

- **Intersphincteric (Type 1- the most common):** The fistula track is confined to the inter-sphincteric plane.
- **Trans-sphincteric (Type 2):** The fistula connects the intersphincteric plane with the ischiorectal fossa by perforating the external sphincter.
- **Suprasphincteric (Type 3):** Similar to trans-sphincteric, but the track loops over the external sphincter and perforates the levator ani.
- **Extrasphincteric (Type 4):** The track passes from the rectum to perineal skin, completely external to the sphincteric complex.

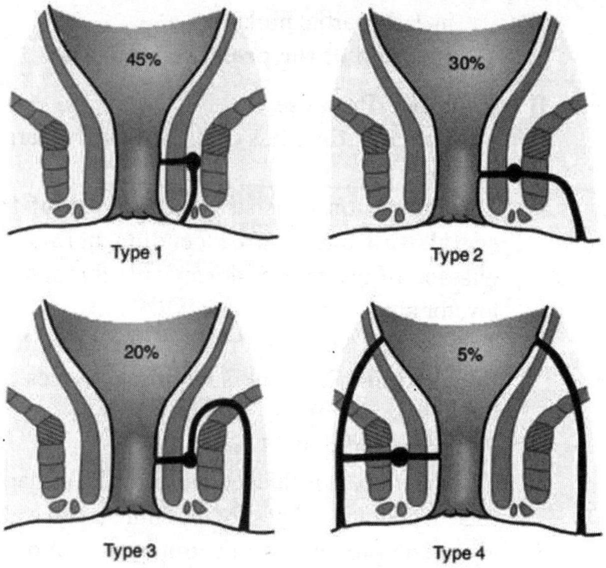

9. **Sacrococcygeal teratoma is associated with:**

A. Meningocele
B. Cardiac defects
C. Hepatic cysts
D. Cystic adenoid malformation

Ans: A. Menigocele

Ref: *Robbins and Cotran Pathologic Basis of Disease: 8th edition*

Explanation:

Sacrococcygeal Teratomas

- **Most common** teratomas of childhood
- Accounts for **40%** or more of cases
- Four times more common in girls
- Approximately 10% of sacrococcygeal teratomas are associated with **congenital anomalies**
  - Primarily defects of the hindgut and cloacal region
  - Midline defects
  - Meningocele and spina bifida
- Approximately **75%** of these tumors are **mature teratomas**, and about **12%** are **unequivocally malignant** and lethal. The remainder is **immature teratomas.**
- Most of the **benign teratomas** are encountered in **younger infants (<4 months)**, whereas children with malignant lesions tend to be older.
- Other sites for teratomas in childhood include:
  - Testis
  - Ovaries
  - Mediastinum
  - Retroperitoneum
  - Head and neck.

ORTHOPAEDICS

1. **Post polio paralysis will lead to following deformity:**
A. FABER B. FADER
C. FADIR D. FABIR

Ans: A. FABER

Ref: Turek's Orthopaedics–Principles and Their Applications, 4th edition, P 529

Explanation:

Post Polio Paralysis

- During the acute and convalescent phases of poliomyelitis the patient lies supine in the so-called **'frog-legged' position** with hips flexed (F), abducted (**AB**) and externally rotated (**ER**); the knees flexed and the feet in equinovarus position.
- Initially this position may be assumed because of the muscle spasm in these muscles.
- Later contractures involving the fascia and inter-muscular septum occur.
- Contracture of the muscles contribute at a later stage.
- With the advent of growth these deformities get worse and adaptive bony changes make correction more difficult.

2. **A patient on colles cast present after two weeks with inability to extend his thumb, the most likely reason is:**
A. Rupture of extensor pollicis longus tendon
B. Compartment syndrome
C. Carpal tunnel syndrome
D. Sudek's osteodystrophy

Ans: A. Rupture of extensor pollicis longus tendon?

Ref: Apley's System of Orthopaedics and Fractures, 9th edition, p 774

Explanation:

- **Rupture of extensor pollicis longus** occasionally occurs a few weeks after an apparently trivial undisplaced **fracture** of the **lower radius.**
- The patient should be warned of the possibility and told that operative treatment is available.

3. **A 75-year-old woman presents with history of tripping and falling in the bathroom and unable to walk or bear weight on her left hip. On examination it was noted that her left lower limb was in an externally rotated position, hip was tender and active straight leg raising was not possible. The most possible diagnosis is:**
A. Fracture neck of femur
B. Osteoarthritis hip
C. Dislocation of hip joint
D. Acetabular fracture

Ans. A. Fracture neck of femur

Ref: Apley's System of Orthopaedics and Fractures, 9th Edition, P 847-848

Explanation:

Fracture Neck of Femur

- Most common site of fractures in the elderly.
- Common in women in the 8th and 9th decades.
- The association with **osteoporosis** is main underlying factor.
- Other risk factors include **bone-losing** or **bone-weakening disorders** such as **osteomalacia, diabetes, stroke (disuse), alcoholism** and **chronic debilitating disease**.
- In addition, old people often have **weak muscles** and **poor balance** resulting in an increased **tendency to fall**.
- The fracture usually results from a **simple fall**; however, in very osteoporotic people, less force is required—perhaps no more than catching a toe in the carpet and twisting the hip into external rotation.
- Occasionally, **stress fractures** of the **femoral neck** occur in **runners** or **military personnel**.
- Not all hip fractures are so obvious. With an impacted fracture the patient may still be able to walk, and debilitated or mentally handicapped patients may not complain at all–even with bilateral fractures.

4. **Most common site of clavicle fracture are all *except:***
A. Junction of middle and outer 1/3
B. Middle 1/3
C. Medial 1/3
D. Lateral 1/3

Ans: C. Meidal 1/3

Ref: Practical Fracture Treatment by Ronald McRae, 4th edition, p 116

Explanation:

Site of Clavicular Fracture

- Clavicular fractures are most common at the junction of the **middle** and **outer 1/3.**

- It is also common throughout the **middle 1/3** and to a lesser extent, the outer 1/3 where the incidence is 18%.
- Fractures at the **medial 1/3** or **medial end** are **uncommon.**

OBSTETRICS & GYNECOLOGY

1. **Least common cause of malignancy in vagina is:**
 A. Choriocarcinoma **B.** Cervical ca
 C. Primary vaginal ca **D.** Endometrial ca

Ans: C. Primary vaginal ca

Ref: Dutta Textbook of Gynecology 5th ed pg 325

Explanation:

PRIMARY VAGINAL CARCINOMA

- Incidence very rare 0.6 per 100000 women [**1%** of genital malignancies].
- Etiology
  - HPV
  - **VAIN** [vaginal intraepithelial neoplasia]
  - Diethyl stilboesterol
  - Irradiation
  - Pessary usage
  - White race
- **Upper 3rd** of vaginal **posterior** wall
- **Most common - Squamous cell ca 90%,** adenoma, melanoma, sarcoma
- Spread-lymphatic, direct and blood borne
- C/F—abnormal vaginal bleeding, foul smelling discharge
- Investigations—cytolgy, colposcopy, biopsy
- Treatment—surgery and radiotherapy

SECONDARY VAGINAL CARCINOMA

- Follows ca of cervix, vulva, urethra by direct spread
- Metastasis in **lower 3rd vagina** or **vault** occurs in choriocarcinoma or endometrial ca
- Commoner than primary ca

2. **PID does not include:**
 A. Cervicitis **B.** Endometritis
 C. Peritonitis **D.** Salpingitis

Ans: A. Cervicitis

Ref: Dutta Textbook of Gynecology 5th Ed pg 124

Explanation:

PELVIC INFLAMMATORY DISEASE (PID)

- Infection of upper genital tract involving
  - Endometrium
  - Fallopian tubes
  - Ovaries
  - Pelvic peritoneum and surrounding structures
- **Cervicitis is not included** in **PID**
- **Risk factors**
  - Menstruating teenagers
  - Multiple sexual partners
  - No OCP use
  - IUCD usage
  - STDs
- **Protective factors**
  - Condoms
  - OCPs
  - Pregnancy
  - Menopause
  - Women whose partner has done vasectomy
  - Husband is azoospermic
- **Causative organisms**
  - Neisseria gonorrhoae
  - Chlamydia trachomatis
  - Mycoplasma hominis
- **Symptoms**
  - Lower abdominal pain
  - Fever
  - Lassitude
  - Excessive vaginal bleeding
  - Purulent vaginal discharge
  - Dyspareunia
- **Fitz-Hugh Curtis syndrome**—Acute salpingitis with perihepatitis causes pain in right hypochondrium
- **Investigations**
  - Discharge sent for stain and culture
  - Leucocytosis
  - **Laparoscopy [Gold standard investigation]**
  - USG
- **Treatment**
  - Doxy 100 mg bd.
  - Erythromycin 500 mg qid.
  - Tetracycline 500 mg qid, Metronidazole 500 mg bd.
  - Azithromycin 1gm single dose, Ofloxacin 400 mg bd for 7 to 14 days.
  - For N. gonorrhoea Ceftriaxone 250 mg deep IM single dose, Ciproflox 500 mg orally single dose.

3. **Highest failure rate is seen in:**
 A. Laparoscopic silastic ring
 B. Irwin method
 C. Pomeroy method
 D. Madlener method

Ans: D. Madlener method

Ref: Dutta Gynecology pg 455, Shaw's Textbook of Gynecology pg 240

Explanation:

FAILURE RATES

Method	Failure Rate
Laparoscopic sterilisation	0.2 to 0.6%
Pomeroy's method	0.1 to 0.5%
Madlener's method	1.5 to 7%
Rhythm method	24 pregnancy rate per HWY
Coitus interruptus	19
Lactational amenorrhoea	2
Condom	14
Diaphragm	20
IUCD	0.1 to 3
OCPs	0.1
POP	1
DMPA and NET injectables	0.3
Norplant	0.1
Vasectomy	0.15
Tubectomy	0.5

4. **Which is not true about pregnancy and TB?**
   A. No difference in prognosis of pregnancy
   B. Congenital TB is rare
   C. Active TB can be transmitted by transplacental route
   D. Concomitant HIV infection increases the risk

Ans: A. No difference in prognosis of pregnancy

Ref: *Dutta Textbook of Obstetrics pg 293*

Explanation:

TUBERCULOSIS IN PREGNANCY

- Incidence —1 to 2%
- **Risk factors**
  - Positive family history
  - Low SE status
  - HIV infection
  - Alcohol
  - IV drug abuse
  - Diabetes
  - Jejunostomy bypass
  - Underweight
- **Diagnosis**
  - Manteaux test
  - Chest x-ray
  - Sputum smear
  - Gastric washings
  - Diagnostic bronchoscopy
  - PCR
- **Congenital TB** is rare– noted in first week of life, **Cavitating hepatic granuloma**, HIV increases risk
- In untreated patients, increased chances of:
  - Preterm labour
  - IUGR
  - Perinatal mortality
- Treatment
  - With no active disease, INH 300 mg/day after 1st trimester for 6 to 9 months.
  - With active disease, INH 300 mg, RMP 600 mg, EMB 2.5 gm, PYZ 2 gm
- **Breast feeding** is **not contraindicated** when mother is taking drugs.
- In active disease baby isolated and given INH prophylaxis 20mg/kg/day for 3 months But if mother is on ATT for 2 weeks there is no need to isolate baby. BCG given as soon as possible.
- **Contraception**—Pregnancy avoided atleast for 2 years. OCPs not used with RMP because of contraceptive failure. Barrier method is used.

5. **Alpha feto protein is decreased in: (Repeat)**
   A. Spina bifida
   B. Down's syndrome
   C. Dead fetus
   D. Abdominal wall deficiency

Ans: B. Down's syndrome

Ref: *Dutta Textbook of Obstetrics pg 106*

Explanation:

MATERNAL SERUM AFP

- AFP is oncofetal protein with molecular weight 70000
- It is produced by **yolk sac** and **fetal liver**
- Highest level of AFP in **fetal serum** and **amniotic fluid** is seen around **13 weeks** and thereafter decreases
- **Maternal serum AFP** reaches a **peak** around **32 weeks**
- **MSAFP level is elevated** in:
  i. Wrong gestational age
  ii. Open NTD
  iii. Multiple pregnancy
  iv. Rh isoimmunisation
  v. IUFD
  vi. Anterior abdominal wall defects
  vii. Renal anomalies
- **MSAFP is low** in:
  i. Down's syndrome
  ii. GTD [Gestational trophoblastic disease]
- Test is done between **15 to 20** weeks

6. **AP diameter is more than transverse diameter in the following:**
   A. Anthropoid pelvis **B.** Android pelvis
   C. Platypelloid pelvis **D.** Gynecoid pelvis

Ans: A. Anthropoid pelvis

Ref: *Dutta Textbook of Obstetrics pg 346*

Explanation:

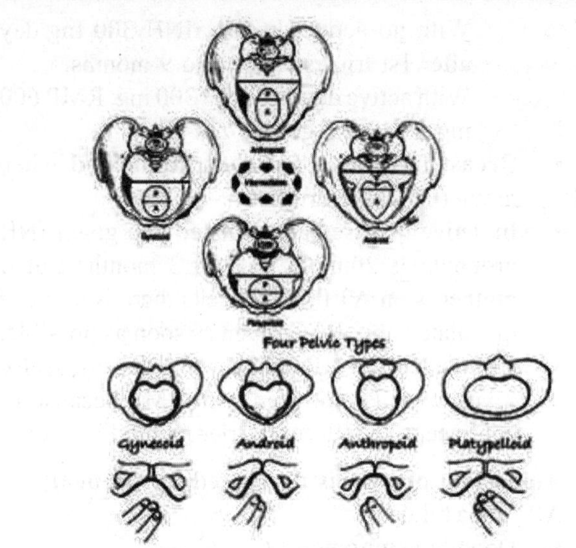

Traditional obstetrics characterizes four types of pelvises:

- **Gynecoid**: Ideal shape, with round to slightly oval (obstetrical inlet slightly less transverse) inlet: best chances for normal vaginal delivery.
- **Android**: Triangular inlet, and prominent ischial spines, more angulated pubic arch.
- **Anthropoid**: The widest transverse diameter is less than the anteroposterior (obstetrical) diameter.
- **Platypelloid**: Flat inlet with shortened obstetrical diameter.
  (See the following table)

7. **In a case of carcinoma cervix, hydronephrosis or renal involvement is seen in:**
   A. Stage 3a B. Stage 3b
   C. Stage 2 D. Stage 4

Ans: B. Stage 3b

Ref: *Shaw's Textbook of Gynecolgy pg 412*

Explanation:

CARCINOMA CERVIX STAGING

Stage I

- Stage I is carcinoma strictly confined to the cervix.
- The diagnosis of both Stages IA1 and IA2 should be based on microscopic examination of removed tissue, preferably a cone, which must include the entire lesion.
- **Stage IA**: Invasive cancer identified only microscopically. Invasion is limited to measured stromal invasion with a maximum depth of 5 mm and no wider than 7 mm.
  – **Stage IA1**: Stage IA1: Measured invasion of the stroma no greater than 3 mm in depth and no wider than 7 mm diameter.
  – **Stage IA2**: Stage IA2: Measured invasion of stroma greater than 3 mm but no greater than 5 mm in depth and no wider than 7 mm in diameter.
- **Stage IB**: Stage IB: Clinical lesions confined to the cervix or preclinical lesions greater than Stage IA. All gross lesions even with superficial invasion are Stage IB cancers.
  – **Stage IB1**: Stage IB1: Clinical lesions no greater than 4 cm in size.
  – **Stage IB2**: Stage IB2: Clinical lesions greater than 4 cm in size.

Stage II

– Stage II is carcinoma that extends beyond the cervix, but does not extend into the pelvic wall.
– The carcinoma involves the vagina, but not as far as the lower third.
– **Stage IIA**: No obvious parametrial involvement. Involvement of up to the upper two-thirds of the vagina.

	Gynecoid (50% of Women)	**Android (23% of Women)**	**Anthropoid (24% of Women)**	**Platyelloid (3% of Women)**
Brim	Sightly ovoid or transversely rounded	Heart-shaped, angulated	Oval, wider anteroposteriorly	Flattened anteroposteriorly, wide transversely
	Round ○	Heart ♡	Oval 0	Flat ⬭
Depth	Moderate	Deep	Deep	Shallow
Sidwalls	Straight	Convergent	Straight	Straight
Ischial spines	Blunt, some-what widely separated	Prominent, narrow interspinous diameter	Prominent, often with narrow interspinous diamater	Blunted, widely separated
Sacrum	Deep, curved	Slightly curved, terminal portion often beaked	Slightly curved	Slightly curved
Subpubic arch	Wide	Narrow	Narrow	Wide
Usual mode of birth	Vaginal Spontaneous Occipitoanterior position	Cesarean Vaginal Difficult with forceps	Vaginal Forceps, Spontaneous Occipitoposterior or occipitoanterior position	Vaginal Spontaneous

– **Stage IAB**: Obvious parametrial involvement, but not into the pelvic sidewall.

Stage III

- Stage III is carcinoma that has extended into the pelvic sidewall.
- On rectal examination, there is no cancer-free space between the tumour and the pelvic sidewall.
- The tumour involves the lower third of the vagina.
- All cases with **hydronephrosis** or a non-functioning kidney are Stage III cancers.
  - **Stage IIIA**: No extension into the pelvic sidewall but involvement of the lower third of the vagina.
  - **Stage IIIB**: Extension into the pelvic sidewall or hydronephrosis or non-functioning kidney.

Stage IV

Stage IV is carcinoma that has extended beyond the true pelvis or has clinically involved the mucosa of the bladder and/or rectum.

- **Stage IVA**: Spread of the tumour into adjacent pelvic organs.
- **Stage IVB**: Spread to distant organs.

8. **Cyst seen in vagina are all *except:***

A. Nebothian cyst B. Gartner's cyst
C. Bartholin's cyst D. Inclusion cyst

Ans: A. Nebothian cyst

Ref: *Shaw's Textbook of Gynecology 15th ed pg 136*

Explanation:

VAGINAL CYSTS

- Vaginal cysts are rare and are located more commonly in **anterior vaginal wall**
- **Gartner's cyst**
  - Arises from remnants of mesonephric duct
  - Lies in anterolateral aspect of vaginal wall
  - Small cyst is asymptomatic
  - Large cyst causes dyspareunia
  - Large symptomatic cysts requires excision
- **Inclusion cyst**
  - Seen in lower end of vagina on its posterior surface.
  - It is caused by tags of mucosa embedding inside the scar that later forms a cyst
- **Bartholin cyst**—Extends into vagina
- **Endometriotic cyst**
  - Bluish bulge in posterior fornix.
  - It is treated with either danazol or surgical excision

A Nabothian Cyst (or Nabothian Follicle)

- It is a mucus-filled cyst on the surface of the **cervix**.
- They are most often caused when stratified squamous epithelium of the ectocervix grows over the simple columnar epithelium of the endocervix (Metaplasia).
- This tissue growth can block the cervical crypts, trapping cervical mucus inside the crypts.

9. **True about amnion are all *except:***

A. No lymph supply
B. Rich blood supply
C. No nerve supply
D. Dilates cervix during labour

Ans: B. Rich blood supply

Ref: *Dutta Textbook of Obstetrics 5th ed pg 37*

Explanation:

AMNION

- Inner layer of fetal membranes
- Amnion can be peeled off the fetal surface of placenta except at the site of insertion of umbilical cord
- **0.02 to 0.5** mm thick
- **No blood or nerve or lymph supply**
- **Functions:**
  - i. Contributes to formation of liquor amnii
  - ii. Prevents ascending uterine infection
  - iii. Dilatation of cervix during labour
  - iv. Steroid hormone metabolism
  - v. Source of glycerophospholipids—Precursors of PG E2 and F2 alpha

10. **Call exner bodies are found in: (Repeat)**

A. Granulosa cell tumour
B. Sertoli leydig cell tumour
C. Gynandroblastoma
D. Thecoma

Ans: A. Granulosa cell tumour

Explanation:

GRANULOSA CELL TUMOUR

- Accounts for 2% of ovarian neoplasms
- Originates from rest of **Primitive granulosa cells**
- **Most common ovarian stromal tumour**
- 2% bilateral, slow growing
- Solid/cystic
- Cut section—yellow/orange due to lipid content
- Histopath
  - Cells polygonal or round with granular eosinophilic cytoplasm with ill defined borders with coffee bean nuclei

- Granulosa cells are arranged in small clusters around a central cavity called call exner bodies
- Tumour marker—**Inhibin**
- Unapposed estrogen secretion→ Endometrial hyperplasia→ Endometrial ca
- C/F—due to **hyperestrogenism**
  - Precocious puberty
  - AUB
  - Postmenopausal bleeding
  - May rupture and cause acute abdomen
- Treatment—Laparotomy and surgical staging, Unilateral salpingooopherectomy
- Chemotherapy
  - **VAC Regimen** [vincristine+adriamycin +cyclophosphamide]
  - **BEP Regimen** [bleomycin, etoposide, cisplatin]

11. Antihypertensive of choice in pregnancy is:

A. Hydralazine **B.** Propranolol
C. Alpha methyl dopa **D.** Labetalol

Ans: C. Alpha methyl dopa

Ref: *Dutta Textbook of Obstetrics, 5th ed pg 506*

Explanation:

See the following table

12. Ventouse is contraindicated in:

A. Preterm **B.** Postterm
C. Prolonged second stage **D.** Cardiac disease

Ans: A. Preterm

Ref: *Dutta Textbook of Obstetrics 5th ed pg 574,580*

Explanation:

Indications of Ventouse

- Prolonged second stage of delivery.
- Fetal hypoxia.
- Severe maternal illness—Cardiac disease, Hypertensive crisis.

Contraindications of Ventouse

- Face, Brow, Breech presentations
- Preterm fetus
- Fetal coagulation disorder
- Fetal macrosomia

13. Invasive mole differs from choriocarcinoma in all the following *except:* (Repeat)

A. Absence of villi
B. No evidence of muscle necrosis
C. Diagnosed <6 months following an abortion
D. Invasive mole follows an abortion or molar pregnancy

Ans: A. Absence of villi

Antihypertensives Used in Pregnancy

	MOA	Side effects	Remarks
Methyl dopa	Centrally acting anti-adrenergic	• Drowsiness • Headache • Postnatal depression • Postural hypotension • Liver dysfunction • Leukopenia • Hemolytic anemia	Contraindicated in patients taking • MAO inhibitors • Lithium • Liver failure • Positive Coombs test
Clonidine	Centrally acting sympathetic inhibitor	• Drowsiness • Dry mouth • Dry eyes • Nausea • Reduced fetal heart rate	Sudden stoppage should be avoided due to pressor effect
Oxprenolol	Beta blocker	• Nightmares	
Labetalol	Alpha and beta blocker	• Worsening asthma • Cough • Nightmares • Bradycardia	Contraindicated in asthmatics Avoided in • Phemochoromocytoma • Heart failure, bradycardia • Peripheral vascular disease • Raynaud's phenomenon
Nifedipine	Calcium channel blocker	• Headache • Edema • Palpitations • Nausea • Dizziness	Metabolised through CYT P450-3A4 - Possible interaction with phenytoin and cisapride
Hydralazine	Peripheral vasodilator	• Flushing • Palpitations • Headache • Nausea	2nd or 3rd line agent. Can cause autoimmune lupus

Ref: Dutta Textbook of Gynecology 5th ed pg 348, Shaw's Textbook of Gynecology 5th ed pg 253

Explanation:

Invasivemole	Choriocarcinoma
Evidence of chorionic villi	Villous formation lost
Follows abortion/mole	Following full term pregnancy
Diagnosed <6 months following an abortion/mole	>6 months to be diagnosed

14. Monoamniotic monochorionic fetus is formed when fertilisation occurs: (Repeat)

A. <2 days **B.** 2 - 8 days
C. >8 days **D.** >2 weeks

Ans: C. >8 days

Ref: Dutta Textbook of Obstetrics 5th ed pg 200

Explanation:

Dizygotic Twins 80% {fraternal, binovular}

- fertilisation of **2 ova by 2 sperms** during single ovarian cycle

Monozygotic twins 20% {identical, uniovular}

- Twinning may occur at different periods after Fertilisation
- Division within 72 hrs—Diamniotic Dichorionic **(30%) - DAD**
- Division **4-8 days** Diamniotic Monochorionic **(66%) - DAM**
- Division **> 8 days**—Monoamniotic Monochorionic **(3%) - DAM**
- Division **> 2 weeks**—conjoined twins **<1% siamese twins**
  i. **Thoracophagus**[Most Common]
  ii. Pyophagus
  iii. Craniophagus
  iv. Ischiophagus

Remember: DAD → DAM → MAM

15. Menopausal flushing is due to:

A. LH **B.** FSH
C. Estrogen **D.** Progesterone

Ans: B. FSH

Ref: Dutta Textbook of Gynecology 5th ed pg 57, Shaw's Textbook of Gynecology 15th ed pg 62

Explanation:

MENOPAUSAL FLUSHING

- Characteristic **vasomotor** symptom of menopause
- **Hot flush** is sudden feel of heat followed by sweating
- **Decreased estrogen** causes **GnRH pulse secretion** lasting for 1 to 10 min
- Thermoregulatory center in association with GnRH—center in hypothalamus is involved in etiology
- Decreased estrogen causes **rebound increase** in secretion of **FSH** and **LH** by anterior pituitary
- FSH level may rise as much as 50 fold and LH 3-4 fold

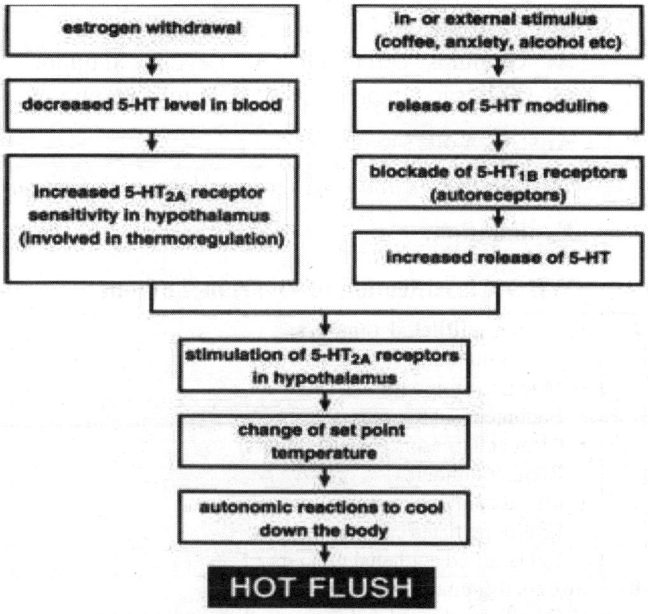

16. Contraindications for OCPs are all *except:* (Repeat)

A. Headache **B.** Jaundice
C. Diabetes **D.** Varicose veins

Ans: D. Varicose veins

Ref: Dutta Textbook of Gynecology 5th ed pg 466

Explanation:

Combination Hormonal Contraceptives

Absolute Contraindications

- Hypersensitivity
- Known/Suspected pregnancy
- Smokers (>15 cigarettes/day) > 35 years old
- Cerebrovascular disease
- Coronary artery disease
- Thromboembolic disorders
  - Pulmonary embolism
  - Myocardial infarction
  - Deep venous thrombosis
  - Stroke
  - Thrombophlebitis
- Known or suspected case of breast cancer
- Undiagnosed abnormal gynecologic bleeding
- Marked impairment in liver function

Relative Contraindications

- Hypertension

- Migraine
- Diabetes mellitus
- Epilepsy
- Obstructive jaundice in pregnancy
- Gallbladder disease
- Surgery with prolonged immobilization
- Sickle cell disease

17. **Sex cord stromal tumors are all *except:***
    A. Granulosa cell tumor **B.** Leydig cell tumor
    C. Yolk sac tumor **D.** Sertoli cell tumor

    Ans: C. Yolk sac tumor

    Ref: *Shaw's Textbook of Gynaecology 15th Edition*

    Explanation:

WHO Classification of Ovarian Tumours

I	**Common epithelial tumours:** • Serous tumours • Mucinous tumours • Endometrioid tumours • Clear cell (mesonephroid tumours) • Brenner tumours • Mixed epithelial tumours • Undifferentiated carcinoma • Unclassified epithelial tumours
II	**Sex cord (gonadal stromal) tumours:** • Granulosa-stromal cell tumours, theca cell tumours • Androblastomas: Sertoli-Leydig cell tumours • Gynandroblastomas • Unclassified
III	**Lipid (lipoid) cell tumours**
IV	**Germ cell tumours:** • Dysgerminoma • Endodermal sinus tumour (Yolk sac tumor) • Embryonal carcinoma • Polyembryoma • Choriocarcinoma • Teratoma • Mixed forms
V	**Gonadoblastoma:** • Pure • Mixed with dysgerminoma or other germ cell tumours
VI	**Soft tissue tumours not specific to ovary**
VII	**Unclassified tumours**
VIII	**Secondary (metastatic) tumours**
IX	**Tumour-like conditions**

Classification of Sex Cord-Gonadal Stromal Tumours by Their Histology

		Cell/tissue normal location		
		Ovary (Female)	**Testicle (Male)**	**Mixed**
Cell/tissue type	**Sex cord**	Granulosa cell tumour	Sertoli cell tumour	Gynandroblas-toma
	Gonadal stroma	Thecoma, fibroma	Leydig cell tumour	Gynandroblas-toma
	Mixed		Sertoli-Leydig cell tumour	Gynandroblas-toma

PAEDIATRICS

1. **Least useful anti-rachitic:**
   A. 1, 25-hydroxy cholecalciferol (calcitriol)
   B. Cholecalciferol
   C. 25-hydroxy cholecalciferol
   D. Calcium

   Ans: B. Cholecalciferol **or D.** Calcium

   Ref: *Nelson's Textbook of Pediatrics. 19th Edition and CRC Desk Reference for Nutrition, Second Edition, By Carolyn D. Berdanier*

   Explanation:

   Sorry, I am not sure of the answer since I could not find the source or references for this question.
   "Nutrients that are required for normal bone growth and developement. Vitamin C, Vitamin D and minerals (Calcium, phosphorous, magnesium, manganese, pottassium . These nutrients are called Antirachitic because they prevent the development of rickets.") *Ref: CRC Desk*

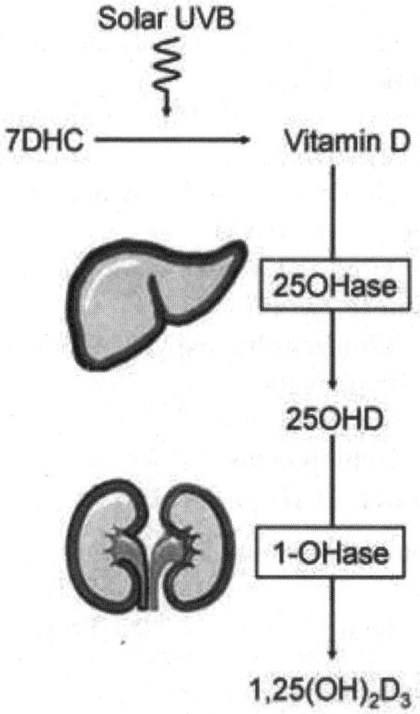

Vitamin D Production

2. **Sub periosteal hemorrhage is seen in: (Repeat)**
   A. Vit C deficiency **B.** Vit A deficiency
   C. Vit E deficiency **D.** Vit B2 deficiency

   Ans: A. Vitamin C deficiency

   Ref: *Nelson's Textbook of Pediatrics. 19th Edition, Page 198*

   Explanation:

   Radiographic Changes in Scurvy

- The typical radiographic changes occur at the distal ends of the long bones and are particularly common at the knees.
- The shafts of the long bones have a **ground-glass appearance** due to trabecular atrophy.
- The cortex is thin and dense, giving the appearance of pencil outlining of the diaphysis and epiphysis (**Pencil thin cortex**).
- **The white line of Fränkel**, an irregular but thickened white line at the metaphysis, represents the zone of well-calcified cartilage.
- The epiphyseal centers of ossification also have a **ground-glass appearance** and are surrounded by a sclerotic ring.
- The more specific but late radiologic feature of scurvy is a zone of rarefaction under the white line at the metaphysis. This zone of rarefaction (**Trumerfeld zone**), a linear break in the bone that is proximal and parallel to the white line, represents area of debris of broken-down bone trabeculae and connective tissue.
- A **Pelkan spur** is a lateral prolongation of the white line and may be present at cortical ends. Epiphyseal separation can occur along the line of destruction, with either linear displacement or compression of the epiphysis against the shaft.
- **Subperiosteal hemorrhages** are not visible using plain radiographs during the active phase of scurvy. However, during healing the elevated periosteum becomes calcified and radiopaque, giving a **dumbbell or club shape** to the affected bone.

3. **Arnold chiari malformation is associated with:**

A. Meningomyelocoele
B. Leptomeningeal cyst
C. Agenesis of corpus callosum
D. Dandy-Walker anomaly

Ans: A. Meningomyelocoele

Ref: *Nelson's Textbook of Pediatrics. 19th Edition*

Explanation:

Arnold Chiari Malformation: Two major subgroups

Type I Chiari Malformation

- It typically produces symptoms during adolescence or adult life and is usually **not associated with hydrocephalus.**
- Patients complain of **recurrent headache, neck pain, urinary frequency**, and **progressive lower extremity spasticity.**
- The deformity consists of **displacement of the cerebellar tonsils into the cervical canal.**
- Although the pathogenesis is unknown, a prevailing theory suggests that obstruction of the caudal portion of the 4th ventricle during fetal development is responsible.
- Other theories include tethering of the cord or additional anomalies (**syrinx**).

The Type II Chiari Malformation

- It is characterized by **progressive hydrocephalus** with a **myelomeningocele.**
- This lesion represents a developmental anomaly of the **hindbrain.**
- Due to failure of pontine flexure during embryogenesis resulting in elongation of the 4th ventricle and kinking of the brainstem, with displacement of the inferior vermis, pons and medulla into the cervical canal.
- Approximately **10%** of type II malformations produce symptoms during infancy, consisting of stridor, weak cry, and apnea, which may be relieved by shunting or by decompression of the posterior fossa.
- A more indolent form consists of abnormalities of **gait**, spasticity, and increasing **incoordination** during childhood.

The Dandy-Walker Malformation

- It consists of a *cystic expansion of the 4th ventricle in the posterior fossa* and *midline cerebellar hypoplasia.*
- It results from a developmental failure of the roof of the 4th ventricle during embryogenesis Approximately *90%* of patients have *hydrocephalus*
- Associated anomalies include *agenesis of the posterior cerebellar vermis and corpus callosum.*
- Infants present with a rapid increase in head size and a prominent occiput.
- Transillumination of the skull may be positive.
- Most children have evidence of long-tract signs, cerebellar ataxia, and delayed motor and cognitive milestones, probably due to the associated structural anomalies.
- Shunting the cystic cavity (and on occasion the ventricles as well) in the presence of hydrocephalus.

4. **LBW is defined as birth weight less than: (Repeat)**

A. 2 kg **B.** 1 kg
C. 1.5 kg **D.** 2.5 kg

Ans: D. 2.5 kg

Ref: *Nelson's Textbook of Pediatrics. 19th Edition*

Explanation:

Some Important Definitions in Neonatology

- **Low birth weight**: Birth weight of less than 2.5 kg irrespective of gestational age
- **Very low birth weight:** Birth weight of less than 1.5 kg irrespective of gestational age
- **Extremely low birth weight:** Birth weight of less than 1.0 kg irrespective of gestational age
- **Neonatal:** First 28 days of postnatal life
- **Preterm:** Less than 37 completed weeks of gestations
- **Term:** After 37 completed weeks of gestations
- **Post term:** After 42 completed weeks of gestations
- **Past Dates:** After 40 completed weeks of gestations
- **Still birth:** Delivering dead fetus after 28 weeks of gestation. (Defn changes with country)
- **Abortion:** Expulsion of products of conception before 28 weeks of gestation.
- **Small for Gestational Age (SGA):** Weight below the 10th percentile for the gestational age
- **Large for Gestational Age (LGA):** Weight above the 90th percentile for the gestational age
- **Appropriate for Gestational Age (AGA):** Weight between 10th and 90th percentile for the gestational age

5. **Alkaline phosphatase level are not elevated in:**
   A. Renal rickets
   B. Nutritional rickets
   C. Hypophosphatasia
   D. Hypophosphatemic rickets

Ans: C. Hypophosphatasia

Ref: *Nelson's Textbook of Pediatrics. 19th Edition*

Explanation:

(See the following table)

ADHR -Autosomal dominant hypophosphatemic rickets

Alk Phos - Alkaline phosphatase

ARHR- Autosomal recessive hypophosphatemic rickets

HHRH- Hereditary hypophosphatemic rickets with hypercalciuria

VDDR- Vitamin D–dependent rickets; XLH, X-linked hypophosphatemic rickets

Hypophosphatasia

- It is defined by **low serum alkaline phosphatase activity**
- This condition **radiographically** resembles **rickets**.
- Autosomal recessive disorder
- Affects mainly the **skeleton** and **teeth**
- Inborn error of metabolism in which activity of the **tissue-nonspecific (liver, bone, kidney)** alkaline phosphatase isoenzyme (TNSALP) is deficient, although activity of the ***intestinal and placental isoenzymes is normal.***
- Some cases appear at **birth**, and diagnosis has even been made **in utero** by **radiographic** examination of a fetus.
- There are 3 different presentations:
  - Lethal neonatal or perinatal form (**Congenital lethal hypophosphatasia**)
  - Severe infantile form
  - Milder form occurring in childhood or late adolescence (**Hypophosphatasia tarda**)

Laboratory Fingings in Disorders Causing Rickets

Disorder	Ca	Pi	PTH	25-(OH) D	1,25-$(OH)_2D$	ALK Phos	Urine Ca	Urine Pi
Vitamin D deficiency	N, ↓	↓	↑	↓	↓, N, ↑	↑	↓	↑
VDDR, type 1	N, ↓	↓	↑	N	↓	↑	↓	↑
VDDR, type 2	N, ↓	↓	↑	N	↑↑	↑	↓	↑
Chronic renal failure	N, ↓	↑	↑	N	↓	↑	N, ↓	↓
Dietary Pi deficiency	N	↓	N, ↓	N	↑	↑	↑	↓
XLH	N	↓	N	N	RD	↑	↓	↑
ADHR	N	↓	N	N	RD	↑	↓	↑
HHRH	N	↓	N, ↓	N	RD	↑	↑	↑
ARHR	N	↓	N	N	RD	↑	↓	↑
Tumor-induced rickets	N	↓	N	N	RD	↑	↓	↑
Fanconi syndrome	N	↓	N	N	RD or ↑	↑	↓ or ↑	↑
Dietary Ca deficiency	N, ↓	↓	↑	N	↑	↑	↓	↑

- The lethal form is characterized by a **moth-eaten appearance** at the **ends of the long bones**, severe **deficiency of ossification throughout the skeleton**, and **marked shortening of the long bones.**
- Patients with mild disease can present with **bowing of the legs** and **variable statural shortening**.
- **Hypercalcemia** is common in the neonatal and infantile forms, and because calcium accumulation by mature chondrocytes does not occur, patients might appear to have rickets.

6. **Suture of skull fuse by:**

   A. 5 years **B.** 1 year
   C. 3 years **D.** 8 years

   Ans: C. 3 years

Ref: *Nelson's Textbook of Pediatrics. 19th Edition. http://www.nlm.nih.gov/medlineplus/ency/article/cranial sutures and Cunningham ML, Heike CL (December 2007). "Evaluation of the infant with an abnormal skull shape". Curr. Opin. Pediatr. 19 (6): 645–51*

Explanation:

Sutures of skull fuse by **22-39 months**. So, **3 years** is the nearest answer.

The infant's skull consists of the:

- **Metopic suture**
- **Coronal sutures**
- **Sagittal suture and**
- **Lambdoid suture**

The **Metopic suture** is supposed to close between **3-9 months** of age.

The **lambdoid, sagittal** and **coronal** sutures are supposed to close between **22 to 39 months** of age.

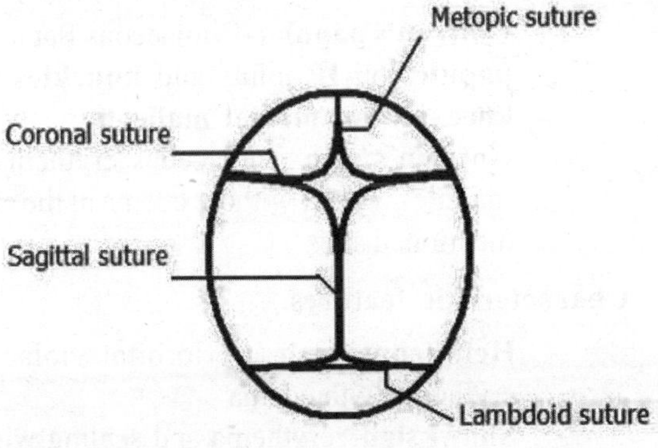

An infant's skull is made up of six separate cranial bones:

- The frontal bone,
- The occipital bone,
- Two parietal bones; and
- Two temporal bones

Important Aspects of Skull Bones, Fontanelle and Growth

- These bones are held together by strong, fibrous, elastic tissues called cranial sutures.
- The spaces between the bones where the sutures are (sometimes known as "**soft spots**") are called **fontanelles**. They are a part of normal development.
- The cranial bones remain separate for about **22-39 months**.
- They then grow together (fuse) as part of normal growth.
- They stay fused throughout adulthood.
- The **posterior fontanelle** (in the back of the head) usually closes by the time an infant is 1 or 2 months old, or may already be closed at birth.
- The **anterior fontanelle** (at the top of the head) usually closes sometime between 9 months and 18 months.
- The sutures and fontanelles are needed for the infant's brain growth and development.
- During childbirth, the flexibility of the fibers allows the bones to overlap so the head can pass through the birth canal without pressing on and damaging the infant's brain.
- During infancy and childhood, the fibers are flexible.
- This allows the brain to grow quickly and protects the brain from minor impacts to the head (such as when the infant is learning to hold his head up, roll over and sit up).
- **Bulging fontanelles** may be a sign of **increased pressure** within the brain.

7. **Incubation period of pertussis is:**

   A. Three days **B.** Three weeks
   C. Two weeks **D.** Four weeks

   Ans: C. Two weeks

   Ref: *Nelson Textbook of Pediatrics, 19th edition*

Explanation:

Pertussis (Whooping cough)

- Caused by Bordetella pertussis.
- Has 3 clinical stages, catarrhal, paroxysmal and convalescent stages.
- The **catarrhal stage** (1-2 wk) begins insidiously after an **incubation period ranging from 3-12 days** with non-distinctive symptoms of congestion and rhinorrhea variably accompanied by low-grade fever, sneezing, lacrimation and conjunctival suffusion.

- As initial symptoms wane, coughing marks the onset of the **paroxysmal stage** (2-6 wk).
- The cough begins as a dry, intermittent, irritative hack and evolves into the inexorable paroxysms that are the hallmark of pertussis.
- **Post-tussive emesis** is common, and exhaustion is universal.
- The number and severity of paroxysms escalate over days to a week and remain at that plateau for days to weeks.
- At the peak of the paroxysmal stage, patients may have more than 1 episode hourly.
- As the paroxysmal stage fades into the **convalescent stage** ($\geq$2 wk), the number, severity, and duration of episodes diminish.
- **Infants <3 mo of age** do not display the classic stages.
- The catarrhal phase lasts only a few days or is unnoticed, and then, after the most insignificant startle from a draft, light, sound, sucking, or stretching, a well-appearing young infant begins to **choke, gasp, gag, and flail the extremities**, with face **reddened**.
- **Cough may not be prominent**, especially in the early phase.
- **Whoop** infrequently occurs in infants <3 mo of age who at the end of a paroxysm lack stature or muscular strength to create sudden negative intrathoracic pressure.
- **Apnea** and **cyanosis** can follow a coughing paroxysm, or apnea can occur without a cough. Apnea may be the only symptom.
- **Apnea** and **cyanosis** both are more common with **pertussis** than with neonatal viral infections, including respiratory syncytial virus (**RSV**).
- The paroxysmal and convalescent stages in young infants are lengthy.
- Paradoxically, in infants, cough and whooping may become **louder** and **more classic** in **convalescence**.
- Convalescence includes intermittent paroxysmal coughing throughout the 1st yr of life, including "exacerbations" with subsequent respiratory illnesses; these are not due to recurrent infection or reactivation of *B. pertussis*.
- **Adolescents** and previously immunized children have foreshortening of all stages of pertussis.
- Adults have **no distinct stages**.
- Classically, adolescents and adults describe a sudden feeling of **strangulation** followed by **uninterrupted coughs, feeling of suffocation**, bursting headache, diminished awareness, and then a gasping breath, usually without a whoop.
- **Post-tussive emesis** and intermittency of paroxysms separated by hours of well-being are specific clues to the diagnosis in adolescents and adults.
- At least 30% of older individuals with pertussis have nonspecific cough illness, distinguished only by duration, which is usually >21 days.
- Signs of lower respiratory tract disease are not expected unless complicating secondary bacterial pneumonia is present.
- **Conjunctival hemorrhages** and petechiae on the upper body are common.

DERMATOLOGY

1. Gottron's papules are seen in:

A. Dermatomyositis
B. Scleroderma
C. Mixed connective tissue disorder
D. Pemphigus vulgaris

Ans: A. Dermatomyositis

Reference: *Connective Tissue Disorders. In: Thappa DM, editor. Essentials in Dermatology, 2nd edn. NewDelhi: Jaypee; 134-47*

Explanation:

DERMATOMYOSITIS

- Connective tissue disorder characterized by **inflammatory myositis** presenting with **proximal muscle weakness** and **cutaneous** manifestations in the form of:

Pathognomonic features:

- **Gottron's papules** – violaceous flat topped **papules** on **IP** joints and **knuckles**; also **knee, elbow, medial malleoli**
- **Gottron's sign**– violaceous erythematous **macules** with or without edema at the above mentioned sites

Characteristic features:

- **Heliotrope rash**– periorbital violaceous erythema with edema
- **Shawl sign**– erythema and scaling with or without poikiloderma over shoulder region
- **Periungual telangiectasia** and dystrophic cuticles
- **Mechanic's hands**– hyperkeratosis, scaling, fissuring and hyperpigmentation over fing-ertips, sides of thumbs and fingers

Compatible features:

- ***Calcinosis cutis***
- ***Poikilodermaa trophicans vasculare***

2. Dennie-Morgan fold is seen in:

A. Atopic dermatitis **B.** Seborrheic dermatitis
C. Contact dermatitis **D.** Dermatomyositis

Ans: A. Atopic dermatitis

Reference: *Thappa DM, editor. Essentials in Dermatology, 2nd edn. NewDelhi: Jaypee*

Explanation:

ATOPIC DERMATITIS

- **Chronic or relapsing dermatitis** characterized by severe pruritus with age at onset between 2-6 months and associated with personal or family history of atopy (asthma, allergic rhino-conjunctivitis, atopic dermatitis)
- Itch that rashes
- **Infants – face, scalp, extensor** of extremities, **trunk**
- **Children** – flexural surface like neck, cubital or popliteal fossa, wrists, ankles
- **Adolescents** and adults – lichenification of **flexures** and **hands**

Hanifin and Rajka Criteria for Eczema Diagnosis

Major Findings (3 or more criteria)

- Pruritus
- Typical morphology and distribution (Flexural lichenification or linearity in adults; facial and extensor involvement – infants and children)
- Chronic relapsing dermatitis
- Personal or family history of eczema

Minor Findings (3 or more criteria)

- Xerosis
- Ichthyosis
- **Palmar hyperlinearity**
- Keratosis pilaris
- Type 1 skin test reactivity
- Elevated IgE levels
- Nipple eczema
- Cheilitis
- Recurrent conjunctivitis
- **Dennie Morgan infraorbital fold**
- **Keratoconus**
- **Anterior subcapsular cataracts**
- Orbital darkening
- Pityriasis alba
- Facial pallor
- Anterior neck folds
- **White dermographism**

3. Herpes zoster patient should be isolated for:

A. 6 days **B.** 3 days
C. 9 days **D.** 12 days

Ans: A. 6 days

Reference: *Thappa DM, editor. Essentials in Dermatology, 2nd edn. NewDelhi: Jaypee. and Park, Preventive and Social Medicine, 28 edn.*

Explanation:

"The period of communicability of patients with varicella is estimated to range from 1 to 2 days before the appearance of rash, and 4-5 days thereafter."
Ref: Park

HERPES ZOSTER (Shingles)

Clinical Features

- More than 2/3rd of patients are above 50 years
- Pain and paraesthesia in the involved dermatome
- The rash is always unilateral
- It begins as closely grouped maculopapules, which rapidly becomes vesicular in 12-24 hours and then pustular in 2-3 days
- The lesions dry up and crust in 7 – 10 days
- Recovery takes about 3-4 weeks or longer
- The common sites of involvement
  - **Thoracic** -53% (**Most Common**)
  - Cervical- 20%
  - Trigeminal- 18%
  - Lumbosacral- 11%
- **Complications**
  - Hypopigmented and Hyperpigmented scars
  - Postherpeutic **Neuralgia**
  - Postherpetic **Anesthesia**
  - Recurrent Zoster
  - **Motor neuron involvement**
  - **Ocular involvement** – Keratitis; Corneal ulcerations, Panopthalmitis, Ocular palsies, Retinal vasculitis and optic neuritis
  - Meningitis
  - Pneumonitis
  - Myelitis

Diagnosis

- **Tzanck smears – Multinucleated giant cells** and epithelial cells with typical acidophilic intranuclear inclusions.

Treatment

- Symptomatic treatment in healthy uncomplicated cases

- Acyclovir- severe zoster (Opthalmic zoster and Ramsay hunt syndrome)

4. **Koilonychia is seen in: (Repeat)**
   A. Iron deficiency anaemia **B.** Hypoalbuminemia
   C. Lead poisoning **D.** Psoriasis

   Ans: A. Iron deficiency anemia

   Reference: *Thappa DM, editor. Essentials in Dermatology, 2nd edn. New Delhi: Jaypee*

   Explanation:

   (See the following table)

5. **Stevens-Johnson syndrome is caused by:**
   A. Herpes simplex **B.** CMV
   C. Chicken pox **D.** Toxoplasma

   Ans: A. Herpes simplex

   Reference: *Thappa DM, editor. Essentials in Dermatology, 2nd edn. NewDelhi: Jaypee*

Explanation: *(See the following table)*

Stevens-Johnson Syndrome (SJS)

- ***Drug induced SJS***
  - Phenytoin
  - Phenobarbitone
  - Sulfonamides
  - Penicillins
  - NSAIDS
- ***Viral Causes***
  - Herpes simplex virus (**Most Common** cause)
  - AIDS
  - Coxsackievirus
  - Viral infections
  - Influenza
  - Hepatitis
  - Mumps
- ***Bacterial causes***
  - Group A beta-hemolytic streptococci

Nail Abnormalities

Nail abnormality	Description	Causes
Koilonychia	Reverse curvature in the longtitudinal and transverse axis	Iron deficiency anemia
Macronychia/Micronychia	Too small or large nails	—
Onycholysis	Distal or lateral separation of the nail from nail bed	Psoriasis, Onychomycosis
Pterygium	Central fibrotic tongue like band from proximal nail fold joins the nail bed dividing the nail proximally into two	Lichen planus
Subungual hyperkeratosis	Excessive collection of squamous debris under the free edge of nail	Psoriasis Onychomycosis
Onychogryphosis	Nail get thickened and grows upwards in a spiral manner	Chronic trauma
Pachynychia congenita	Hypertrophy of nails associated with nail bed and hyponychial hyperkeratosis	—
Beau's lines	Transverse grooves on nails	Temporary cessation of nail formation Chemotherapy Hypocalcemia Nail infection Coronary occlusion Malnutrition
Terry's nail	Nail is white proximally but normal distally	Congestive cardiac failure Cirrhosis Diabetes mellitus
Pitting	Punctate erosions on nail surface	Psoriasis Alopecia areata
Red Lunulae	Nails show erythema of lunula	Psoriasis (Dotted red lunula) Congestive cardiac failure CirrhosisSLE
Splinter hemorrhages	Longtitudinal hemorrhages in nail bed	Psoriasis Dermatitis Fungal infections Infective endocarditis SLE Mycosis fungoides Rheumatoid arthritis
Mees lines	Whitening or discoloration of the nail in bands or "stria" that run parallel the lunula (nail base)	Cirrhosis Chemotherapy Heavy metal poisoning (Arsenic, Thallium) Trauma
Muehrcke's nails	White lines (leukonychia) that extend all the way across the nail and lie parallel to the lunula (half moon)	Non-specific Assc with decreased protein synthesis Hypoalbuminemia Nephrotic syndrome

- Diphtheria
- Brucellosis
- Lymphogranuloma venereum
- Mycobacteria
- Mycoplasma pneumoniae
- Ricketsial infections
- Tularemia

- It is common in **children** and **young adults**
- The disease is preceded by a nonspecific prodrome with **fever**, **myalgia**, **rhinitis** and **cough**
- Skin lesions occur abruptly and are **purpuric macules**, **atypical target lesions** and **papules**
- **Bullous lesions** may occur in **oral**, **genital** and **anal** mucosa
- **Ulcerative stomatitis** with hemorrhagic crusting is the most characteristic feature
- **Corneal erosions** may lead to **symblepharan**, **synechiae** and **opacities**
- Constitutional symptoms may be severe during active stages
- The treatment includes supportive care and steroids.

SJS Vs TEN

- **SJS** – Mucosal erosions and epidermal detachment **below 10%**
- **Toxic epidermal necrolysis (TEN)**– Mucosal erosions and epidermal detachment **more than 30%**

6. Exfoliative dermatitis is seen in:

A. Eczema
B. Epidermolysis bullosa
C. Dermatitis herpetiformis
D. Vitiligo

Ans: A. Eczema

Reference: *Thappa DM, editor. Essentials in Dermatology, 2nd edn. NewDelhi: Jaypee*

Explanation:

Erythroderma

- Also known as **Exfoliative dermatitis**, **Dermatitis exfoliativa** and **Red man syndrome**
- It is an inflammatory skin disease with erythema and scaling that affects nearly the entire cutaneous body surface area (usually **> 90%)**
- **Common causes are:**
  - Idiopathic
  - Drug allergy
  - Seborrheic dermatitis
  - Contact dermatitis
  - Atopic dermatitis (Eczema)
  - Lymphoma and leukemia
  - Psoriasis
  - Dermatomyositis
  - Lichen planus
- **Drug induced**
  - Phenytoin
  - Carbamazepine
  - Cimetidine
  - Lithium
  - Gold
  - Chloroquine
  - Isoniazid
  - Mercury
- **Sezary syndrome** – Erythroderma, general lymphadenopathy and atypical cells in peripheral smear (>10%)

7. Typical lesion in hard chancre is:

A. Painless and indurated
B. Painful and indurated
C. Painless and non-indurated
D. Painful and non-indurated

Ans: A. Painless and indurated

Ref: *Thappa DM, editor. Essentials in Dermatology, 2nd edn. NewDelhi: Jaypee*

Explanation:

Primary Syphilis

- **Painless chancre** (Primary Chancre/Hunterian Chancre/Hard Chancre)
- Typical chancre is round or oval ulcer, 1-2 cm across, has indurated margin, clear base and without any exudate
- Moderate enlargement of inguinal lymph nodes
- Nontender, nonsuppurative, **firm**, shotty (**Indolent bubo**)
- Relapse of primary syphilis extremely rare **(Chancre Redux)**

Secondary Syphilis

- Lesions are due to hematogeneous dissemination of treponomes
- Flu like symptoms - malaise, loss of appetite, fever, headache, stiff neck, myalgia and arthralgia
- Skin manifestation are termed as **'Syphilids'**, are asymptomatic, polymorphous, variegate, bilateral and symmetrical
- Evanescent macular rash involving entire trunk, extremities and palms and soles
- Papular lesions demonstrate **ollendor fsign**
- Even nodules may appear; They may be pustular but **never vesicular**
- **Condylomata lata:** The moist, smooth surfaced warty intertriginous plaques (Most Infectious Lesion)

- Generalised lymphadenopathy: especially epitrochlear lymph nodes
- **'Moth eaten alopecia'** in scalp

Tertiary Syphilis

- Gummatous: Non tender, pink to dusky red nodules or plaques that vary in size
- Cardiovascular and neurosyphilis

8. **Apple jelly nodules on diascopy is seen in:**
 A. Lupus vulgaris **B.** Tinea versicolor
 C. Erythrasma **D.** Vitiligo

Ans: A. Lupus vulgaris

Ref: *Principles of Diagnosis in Dermatology. In: Thappa DM, editor. Essentials in Dermatology, 2nd edn., New Delhi:Jaypee Brothers Medical Publishers (P) Ltd 2009;16-30*

Explanation:

Lupus Vulgaris

- It is a type of **progressive cutaneous tuberculosis**
- Occurs in people with moderate to high immunity
- **Single plaque** composed of grouped **redbrown papules** with peripheral extension on one side and scarring on the otherside.
- On diascopy of active edge-translucent **pale brownish yellow or apple jelly colour** in the periphery–**apple jelly nodules**– **granulomatous nodules**
- **Diascopy/vitropression**:
  - Compression with a glass slide
  - Differentiating **purpura** (no blanching) from **erythema** (blanches)
  - Differentiating **nevus anemicus** (margins blurred) from **nevus depigmentosus** (no change)

ANAESTHESIOLOGY

1. **Which of the following agents can be safely used in asthma? (Repeat)**
 A. Thiopentone **B.** Ketamine
 C. Etomidate **D.** Propofol

Ans: B. Ketamine

Ref: *Miller's Anesthesia, 7th edn. & Ajay Yadav*

Explanation:

Ketamine

- Causes **Dissociative anesthesia**
- Phencyclidine derivative
- **NMDA receptor agonist**
- **Anesthetic properties**
  - Onset of Action: 30 – 60 seconds
  - Early regain of consciousness after 15–20 min due to **Redistribution**
  - Elimination half life: 2-3 hours
  - **Strong analgesic property**
  - Metabolised in **Liver** and products excreted in **urine**
  - Not a muscle relaxant
- Primary site of action – **Thalamo-neo-cortical projections**

Cardiovascular system

- Increases arterial BP
- Increases heart rate and
- Increases cardiac output
- IV agent of choice in **Shock**

Respiratory system

- **Potent bronchodilator**
- Good induction agent for asthmatics
- **Upper airway reflexes remain largely intact**
- Increases salivatory and tracheo bronchial secretions
- Using glycopyrollate or atropine becomes necessary

Central Nervous system

- **Increases intracranial pressure** and can precipitate **seizures**
- **Emergence reactions:**
  - These are seen at emergence
  - Vivid dreaming
  - Illusions
  - Extracorporeal experiences like floating
  - Excitement
  - Confusión
  - Euphoria
  - Fear
- **Hallucinations:**
  - Auditory and visual hallucinations (Most Common side effect of ketamine)
  - Treated with benzodiazepine

Other Systems

- **Eye**:
  - Increase intraocular tensión
  - Pupils dilate moderately
  - Nystagmus
- **GIT**
  - Increases intragastric pressure
  - Salivary secretions increased
- **Muscluar**
  - Increases muscle tone
  - Increased non-puposeful movements

Dose

Can be given IV, IM, oral, rectal and intrathecal route
IV – 2 mg/kg
IM- 5-10 mg/kg

Advantages

- **Induction agent of choice in:**
  - Asthmatics
  - Shock **(HYPOTENSION)**
  - Children (Now Sevoflurance is DOC)
  - Constrictive pericarditis
  - Cardiac tamponade
- Can be used as **Sole** agent
- Can be used safely at remote places and in inexperienced hands since does not depress heart or respiration
- Preferred agent when patient is in **Full Stomach** (Preserves laryngo-pharyngeal reflexes)

Contraindicated in:

- Head injury
- ICSOL
- Eye injury
- Opthal pathology
- Ischemic heart disease
- Vascular aneurysm
- Psychiatric diseases
- Drug addicts
- Hypertensives

2. **Which anaesthetic agent does not affect blood flow to liver?**

   A. Halothane **B.** Isoflurane
   C. Enflurane **D.** Sevoflurane

Ans: D. Sevoflurane

Ref: *Miller's Anesthesia, 7th ed.*

Explanation:

*"All volatile anesthetics decrease hepatic blood flow, but **desflurane** and **sevoflurane** have the least significant effect on total hepatic blood flow and hepatic oxygen delivery, whereas halothane induces the most profound reductions in hepatic blood flow."* *(Ref: Miller)*

Effects of Anesthesia on Liver Blood Flow

- All anesthetics and techniques that decrease cardiac output produce at least proportional decrements in total hepatic blood flow.
- In addition, some anesthetics have more specific effects on hepatic blood flow that either mitigate or accentuate these changes.
- **Halothane** anesthesia usually **decreases** hepatic blood flow to a greater extent.
- **Isoflurane increases** hepatic artery blood flow.
- **Regional anesthesia** may **decrease** hepatic blood flow.
- The extent to which subarachnoid block decreases hepatic blood flow depends on the level of the block.
- A **T4 level** of anesthesia results in a **20%** reduction in liver blood flow, which closely parallels the decrease in systemic blood pressure.

3. **Post operative shivering is treated with:**

   A. Diazepam **B.** Antihistaminics
   C. Anticholinergics **D.** Pethidine

Ans: D. Pethidine

Ref: *Miller's Anesthesia, 7th edn. and Internet*

Explanation:

Post Operative Shivering

- It is commonly seen (incidence - 3.5%) due to fall in core temperature.
- Risk factors as:
  - Age > 6 years
  - Prolonged duration of surgery
  - Use of an intravenous induction agent
- It is also commonly seen after **halothane** anaesthesia.
- Intravenous **pethidine** (0.35 - 0.5 mg/kg) and **clonidine** (1.5 mcg/kg) has been widely studied in adults. Therefore, it has become most recommended treatment options in children.
- A single intravenous dose of **dexmedetomidine** (0.5 mcg/kg) has been found to be as effective as pethidine in controlling shivering.
- **Oxygen therapy** and **forced air warming** of the child.

RADIODIAGNOSIS AND RADIOTHERAPY

1. **Investigation of choice in subarachnoid hemorrhage:**

   A. Noncontrast CT **B.** Contrast CT
   C. MRI **D.** Lumbar puncture

Ans: D>A

Ref: *Harrison's Principles of Internal Medicine, 18th ed.*

Explanation:

Investigation for Subarachnoid Hemorrhage

- The hallmark of **aneurysmal rupture** is **'blood in the CSF'**.

- More than **95%** of cases have enough blood to be visualized on a high-quality **noncontrast CT** scan obtained **within 72 h.**
- If the scan fails to establish the diagnosis of SAH and no mass lesion or obstructive hydrocephalus is found, a **lumbar puncture** should be performed to establish the presence of subarachnoid blood.
- Lysis of the red blood cells and subsequent conversion of hemoglobin to **bilirubin** stains the **spinal fluid yellow** within **6–12 h.**
- This **xanthochromic spinal fluid** peaks in intensity at **48 h** and **lasts for 1–4 weeks**, depending on the amount of subarachnoid blood.

2. **Following is used in PET scan:**
   A. FDG **B.** DTPA
   C. MAG-3 **D.** I ^{131}

   Ans: **A.** FDG

Ref: Radiology by Wolfgang Dahnert 5th ed; pg 1113

Explanation:

*"**Fluorine-18 Fluorodeoxyglucose (FDG)** is the most common positron-labeled radiotracer in positron emission tomography (**PET**). In most tissues, including cancer, there is little phosphatase activity. The intracellular metabolite, FDG-6-phosphate cannot undergo further conversions and is therefore trapped inside the cell. FDG is useful in staging and metastasis of Renal cell cancer by PET."*

(Ref: Wolfgang)

Positron Emission Tomography (PET)

- It is a nuclear medicine imaging technique that produces a three-dimensional image or picture of functional processes in the body.
- The system detects **pairs of gamma rays** emitted indirectly by a **positron-emitting radionuclide (tracer)**, which is introduced into the body on a biologically active molecule. Three-dimensional images of tracer concentration within the body are then constructed by computer analysis. In modern scanners, three dimensional imaging is often accomplished with the aid of a CT X-ray scan performed on the patient during the same session, in the same machine.
- If the biologically active molecule chosen for PET is **FDG**, an analogue of **glucose**, the concentrations of tracer imaged then give tissue metabolic activity, in terms of regional glucose uptake.
- The electron-positron **decays** result in **two 511 keV gamma photons** being emitted at almost **180 degrees** to each other; hence, it is possible to localize their source along a **straight line of coincidence** (also called the **line of response**, or **LOR**).
- A **collimator** is a device that narrows a beam of particles or waves. Lead collimators are used in X-rays and linear accelerators.

3. **Rotting fence post appearance of femur is seen in:**
   A. Fibrous dysplasia
   B. Hyper parathyroidism
   C. Pagets disease
   D. Fracture neck of femur

   Ans: **B.** Hyperparathyroidism

Ref: *Harrison's Principles of Internal Medicine, 18th ed. and Internet Source*

Explanation:

Renal Osteodystrophy

- CRF leading on to hyperparathyroidism
- **Signs of chronic renal failure**
  - Findings of osteomalacia
  - Hyperparathyroidism
  - Bone sclerosis
- **Rugger jersey spine**
- **Rotting fence post appearance**: Due to Rickets + Hyperparathyroidism
- In children, **metaphyseal** changes resembling rickets are seen, which together with **cortical** erosions can give rise to the so-called 'rotting fence-post' appearance, particularly at the **femoral neck.**
- **Looser's zone**

4. **Mega voltage therapy consists of:**
   A. Greater than 1000 k volts **B.** 500-1000
   C. Less than 500 **D.** More than 2000

   Ans: **A.** Greater than 1000 k volts

Ref: *Internet source*

Explanation:

- **Megavoltage X-rays** are produced by **linear accelerators**
- Operates at voltages in excess of **1000 kV (1 MV) range**, and therefore have an energy in the **MeV range**
- Beams with the voltage range of **4-25 MV** are used to treat patients because they penetrate well to deep sites within the body.

5. **T_D 50 for kidney is:**
   A. 2000 cGy **B.** 3000 cGy
   C. 2800 cGy **D.** 2400 cGy

   Ans: **C.** 2800 cGy

Ref: Emami B, Lyman J, Brown A, Coia L, Goitein M, Munzenrider JE et al.Tolerance of Normal tissue to therapeutic Irradiation. Int J Radiat Oncol Biol Phys. 1991 May 15;21(1):109-22

Explanation:

- What is **TD 5/5**? (Also known as **T_D5)**
  Tolerance dose that within 5 years will cause a minimal 5% complication rate (**Acceptable**)
- What is TD 50/5? (Also known as **T_D50)**
  Tolerance dose that within 5 years will cause a maximal 50% complication rate (**Unacceptable**)

Normal Whole Organ Tissue Tolerances (cGy)

Organ	TD 5/5 Whole	TD 50/5 Whole
Bladder	6500	8000
Brain	4500	6000
Colon	4500	5500
Esophagus (stricture,perforation)	5500	6800
Femoral head	5200	6500
Heart (pericarditis)	4000	5000
Kidney	**2300**	**2800**
Larynx (edema)	4500	8000
Liver	3000	4000
Lung	1750	2450
Parotid gland	3200	4600
Rectum (severe proctitis, necrosis, fistula, stenosis)	6000	8000
Retina	4500	6500
Skin	(100 cm^2) 5000	(100 cm^2) 6500
Spinal cord	(20 cm) 4700	–
Small intestine (obstruction, perforation)	4000	5500
Stomach (ulceration, perforation)	5000	6500
Thyroid	4500	8000

6. **Which technetium is most commonly used in bone pathology? (Repeat)**
   A. 99m Tc MDP
   B. 99mTc Sestamibi
   C. 99m Tc Exametazime
   D. 99m Tc Pyrophosphate

Ans: A. 99m Tc MDP

Ref: *Bracco, Kit for the Preparation of Technetium Tc 99m Medronate. 2006, Bracco Diagnostics Inc.: Princeton, NJ 08543.*

Also Refer 2011 Radiology section; Question on Radioisotopes.

Explanation:

Technetium (99mTc) medronic acid is a pharmaceutical product used in nuclear medicine to localize **bone metastases** as well as other diseases that can alter the normal osteogenesis in bone.

99mTc-medronate

- Aka 99mTc-methylene diphosphonate, or 99mTc-MDP
- FDA approved imaging agent to investigate **extra-skeletal osteogenesis (Metastasis)**

7. **Half life of I 131 is: (Repeat)**
   A. 13 days **B.** 8 days
   C. 2 days **D.** 12 hours

Ans: B. 8 days

Ref: *Internet Source*

Explanation:

Refer JIPMER 2012 Radiology.

PSYCHIATRY

1. **Catatonia is most commonly seen in:**
   A. Dementia
   B. Schizophrenia
   C. Depression
   D. Dissociative disorder

Ans: C. Depression

Reference: *Kaplan & Sadock's Synopsis of Psychiatry. 10th edition*

Explanation:

CATATONIA

It is a syndrome characterized by the following "set" of signs and symptoms:

- Stupor / excitement
- Mutism
- Rigidity / posturing
- Waxy flexibility
  – Catatonia has several causes as listed in the options, but the most common cause is **organic**, followed by **mood disorders** like **depression.** (Note– Though dementia is an organic syndrome, it accounts least for the occurrence of catatonia)

Causes of Catatonia:

1. **Organic (where oculo-vestibular reflex is absent, doll's eye movements present and abnormal EEG)**

- Stroke (Pons)
- Tumors (midline)
- Herpes simplex infection

2. **Functional (Opposite of organic)**
- Depression
- Schizophrenia.

Differential Diagnosis
- Coma
- Conversion/Dissociative disorders
- Malingering.

Key features that differentiate **psychotic vs mood disorder** presenting with **catatonia**:

Schizophrenia spectrum	Mood disorder spectrum
Affect-apathy Catalepsy Stereotypy	Depressed affect Reactive to emotional stimuli

- Catatonia – was coined by "Kahlbaum"
- Psychological pillow is one of classical features of catatonia
- Drug of choice- **Lorazapam**
- Treatment of choice- **ECT**.

2. **The following has least anti-cholinergic side effects:**

A. Clomipramine **B.** Desipramine
C. Imipramine **D.** Trimipranine

Ans: B. Desipramine

Ref: *Kaplan & Sadock's Synopsis of Psychiatry. 10th edition. P.1109 and Kishore-Kumar R et al. Desipramine relieves postherpetic neuralgia. Clin Pharmacol Ther. 1990 Mar;47(3):305-12*

Explanation:

"Desipramine has the least anticholinergic and sedative effects of the tricyclic anti-depressant agents."

All are tricyclic amine used to treat
- Depression (Unipolar, NOT Bipolar since the risk of 'switch' is high)
- OCD (Clomipramine)
- Pain syndromes (Amitriptaline)
- Nocturnal enuresis (Imipramine)
- Acid peptic disease (Doxipin)

Mechanism of action: They block the transporter proteins of Nor-epinephrine and Serotonin, thereby elevating the level of both at synaptic cleft → enhanced activity of these neurotransmitters → mood elevation/reduction of anxiety.

Side-Effects are:

Anticholinergic Side-Effects
- Dry mouth
- Tachycardia
- ↑ QT interval
- Heart block
- Constipation
- Precipitation of angle-closure glaucoma
- Orthostatic hypotension

The other drugs related to them are:
- **Tetracyclics**-Amoxapine, Mirtazapine, Mianserine
- **Monoamine oxidase inhibitors (MAOIs)**

1. Irreversible monoamine oxidase inhibitors: Selegiline, Tranycypromine
2. Reversible monoamine oxidase inhibitors: Moclobemide, Pirlindole

3. **Systematic desensitization is:**

A. Passive avoidance **B.** Active avoidance
C. Sudden exposure **D.** Graded exposure

Ans: D. Graded exposure

Ref: *Kaplan & Sadock's Synopsis of Psychiatry. 10th edition*

Explanation:

Systematic Desensitization

It is a type of '**Behavior therapy**' (which in turn is a type of **Psychotherapy**).
It is based on the principle of "**Respondent Conditioning**".
It was first elaborated by **Wolpe**.
It is used to treat 'Phobias' (Specific and Social).
It consists of three steps: [**HCG**-pneumonic]

1. **Hierarchy chart** (where anxiety/fear provoking stimuli are identified and charted from lowest to highest level of potency in inducing the anxiety/fear).
2. **Coping skills** (learning to relax by various methods like – paced breathing exercises, Jacobson's progressive muscle relaxation, applied relaxation by meditation).
3. **Graded exposure** (applying the relaxation techniques after exposing oneself to the anxiety/fear provoking stimuli in graded manner, i.e., from weakest stimulus to strongest stimulus).

Other Forms of Exposure Therapy

1. **Flooding**-sudden exposure and making one to cope up at one go.
2. **Virtual Reality Exposure** – useful for PTSD.
3. **ERP- Exposure and Response Prevention**– Unlike other exposure therapies, here, the escape is not allowed completely and even in between the sessions. Used in OCD.

Psychotherapy
- It is one of three forms of therapy (the other two are – chemical, i.e., drugs and physical, ie., ECT, Psychosurgery, VNS, rTMS).

- It involves patient–therapist co-operation and usually conducted in sessions.
- The following is an outline of psychotherapies practised worldwide.

1. **Supportive psychotherapy** (often termed as counseling), is the most widely used method
2. **Cognitive therapy** (for depression, anxiety disorders, eating disorders, sexual disorders)
3. **Behavior therapy** (anxiety disorders like OCD, Childhood behavioral problems).
4. **Cognitive-Behavior therapy (CBT)**- Highly useful and often an alternative to substance abuse (a special form called Motivation Enhancement Therapy used here), depression, anxiety disorders, eating disorders, sexual disorders.
5. **Dialectical**– Behavior therapy– useful for BPD (Borderline personality disorder)
6. **Psychoanalytical/Psychodynamic therapy**– not used as before, however useful in conversion/dissociative disorders

4. Anxiety is different from fear in that it is:

A. Known B. External
C. Vague D. Non-conflictual

Ans: C. Vague

Ref: Kaplan & Sadock's Synopsis of Psychiatry. 10th edition. P.579

Explanation:

Anxiety	Fear
Response to an unknown stimulus	Known stimulus
Stimulus is internal	External
Stimulus is vague	Definite
Stimulus is conflictual	Non-conflictual

5. All are true regarding Ganser's syndrome *except:*

A. Involuntary
B. Psychotic symptoms present
C. Memory symptoms present
D. Appropriate answers

Ans: A. Involuntary

Ref: Bhatia's Textbook of Psychiatry. P.185

Explanation:

Ganser's Syndrome

- It is a **voluntary** production of **psychotic, memory symptoms** and **approximate answers.**
- It is common in **males,** especially seen in **prison inmates/ hospitalized persons.**
- It is a form of **malingering** (voluntary and willful production of symptoms with the aim of *materialistic gain*) [Note– voluntary production of symptoms for *immaterial gains– Factitious disorder*].
- E.g., if a female complains of headache to get money from her husband and spending it on movies – malingering. If the female complains of headache get attention and affection from her ever-running husband- factitious disorder.
- **Approximate answers**-Vorbeireden.
- **Verbegeration**-meaningless repetition of words (syn. *Cataphasia*).
- **Neologism**- new word with only self-referential meaning.
- **Word salad**- mixing up of syllables resulting in un-understandable words.
- All three are seen in **Schizophrenia.**

6. Regarding etiology of autism all are true *except:*

A. Fragile- X- syndrome B. Tuberous sclerosis
C. Down's syndrome D. Phenylketonuria

Ans: C. Down's syndrome

***Ref:** Kaplan & Sadock's Synopsis of Psychiatry. 10th edition*

Explanation:

Autism

It is a syndrome characterized by the triad of:
1. Poor language development
2. Un/under-development of communication
3. Restricted, repetitive movements/ behaviors/ interests.

The spectrum is called as **"Pervasive Developmental Disorders (PDD)".**
Autism is the classical disorder of such spectrum.
The word was coined by 'Kanner'.
It is associated with mental retardation (part of the autism) and seizures.

Autism	• Typically seen before 2-3 years • Impaired language development • Communication development • Stereotypy
Atypical autism	• Symptoms appear after 3 years • Profound mental redartaion
Asperger's syndrome	• Male • Language development normal • Similar to autism
Rett's syndrome	• Females • Normal development till 6 months of age • Followed by deceleration of head growth • Stereotypy
Childhood disintegrative disorder	• Normal development till 2-3 years • Followed by loss of acquired skills of lan guage, communication

7. Auditory hallucinations are seen in *except:*

A. Schizophrenia
B. Acute and transient psychotic disorder
C. Delirium tremens
D. Panic disorder

Ans: D. Panic disorder

***Ref:** Kaplan & Sadock's Synopsis of Psychiatry. 10th edition*

Explanation:

- Hallucination is a perceptual pathology where perception occurs without real, external stimuli/ objects. (The other is *Illusion– where objects are present but perceived otherwise. E.g., rope perceived as snake*).
- The presence of hallucination is suggestive of psychosis.

Psychotic Symptoms are:

1. Hallucinations
2. Delusions
3. Extreme excitement
4. Extreme retardation

Psychotic symptoms occurs in:

1. Delirium
2. Schizophrenia, Acute and transient psychotic disorder, Psychosis (NOS)
3. Mania, Severe depression

Hallucinations occurs in several modalities:

1. Visual (suggestive of organicity)
2. Auditory (non-specific)
3. Olfactory (suggestive of organicity)
4. Gustatory (suggestive of epilepsy)
5. Somatic (suggestive of schizophrenia)

Pseudo-hallucinations- Which occurs in mind, not from outer space.

Functional hallucinations- Hallucinations present only with real stimulus (but both are perceived differently at the same time e.g., tap water sound and voices).

Causes of Auditory Hallucinations

- Schizophrenia
- Psychotic Disorders
- Delirium tremens
- Mood Disorders
- Intense stress
- Sleep deprivation
- High caffeine consumption

8. Nihilistic delusions seen in: (Repeat)

A. Depression **B.** Mania
C. Schizophrenia **D.** OCD

Ans: A. Depression

***Ref:** Kaplan & Sadock's Synopsis of Psychiatry. 10th edition*

Explanation:

- Delusion is one of the psychotic symptoms seen in several disorders (see previous question).
- Delusion is false, unshakable belief held with extraordinary conviction.
- **Nihilistic delusion** is a type of delusion, characterized by a false belief that everything **will come to an end** including **one's life** or **lost everything including one's body parts.**
- It is seen in **severe depression.**
- **Hypochondriac delusion** is a false belief that one has an incurable illness.

Cotrad syndrome: Presence of both nihilistic and hypochondriac delusions, seen in severe depression.

Other delusions seen in depression are:

1. Delusion of hopelessness/helplessness/ worthlessness.
2. Delusion of guilt (marker of suicidality).

Mania – Delusion of grandiosity

Schizophrenia – Bizarre delusions, delusion of persecution/reference.